Race and Medicine in Nineteenth- and Early-Twentieth Century America

Race and Medicine in Nineteenth- and Early-Twentieth-Century America

Todd L. Savitt

THE KENT STATE UNIVERSITY PRESS
KENT, OHIO

Library of Congress Catalog Card Number 2006016314
ISBN 978-0-87338-878-8 (cloth)
ISBN 978-1-60635-512-1 (paperback)
ISBN 978-1-61277-990-4 (epub)
ISBN 978-1-61277-991-1 (epdf)
Manufactured in the United States of America

The Library of Congress has cataloged the hardback edition as follows:
Savitt, Todd Lee, 1943–
Race and medicine in nineteenth- and early-twentieth-century America / by Todd L. Savitt.
p. ; cm.
Includes bibliographical references and index.
ISBN-13: 978-0-87338-878-8 (hardcover : alk. paper) ∞
ISBN-10: 0-87338-878-x (hardcover : alk. paper) ∞
1. African Americans—Health and hygiene—Southern States—History—19th century.
2. African Americans—Medical care—Southern States—History—19th century.
3. Sickle cell anemia—Southern States—History—19th century.
4. Racism—Southern States—History—19th century.
I. Title.
[DNLM: 1. African Americans—history—United States. 2. Delivery of Health Care—history—United States. 3. Anemia, Sickle Cell—history—United States. 4. Education, 20th Century—United States. 5. History, 19th Century—United States. 6. History, 20th Century—United States. WA 11 AA1 S267r 2006]
RA448.5.N4S28 2006
362.1089'96073—dc22 2006016314

British Library Cataloging-in-Publication data are available.

For Madison, Mitchell, and Jeremy

Contents

Preface

This collection of papers comprises a major portion of the writing I have done in the field of African American medical history. My work falls into three general areas: diseases and disorders of African Americans, blacks as patients during the antebellum and Reconstruction periods, and the education and medical practice of physicians of color in the late nineteenth and early twentieth centuries. For the most part, the subjects I write about have followed a logical, if not apparent, progression. After completing a book on slave health, *Medicine and Slavery: The Diseases and Health Care of Blacks in Antebellum Virginia* (1978), I published several articles based on information not included in that book, relating to slave life insurance, medical experimentation on slaves, and diseases such as crib death, elephantiasis, and sickle cell anemia. It then seemed fitting to investigate the health and health care of former slaves following emancipation. I began that project but kept stumbling on African American physicians (such as Alexander Augusta, the physician who ran the Freedmen's Bureau hospital and dispensary in Savannah, Georgia) and wondered where these physicians came from and where they had obtained their medical training. Those questions led me from postbellum black health to medical education for African Americans. Between 1868 and 1900 some fourteen medical schools dedicated to the training of African American physicians were founded. I decided to learn as much as I could about those schools. That study led me to the question of what happened when newly minted physicians of color attempted to enter the essentially white medical profession of the late nineteenth and early twentieth centuries and, finally, to the issue of professionalization among black physicians, including the establishment of black medical journals and medical societies. My writings, then, basically trace (with some gaps) the story of African Americans and medicine in the South from colonial times to the early twentieth century.

I have revised the content of articles to update language and medical information, correct factual errors, clarify or embellish statements, standardize referencing format in the endnotes, and include citations in the references to recent scholarship where appropriate. I have also written introductions to the three articles on sickle cell anemia and the seven articles on the history of medical education for African Americans to reduce repetition of the same information in the articles themselves. Not all illustrations and tables that appeared in the original articles have been reproduced in the current volume. Readers wishing to view them should consult the original articles. Similarly, several charts that did not appear in the original articles have been added to the current volume.

Diseases and Disorders of African Americans

CHAPTER 1

Smothering and Overlaying of Virginia Slave Children

A Suggested Explanation

Infant mortality in antebellum Virginia was extremely high. During the 1850s, between 16 and 20 percent of all deaths in the state occurred among children under the age of one year. The major causes of death included croup (much of which was probably diphtheria), diarrhea and dysentery, whooping cough, pneumonia, scarlet and other types of fever, and suffocation (also referred to as smothering and overlaying).[1] Since the 1850s medical science has substantially reduced the incidence of all but two of these diseases—pneumonia (which is today responsible for up to 27 percent of infant deaths between one and eleven months)[2] and suffocation.[3] With regard to the latter there is strong evidence to indicate that many deaths that physicians and planters of the 1850s ascribed to suffocation, smothering, and overlaying (almost always among the enslaved) were actually cases of what is now known as Sudden Infant Death Syndrome (SIDS) or "crib death." The Second International Conference on Causes of Sudden Death in Infants (1970) defined SIDS as "the sudden death of any infant or young child which is unexpected by history, and in which a thorough postmortem examination fails to demonstrate an adequate cause for death."[4] This is still the most accepted definition, though there has been much discussion and disagreement about it over the years.[5] In 1999, SIDS was still the leading killer of children between twenty-eight days and eleven months of age, accounting for 26.5 percent of deaths.[6]

Typical historical cases of presumed overlaying share several of the unmistakable hallmarks of SIDS. Compare a twentieth-century physician's description of the latter with an overseer's and a planter's remarks on the former:

An apparently thriving two-month-old boy is found dead face down in his crib. Except for a brief mild rhinorrhea during the previous week, the child had been in excellent health from birth. At a routine well-baby check by the family doctor a few days prior to the event, he appeared robust and free of problems. On the night of the death, he took his formula eagerly and was put down in his crib about 10 P.M. His mother looked in before retiring; he was sleeping peacefully on his abdomen with his face to the side. When found at 6:30 A.M., he had obviously been dead for several hours.[7]

I [Nathaniel Ryan, overseer] am sorry to inform you [Edmund Hubard, slave owner] that Matilda has lost her youngest child she over laid it, it was well and hearty when she went to bed and found it dead sometime in the night.[8]

Last week [wrote Robert Hubard to his brother, Edmund] Tilla overlaid/ when asleep/and killed her youngest child—a boy 6 or 7 months old. This was no doubt caused by her own want of care and attention.[9]

Most people, both today and 120 years ago, automatically assume that the fault lies with the parent and that the death is preventable. These are false assumptions. Physicians now know that children cannot be smothered as long as there is any circulating air available, even when the infant is beneath the covers or wedged against the sleeping mother.

(Studies published since the mid-1970s have revised this thinking. Commenting on that earlier view, a SIDS expert wrote in 2001, "It is now recognized that occasionally infants can be overlaid, especially by a drug-affected or exhausted parent, or by a young sibling, that infants can suffocate under pillows or bedclothes, and that although rare, intentional suffocation of infants also occurs."[10])

In addition to this descriptive similarity between SIDS and overlaying, there is a remarkable epidemiological correspondence, in both age and seasonal variation. Crib death does not occur among children of all age groups. Those younger than two weeks and older than one year are almost entirely spared; those between two weeks and four months are prime victims. (The recent "back to sleep" campaign educating parents to put their infant children to sleep on their backs has resulted in a significant reduction in SIDS deaths, particularly in the highly susceptible two-to-four-month-old age group.[11] In two studies, conducted in King County [Seattle], Washington [1972], and Richmond, Virginia [1968], 85 percent and 63 percent, respectively, of the victims were between one and four months old. The majority of these deaths occurred during the colder six months of the year (October through March).[12]) The figures obtained from an analysis of the manuscript register of deaths for twenty-six Virginia counties between 1853 and

1860 corroborate the King County and Richmond studies. Of the 226 children whose demise the parent or slave owner attributed to overlaying, smothering, or suffocation, 54 percent were between one month and four months of age. Fifty-six percent of the deaths occurred between October and March.[13]

The relative incidence of purported overlaying was much lower in antebellum Virginia (about 4 percent of infant deaths) than that of SIDS in present-day America (26.5 percent of infant deaths between two weeks and eleven months of age) for several reasons. Because people did not understand the cause of sudden infant death, they usually classified it as "unknown" in most mortality lists. Even today we cannot explain this phenomenon of unexpected death in young babies, but rather than lump it with other unknown causes of death, medical scientists have provided us with the descriptive term "Sudden Infant Death Syndrome."[14] Another important factor was the marked underreporting of white suffocation deaths (only about 2 percent of the total from this cause), probably due in part to the social stigma associated with child smothering. White parents and physicians likely attributed many sudden deaths among these children to teething, pneumonia, and, most often, to "unknown causes." Though present studies indicate that African Americans do in fact have a higher incidence of SIDS than whites (129 vs. 50 deaths per 100,000 live births in 1999 for children twenty-eight days to eleven months of age)[15] and that all members of lower socioeconomic groups regardless of race also exhibit an increased incidence of SIDS (probably owing to poorer sanitary conditions and overcrowding),[16] the figure for antebellum Virginia blacks (98 percent, or 229 of 232 smothering deaths) is much too high. It is interesting to note that in the latest available Department of Health, Education and Welfare national survey (in the late 1960s), underreporting continues to be a problem. Less than half of the estimated infant deaths attributable to SIDS (based on recent epidemiological studies) were classified as such on 1968 death certificates. Among the reasons for this were the lack of acceptance of SIDS as a disease entity and the subjectivity on the part of the local certifier, a condition remarkably similar to that which existed in antebellum Virginia.[17]

Smothering was not a problem confined solely to the plantation, though one early Southern writer asserted that the peculiarities of the slave system increased its incidence: "Not a few [babies] are overlaid by the wearied [slave] mother, who sleeps so dead a sleep as not to be aware of the injury to her infant."[18] Overlaying occurred in the North as well, but it was reported with much less frequency, again no doubt due to social pressures, as was the case in European countries.[19]

Certainly not all cases of suffocation among enslaved children can be attributed to crib death. Nineteenth-century physicians rarely performed autopsies and probably misdiagnosed a percentage of all their cases simply because they lacked the requisite knowledge. In addition, some enslaved mothers did actually commit infanticide,[20] though without their master's knowledge. The information presented here, however, indicates that the majority of infant deaths attributed to suffocation, smothering, and overlaying in antebellum Virginia (and the rest of the nation) were actually cases of SIDS.[21]

CHAPTER 2

Filariasis (Elephantiasis) in the United States

The coming of the European to North and South America after 1492 resulted in biological and cultural changes on both sides of the Atlantic, changes that one writer has termed "The Columbian Exchange." In addition to such items as foods, animals, and plants, several infectious diseases were exchanged, including smallpox and tuberculosis, which ravaged the Native American population, and perhaps syphilis, which afflicted many Europeans.[1] A similar exchange of disease agents occurred in Africa during the European age of exploration, as whites and blacks met and traded along the African coast. Various "fevers" (including yellow fever and malarial fevers) and parasitic infestations unknown in Europe plagued whites, while black Africans suffered from pneumonia, tuberculosis, measles, and other disorders not commonly found in the tropics. With the development of slavery in the Americas and the transportation of large numbers of blacks to both North and South America, the "African Exchange" soon became important in the New World. Several African tropical diseases appeared and lingered in the Americas as legacies of the slave trade.

Among the many transmissible infections that Africans carried with them to the New World were malaria in its various forms, yellow fever, smallpox, yaws, leprosy, guinea worm, filariasis, ascariasis, tapeworm, hookworm, and trypanosomiasis. Some of these infections disappeared with the first generation of imported slaves; others took firm root and lingered through the nineteenth century and on to the present. No part of the New World entirely escaped the new African infections. Even the American South, though not tropical, had a warm enough climate throughout much of the year to support the growth and permanent residence of a number of disease agents brought from Africa. One nental North America—existed there until the 1920s. Elephantiasis was reported throughout the South and even in several Northern states in the eighteenth, nineteenth, and twentieth centuries. Sporadically cases also occurred outside of Charleston, but usually among persons who had lived in or visited known areas of endemic filarial infection. In the United States only Charleston seems to have harbored a large enough population of infected persons to sustain the filarial life cycle for many generations.

Wuchereria bancrofti is endemic to both east and west Africa in precisely those areas tapped by slave traders from Europe and America.[6] Manifestations of bancroftian filariasis began to appear among slaves taken to the West Indies soon after the beginning of the slave trade. The island of Barbados in particular early became an endemic focus of filarial infection. In Barbados elephantiasis was originally confined to the slave population, but, beginning about 1704, infection spread to an increasing number of white and creole residents. So common was the disorder that it became known in the English-speaking New World as "Barbados-leg." Throughout the nineteenth century and into the twentieth, Barbados (and several other West Indian islands) remained an endemic focus of filariasis.[7]

On the North American continent, Charleston, because of certain special factors, became a major center of filarial infection. As a primary port of entry for enslaved people from the West Indies during colonial times, Charleston constantly received persons infected with the parasite. Slaves also passed through and spread *Wuchereria bancrofti* in other port towns of North America at this time, but it is uncertain whether filariasis ever became endemic anywhere but Charleston. Charleston and the surrounding Low Country possessed one of the highest densities of blacks of all the continental colonies. Enslaved people imported to South Carolina—many carrying microfilariae in their blood—usually remained in Charleston or the vicinity and were not dispersed to widely scattered plantations as occurred in the other large slave-owning colony, Virginia.[8] Also, the *Culex quinquefasciatus* mosquito occurred mainly in South Carolina, and not to any great extent in lands to the north.[9] Even when numbers of infected slaves were brought into New York, Philadelphia, or Boston, *Wuchereria bancrofti* could not have been transmitted to new human hosts without the proper intermediate insect. The presence of the *Culex quinquefasciatus* mosquito together with great concentrations of *Wuchereria bancrofti* carriers ensured the Charleston area of a constant supply of infected humans and mosquitoes sufficient to maintain the filarial life cycle. A sizable reservoir of infected human hosts was necessary because (a) not all microfilariae ingested by a mosquito survive residence in the insect's body; (b) unlike the malarial parasite that multiplies within the mosquito's body, microfilariae simply grow in size, not number, in the intermediary host; and (c) once settled in a human lymphatic vessel, adult worms cannot reproduce without a member of the opposite sex in that same location. It usually requires multiple bites of mosquitoes carrying *Wuchereria bancrofti* to obtain infestations in humans sufficient for the production of microfilariae.[10] With a constantly replenishing supply of human carriers from the West Indies passing through or settling in Charleston during the colonial period, conditions were ideal for that town to become an endemic focus of *Wuchereria bancrofti*.

A further reason for Charleston's unique position as a haven for filarial worms was its close ties with the major West Indian focus of this disease—Barbados. South Carolina was settled and initially developed in large part by whites and enslaved people transplanted from that island. The two colonies retained economic and social relations throughout their early histories and into the nineteenth century. As a result, black and white Barbadian emigrants and merchants simply transferred *Wuchereria bancrofti* from one hospitable environment to another.[11]

There is not enough evidence to designate an exact time at which the filarial worm became able to sustain itself in the Charleston area without periodic reinforcements from the West Indies or Africa. The establishment of the infection at Charleston must have occurred some time before cessation of the slave trade in 1808. It was not until 1886, shortly after *Wuchereria bancrofti* was discovered and associated with elephantiasis and chyluria, that medical scientists first recognized the endemicity of that parasite in Charleston and the Low Country of South Carolina. Before 1886, Charleston residents had known that cases of elephantiasis and chyluria occurred regularly in their city, but had been unaware of Charleston's uniqueness in this respect.

Among the early descriptions of elephantiasis in the American colonies is the following, excerpted from Bernard Romans's 1775 book *A Concise Natural History of East and West Florida*. For twenty years Romans had lived in Georgia and the Floridas and traveled through the Carolinas. Though he did not state precisely where he observed cases of elephantiasis, the context of his excellent and accurate description indicates that the probable locale was coastal South Carolina and Georgia:

> A loathsome disease appears some times among the Negroes after severe acute disorders, especially if the patient has been obliged to keep his bed long, likewise after a violent exercise has brought on a surfeit: this is called the *Elephantiasis* from the swelling of the feet and legs; it is most frequently seen to affect one leg only; in the first stages of this disorder the patient becomes wretched through excessive lassitudes which bring on an emaciation of the body, then the corrupted juices subside into the leg or legs and feet, these swell, the skin becoming distended, shines and shews the distended veins every where below the knee; now the skin by degrees loses its gloss and becomes unequal and something scaly; after this chaps make

> their appearance, the glands are stretched and the scales are daily enlarged, appearing as hard and callous as the hide of an Alligator, notwithstanding which the slightest prick of a pointed instrument will cause the blood to exude; this disease affects neither the appetite nor the digestive powers of the body, on the contrary the patient in this and chearfulness [*sic*] of spirits resembles the healthiest of men, and the inconvenience of his heavy leg only prevents his ability for the more laborious part of his duty.[12]

Subsequent cases of elephantiasis appearing in the medical literature often originated from this same area. Those that did not may have been nonfilarial in etiology, or imported from outside the United States, or the result of small endemic foci in other slave port cities. Disorders other than filariasis can also cause gross swelling of the scrotum, labia, or lower extremities. Bacterial or accidental mechanical obstruction of lymphatics may result in such elephantoid symptoms.[13] There is no way to know whether the cases reported before the days of routine blood examinations (1880s) were truly filariasis. Patients with elephantiasis and chyluria in and around Charleston most likely harbored the parasites, because we know from later microbiological studies that *Wuchereria bancrofti* was endemic there. But how does one explain the several cases in Georgia and Louisiana? Though public health surveys in 1915 and 1918 failed to turn up endemic cases of filariasis in Savannah or New Orleans, probably *Wuchereria bancrofti* was brought into these towns during the eighteenth and nineteenth centuries but did not survive. Both cities had had sizable slave populations and served as ports of entry for imported African and West Indian slaves. But there are no early records suggesting that either town ever harbored large numbers of individuals with elephantiasis or chyluria.[14]

The first case to appear in the nineteenth-century Southern[15] medical literature is a good example of the problem. Nelson, a thirty-eight-year-old slave belonging to Mr. J. F. Piseros of St. Charles Parish, Louisiana, was taken to New Orleans in June 1837 for treatment of an enormously enlarged scrotum (see figure 1). No other patient history was presented in the report except that the enlargement had begun some ten years earlier. A lithograph of Nelson before and after the successful operation to remove his huge burden accompanied the article. The physician's language throughout the report indicated that it was one of the first cases of elephantiasis he and his colleagues in New Orleans had seen. There was no mention of other persons with the disorder living in St. Charles Parish, so it is difficult to draw any conclusions as to the origin of Nelson's disorder.[16] Similarly, the three cases of elephantiasis that Dr. Joseph Jones observed among whites in New Orleans during the 1870s are doubtful but possible instances of *Wuchereria bancrofti* infection. Jones provided little background information on which present-day readers might base a diagnosis, and he failed to mention

African parasite that became endemic in a portion of the South was the filarial roundworm, *Wuchereria bancrofti*, causative organism of elephantiasis.[2]

Wuchereria bancrofti has a life cycle that involves both an intermediate insect and a final human host. Adult worms live in the lymphatic vessels and lymph nodes of humans, causing an inflammatory response, growth of connective tissue within the vessels, and the eventual development of lymphatic obstruction and varicosities. The closing off of the lymphatic circulation produces the well-known scrotal, labial, or leg and foot swelling so characteristic of elephantiasis. Many other manifestations of chronic filarial infection may also occur. One such symptom is chyluria, the discharge of milky urine that is caused by the rupture of an obstructed lymphatic vessel into the urinary tract. Chyluria and scrotal, labial, or lower leg enlargement actually occur only in the later stages of filarial infections. Periodic attacks of glandular pain, scrotal or labial swelling, and general malaise, over the course of many years, are the most common early signs of filariasis.[3]

The long time lapse between initial filarial infection and the appearance of severe symptoms was deceptive to slave traders and prospective buyers. Infected enslaved people brought to the North American colonies might have appeared perfectly healthy upon departure from western Africa or the West Indies, and also upon sale to a planter. Only years later, perhaps after many puzzling episodes of pain in the groin or glands, would elephantiasis or chyluria develop.

Though carried to the New World, *Wuchereria bancrofti* might have disappeared like *Trypanosoma gambiense*, the parasite causing African sleeping sickness, had no suitable insect vector been available to transmit it from one human being to another. In the case of sleeping sickness, which many Africans did bring with them to the Americas, the absence of its carrier, the tse-tse fly, in the New World, prevented establishment of the disease here.[4] The parasite causing elephantiasis was more fortunate. Throughout the West Indies and the Americas lives a mosquito, *Culex quinquefasciatus* (also known as *C. fatigans*), which, when it draws blood from a person infected with *Wuchereria bancrofti*, is capable of supporting the growth of several microfilariae, the offspring of adult worms. Thus when the microfilariae, produced by worms situated deep in the human lymphatic system, escaped into the blood stream, they could then pass on to, and survive in, the body of the mosquito. At the insect's next blood meal, filarial larvae escaped through the mosquito's proboscis onto human skin. They penetrated through the bite wound and entered the lymphatic system where they developed to adulthood in about a year. If the adult filaria worm settled in the same lymphatic as another of the opposite sex, the two worms mated, new microfilariae were produced, and the life cycle was repeated.[5]

Filariasis has usually been associated in this country with Charleston, South Carolina. A major endemic focus of the disease—perhaps the only one in conti-

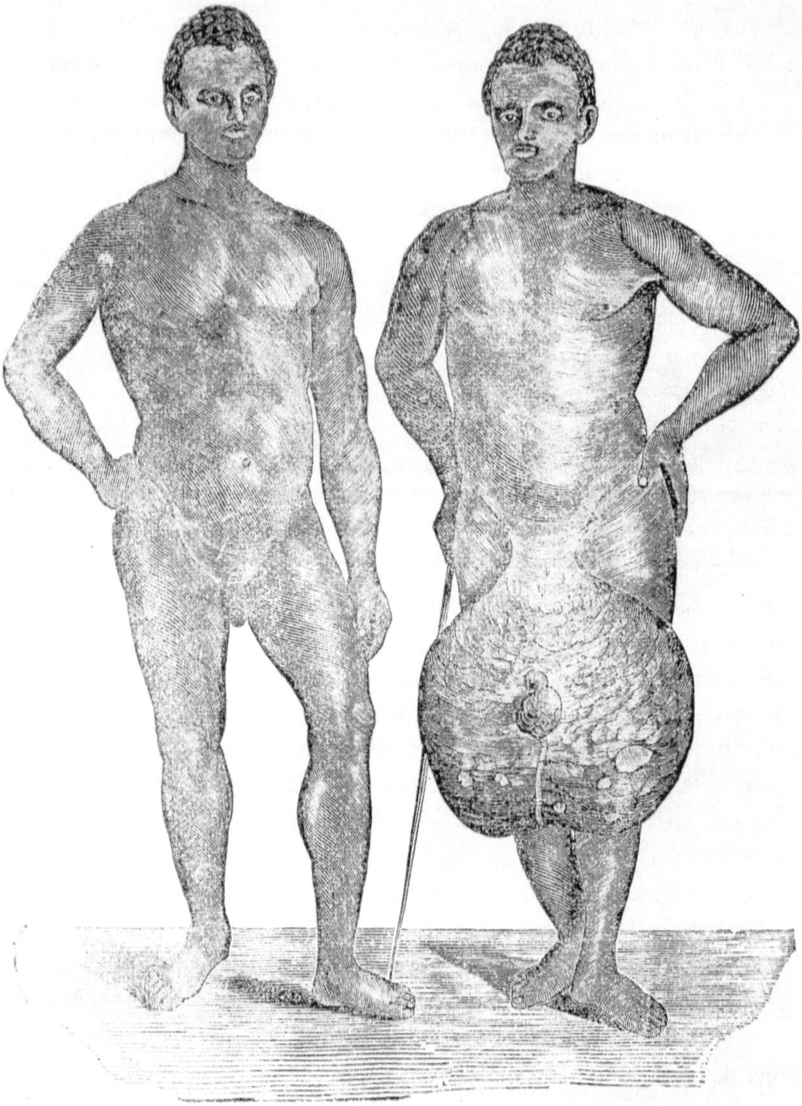

Fig. 1. A case of elephantiasis in a Louisiana slave, from J. M. W. Picton, "A Case of Elephantiasis Scroti, With Successful Operation," *New Orleans Medical and Surgical Journal* 2 (1845–46): 316–21. The surgery was performed by Dr. Picton on October 3, 1837. The patient is pictured here before the operation (right) and after.

any other local cases in an extensive review of the subject some nine years later. More easily explainable are Jones's six reported cases of elephantiasis (four of the foot and leg and two of the scrotum) observed among slaves on coastal Georgia cotton, rice, and sugar plantations during the 1840s and 1850s. This area, part of the Charleston-influenced Low Country, had large areas of marsh where mosquitoes bred readily and many slaves whose parents and grandparents had come from the West Indies and Africa. Spread of the filarial infection under these favorable conditions was likely.[17] The occurrence of three other reported cases of elephantiasis in the inland Georgia towns of Atlanta, Columbus, and Lawrenceville is difficult to explain as *Wuchereria bancrofti* infections. None of the three towns was a likely focus for filariasis, and none produced subsequent reported cases of elephantiasis. Neither was Charleston mentioned as a previous residence of any of the three patients whose case histories were given.[18]

The pre-1886 evidence for filariasis in Charleston is very convincing. Mention of elephantiasis by physicians occurred with some regularity, thereby suggesting that the cases of elephantiasis were not isolated phenomena of traumatic or bacterial origins. For each year between 1855 and 1858, for example, one black Charleston resident succumbed to elephantiasis.[19] Chyluria occurred frequently enough for Dr. Charles Witsell of Ashepoo, South Carolina, in the Low Country near Charleston, to describe its pathology and treatment in 1855. Witsell stated that Dr. Dickson of Charleston had also seen several cases of "chylo-serous urine."[20]

Some South Carolina physicians mentioned or described individual cases of elephantiasis. In 1849, Dr. William F. Holmes reported in an article on the treatment of pneumonia that a slave, Peter, suffering from pneumonia, was also "the subject of elephantiasis."[21] In 1855, a medical student, Clarence A. Fripp of Beaufort, South Carolina (on one of the Sea Islands along the coast, heavily populated with slaves), had seen enough local cases of elephantiasis to justify writing his M.D. thesis on the disease: "Our attention," he wrote, "has been directed into this channel, from having seen several cases & being impressed with the idea that, through causes neither appreciable, nor within our controul [*sic*], this disease formerly so rare, is now becoming far more frequent."[22] Fripp noticed that elephantiasis occurred much more often "among the negros [*sic*] and mulattoes than the whites" in that area; in fact, of the several cases he had seen, none were among whites.[23] He gave a general description of the disease and then mentioned specifically a case he had observed of a man whose scrotum "was so hypertrophied, as to hang below the knees involving the prepucial folds of the penis in one colossal mass of immense height."[24]

Two other antebellum cases of elephantiasis in the Charleston area appeared in the medical literature. Dr. F. Galvez listed the name of Dr. Middleton Michel of Charleston in a "Statistical Table of the Different Operations for Elephantiasis of the Scrotum, Performed in Different Parts of the World." Though no report of the procedure Dr. Michel performed is extant, Dr. Galvez stated that the patient had been cured.[25] In February 1860, Dr. T. L. Ogier of Charleston presented a case history of elephantiasis to the South Carolina Medical Association. The patient, he reported, a twenty-six-year-old bondsman, desperately wished for relief from the discomfort of a greatly enlarged leg and foot. His owner agreed. Ogier succeeded in reducing the swelling by ligating the femoral artery, though, as in all radical "cures" of elephantiasis, the results may not have been permanent.[26]

Elephantiasis continued to plague Charlestonians at the rate of several cases annually in the years following the Civil War. Throughout the 1870s and early 1880s both whites and blacks fell ill or died from the disorder, and a few people reported "chylous urine." In 1870, though no deaths occurred, city health officers treated three whites and four African Americans for elephantiasis at the city hospital or at home. Three years later public health officials attributed two deaths to elephantiasis—one white and one black—and were treating seven active cases—six black and one white. In 1883, three deaths of persons with elephantiasis occurred.[27] By 1885, the frequent occurrence of chyluria and elephantiasis among Charlestonians had aroused enough concern among local physicians to have the matter discussed at the annual meeting of the State Medical Society.[28]

Also in 1885, a physician interested in the newly discovered relationship of human filarial infestations to elephantiasis and chyluria came to Charleston. During the previous year, Dr. John Guitéras had treated four Cubans in Key West, Florida, for *filaria sanguinis hominis* (microfilariae in the blood), and now wished to examine Charlestonians for the presence of these parasites. His reasons for undertaking such an investigation were compelling: "I was told that this disease [chyluria] and elephantiasis were not rare in the city. I also found that mosquitoes were very plentiful during the summer and fall; that cistern water was in general use, and that no filters were to be found for sale in the shops. These observations, together with the fact that Charleston has been for many years in constant intercourse with the West Indies, induced me to be on the lookout for filaria."[29] Guitéras was assisted in his work by several physicians, two of whom, J. J. Edwards and W. D. Bratton, had been examining the blood of suspected filarial carriers since 1882 or 1883, but without observing microfilariae.[30]

Microfilariae were seen first in the blood of a mulatto woman, a native of Charleston, suffering from chyluria in 1886. Over the next four years twenty-two Charlestonians—fifteen blacks and seven whites—were found to harbor microfilariae in their blood. One was a one-hundred-year-old woman who had been brought from Africa in a slave ship.[31] Manifestations of filarial infection continued to appear among Charleston area residents throughout the 1890s and early 1900s.[32] Writers of textbooks and articles on tropical diseases now began to include Charleston in the list of areas where filariasis was to be found.[33]

Not until 1914 did a large-scale statistical study reveal the extent of the problem in Charleston. Dr. Francis B. Johnson, clinical pathologist at the Medical College of South Carolina in Charleston, disclosed that he had discovered microfilariae in the blood of 19.25 percent of 400 routinely cultured hospital and clinic patients. Still more startling was the finding that only a fourth of those infected showed symptoms of filariasis—the remaining three-fourths were carriers.[34] Another study, performed a year later in Charleston's "Old Folks' Home," revealed that thirteen of the residents there (35 percent) had microfilariae in their blood.[35] Dr. Johnson also questioned about two-thirds of Charleston's physicians regarding the number of filariasis cases they had seen in their practices. The physicians reported having noted 494 cases, including 244 of chyluria, 213 of elephantiasis, 8 of the two combined, 4 of other symptoms, and 25 not stated.[36]

After 1886, American physicians throughout the South began searching for other concentrations of filarial infection. Cases were reported from many towns but none were more than isolated phenomena.[37] Finally, in 1917, Dr. Edward Francis of the U.S. Public Health Service undertook a filarial survey of nine southern towns with climatic conditions and mosquito species similar to Charleston's, in order to discover the true extent of the problem.[38] Interestingly, only 9 of 1,470 individuals tested showed microfilariae in their blood, and these 9 had "histories either of having been born and raised in Charleston or of having been born in Cuba which is a well-known filarial focus."[39] Charleston was the only endemic focus of filariasis in the United States at that time.

The upshot of Johnson's and Francis's reports was an intensive mosquito control campaign during the early 1920s to eradicate filariasis from Charleston. In 1924, it was necessary to conduct only thirty-six blood tests at the city hospital for filariasis; this number was reduced to four the following year,[40] and to zero by 1930.[41] When a group of Mexican scientists visited Charleston in the late 1920s to study the filarial problem, the city health officer was unable to show them a single case. In 1949, a leading parasitologist reported, "In the United States the one previously known endemic area, that around Charleston, South Carolina, has become filaria-free."[42] One of the consequences of the "African Exchange"—filariasis—now became only a memory in the United States.

CHAPTER 3

Race, Medicine, and the Discovery of Sickle Cell Anemia

Introduction

In the November 1910 issue of the *Archives of Internal Medicine*, Dr. James B. Herrick of Chicago reported on "Peculiar Elongated and Sickle-Shaped Red Blood Corpuscles in a Case of Severe Anemia."[1] Three months later, in the February 1911 issue of the *Virginia Medical Semi-Monthly*, an author identified erroneously as "R. E. Washburn" (it should have read "B. E. Washburn") published a case report citing Herrick's article and using precisely the same descriptive title as Herrick.[2] These two reports, appearing in the medical literature within the space of a few months, introduced modern medicine to the disorder that came to be known as sickle cell anemia (SCA).[3] The articles were recognized by subsequent researchers in the field as the first published notices of the new disorder and served as models for the two other case reports of SCA that appeared in the medical literature (in 1915 and 1922) before more intensive studies of the disease began in the early 1920s.[4] By the mid-1920s, enough patients with this distinctive form of anemia had been studied for physician-researchers to note the disease's hereditary pattern and natural history.[5]

Herrick's and Washburn's pathbreaking case reports are of historical interest not only for the information they convey about a newly discovered and quite important medical condition but also for the glimpse they provide into medicine and society at the turn of the twentieth century. Specifically, the stories behind the two cases—of the lives of the physicians and patients involved, the circumstances that brought the physicians and patients together, and the events that led to publication of the two articles—reflect the excitement and competitiveness of medical science in early-twentieth-century America and the varying economic and social status of people of color in the United States at the time. Though the medical literature for sixty years following these first reported cases of SCA demonstrates the interest some medical scientists and practitioners took in the disease, SCA was not well-known to the general public, white or black, as late as the early 1970s. The following three papers in this section describe in detail the discovery of the first and second cases of SCA, discuss the striking differences in authorship and patient background between the first two published cases, and attempt to explain the slow dissemination of information about this disease among whites and blacks in the United States over the next half-century.

CHAPTER 4

Herrick's 1910 Case Report of Sickle Cell Anemia, Chicago, Illinois

Co-authored with Morton F. Goldberg, M.D.

When the SS *Cearense* docked in New York on September 15, 1904, after an eight-day voyage from Barbados, one of its passengers had a medical problem. A sore on the ankle of a twenty-year-old Grenadian, Walter Clement Noel, had become quite painful. He sought help from a physician after clearing customs and immigration. Within a week, time and the iodine applied by his physician healed the wound, leaving a scar similar to others on his limbs.[1] He continued his journey, now over land, to Chicago.

Around Thanksgiving Day, Noel, now a first-year dental student at the Chicago College of Dental Surgery (CCDS), developed severe respiratory problems. He coped with these symptoms until the day after Christmas, when he walked, weak and dizzy,[2] across the street from his lodgings to Presbyterian Hospital.[3] There Dr. Ernest E. Irons, a twenty-seven-year-old intern, obtained a history and performed routine physical, blood, and urine examinations (see figure 2).[4] He noticed that Noel's blood smear contained "many pear shaped and elongated forms—some small," and alerted his attending physician, James B. Herrick, of the unusual blood findings. In his next blood examination report, on December 31, Irons drew a rough sketch of these erythrocytes (see figure 3).[5]

For the next two and a half years Herrick and Irons followed Noel through several episodes of severe illness as he continued his dental studies. Though the two physicians performed numerous tests, consulted with colleagues, and searched the medical literature for similar cases, they never could confirm a diagnosis for Noel's illness. Finally, in May 1910, three years after losing track of their patient, Herrick presented the case to the Association of American Physicians in Washington, D.C.,[6] and published it, still undiagnosed, in the November 1910 issue of

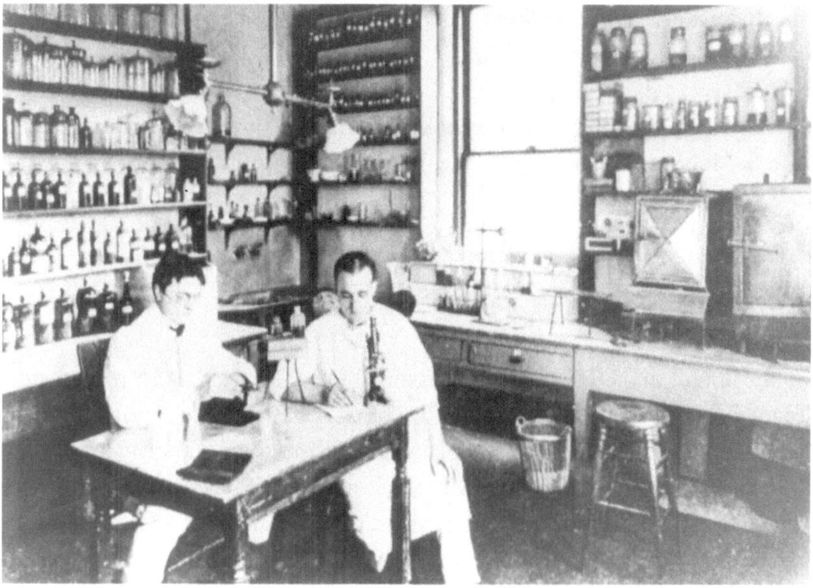

Fig. 2. A laboratory at Presbyterian Hospital, Chicago, ca. 1905. Picture from *Presbyterian Hospital, 22nd Annual Report* (1905) (available in Rush-Presbyterian–St. Luke's Medical Center Archives, Chicago).

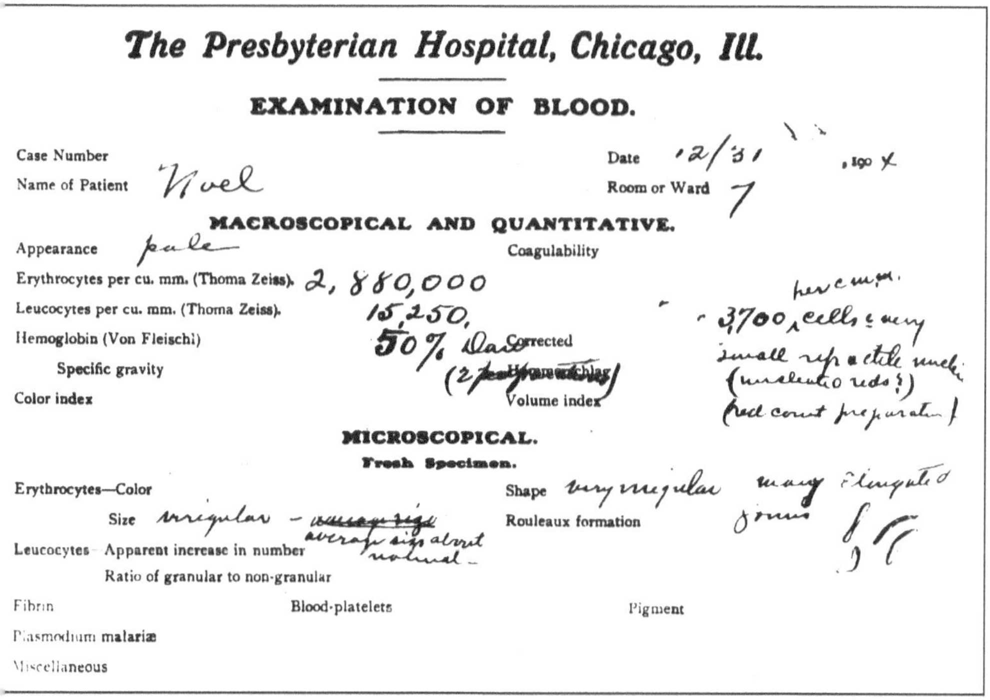

The Presbyterian Hospital, Chicago, Ill.

EXAMINATION OF BLOOD.

Case Number Date 12/31, 1904
Name of Patient Noel Room or Ward 7

MACROSCOPICAL AND QUANTITATIVE.

Appearance pale Coagulability
Erythrocytes per cu. mm. (Thoma Zeiss). 2,880,000
Leucocytes per cu. mm. (Thoma Zeiss). 15,250, 3700 cells per c.mm. very small refractile nuclei (nucleated reds?) (red count preparation)
Hemoglobin (Von Fleischl) 50% Dare Corrected
Specific gravity Hæmatochlar
Color index Volume index

MICROSCOPICAL.

Fresh Specimen.

Erythrocytes—Color Shape very irregular many elongated forms
Size irregular — average size about normal Rouleaux formation
Leucocytes—Apparent increase in number
Ratio of granular to non-granular
Fibrin Blood-platelets Pigment
Plasmodium malariæ
Miscellaneous

Fig. 3. Ernest Irons' blood examination report on Walter Clement Noel, December 31, 1904, describing and depicting the oddly shaped red blood cells. From the James B. Herrick Papers (available in University of Chicago Library, Manuscript Division).

the *Archives of Internal Medicine*.[7] Following time-honored medical tradition, the patient's name was not revealed.

Noel's was the first recorded and documented case of sickle cell anemia in Western medicine. The discovery took place during a time of change in medicine and in American race relations. The main characters of the story exemplify this transitional period.

Chicago Medicine, 1904

At the time of the actual discovery, December 1904, Chicago was a growing center of medicine and of medical education. The city boasted some nationally known practitioners, medical educators, and researchers, including Frank Billings, Nicholas Senn, Ludvig Hektoen, John B. Murphy, Daniel Hale Williams, Christian Fenger, and Arthur Dean Bevan. The American Medical Association made its headquarters there. Just west of the downtown area stood a medical district of several square blocks housing a number of medical and dental schools and hospitals.[8]

Both James Bryan Herrick (1861–1954) and Ernest Edward Irons (1877–1959) lived and worked in that medical district. Herrick, who had already earned a reputation for his teaching, publications, and medical skills, served as an attending physician at both Presbyterian and Cook County Hospitals and as professor of medicine at Rush Medical College. A native of nearby Oak Park, Illinois, and an 1888 graduate of Rush, Herrick practiced internal medicine in Chicago after his internship at Cook County Hospital. During the 1890s and early 1900s he published numerous articles, often case reports based on his wide experience in medical practice. Throughout those years he maintained a keen interest in diagnostic techniques and wrote a short textbook in 1895, *Handbook of Medical Diagnosis for Students*. Always a student himself, Herrick was studying chemistry every morning that fall and winter of 1904 in courses at the University of Chicago. In later years his research into angina pectoris and coronary occlusion would win him national attention and a number of awards.[9]

Irons, a native of Council Bluffs, Iowa, had graduated from Rush Medical College in 1903 and was now completing his internship under Herrick at Presbyterian Hospital. His primary interests were infectious diseases and bacteriology. He earned a Ph.D. in bacteriology at the University of Chicago in 1912 and national recognition for his studies on focal infections. From 1923 to 1936 Irons served as dean of his medical alma mater and in 1949–50 as president of the American Medical Association.[10]

The two men were quite close.[11] Irons took a room in the Herricks' home, just a few blocks from the medical district, and, from 1904 to 1908, shared Herrick's downtown private office.[12]

Herrick had an interest in blood and blood disorders. In 1892, asked by Dean C. W. Earle of Northwestern University to head the school's medical clinic, Herrick insisted first on a "good microscope" and the latest hemocytometer and hemometer.[13] At the May 1895 meeting of the Illinois State Medical Society, an organization in which he was active,[14] Herrick heard a paper reinforcing his belief in the usefulness of microscopic blood examinations.[15] Two years later, he presented a paper in Philadelphia on lymphatic leukemia, attracting the attention of Richard C. Cabot, the famous Boston physician. Cabot even asked Herrick for the names of Chicago's experts on blood and for Herrick's comments on the hematologic aspects of Cabot's own writings. During the fall and winter of 1904, Herrick was again thinking about hematology. In October he presented a talk to members of the West Side branch of the Chicago Medical Society, introducing a lecture series on diseases of the blood. He titled his discussion, "The Practical Value of Blood Examinations."[16] Both he and his intern Irons knew how to prepare their own blood specimens for microscopic studies and how to interpret the results.

Fifty years earlier the two could not have performed such procedures. Knowledge of blood disorders based on red blood cell counts, altered red blood cell morphology, and changes in hemoglobin content grew rapidly during the latter half of the nineteenth century. Discussions by Rudolph Virchow and others on the significance of blood cells as well as subsequent discoveries by Robert Koch and Paul Ehrlich of effective methods of staining tissues on microscopic slides offered physicians a variety of ways to measure and observe blood components.[17] In the first decade of the twentieth century, medical writers were recommending for every newly hospitalized patient a routine hematologic examination, including a blood cell count, microscopic study of both fresh and fixed blood stained with Ehrlich's triacid stain, and measurement of hemoglobin content.[18] These textbooks and articles discussed several types of anemias and leukemias, disturbances in blood's appearance and measurement due to infection or foreign substances, and the use of special stains to demonstrate hidden blood disorders. Hematology, though not a specialty, had become an integral part of medicine.

Integration had begun to occur on another medical front as well. Walter Clement Noel could not have come to the United States to study dentistry in 1904 had not race relations begun to change around the nation. Emancipation of slaves after the Civil War had posed terrible medical problems but also opened great opportunities for blacks. With a large, generally impoverished, rural African American population in great need of medical care and a white Southern medical profession reluctant to provide that care without payment, the call for black health professionals grew steadily. In answer to that call, a few medical schools in the North occasionally admitted black students, and Northern missionary associations dedicated to providing a basic education for the newly freed slaves established a handful of medical schools including Howard and Meharry. Within a generation, some newly minted African American physicians founded private (proprietary) medical schools similar to those proliferating in white America during the pre–Flexner Report days. Schools for training black nurses, dentists, and pharmacists also opened their doors.[19] By the turn of the century black health professionals were practicing not just in the South but in increasing numbers in the North.[20]

Chicago drew its share of these practitioners, along with many African American workers attempting to escape the racism and poverty of the rural South. Black America's most renowned physician and surgeon, Daniel Hale Williams, lived in Chicago and operated Provident Hospital with several other African American physicians, staffing it with black nurses and nursing students.[21] Between 1900 and 1910, the black professional population of Chicago was growing, in part because several of the local medical schools accepted blacks as students during this unregulated era of keen competition for pupils.[22] It was this magnet of educational opportunities for blacks that attracted Walter Clement Noel to Chicago from his West Indian home.

Who Was Walter Clement Noel?

Some 2,500 miles from Chicago and about one hundred miles from Venezuela lies the island of Grenada. In 1904, the colony, just twelve miles wide by twenty miles long, belonged to Great Britain; the British and French had traded ownership several times since Grenada's first white settlement in 1650. Though English in government, language, and customs, Grenada retained evidence of its French and African heritages, including an abundance of families with French surnames and people of mixed racial background. Census takers in 1901 counted 63,438 citizens, most living in rural areas. Tropical agricultural crops grown on numerous estates throughout the island were the mainstay of the economy. Most business people and professionals lived and worked in St. George's, the capital (population 5,184 in 1901).[23]

Born June 21, 1884,[24] and raised on Duquesne Estate in the mountainous bush country of St. Patrick's Parish at the north end of the island, Walter Clement Noel grew up in an agricultural setting. His boyhood home, the foundations of which may still be seen, sat atop a hill overlooking the plantation lands in an area of the estate aptly known as Prospect.[25] Noel's family was wealthy. His mother, Mary Justina Noel (d. 1936), owned the estate, inherited with other property from her father, who had migrated from Dominica, British West Indies.[26] Noel's father, John Cornelius Noel (1849 or 1850–1886),[27] came from a landholding family on the eastern side of Grenada, near Grenville.[28] The family could well afford to pay for Noel's education, when, in June or July of 1904, after completing studies at

Harrison College in Barbados,[29] he decided to become a dentist and to study in the United States.

He was not alone in this desire. Other black West Indians also enrolled in American dental and medical schools, especially those founded in the South to provide professional education for blacks.[30] One such man, Oliver Charles Arthur, had returned to Grenada in 1901 or 1902, after studying for three years at Howard University Dental School.[31] Arthur opened offices in St. George's and Grenville as the only licensed and professionally educated dentist on the island.[32] Five years older than Noel, Arthur may have encouraged the younger man to pursue a career in dentistry. He wrote letters and sent college transcripts[33] on Noel's behalf, not to one of the Southern black institutions, but first to an unidentified dental school in Pennsylvania and then, when Noel decided on Chicago, to Truman Brophy, dean at CCDS, one of the leading dental schools in the nation.[34] Once the final arrangements had been made, Noel's mother also wrote a note to Dean Brophy, from Duquesne, just three weeks before her son's departure: "I will be very glad if you would take an interest in him, and see that he does his work, especially as he is a stranger."[35]

On arriving in Chicago, Noel, with less than seventy dollars in his pocket,[36] found rooms at 618 West Congress Street,[37] just one block and around the corner from CCDS, in the heart of the medical district. On Wednesday evening, October 5, 1904, he first saw his classmates and faculty, assembled for opening exercises. Though other persons of color were studying medicine, dentistry, and nursing in Chicago at the time, he was probably the only black person at CCDS, and one of several foreign students (others came from Europe, Asia, and Canada).[38]

Less than three months later Noel was admitted to Presbyterian Hospital.[39] After intern Irons reported the unusual findings in Noel's blood to his attending physician, Dr. Herrick, the two doctors performed and repeated tests on the patient's sputum, stool, urine, and blood, searching for an explanation. Their differential diagnosis included hookworm disease, yaws, syphilis, ground itch, malaria, intestinal parasites, and the effects of coal tar medicinal preparations.[40] None fit the clinical picture. Noel slowly recovered his strength and overcame the respiratory infection. His physicians discharged him on January 22, 1905, still without a clear diagnosis.

Noel returned to school. A full year elapsed before he again sought Irons's and Herrick's medical attention. He was admitted twice in 1906 to nearby Frances E. Willard National Temperance Hospital: for a few days in January 1906 for bronchitis, and for two months starting in late December (December 26, 1906, to February 26, 1907) for a "'bilious' attack" and "muscular rheumatism."[41] (He probably participated in the "Students' Sick Benefit Fund," a medical care program sponsored by CCDS[42] that permitted students, for one dollar per year, to obtain medical attention at one of four nearby hospitals: Presbyterian [affiliated with

Rush Medical College], Homeopathic, West Side, and Frances E. Willard National Temperance [sponsored by the Chicago-based Women's Christian Temperance Union].) Irons cared for him on both occasions, and between those hospitalizations visited the young man twice (in March 1906, for bronchitis, and in May, for knee joint problems) at his new lodging, 534 Monroe Street, not far from where Irons and Herrick lived. Irons kept clinical notes each time and passed them on to Herrick for his file. Irons saw Noel one last time, in April 1907, to discuss progress made since his February discharge from Frances Willard Hospital. Noel reported feeling much better at that time, except for some lingering shortness of breath.[43]

And then he disappeared. Herrick wrote in 1910, "Since then I have never seen or heard from him."[44]

Discussion

During the two and a half years they knew Noel, Herrick and Irons remained interested in his case. They made extra efforts to determine the root of the young man's problem, followed the course of his disease after discharging him from Presbyterian Hospital, and visited him at home when he was sick. Several possible factors, in addition to the medical uniqueness of the case, help explain Herrick's and Irons's concern.

In his article Herrick twice commented about Noel's race and his mental abilities, calling him "an intelligent Negro" and "bright and intelligent." His use of those two phrases suggests that he found Noel different from other patients of color he had encountered. Blacks whom Herrick treated at Cook County Hospital, the large charity institution in Chicago where he also served as attending physician (in addition to the private Presbyterian Hospital), often had recently migrated from the South and were in poor financial situations with little education. He likely saw few black patients in his private practice. So the well-educated and well-heeled Noel, a dental student with a West Indian English accent, differed from Herrick's previous experience with black patients. The young man probably provided a good, clear history and answered medical questions easily. Furthermore, Herrick and Irons were based in a private hospital rather than Chicago's busy and crowded public facility, Cook County Hospital, so they could make extra efforts to help him.

In addition, Noel's blood findings were interesting. So interesting that, in late 1905 or early 1906, Herrick read articles cited in the *Journal of the American Medical Association*'s "Current Literature" section and in German medical journals (he had just spent several months studying in Germany) on yaws, hookworm disease, and alterations in red blood cell morphology. He scribbled down on several pieces of loose paper (one of which was the backside of a daily calendar sheet for September 10, 1905) references to four medical journal articles that seemed promising. Though none of the articles satisfactorily answered Herrick's questions about Noel's condition, one of them, written in German by M. Löwit, apparently gave him a descriptive term he later applied to the odd cells present in the patient's blood smear: *sickle-shaped* (*sichelförmiger*). The references to these articles sat in Herrick's file, along with Irons's notes from visits to the patient through 1907 and with key documents from Noel's Presbyterian Hospital visit.[45]

For several more years, amid their other activities, Irons and Herrick thought about the strange case. Neither met other physicians who had encountered patients with a similar condition. In a 1954 obituary notice about his mentor, one of their only direct published references to the discovery of sickle cell anemia besides Herrick's 1910 case report, Irons stated, "We had never seen anything like this before and Dr. Herrick delayed his report until all sorts of tests to exclude artefacts [*sic*] were repeated again and again."[46] Herrick even consulted with his colleague Ludvig Hektoen, the highly regarded pathologist and bacteriologist, and tried some experiments to produce sickled cells in vitro, but to no avail.[47] Ultimately stumped by the case, Herrick presented it unsolved in 1910.

Irons played a crucial but less visible role than Herrick in the story. He noticed the strange blood cells after doing the initial blood smear, sketched them, and brought the findings to his attending physician's attention. He followed the patient's course over the next two years, visiting him at home and in the hospital, and turned his notes over to Herrick. Herrick described some of these activities in his 1910 presentation and article, but Irons received none of the subsequent recognition for helping to discover sickle cell anemia. Herrick appears to have directed the handling of the case, performed the search for references, and worked through and written up the results. He therefore has received the credit.

The paper he published was a case study, like many of Herrick's other previous writings. By the time he wrote it, his interests had begun to focus on angina pectoris and coronary occlusion, and Irons's interests had turned to his Ph.D. studies on focal infections. Though neither man pursued the case or its implications for hematology, both physicians and their patient had already made their marks on history.

Herrick and Irons were men of their times, open to the new ideas and techniques of medicine being taught in the classroom, described in medical journals, and discussed at medical conventions and local medical society meetings. They applied this new knowledge and technology as best they could in their pursuit of an explanation for Noel's unusual blood problem, even searching the world medical literature for pertinent articles. The end product of their work, publication of a case study, stimulated other physicians to notice similar instances in their own practices and to publish that information. These case studies generated enough information and curiosity about the sickling phenomenon for physicians to begin conducting full-blown clinical and laboratory studies. By the late 1920s sickle cell anemia had become a recognized medical entity. By the 1950s it had great importance for medicine as the first identified molecular genetic disease.[48]

Noel, of unusual national background (Grenada, West Indies) for Herrick and Irons, was an English-speaking black man studying dentistry with whites in the United States. He may have been the only black person at CCDS, but others attended integrated or all-black dental, medical, nursing, and pharmacy schools in Chicago and elsewhere. Noel's experience exemplified the racial changes occurring in American society and American medicine.

Epilogue: What Happened to Noel?

Herrick's comment in 1910, "Since then [April 1907] I have never seen or heard from him," seems odd in light of what he and Irons knew of their West Indian patient. Perhaps Noel failed to tell them in April 1907 that he was about to graduate from dental school at the end of the following month. But Herrick and Irons should have assumed that his disappearance was related to his student status and inquired at CCDS, directly across the street from Rush Medical College.

Despite his serious and lengthy illnesses between December 1904 and February 1907, Noel completed his work sufficiently well to graduate with his class on May 28, 1907.[49] He returned to Grenada and opened an office in the heart of St. George's on the ground floor of a building his mother owned (corner of Young and Government streets). He lived upstairs.[50]

Little is known of Noel's life during these years. In 1987, one of his former patients recalled leaving her convent school one day as a sixteen-year-old pupil (with an escort) and walking the few steps to Noel's office, where he pulled her aching tooth. She described Noel as smartly dressed, healthy looking, and plump, with dark coffee-colored skin, a "round, fat face and a good body."[51] He owned his own dental equipment and, by 1915, had hired a young man in the office as his assistant.[52] Noel never married.

On May 2, 1916, some nine years after his return to Grenada, Walter Clement Noel died in his home/office at age thirty-two. Eldon Marksman, his assistant, reported the death, which Dr. G. W. Paterson certified as having been caused by "asthenia from pneumonia."[53] According to family members, Noel, who enjoyed going out, had gone to a "race meeting" (horse race) in Grenville, across the mountains on the other side of the island, and returned, all in one day. He had then taken a bath, caught a chill, developed pneumonia, and died.[54]

Noel could not have been a healthy man. He had suffered several bouts of illness before he left home for Chicago in 1904 and again during his stay there.

He died young, of pneumonia, a disease not uncommon in those with sickle cell anemia. Furthermore, Noel wrote a will about a year before he died, indicating that he probably had some concerns about the status of his health.[55]

Noel was buried in the Catholic cemetery behind the church in Sauteurs overlooking the Caribbean. He and his sister, Jane, who had died at age twenty-four ("asthenia from pulmonary tuberculosis"), shared a grave next to their father, who had died some thirty years earlier at age thirty-six ("disease of the kidney" [Noel had told Herrick he had died of an "accident"]).[56] Could each of them (as well as a deceased sister born in 1875) have been victims of sickle cell anemia? Perhaps. But Noel never knew that his former physician, Herrick, had presented and then published his case history or that he was the first patient with a recorded, documented case of sickle cell anemia.

CHAPTER 5

Washburn's 1911 Case Report of Sickle Cell Anemia, Charlottesville, Virginia

In February 1911, the *Virginia Medical Semi-Monthly* published a case report of a Campbell County, Virginia, patient then at the University of Virginia Hospital, admitted with unusual-looking red blood cells.[1] That report constituted the second recorded case of sickle cell anemia in the medical literature. This chapter brings to life the characters involved in that second case report and the setting in which the event occurred, contrasting the people, setting, and outcome of that report with those in the first case report.

Benjamin Earl (sometimes spelled Earle) Washburn was a fourth-year medical student at the University of Virginia (UVa) when he wrote his article about Ellen Anthony, the second reported sickle cell patient in the medical literature. These two young people's lives intersected for a few months during the winter of 1910–11 and then moved in different directions, never to cross again, just as had occurred with the first sickle cell patient and his physicians.[2] For Washburn, Ellen Anthony was an "interesting case."[3] For Anthony, Benjamin Washburn was probably just another of the many students, interns, and attending physicians she saw during long months spent as a patient in the wards of the UVa Hospital. Would they have remembered each others' names a year later? Though they had a short-term common interest—Ms. Anthony's health—Washburn and Anthony, approximately the same age, were worlds apart.

Washburn was born on December 29, 1885, and raised in western North Carolina, in and around the small town of Rutherfordton. The eldest child of John Rutherford Washburn, a merchant, and Camila Miller, Benjamin Washburn had two brothers and three sisters. Though the family was not wealthy, owing to a number of unfortunate business deals John Washburn made when his children were growing up, the Washburn parents valued education and managed to send all their children to college. As a teenager, Ben Washburn worked in Rutherfordton after school and during summers to save enough money to pay for his first undergraduate year at the University of North Carolina (UNC). During his college years he earned money by tutoring; typing notes, lectures, and theses for students and professors; working at the UNC library for Librarian Louis Round Wilson; and serving as secretary to C. Alphonso Smith, a nationally known professor of English literature. Washburn also used his earnings to help defray his brothers' and sisters' college expenses whenever he could.[4]

During his years at UNC (1902–6), Washburn earned a reputation (retained in graduate and medical schools) for being a reader and lover of literature.[5] As campus yearbook editors characterized him in the 1906 *Yakety Yak*, "[H]e has distinguished himself . . . by passing off a large number of hours without opening a text-book, and by reading every book in the library. It is said that ten men are necessary to turn the leaves when he reads."[6] His UNC library job allowed him to become acquainted with, by his own estimate, "at least 90 percent of the academic student body and many of those in the professional departments."[7] Among the contacts he made was a number of future prominent North Carolinians, contacts that served Washburn well throughout his life.

Upon graduating from UNC in 1906, Washburn thought he would become a teacher. A year as principal of a rural school in Wilson Mills, North Carolina, near Smithfield, convinced him otherwise, and he returned to UNC the following year as a graduate student to pursue his interest in literature. Recognizing that a master's degree in English would inevitably lead him back to teaching, the profession he had just left, Washburn considered and rejected possible careers in law and pharmacy. He ultimately selected medicine because, as he stated in his autobiography, UNC allowed him to apply credits he had earned from undergraduate biology, chemistry, and physics courses toward his M.D. degree and to use that time to take graduate courses in English.[8]

Washburn could thus remain a matriculant at the UNC medical school for two years, take English courses toward a master's degree, and also earn tuition and expense money by working at the UNC library, doing secretarial work for Professor Alphonso Smith, and taking in typing. Despite all these responsibilities and activities, Washburn touched his fellow medical students enough that they selected him historian of his first year class and then president of his second.[9] He wrote a master's thesis under Smith, an expert on literature of the American South, on the subject of the use of African American dialect in the Uncle Remus stories.[10]

Because the UNC medical school's clinical program in Raleigh had a poor reputation (and would soon close under pressure from the American Medical Association and the 1910 Flexner Report), Washburn could not complete his medical education in North Carolina.[11] Professor Smith had just accepted a position at the University of Virginia and offered his young assistant an opportunity to help him on a large book project if he transferred to that institution. Smith also suggested that Washburn would probably encounter little difficulty securing a position at the UVa library given all his experience at UNC. The medical school at Charlottesville had earned a high rating from the American Medical Association's (AMA) Council on Medical Education, further inclining Washburn to apply for admission there.[12]

Though he lacked sufficient funds to pay for a UVa education, Washburn decided that he could earn the money during summers and with outside jobs during the year. Through a series of fortuitous occurrences, he found a way to support himself for two years at UVa by working in the university library, then housed in the campus' famous Rotunda building, designed by Thomas Jefferson.[13] He could now make plans to complete his medical studies at UVa in the fall of 1909. It was on the wards of UVa's teaching hospital that medical student Benjamin Washburn met patient Ellen Anthony.

Ellen Anthony was born about 1885, though no available county or state documents record that event.[14] She grew up in the rolling farmland and wooded hills of Campbell County, Virginia, around Evington and Lynch Station.[15] White families with the surname Anthony owned property in that area dating back in some cases to colonial times.[16] It is probable that the several African American families with the surname Anthony, including Ellen Anthony's, were once owned as slaves by some of the white Anthonys.

Entries in the UVa Hospital admissions books between 1907 and 1911 identify Ellen Anthony's father as Richard Anthony,[17] though no Richard Anthony with a daughter named Ellen appears in any of the appropriate manuscript censuses for Campbell County.[18] The only available information concerning Richard Anthony derives from a few words in Washburn's 1911 case report: "The patient's father . . . is now an old man and has been in bad health for many years. He suffers with rheumatism and kidney disease."[19] Of the remainder of Ellen Anthony's family almost nothing is known. Washburn's 1911 article states that the patient's mother "died about twenty years ago," her four brothers and three of her sisters died in childhood, and her one remaining sister "died in a New York hospital last June, of some brain trouble."[20] Interviews conducted among members of the African American and white communities of southern Campbell County (including Leesville, Altavista, Lynch Station, and Evington) during the summer and fall of 1993 produced only one person who remembered or knew anything about Ellen or Richard Anthony.[21]

Ellen Anthony worked, when she was able, as a cook and housemaid.[22] Of her childhood and education no information is available save that she told Washburn she had been sickly all her life, enduring bouts of pneumonia, pleurisy, severe abdominal pain, malaria-like symptoms (chills and fever), chronic left-sided chest pain, frequent nosebleeds, shortness of breath on exertion, night sweats, constipation, and indigestion.[23] We know Ellen Anthony primarily through her illnesses.

Some five years before Anthony encountered Washburn on the wards, about 1905 or 1906, she developed the medical problems that eventually took her to Charlottesville for her first admission to the UVa Hospital. Anthony found that any slight exertion caused her dizziness and shortness of breath as well as foot and ankle swelling. Once, when she knocked the skin off her left shin, a tenacious ulcer formed and became infected. At a later date an ulcer developed on her right leg, though she did not recall having hurt it. When severe, sharp, stabbing abdominal pains radiating from her left side to the region of her liver became increasingly frequent, she finally sought medical help.[24]

Washburn's 1911 article does not identify Anthony's local physician, and no medical records of physicians from the Evington/Lynch Station area of Campbell County are extant, but a notation in the UVa Hospital admissions book for Ellen Anthony's second admission (March 30, 1908) names "Dr. J. S. Irving" as her physician.[25] J. Sinkler Irvine was, according to the 1909 *American Medical Directory*, the only physician practicing in Evington, Virginia, population 103. He graduated from the University of Louisville Medical Department in 1891 and received his medical license in 1895. Mrs. Anna Keller, Irvine's daughter, remembered, during a May 1993 telephone interview, her father's horse-and-buggy physician days at the turn of the century, but had no recollection of hearing about Ellen Anthony. Her father treated everyone in the area in those days, she said, but none of his patient records survive.[26] Extrapolating from these scanty facts, one can conclude that Anthony, like other poor black and white residents of the area, probably turned to Dr. Irvine for medical attention after all home treatments and suggestions from relatives and friends had failed. Her abdominal crisis in the autumn of 1907 must have taken Anthony to Dr. Irvine, for shortly thereafter, Anthony was in Charlottesville as a patient at the new UVa Hospital.

The UVa Hospital had opened its doors for surgical procedures in 1901 and for the accommodation of twenty inpatients in 1902. In 1905, thirty more beds had been added, and in November 1907, another fifty were added, boosting the hospital's capacity to one hundred. As the purpose of establishing a hospital at the University of Virginia had been to provide medical and surgical care for charity patients and clinical experience for medical students, eighty of those one hundred beds were devoted to indigents, equally divided among black males, black females, white males, and white females. Ward C, designated for public (i.e., nonpaying) African American female patients, was located in the south wing of the basement, the same floor as the public black male ward and the dining rooms, kitchen, and store rooms.[27]

Dr. Irvine reportedly knew a number of physicians at the UVa Hospital, because he had begun his medical training there before transferring to the University of

Louisville to complete his M.D. degree.[28] Ellen Anthony's severe and puzzling symptoms, combined with the charity mission of the UVa Hospital and Dr. Irvine's acquaintance with the university's medical school, may have induced him to send his patient to Charlottesville. Anthony was admitted before September 1, 1907, the beginning date of the hospital's first admissions register, and discharged in December of that year, "feeling much improved," according to Washburn's information.[29] The hospital register books indicate that for all her admissions Anthony was classified as a free or public patient assigned to Ward C.

Just three months following her discharge, on March 30, 1908, the young woman was back in the hospital, admitted again by Dr. Irvine, and suffering once more from severe abdominal pain and other symptoms. She was quickly transferred from the medical to the surgical service where she underwent an operation to remove a number of gallstones. Anthony remained in the hospital through mid-June, a period of some eighty days, and then returned home "well," according to the entry in the hospital record book.[30]

She remained out of the hospital for almost a year, until April 1909, when she was yet again admitted with severe left-sided pain. Routine blood smears revealed, according to Washburn's 1911 summary of Anthony's chart from that 1909 hospital stay, "poikilocytes [red blood cells of irregular shape] in a variety of shapes, the most common variety being of a crescent shape," though that term "crescent" does not appear in the hospital record book for that admission. Unfortunately, Anthony's chart, along with all of the earliest UVa Hospital patients' charts, is missing.[31] Were that chart available, it might reveal more details about an incident that could have changed the early history of sickle cell anemia and given credit for discovery of the disease to physicians at the University of Virginia in 1909.

According to the distinguished hematologist Russell L. Haden (1888–1952), who grew up near Charlottesville and received his undergraduate and master's degrees from UVa in 1910 and 1911, respectively, clinicians at the UVa Hospital were sufficiently puzzled and intrigued by Ellen Anthony's unusual blood smear in 1909 that they sent it to pathologists at the Johns Hopkins University Hospital for identification.[32] The Hopkins pathologists, Haden recounted, interpreted the smear as an unusual instance of pernicious anemia rather than as evidence of a new blood disease worthy of further investigation and reporting in the medical literature. As a result, no one at UVa wrote about the Anthony case until after Herrick's 1910 report apparently startled the Charlottesville physicians into identifying Anthony's medical problem as a case of this newly recognized form of anemia. UVa physicians could possibly have been the first to report sickle cell anemia, though Herrick and Irons noticed the unusually shaped blood cells in 1904, but they waited almost six years to publish their case history.

Anthony's regimen during her two-month stay at UVa Hospital included bed rest and potassium iodide. She left in early June 1909 without the severe pains in her side, but also without a clear diagnosis of her condition.[33] For three weeks she felt fine, but then began an almost three-month siege of symptoms including pains in her left side that kept her in bed, shortness of breath, night sweats, and "sleep starts." Leg ulcers, one of Anthony's constant complaints from the time the illness first began in 1905 or 1906, enlarged and also caused her much pain.[34] She finally had to return to Charlottesville for her fourth UVa Hospital admission on September 18, 1909,[35] just a few weeks after the arrival in town of the other principal character in this story, Benjamin Earl Washburn.

Early one morning during the first week of September 1909, Washburn, now a transferring third-year medical student from the University of North Carolina, obtained his first view of the UVa grounds and the hospital that Ellen Anthony already knew so well. Having ridden on the night train from Charlotte, North Carolina, to save money, he arrived in Charlottesville, sleepless, at 7:00 A.M. Over the next several days he made his living, dining, and student employment arrangements and was ready to begin classes and his clinical clerkship as soon as the other medical students returned from summer break.[36]

When the term began, Washburn's medical school class of nineteen was divided into two sections for clinical work, each spending half the year on the surgical service and half on the medical. As third-year students, they saw patients both in the hospital and in the dispensary (outpatient clinic). Though no corroborating evidence is available, Washburn must have encountered Ellen Anthony on the wards during this year of medical training. Anthony was quite sick and took a long time to recover. She spent 284 days in the hospital, giving medical students ample opportunity to meet her and to study her case. Washburn described Anthony's medical findings from this admission in great detail in his 1911 article, indicating that he had access to her chart and probably had examined her several times during his time on the wards. He mentioned the "crescent-shaped poikilocytes" again as well as iron and arsenic treatments for her anemia.[37]

Though Anthony recovered sufficiently to go home on July 9, 1910, after more than nine months in Charlottesville, she had to return to the hospital just one hundred days later. Washburn briefly described those hundred days at home in his 1911 article, offering readers some insight into the frustrating life Anthony must have led at this time:[38]

> The patient left the hospital June 27, 1910 [according to the hospital record book, it was July 9, 1910], feeling much stronger and with the ulcers on her legs healed. She obtained employment as a cook. After working for about a month, the ulcer on her left leg broke down. She also had headaches, which were worse in the morning; and the pain in her left side returned. These troubles, together with general weakness, made it impossible for her to do regular work, and since August, she has been unable to do any

kind of work, as exertion made her short of breath and caused her ankles to swell. She returned to the hospital, October 25, 1910.

By October 1910 Washburn had entered his fourth year of medical school. As during the third year, his class was divided in two, each group spending half the year on the medicine service and half on the surgical. Washburn rotated through medicine first and was assigned to Ellen Anthony when the young woman was admitted for the fifth time to Ward C on October 25. Within a few weeks of this admission, James B. Herrick in Chicago published his report describing "peculiar elongated and sickle-shaped red blood corpuscles in a case of severe anemia" in the *Archives of Internal Medicine.*[39]

When Washburn and his instructors at the UVa Medical Department actually read Herrick's article is unknown, but an ambiguous entry in the UVa Hospital admissions register at about that time raises some questions about Anthony's care. The entry for Ellen Anthony's fifth stay at UVa Hospital shows that she was discharged on November 15, 1910, after only twenty-two days in the hospital. A second discharge date of April 1, 1911, also appears in that same record. There are several possible reasons for this curious insertion in the admission register. Perhaps the hospital authorities meant to discharge Anthony on November 15th and got as far as entering the information in the record book before they realized that she was not really well enough to go home and so kept her in the hospital. Or perhaps Anthony actually left the hospital but returned hours or days later because she was so sick. Or perhaps the November issue of the *Archives of Internal Medicine* arrived about the 15th of November, after the hospital staff had decided to discharge or already had released Anthony. Suddenly someone, possibly Washburn, recognized the similarities between Herrick's published case and Ellen Anthony's medical problems and wished to investigate her condition further. Perhaps there was even some thought of earning the distinction of reporting the second case of "peculiar elongated sickle-shaped red blood cells" in a patient with severe anemia. Whatever the reason for her readmission in November, Anthony must have been sick enough to be a patient in the hospital, because she remained there until the following April.

Available records do not identify the person in Charlottesville who first recognized the similarities between Herrick's patient Walter Clement Noel and Washburn's patient Ellen Anthony, though, as mentioned, some physicians at the medical school were well aware of Anthony's atypical blood cells from her 1909 admissions. Washburn did not comment on this matter in his 1911 article or in his autobiography. He did state, however, that the idea of writing a history of the Anthony case and submitting it to a medical journal came from his professor of medicine, Dr. John Staige Davis Jr.: "Upon the suggestion of Dr.

Davis and with his help, I prepared a report, illustrated with photomicrographs of blood smears."[40] Davis, professor of medicine, son of an early professor of anatomy at UVa,[41] and Washburn's favorite instructor,[42] had, according to the hospital record book, served as Anthony's physician during her earlier stays in the hospital. He was also a member of the editorial board of the *Virginia Medical Semi-Monthly*,[43] published in Richmond. It was the logical journal for a University of Virginia medical student to approach for expeditious publication of the second case report of a newly discovered disease. The report quickly appeared. It was submitted after January 8[44] and published in the February 10, 1911, issue, just three months after Herrick's article.

Washburn refers to Herrick's article at the beginning of his own, reviewing in two long paragraphs the earlier case's salient features and quoting Herrick's justification for publishing the case at all: "This case is reported because of the unusual blood findings, no duplicate of which I have ever seen described."[45] A brief third paragraph then explains Washburn's publication: "There is a patient in the medical ward of the University of Virginia Hospital, with a somewhat similar history, whose blood shows the same, if not more marked, characteristics as in the case reported by Herrick. This patient has been under observation, at intervals, since 1907."[46] The next three pages are packed with the history and present medical situation of Ellen Anthony (not named in the article, of course), whose initial admission to UVa Hospital occurred at about the time Herrick lost track of his patient in Chicago. Washburn tells of previous admissions; blood, urine, stool, and sputum examinations; treatments; physical examination findings; and the patient's course during each hospital stay. Similar to Herrick's article, this paper also contains a photomicrograph, prepared by Washburn's classmate Frank P. Smart,[47] illustrating the crescent-shaped red cells in Anthony's blood.

Amid the abundance of medical particulars about physical findings and symptoms, Washburn occasionally includes details that remind readers of the human being behind the clinical descriptions:

> She states, that she has never had good health. (p. 490)
>
> The patient is a cook and has always done house work. In September 1910, she weighed 115 pounds, but has fallen off since that time. (p. 490)
>
> The patient is a fairly well developed negro woman, with facies characteristic of her race, and looks intelligent. (p. 492)
>
> [T]he teeth are few in number, decayed, and in a very bad condition. (p. 492)

The paper closes as inconclusively as did Herrick's, with a positive statement about the patient's current health ("general condition is much improved and she feels much better than when she entered the hospital"[48]) and a noncommittal comment about the disease process ("The facts do not seem to warrant a diagnosis as to the cause of the condition"[49]). Neither Washburn nor Herrick ever published follow-up reports on their patients; in their autobiographies, neither devoted more than a few sentences to their articles reporting the first cases of sickle cell anemia.

Ellen Anthony finally left the UVa Hospital from her fifth and, as it turned out, historic admission, on April 1, 1911, but not for the last time. She returned to the hospital at least eight more times between August 22, 1911, and May 14, 1918, with the same familiar complaints on each occasion. Dr. Irvine remained her local physician, while Dr. Davis continued to supervise her care at the hospital. Admissions books through July 1922 do not record further hospital contact with Ellen Anthony beyond 1918, nor do local and state mortality records mention the death of Ellen Anthony. She was unrecognized in the state's public records throughout her life.

Benjamin Earl Washburn's life after publication of his article on sickle cell anemia is, in contrast, well documented. He earned his M.D. degree from the University of Virginia in 1911 and served a six-month internship at James Walker Memorial Hospital in Wilmington, North Carolina, before returning to his native Rutherford County for a fourteen-month stint as a country doctor in the South Mountains.[50] Public health medicine and medical care to underserved populations then became his life's work. Washburn joined the Rockefeller Sanitary Commission's hookworm campaign in his native state, served as health officer for Nash County, North Carolina, then spent the remainder of his career with the Rockefeller Foundation's International Health Division in the West Indies. Retiring to Rutherford County in 1939, he continued working for local and state health agencies and the community hospital in Rutherfordton. He died in 1980.[51]

The first two articles describing cases of sickle cell anemia contain similar kinds of medical information, but the articles differ quite starkly in the matter of crediting scientific discovery. The early twentieth century continued the great era of medical discovery that had begun in the late nineteenth century with the advancement of bacteriology and laboratory studies.[52] Physicians and scientists were uncovering and naming new bacteria, studying basic pathology and physiology, and learning about normal and unusual components of blood. Individuals worked hard to gain the distinction of being called the discoverer of a bacterium or of a medical condition. In the instance of sickle cell anemia, credit for detecting and describing the first case went not to the physician who initially treated the patient and noted the abnormality, Ernest E. Irons, but to his attending physician, James B.

Herrick, while credit for reporting the second case went not to the senior physicians who had worked with the patient previously but to a fourth-year-medical student assigned to the patient on her fifth admission.

Why did John Staige Davis Jr., the attending physician and professor who oversaw Ellen Anthony's care at the UVa Hospital, allow credit for describing the second case of a newly recognized disorder to go to a medical student? Herrick, in a similar situation at Rush Medical College and Presbyterian Hospital in Chicago, gave only a passing nod in his 1910 article to his resident and protégé Irons, who actually first saw the patient Walter Clement Noel, recognized the oddly shaped red blood cells, and treated Noel for his medical problems over a three-year period. Herrick, as senior attending physician on the case, took a leadership role in pursuing further information about the medical findings and in writing the report and presenting it at professional meetings. Extant records do not indicate why Irons did not receive equal credit with Herrick in those presentations and the resultant article on Noel's case of sickle cell anemia.[53]

Perhaps it was Benjamin Washburn who first saw Herrick's article in the *Archives of Internal Medicine* and recognized the similarities to the case of Ellen Anthony. If so, and Washburn pointed out the unique medical situation to his attending, then Davis apparently was the kind of person who had no need to claim even partial credit for a discovery that was not technically his. Or perhaps Davis was the one who noticed the similarities in the two cases but wanted to allow a younger person to shine. Whatever the reason, Washburn had one advantage over his classmates: his writing and typing abilities, developed in the bachelor's and master's programs in English at UNC, were well-known at the Charlottesville medical school. Washburn's classmates and teachers were well aware of the quality of his patient histories and of the way he typed them: "I was commended for them [the patient histories] upon a number of occasions," he reported in his autobiography.[54] Davis knew that Benjamin Earl Washburn could be trusted to write a good case report.

Finally, the contrast between the first two sickle cell anemia patients reported in the medical literature bears comment. While opportunities in the United States for aspiring persons of color (American and West Indian) to study and enter medicine, dentistry, and law were increasing during the late nineteenth and early twentieth centuries, segregation in the South was becoming more rigid and formalized.[55] Some African American men and women felt the need to migrate to the North or to Southern cities in search of better jobs. Large numbers of black people, however, remained in their rural or small-town homes, eking out a living in agriculture, unskilled labor, or domestic service.

Walter Clement Noel, a man of color, was, in many ways, the social and professional equal of his physicians, Herrick and Irons.[56] Noel came from a prosperous family on the island of Grenada, a British colony in the Caribbean. He attended a private school in Barbados and was, when he fell ill in the United States, a student at the Chicago College of Dental Surgery. He was unlike the majority of black patients his physicians usually saw in practice. The fact that Noel was well-educated and well-spoken may have stimulated Herrick's and Irons' interest in discovering the nature of the young man's illness. Noel may have even assisted them in thinking through the problem. When Herrick and Irons lost track of Noel, it was because their patient had returned to his West Indian homeland to practice his chosen profession of dentistry. Members of his family were landowners and known figures on an island where most residents, largely people of color, lived in poor circumstances with little opportunity for advancement.

Ellen Anthony, in contrast to Noel, was typical of many African Americans of her day. She appears to have grown up poor, had little education, earned little money, and was thus quite different, economically and socially, from her physicians, including the medical students who treated her. In Virginia's racially segregated society of the late nineteenth and early twentieth centuries, Anthony remained a relatively anonymous citizen. Public records reported neither her birth nor her death, as was also true of her father and the rest of her family. Whereas Walter Clement Noel's history is easy to trace from family, school, and official government sources, almost nothing is available on Ellen Anthony from any sources, written or oral. How ironic, considering that the disease from which she suffered and which was first discovered in her and in a West Indian dental student became one of the most studied in medicine.

CHAPTER 6

Sickle Cell Anemia

The Invisible Malady

In the sixty years following publication of Dr. James B. Herrick's 1910 case description of a twenty-year-old West Indian professional student with leg ulcers, anemia, joint and abdominal pains, and a "large number of thin, sickle-shaped and crescent-shaped" red blood cells,[1] hundreds of researchers published articles in professional journals on all aspects of what came to be known as sickle cell anemia (SCA).[2] Yet in 1969, John C. Lane, a high school science teacher and master's degree candidate, and Robert B. Scott, a hematologist, wrote an article for the Public Health Service's journal, *Public Health Reports*, which pointed out that only three of ten black adult residents of Richmond, Virginia (and, by implication, the rest of the country), had ever heard of SCA. Furthermore, when the authors adjusted this figure for the educational level of their sample (the population surveyed included more highly educated persons than did the population as a whole), they found that fewer than 20 percent of adult African Americans knew of SCA.[3] Other researchers performing studies similar to that of Lane and Scott had like findings. Only 5 of 150 black military recruits at an army base in Texas were aware of sickle cell states; 47 percent of Boston parents whose children (650 of them) had been screened for SCA had heard of the disease, but none knew it was passed on from generation to generation; and about 70 percent of 147 Seattle parents whose children had been screened for SCA believed that people with sickle cell trait suffer such physical problems as lack of energy, weakness, limb pain, and frequent colds.[4] Not only was SCA barely recognized among African Americans, but it was also regularly passed over by Congress when it came time each year to allocate research funds.[5] How could a condition that commonly caused chronic illness and death among black children, and was therefore of great importance to the entire nation, be ignored for so long by both blacks and whites? The answers to this question are not clear, but several are suggested in a study of the history of the disease, of blacks, and of public health in America.

Sickle Cell before 1910

Though Western medicine did not discover SCA until Herrick's report in 1910, the condition had actually existed for centuries, first in Africa and the southern Mediterranean area, and later, transported by enslaved blacks, in the West Indies, South America, and the United States. African tribes in Ghana, Nigeria, and the Cameroons had known of the disease and had named it centuries earlier. Oral tradition had kept knowledge of SCA and its hereditary character alive for each succeeding generation.[6] Early white physicians of enslaved Africans in the Americas may have simply ignored or perhaps never heard this oral tradition. With the breakup of African tribal groups in America and the social and psychological dislocations caused by the slave system, it is probable that oral knowledge of what is now called sickle cell disease did not last many generations.

But the sickle cell gene was certainly present in the black population of early America. Its history is intimately tied to another important worldwide disease—malaria. Malaria was the plague of the American South from early slavery times to the 1930s. The disease struck whites and blacks alike, incapacitating them for weeks during the attacks, and weakening them for months thereafter. Relapses often occurred as a microscopic parasite, *Plasmodium,* lingered in the bloodstream and internal organs. Not only did malaria render life generally unpleasant, but it also hindered industrial advancement owing to a sickly labor force.[7] The unpredictability of the disease was a source of great frustration to planters during important seasons. Unfortunately for the slave owner, harvest time for many crops—late summer and early fall—coincided with the period of greatest activity for the mosquito vector of malaria. And since malaria was endemic throughout much of the slaveholding South, it posed a constant threat to health year in and year out.[8]

Devastating as malaria was to residents of the South, it seemed to spare many blacks, planters and physicians noted as far back as the seventeenth century. This trend was first observed on the huge rice plantations of the South Carolina Low Country between Charleston and Savannah, and later throughout all the slave states. Racial theories regarding the medical differences between whites and blacks sprung up around such observations as these and around other apparent physiological distinctions. These theories later became incorporated into the proslavery argument of the pre–Civil War era.[9] Today it is known that people carrying at least one sickle cell gene are resistant to the inroads of the most virulent form of malarial parasite, *Plasmodium falciparum*, but people in earlier times could only speculate on the apparent immunity of persons of African descent. It has been estimated that at least 22 percent of Africans brought to this country possessed a sickle cell gene (and another 20 percent had the gene of G-6-PD disease, which also confers immunity to malaria).[10]

Aside from the testimony of some planters and physicians that many enslaved blacks appeared to be immune to malaria, there is little concrete evidence to show that the diseases associated with sickle cell genes occurred in the antebellum South. Some pre–Civil War records do hint, however, at probable instances of these diseases, though the ambiguity of their symptoms makes them difficult to positively identify. First, many planters complained of the high rate of spontaneous abortion among their enslaved women.[11] Since young women with either sickle cell anemia or sickle cell–Hemoglobin C disease (another genetic condition related to SCA) are known to have a higher rate of miscarriage than other women, the presence of these diseases among bondswomen probably accounted for a portion of the spontaneous abortions noted.[12] Second, all the abnormal hemoglobin diseases produce mild to severe joint pains that were probably labeled rheumatism by planters, physicians, and bondspeople alike. No doubt older adults normally experienced such pains, especially during damp weather, but when children suffered from them, the cause in some cases must have been SCA. Third, a partial reason for the notoriously high mortality rates among enslaved children in the antebellum South was the fact that about half of the children with SCA probably died before reaching the age of twenty.[13] Fourth, in partial explanation of the extreme sensitivity of blacks to all infections of the lungs noted by planters and physicians,[14] studies indicate that sickle cell anemia and sickle cell–Hemoglobin C disease predispose individuals to severe pneumococcal infections.[15] Fifth, the occurrence of chronic leg ulcers among enslaved blacks also hints at the existence of sickle cell disease.[16] Finally, a case described by a Charleston physician in 1834 of a bondsman who suffered frequently from fevers in the summer and respiratory ailments in the winter and who, upon autopsy, was found to be lacking a spleen, led one modern physician to speculate that this might have been a case of sickle cell anemia.[17] SCA was certainly present in this country prior to the Civil War.

Medicine Learns about Sickle Cell Anemia

In the thirty-five years before Herrick's 1910 description of "peculiar elongated and sickle-shaped red blood corpuscles in a case of severe anemia," several other reports of cases that may have been SCA appeared in the world medical literature.[18] These reports were largely ignored. In contrast, Herrick's announcement, perhaps because of its completeness and accuracy (it even included photomicrographs of blood smears), was soon confirmed by similar cases in other parts of the country. As described in the previous chapter, Benjamin E. Washburn, a fourth-year medical student at the University of Virginia in Charlottesville, published the second case of sickle-shaped red blood cells, this time in an anemic female patient.[19] Recognition of the sickled cells did not aid in treatment of the condition, but medical science was now on its way to a better understanding of it.

At first, advancement was slow. Though the first two cases were reported within a year of each other, the next two did not appear until 1915 and 1922, respectively.[20] Two physicians, one at Johns Hopkins in Baltimore, the other at the University of Georgia Medical Department in Augusta, then became quite interested in SCA and began intensive investigations that brought much new information to light. Up to mid-1923, the condition was thought to be rare, probably confined to blacks, and familial in its transmission. Papers presented orally and then published that year by Virgil P. Sydenstricker of Augusta and John G. Huck of Baltimore confirmed at their respective clinics the previously suspected racial and familial nature of SCA. Both physicians had begun screening clinic patients (and their families when warranted) for the disease many months earlier by testing for sickling in sealed blood smears. These investigations, which ultimately included several autopsies, clearly established SCA as a clinical entity common enough to warrant further research.[21]

Now other medical investigators initiated studies of SCA's incidence. The results continued to surprise physicians: 6.6 percent of 858 black patients at a Birmingham, Alabama, hospital, 7.5 percent of 400 black children in a Detroit hospital, and 6.3 percent of 300 black patients in Barnes Hospital, St. Louis, showed positive sickling tests.[22] Commenting on the elevated frequency, a University of Pennsylvania physician wrote, "Such an unexpectedly high incidence should challenge one to a clearer knowledge and more ready recognition of this condition."[23]

But clearer knowledge of SCA was an elusive goal. The confusion over its nature and etiology was illustrated early on by the differences between the research of Sydenstricker in 1923 and Huck in 1924. It was the former's observation that the sickling condition occurred in two forms: active and latent. The active type was characterized by anemia, joint and muscle pain, severe abdominal discomfort, and often leg ulcers. These symptoms remitted and recurred at uneven intervals throughout an individual's lifetime. Patients with latent SCA presented with no symptoms of anemia, but always had a history of rare rheumatic attacks, abdominal pain, and other complaints. These people were generally healthy, though, said Sydenstricker, "scleral discoloration [characteristic, he claimed, of SCA] is always present"; leg ulcers appeared occasionally; and other minor physical signs could be discerned.[24] Huck divided his cases into three groups: symptomless, mild, and severe. Those persons whose blood sickled after twenty-four hours in sealed preparations but who suffered no ill effects from the disease, he placed in the "symptomless" category—a classification Sydenstricker omitted. "Mild" SCA patients were only occasionally affected with symptoms, while those in the last ("severe") group were rarely symptom free. On one point they both agreed—any person with a positive sickle cell test could pass from one state of the disease to another at any time in his or her life. This belief persisted until the late 1950s.

Thomas B. Cooley and Pearl Lee, the Detroit physicians who in 1925 first described thalassemia, helped clarify the problems of SCA classification in 1926. They studied the blood of all black children (400) admitted to Children's Hospital of Michigan (Detroit) for sickle cells over a ten-month period, and then observed those with a positive sickle cell test for evidence of anemia. Their results indicated that "the presence of sickle cells in the blood does not in itself imply any essential anemia, active or latent." They found that most in vitro sicklers lived normal lives and had no greater incidence of anemia, joint or abdominal pains, or leg ulcers than black children with negative sickle tests. None had discolored sclerae. A positive sickle test did not mean one suffered from SCA. Cooley and Lee proposed labeling the disorder suffered by persons with hemolytic (destruction of red blood cells) anemia "sickle cell anemia," and calling the symptomless state "sicklemia." (They were also the first to suggest in writing that medical researchers in Africa might "perhaps find a tribe in which sicklemia is the rule, and from which the condition was imported to this country.")[25] The following year, 1927, two researchers from Indiana, E. Vernon Hahn and Elizabeth B. Gillespie, introduced the term "sickle cell trait" that was soon used to describe "asymptomatic" (Huck) and, sometimes (wrongly), "latent" (Sydenstricker) cases. For some years, the confusing terms "sicklemia," "sickle cell trait," "active," and "latent sickle cell anemia" were used, along with others such as "drepanocythemia" and "meniscocytosis," undoubtedly causing difficulties among the patient population and, conceivably, among clinicians.[26]

The relationship between "sickle cell trait" and "sickle cell anemia" also remained unclarified until the 1950s. Most researchers from the 1920s on accepted the idea that sickling was an inherited characteristic passed on to offspring in Mendelian dominant fashion.[27] According to this theory, the sickle cell gene "had a variable expression which was more pronounced in some individuals, producing sickle cell anemia, and weaker in others, resulting in what is now termed the sickle cell trait."[28] In other words, it required the sickle cell gene of only one parent to produce the condition in offspring, although it was uncertain whether the trait or the disease would express itself. Controversy arose here over the question of transformation from trait to disease. Until the mid-1930s many researchers felt that a person with the asymptomatic or latent (trait) form could at any time develop active sickle cell anemia. However, some found no evidence to support the claim that "every case of sicklemia [trait] is potentially one of sickle cell anemia."[29] In 1933, L. W. Diggs and coworkers in Memphis demonstrated convincingly that the trait and the disease were separate entities. It was not until 1949 that two medical investigators working independently, James V. Neel at the University of Michigan and E. A. Beet in Northern Rhodesia, demonstrated that sickle cell genes from both parents were required to produce anemia, while the gene from only one parent was necessary to produce the trait.[30] Transformation from trait to disease or vice versa could not occur.

This summary of the early research on SCA has excluded many reports that helped elucidate the disease's pathology, symptomatology, treatment, and complications. These contributions were by no means unimportant, but they have been described elsewhere[31] and are not essential to an understanding of dissemination of SCA information among African Americans. Suffice it to say that by the 1950s the nature of the sickle cell phenomenon was fairly well defined. Between 1933 and the 1950s, further studies using more sensitive tests had shown that the incidence of sickled cells in peripheral blood smears was closer to 10 percent of all African Americans than to the 7 percent previously accepted.[32] That SCA was more a problem of children than of adults had become apparent in the late 1920s and early 1930s, as the number of cases recognized increased. Physicians during this period also noted that patients usually died of intercurrent infection (owing to weakened body resistance to invading bacteria and viruses) and not of the anemia.[33] Studies in the late 1940s demonstrated the higher risk factor that women with SCA encountered during pregnancy and childbirth.[34] Linus Pauling's revelation in 1949 that sickle cell anemia was caused by an alteration in the usual structure of the hemoglobin molecule started a new era in sickle cell research.[35]

Response of the Medical Community to Sickle Cell Anemia

What effect did the discovery and eventual understanding of SCA have on the black population of this country, and what significance did the medical community place on the disease? In general, after an initial flurry of statements by several physicians in the mid-1920s regarding the need to improve recognition and understanding of SCA, most people other than victims of the disease and their physicians, as well a few medical researchers, ignored or knew little about sickle cell disease until the late 1950s. Then a growing black awareness of SCA and the increasing publicity that SCA investigators received with each new development gradually brought the disease to people's consciousnesses. Despite the development of better screening tests and additional information about SCA, it was not until the early 1970s that sickle cell research was federally funded and encouraged, that genetic screening and counseling programs were established, and that public education campaigns were inaugurated.[36] Dr. C. Lockard Conley, a hematologist and historian of the condition, commented in 1980 that "studies of sickle-cell anemia have had an enormous impact, initially more on biological science than on clinical medicine."[37] What Dr. Conley did not say was that these studies generally remained the knowledge of relatively few people and provided little aid or useful information to the general African American or sympathetic white populations until recently.

Back in 1923, after Sydenstricker and Huck had elucidated the racial and familial components of the disease, few medical or laypeople commented on its significance. One who did was W. A. Mulherin, an associate of Sydenstricker in Augusta: "Very little has been known about it, therefore it has not been looked for, and in consequence has not been found. It is of industrial, as well as medical, importance. Efficiency is lowered in the adult and total disability is the result of recurrent attacks. In families where it exists infant and child mortality runs very high."[38] He (and others)[39] also felt that Southern physicians had a special commitment to attend to sickle cell diseases, as that region had the largest African American population in the nation: "As we have a plentiful supply of Negroes with us in the South, it is important that we acquaint ourselves with this disease. I am quite convinced there is more . . . [sickle cell] anemia in the South than is at present realized. It is therefore a Southern problem for us to work out."[40]

Cooley and Lee and others soon demonstrated that with the large post–World War I black migration to urban areas of the North, SCA was not a regional but a nationwide problem. They concluded their 1926 report on SCA in Detroit with the following question: "If . . . sicklemia is a dominant Mendelian characteristic [it is not], and it is now as common as it seems to be in Detroit, shall we not in a few generations have a Negro population, the majority of whom show this peculiarity, and will not 'sickle cell anemia' then be a common condition?"[41]

The biggest difficulty for physicians was recognizing the disease. Because its manifestations resembled, depending on the patient, rheumatic fever, acute abdominal disorders, tuberculosis, pernicious anemia, and other diseases, the diagnosis of SCA was not always obvious. Those researchers who discussed this problem urged their colleagues to examine fresh blood smears in any disease of doubtful etiology in a person of color.[42] Reported in 1926, the case of R. H. B., a thirty-three-year-old black male farmer, was typical. He had suffered few symptoms of SCA until about age twenty-one. From then until his admission to the Memphis Veterans' Hospital in 1925, twelve years later, no physician correctly diagnosed his condition. Fortunately for him, SCA was, as described earlier, receiving increased attention in the medical community at about the time he was a patient in Memphis, so this time the diagnosis was made correctly.[43] In another case, T. J., a black St. Louis woman, had her first sickle cell crisis at age eight in 1928. It was misdiagnosed as acute rheumatic fever. Not until some years later was the true ailment recognized. (She lived to age forty-eight.)[44] Dr. George S. Graham of Birmingham emphasized the importance of diagnosis in comments he delivered at an American Medical Association meeting in 1932: "I have seen two cases in which the acute abdominal symptoms had led to the removal of normal appendixes. Here is perhaps the most practical aspect of the whole problem, and it should be emphasized that in dealing with the Negro patient one should always keep the disease in mind."[45] The problem of SCA identification was not confined to white physicians, as this 1945 editorial from the *Journal of the National Medical Association* (organ of the predominantly black National Medical Association) demonstrates:

> This disease is of the utmost importance to the colored physician and surgeon. There are frequent abdominal crises which may mislead the best surgeon into operating for some acute surgical condition when the real diagnosis is sickle-cell anemia. Such trauma, combined with an inhalation anesthetic, is certain to spell the doom of the patient. . . . The surgeon must not be caught unawares by this condition. The medical man, also would do well to look for this trouble in many unexplained and obscure ailments. Ulcer of the legs is another condition in which sickle-cell anemia may be a causative agent. This condition must be kept in mind constantly and an occasional life would be saved if the laboratory were always informed to look out for sickle-cell anemia.[46]

Knowledge of Sickle Cell Anemia in the Black Community

During the 1920s, 1930s, and 1940s members of both races in medicine and in community organizations were keenly aware of the severe health problems of African Americans. In 1915, Booker T. Washington introduced National Negro Health Week as an annual education and self-improvement campaign.[47] The emphasis, however, was always on tuberculosis, maternal and childhood mortality, malaria (in the South), syphilis, and respiratory diseases—problems much more visible and therefore threatening to African Americans. Given the rising interest and increasing recognition of SCA in the medical community, how did this condition elude discussion? No articles or papers describe physicians' explanations of SCA to their patients. What were people told, if anything, about the inheritability of SCA? Were they counseled in any way? What kind of information did they pass on to their children, their friends, their relatives about this unique condition? What ideas were current in the black community about SCA?

Answers to these questions are difficult to find. None of the widely circulated African American magazines or newspapers, and none of the Public Health Service publications or other white print media, appear to have even mentioned SCA as a disease of significance among blacks. Only the African American pathologist Julian Lewis, in his 1942 landmark publication *The Biology of the Negro*, discussed SCA, and he did so in a clear, understandable manner. S. J. Holmes failed to mention SCA in his otherwise thorough 1937 book *The Negro's Struggle for Survival: A Study in Human Ecology*, as did Gunnar Myrdal in *An American Dilemma*, his monumental synthesis of black problems in the United States (which included chapters on health), published in 1944. SCA was also missing from lengthy special "black health" issues of the *Journal of Negro Education* in 1937 and 1949.[48] And yet, in the highly specialized medical journals of the period, physicians were writing about SCA's surprisingly high incidence and its dangers. Even the *Journal of the National Medical Association* urged black physicians to do research on SCA, especially because "nearly all the information that we have about the condition has been obtained by scientists of other races."[49]

This lack of public awareness began to change in the 1950s. *Scientific American* ran two articles, one in 1951 and one in 1956, describing both Pauling's discovery of an alteration in the normal hemoglobin molecule and Anthony C. Allison's correlation of the sickle cell states with malarial immunity.[50] But *Scientific American* reached relatively few African Americans. The *Negro Digest* published a rather sensationalized, often misleading article on SCA about 1953 (which was reprinted some ten years later). Nothing more appeared in print until the latter part of the decade, when the new medical findings began to filter down into other popular magazines. The *American Mercury* ran an article in 1959 explaining the importance of sickle cell blood tests and the nature of the disease. And *Ebony* published a story that year by an African American college student on the difficulties of life with SCA. *Time* picked up this story a few weeks later, relaying the information to an even larger audience.[51] The small number of other articles in black-oriented and white-oriented magazines and newspapers during the 1960s increased some (primarily white) people's awareness of the sickle cell condition.[52] In fact white opponents of the civil rights movement in the 1950s and 1960s got plenty of publicity out of the sickle cell issue, using it to demonstrate Caucasian genetic superiority and the need to send blacks back to Africa where the genetic defect would again protect against malaria.[53] But still, by 1969, when Lane and Scott's article appeared, fewer than two in ten of the adult population directly affected by SCA—African Americans—knew of it.

Several reasons for this lack of awareness should now be apparent. Medically, other diseases had greater morbidity and mortality among African Americans than did SCA. Necessity dictated that reducing the incidence of tuberculosis, syphilis, maternal and childhood diseases, and malaria took precedence over SCA. So both the black and white communities, and medical and political leaders, failed to mention this condition in their health education campaigns. Prior to 1949 neither the exact nature of the inheritance pattern nor the underlying cause of the disease (molecular defect) was understood, barring dissemination of useful knowledge to the lay community. In addition, SCA was a hopeless disease, having no reliable treatment. What good would it have done to publicize SCA among African Americans? Still, there is little evidence to suggest that governmental, medical, or local community groups even considered those questions or debated the need for an education or awareness campaign based on the knowledge of SCA then available.[54]

There are other equally if not more compelling arguments than these for Americans' lack of awareness of SCA. Until relatively recently, African Americans have been, for the most part, socially and politically invisible. Both as slaves and as free people, they have had little voice in affairs that affected them directly. Only, for instance, when epidemic diseases threatened to spread from black to white victims did nineteenth-century public officials act to protect the entire population. Persons of color were routinely ignored or, as in National Negro Health Week, told what was important and what was not. The civil rights movement of the 1950s and 1960s changed that, however. As part of their quest for self-awareness and self-identity, African Americans rediscovered SCA. But not until the 1970s.

Dr. Scott published an editorial in the *New England Journal of Medicine* a few months after his initial article in *Pubic Health Reports* appeared, and then published an article in the *Journal of the American Medical Association* several months later.[55] In these pieces he argued that voluntary and federal agencies contributed little to SCA research when compared with what they allocated for other less frequently encountered conditions, because Americans did not realize the "real importance of the disease as a community problem."[56] He cited statistics showing that SCA occurs in about 1 of every 500 black births, compared with, for example, 1 of every 2,500 births for diabetes mellitus. Though a few physicians from the 1920s through the 1940s noted a sense of social responsibility toward sufferers of SCA, and several African American physicians tried to alert the black community about the dangers of SCA,[57] most physicians, white and black, seem to have worked on their own research or ignored the problem entirely. But shortly after Scott's editorial, other editorials as well as letters to the editor and articles appeared in medical journals deploring the apparent lack of interest in SCA on the part of the American people and government. Television editorials and news stories as well as a statement by President Nixon in his February 1971 health message brought SCA into the national spotlight. Congress then began voting funds to support sickle cell research and awareness programs.[58] What had once been an unknown disease with manifestations silently influencing the lives of white and black Southerners now became a recognizable badge of purported black identity and a subject of explosive national importance that raised a new set of social and political problems.[59]

Health and Health Care during Slavery and Reconstruction

CHAPTER 7

Black Health on the Plantation

Sickness and death were constant worries of nineteenth-century Americans, especially in the disease-ridden antebellum South, where, by 1860, more than 4 million blacks, most of them enslaved, composed much of the work force. Their presence created a special situation for two reasons: first, whites, responsible for slave medical care, in large part dictated the living and working conditions that promoted or destroyed blacks' health; second, some white Southerners claimed (and many others believed) that blacks were medically different from whites and so in need of special treatment. This chapter will look at the three groups of Southerners most directly involved in issues of black health and care of slaves—owners, physicians, and the enslaved themselves—and consider their relationships to the special problem of slavery.[1]

The first section discusses how Southern physicians used their own and others' observations of black medical differences to develop both a partial rationale for enslaving blacks in the American South and a special approach to their medical care and treatment. The second section describes the various ways in which the living and working conditions of the enslaved on plantations and farms affected black health. Finally, the third section examines the various forms of medical care that owners, physicians, and the enslaved themselves provided under this unique labor system known as "the peculiar institution."

Were Blacks Medically Different from Whites?

"Scarcely any observant medical man, having charge of negro estates, fails to discover, by experience, important modifications in the diseases and appropriate treatment of the white and black race respectively."[2] Thus wrote the editor of a prominent Virginia medical journal in 1856, in an attempt to impress upon the state's physicians the importance of providing adequate health care to the enslaved. He could very well have been speaking to all Southern physicians, many of whom believed that medical differences existed between blacks and whites. The issue was of both practical and political importance: it involved not only the health care of an entire group in the South—persons of color—but also the partial justification for enslaving them.

Physicians who treated diseases of the enslaved in the South had a pecuniary and professional concern with the subject. Their recorded opinions in medical, commercial, and agricultural journals, as well as in personal correspondence, attest to the seriousness with which they approached issues of black health. Some politically minded physicians were also resolutely committed to explaining the Southern position on slavery. In publications for the medical, commercial, and lay public, men such as Josiah Clark Nott of Mobile and Samuel A. Cartwright of New Orleans used their knowledge derived from black medical care to rationalize the necessity and usefulness of slavery. These apologists for the peculiar institution, in order to prove that slavery was humane and economically viable in the South, argued that blacks had immunity to certain diseases that devastated whites. Slave owners, they said, did not sacrifice blacks every time they sent them into the rice fields or canebrakes. Nor could physicians adequately treat blacks without knowledge of their anatomical and physiological peculiarities and disease proclivities. Blacks were medically different from whites, they asserted.

In certain obvious physical ways blacks did vary greatly from whites. Old South writers particularly commented on facial features, hair, posture and gait, skin color, and odor. One school of American scientists spent much time and effort investigating cranium and brain size, as well as other characteristics, in part to discover whether blacks were inferior to whites. Physicians, slave owners, and other interested persons also detected distinctions in the physical reactions of whites and blacks both to diseases and to treatments. Their observations were often accurate, but at times they allowed racial prejudice to cloud their views. These observers remarked particularly about the relative immunity of blacks to Southern fevers, especially intermittent fever (malaria) and yellow fever; blacks' susceptibility to intestinal and respiratory diseases; and their tolerance of heat and intolerance of cold. Black children, they noted, died more frequently of marasmus (wasting away), convulsions, "teething," and suffocation or overlaying than did whites.[3]

One of the most fascinating subjects of Old South medical authors was black resistance to malaria, the focus of constant comment during the antebellum period because blacks' resistance to it appeared to vary from region to region, plantation to plantation, and individual to individual. In dispute was the degree of susceptibility and the virulence of the disease in blacks: Could blacks acquire some resistance to malaria by living in constant proximity to its supposed source? Were some blacks naturally immune? Did blacks have milder attacks of the disease than whites?

Modern science has answered many of the questions of immunity and prevention of malaria with which doctors and planters struggled in the antebellum period. Several factors contributed to the phenomenon of malarial immunity. Many of the enslaved did possess an inherited immunity to one or another form of malaria. But whites and blacks without natural resistance to a particular type of *Plasmodium* (the organism that causes malaria) could acquire malarial immunity or tolerance only by suffering repeated infections of the disease over several years, as was noted by the author of an article in the *New Orleans Medical News and Hospital Gazette* (1858–59). For this to occur, one of the four species of *Plasmodium*—*falciparum, vivax, malariae,* and *ovale*—had to be present constantly in the endemic region, so that with each attack a person's supply of antibodies was strengthened against further parasitic invasions. Interruption of this process, such as removal to nonendemic areas for the summer (when exposure to the parasite was useful in building immunity) or for several years (during schooling or travel), prohibited the aggregation of sufficient antibodies to resist infection. In truly endemic areas, acquiring immunity this way was a risky affair: unprotected children struggled for their lives, adults suffered from relapses of infections contracted years before, and partially immune adults worked through mild cases. It is no wonder, then, that enslaved people sold from, say, Virginia, where one form of malaria was prevalent, to owners on a Louisiana bayou or South Carolina rice plantation, where a different species or strain of *Plasmodium* was endemic, had a high incidence of the disease. Even enslaved adults from Africa had to go through a "seasoning" period, because the strains of malarial parasites in this country differed from those in their native lands.

Generally speaking, most cases of malaria in the upper South and in inland piedmont areas were of the milder *vivax* type, whereas *vivax* coexisted with the more dangerous *falciparum* malaria in coastal and swampy inland portions of both the lower and upper South. Rare pockets of the *malariae* type (quartan fever) were scattered across the South. *Ovale* malaria appears not to have been present in the United States. Of course, epidemics of one type or another could strike any neighborhood and bring sickness and death even to those who had acquired resistance to the endemic variety. *Plasmodium falciparum* usually caused such epidemics, especially in the temperate regions of the South.[4]

The major reason for black resistance to *vivax* or *falciparum* malaria relates not to acquired protection, but to selective genetic factors. At least three hereditary conditions prevalent among blacks in parts of modern Africa appear to give their bearers resistance to malaria. Medical research indicates that the red blood cells of persons lacking a specific factor called "Duffy antigen" are resistant to invasion of *Plasmodium vivax*. Approximately 90 percent of West Africans lack Duffy antigens, as do about 70 percent of African Americans. This inherited, symptomless, hematologic condition is extremely rare in other racial groups. All evidence points to the conclusion that infection by *Plasmodium vivax* requires the presence of Duffy-positive red blood cells. Because most blacks do not possess this factor, they are immune to *vivax* malaria. It can be safely assumed that the vast majority of American slaves and free blacks were therefore resistant to this form of the disease.

Some antebellum persons of color had additional protection against malaria resulting from two genetic hemoglobin conditions, sickle cell disease (a form of anemia) and sickle cell trait (the symptomless carrier state of the sickling gene). People with either of these conditions had milder cases of, and decreased risk of mortality from, the most malignant form of malaria, *falciparum*. Many of those who had sickle cell disease died from its consequences before or during adolescence; however, blacks who had sickle cell trait lived entirely normal lives and could then transmit the gene for sickling to their offspring. Because people with the trait had one normal gene and one variant gene for sickling (in contrast to those with the disease, who had two of the sickling genes), their offspring could inherit sickle cell anemia only when each parent contributed a gene for sickling. Because the sickle cell condition was not discovered until 1910, physicians in the antebellum South were unaware that this was one reason why some enslaved people on plantations appeared to be immune to malarial infections. One other genetic condition with a high incidence within the former slave-trading region probably affords some malarial resistance: deficiency of the enzyme glucose-6-phosphate dehydrogenase (G-6-PD deficiency).

It is impossible to provide an exact calculation of the prevalence of sickle cell and G-6-PD deficiency gene among antebellum Southern blacks. An estimate might be ventured, however, on the basis of known gene frequencies among present-day African Americans and those Africans residing in former slave-trading areas. One leading medical authority on abnormal hemoglobins has estimated that at least 22 percent of the Africans first brought to this country possessed genes for sickling. Other medical scientists have determined that approximately 20 percent of West Africans have genes for G-6-PD deficiency. Overall, then, a conservative estimate would be that approximately 30 to 40 percent of newly arrived slaves had one or both of these genes. Evidence points to a higher than expected frequency of the G-6-PD gene in patients having sickle cell disease, which might reduce this estimate by a few percentage points. Thus, a large proportion of blacks were immune to the severe effects of *falciparum* malaria and the less virulent *vivax* malaria, facts which planters and physicians in the South could not help but notice.

As with malaria, planters and physicians speculated publicly on blacks' intolerance of cold climates but could never adequately prove their contentions. It was the confirmed opinion of many white Southerners that blacks could not withstand cold weather to the same degree as whites because of their dark skin and equatorial origins. Their major concern was that blacks seemed less able to resist and tolerate respiratory infections than whites. Since the germ theory of disease was years in the future, these men and others explained their observations with a combination of then current though not universally accepted medical, anthropological, and scientific logic—and occasionally with unfounded theories. Blacks—natives of a tropical climate—white observers reasoned, were physiologically ill suited for the cold winter weather and cool spring and fall nights of the temperate zone. They breathed less air, dissipated a greater amount of "animal heat" through the skin, and eliminated larger quantities of carbon via liver and skin than whites. In addition, the exposure of enslaved blacks to the elements for much of the year placed a strain on heat production within the body. One medical extremist, Samuel A. Cartwright of New Orleans, even claimed that inefficient functioning of blacks' lungs caused "defective atmospherization of the blood." Some noted that the enslaved often slept with their heads (rather than their feet) next to the fire and entirely covered by a blanket; this was seen as proof that they required warm, moist air to breathe and to survive in this climate. Blacks were, these men concluded, physiologically different from whites.

Even today there is some confusion among medical authorities regarding the susceptibility of blacks to severe pulmonary infections. Some claim a racial or genetic predisposition while others deny it. Historically, blacks have shown a higher incidence and more severe manifestations of respiratory illness than have whites. Explanations for this phenomenon are numerous. First, black Africans did not experience bacterial pneumonias until the coming of whites. The entire newly exposed population was thus exquisitely sensitive to these infections and developed much more serious cases than whites, who had had frequent contact with the bacteria since childhood. Second, black African laborers who today move from moist tropical to temperate climates (e.g., to the gold mines of South Africa) contract pneumonia at a much higher rate than whites. Though the incidence of disease decreases with time, it always remains at a more elevated level than among whites. The same phenomenon probably operated during slavery. At first the mortality rate from pneumonia among newly arrived enslaved people was probably inordinately high, but with time the figure decreased somewhat, though it remains higher than in whites. Third, there appears to be a close relationship between resistance to pulmonary infection and exposure to cool, wet weather.

The enslaved, who worked outdoors in all seasons and often lived in drafty, damp cabins, were therefore more likely to suffer from respiratory diseases than their owners. Fourth, poor diet, a common problem for the enslaved, predisposes people to infections such as pneumonia and other respiratory problems.[5] Finally, overcrowding and unsanitary living conditions increased the incidence of respiratory diseases. Enslaved people living in small cottages or grouped together in a large community, where intimate and frequent visiting was common, stood a greater chance of contracting airborne infections than did more isolated whites. Undoubtedly, all these factors combined to increase the occurrence of respiratory illness among Southern blacks.

The most serious nonfatal manifestation of cold intolerance was frostbite. At least one proslavery apologist claimed that the Negro race was more susceptible than whites to this condition: "Almost every one has seen negroes in Northern cities, who have lost their legs by frost at sea—a thing rarely witnessed among whites, and yet where a single negro has been thus exposed doubtless a thousand of the former have."[6] The condition was a serious one, especially for slave owners who stood to lose the labor of valuable workers.

Blacks are in fact more susceptible to cold injury than whites. Studies conducted during and after the Korean War indicate that the adaptive response of blacks to cold exposure is poorer than that of whites in the following ways: blacks' metabolic rates increase more slowly and not as much as those of whites; their first shivers (one of the body's defensive responses to cold) occur at a lower skin temperature than for whites; and their incidence of frostbite is higher and their cases more severe than those of whites. Even after blacks have acclimated to cold (and they do so in a manner physiologically similar to whites), they are then only slightly less liable to sustain cold injury than they had been previously. Those antebellum observers who warned against overexposure of enslaved blacks to cold were essentially correct.

Racial differences in tolerance to heat exist but may be modified under certain conditions. Again, antebellum observers agreed that blacks, having originated in an area known for its heat and humidity, were ideally suited for labor in the damp, warm South. One Northern physician, John H. Van Evrie, explained blacks' resistance to heat in both religious and physiological terms: "God has adapted him, both in his physical and mental structure, to the tropics. . . . His head is protected from the rays of a vertical sun by a dense mat of wooly hair, wholly impervious to its fiercest heats, while his entire surface, studded with innumerable sebaceous glands, forming a complete excretory system, relieves him from all those climatic influences so fatal, under the same circumstances, to the sensitive and highly organized white man. Instead of seeking to shelter himself from the burning sun of the tropics, he courts it, enjoys it, delights in its fiercest heats."[7]

Modern medical investigators would not agree with Van Evrie's reasoning. But they have discovered that under normal living conditions, blacks in Africa and the United States are better equipped to tolerate humid heat than whites. However, both groups possess the same capacity to acclimatize to hot, humid conditions. The physiological mechanisms by which the human body acclimatizes to heat can be readily observed and measured. Increased external temperature causes the body to perspire more, resulting in a greater evaporative heat loss, a decline in skin and rectal temperatures, and a drop in the heart rate from its initially more rapid pace. When whites and blacks are equally active in the same environment over a period of time, there is little difference in heat tolerance.

From this information it can be assumed that in the Old South enslaved and free blacks possessed a higher natural tolerance to humid heat stress than did whites. In addition, blacks became quickly acclimatized to performance of their particular tasks under the prevailing climatic conditions of the region. This natural and acquired acclimatization enabled black laborers to withstand the damp heat of summer better than whites, who were unused to physical exertion under such severe conditions. White farm and general laborers, however, also must have adjusted to the heat and fared as well as blacks. One physiological difference between Caucasians and Negroes that might have affected work performance in the hot, humid South was the latter's inherent ability to discharge smaller amounts of sodium chloride and other vital body salts (electrolytes) into sweat and urine. Excessive loss of those salts leads to heat prostration and heatstroke. Thus conservation of needed electrolytes gave slaves an advantage over laboring whites, whose requirements for replacements of the substances were greater. In the case of heat tolerance, then, white observers were correct in noting a racial difference, but they tended to ignore the fact that many whites did become acclimatized to the hot, humid environment.[8]

Whites detected, or thought they detected, distinctive variances in black susceptibility to several other medical conditions common in the antebellum South. Many believed that enslaved women developed prolapsed uteri at a higher rate than white women, though modern anatomists have shown that blacks are actually less prone to this affliction than whites. Observers also noted that the enslaved were frequent sufferers of typhoid fever, worms, and dysentery, though we now know that the reason for this high prevalence was environmental rather than racial or genetic. Blacks did, however, have a greater resistance to the yellow fever virus than whites.[9]

One disease that drew great attention because of its frequency and virulence was consumption (pulmonary tuberculosis), a leading cause of death in nineteenth-century America for members of both races. A particular form of the disease—characterized by extreme difficulty in breathing, unexplained abdominal pain around the navel, and rapidly progressing debility and emaciation, usually resulting in death—struck blacks so commonly that it came to be known as Negro Consumption or *Struma Africana*. In all likelihood most of the cases that white Southerners described as Negro Consumption were miliary tuberculosis, the most serious and fatal form of the disease known, in which tubercles occur in many body organs simultaneously and overwhelm what natural defenses exist. The reason that rapidly fatal varieties of the disease (so-called galloping consumption) afflicted blacks more frequently than whites may be related to the fact that Caucasians (like Asians) had suffered from tuberculosis for many hundreds of years and had developed a strong immune response to the infection, whereas black Africans (as well as Native Americans and Eskimos) had been exposed to tuberculosis only since the coming of whites and had not yet built up this same effective resistance. Others have discounted racial immunity as an explanation and have argued that, as a "virgin" population, blacks were highly susceptible to serious first attacks of tuberculosis. Additional factors such as malnourishment, preexisting illness, or general debility also contributed to the apparent black predisposition to tuberculosis.

Neonatal tetanus (also called *Trismus nascentium*) was a common cause of death among enslaved newborns throughout the South. Slave owners and physicians, few of whom recognized that it was caused by the improper handling of the umbilical stump, often discussed it in their writings. It still kills large numbers of children in underdeveloped countries. *Clostridium tetani*, the same bacterium that causes tetanus in older children and adults, infects newborns through unwashed and frequently touched umbilical stumps. In a typical antebellum case, related by Dr. Albert Snead of Richmond to his colleagues at a medical society meeting in 1853, an eight-day-old black child first refused her mother's breast and gave a few convulsive hand jerks. Soon the baby's entire muscular system was rigid, with her head bent back, fists and jaws clenched, and feet tightly flexed, as the bacterial toxin affected her central nervous system tissue. In this case, death from suffocation owing to respiratory muscle paralysis did not intervene until the eighteenth day (though it usually occurs within seven to ten days).[10]

One cause of death not considered a disease that seemed to occur almost exclusively among the enslaved population was "smothering," "overlaying," or "suffocation." Observers assumed that sleeping mothers simply rolled onto or pressed snugly against their infants, cutting off air supply, or that angry, fearful parents intentionally destroyed their offspring rather than have them raised in slavery. Modern medical evidence strongly indicates that most of these deaths may be ascribed to a condition presently known as Sudden Infant Death Syndrome (SIDS) or "crib death," which, for reasons yet unexplained, affects blacks more frequently than whites.[11]

The previously discussed diseases and conditions represent only some of several that whites noted affected blacks and whites differently. Others are difficult to trace back to slavery times, either through direct records or by implication through comparative West African medicine. Among those not mentioned, the most important is hypertension (high blood pressure). Others include polydactyly (six or more fingers per hand), umbilical hernia, certain cancers, and toxemia of pregnancy. At the same time, blacks are much less susceptible to hookworm disease, cystic fibrosis, and skin cancer than whites. Though blacks are not the only racial or ethnic group possessing increased immunity and susceptibility to specific diseases, they were the only group whose medical differences mattered to white residents of the Old South. Reports of black medical "peculiarities" appeared regularly in periodicals and pamphlets, presumably to alert Southern physicians to problems they might encounter in practice. Agricultural and medical journal articles and medical student dissertations also discussed racial differences in responses to medical treatments. Most writers agreed that blacks did not withstand the depletive therapies of the day (bleeding, purging, vomiting, blistering) as well as whites.

Despite many writings on the subject of black diseases and treatments, no comprehensive discussion existed in any standard textbook for student doctors or practitioners. Some articles on the subject of treatment provided vague information, such as "the Caucasian seems to yield more readily to remedies . . . than the African," or "it is much more difficult to form a just diagnosis or prognosis with the latter [African] than the former [white], consequently the treatment is often more dubious."[12] In 1855 an editor of the *Virginia Medical and Surgical Journal* suggested that a Virginian write a book on "the modifications of disease in the Negro constitution." The subject, he proclaimed, stood "invitingly open"; no medical student "fresh from Watson or Wood [textbooks of the day], with his new lancet and his armory of antiphlogistics" had been properly trained to treat many of the diseases to which the black man was subject: "Has he been taught that the African constitution sinks before the heavy blows of the 'heroic school' and runs down under the action of purgatives; that when the books say blood letting and calomel, the black man needs nourishment and opium?"[13] Other Southern medical writers put forth similar pleas for medical school courses and books on black medicine. Northern textbook authors and professors at Northern medical schools, they asserted, could not and did not accurately or adequately discuss diseases afflicting blacks in the South.[14]

John Stainbach Wilson, a physician in Columbus, Georgia, who had spent years practicing medicine in southern Alabama, came closest to actually producing a textbook on black health. Its advertised title indicated the wide scope of the proposed contents: *The Plantation and Family Physician; A Work for Families Generally and for Southern Slaveowners Especially; Embracing the Peculiarities and Diseases, the Medical and Hygienic Management of Negroes, Together with the Causes, Symptoms, and Treatment of the Principal Diseases to Whites and Blacks.* But apparently the outbreak of hostilities in 1861 interrupted Wilson's plans. It was not until more than one hundred years later, in 1975, that a book titled *Textbook of Black-Related Diseases* was finally published, written this time by black physicians.[15]

For Southern whites, black medical problems and health care had political as well as medical ramifications. Men such as Cartwright, Nott, and Wilson, advocates of what historians have labeled "states-rights medicine," were writing for a sectional audience that wished to hear that blacks were distinct from whites. This was, after all, a part of the proslavery argument. Medical theory and practice were still in such a state of flux in the late eighteenth and early nineteenth centuries that there was little risk of any true scientific challenge to a medical system based on racial differences. Observers were correct in noting that blacks and whites showed differing susceptibilities and immunities to some specific diseases and conditions. They capitalized on these differences to illustrate the inferiority of blacks to whites, to rationalize the use of the "less fit" racial group as slaves, to justify subjecting enslaved blacks to harsh working conditions in extreme dampness and heat in the malarial regions of the South, and to prove to their critics that they recognized blacks' special medical weaknesses and took these failings into account when providing for their human chattel. But in terms of an overall theory of medical care predicated on racial inferiority, the issue was a false one. It is instructive to note here, for example, that no writer ventured beyond vague and cautious statements about bleeding or purging blacks less often than whites. None presented an account of the amount of blood loss or the dose of medicine that was optimal for blacks. Remarks on the subject were always couched in terms that placed whites in a position of medical and physical superiority over blacks, perfect for Southern sectional polemics and useless to the practitioner.

Living and Working Conditions

The state of enslaved people's health depended not only on disease immunities and susceptibilities but also on living and working conditions. How whites in the slaveholding South provided for sanitation, housing, food, clothing, and children's and women's special needs, and how they worked and disciplined their human chattel, necessarily affected the health of their black work force.[16] (See Appendix, Table 1.)

Most enslaved people lived on plantations or farms in a well-defined area known as the "quarters." Here was an ideal setting for the spread of disease, similar to the situation in antebellum villages and urban areas. What might have

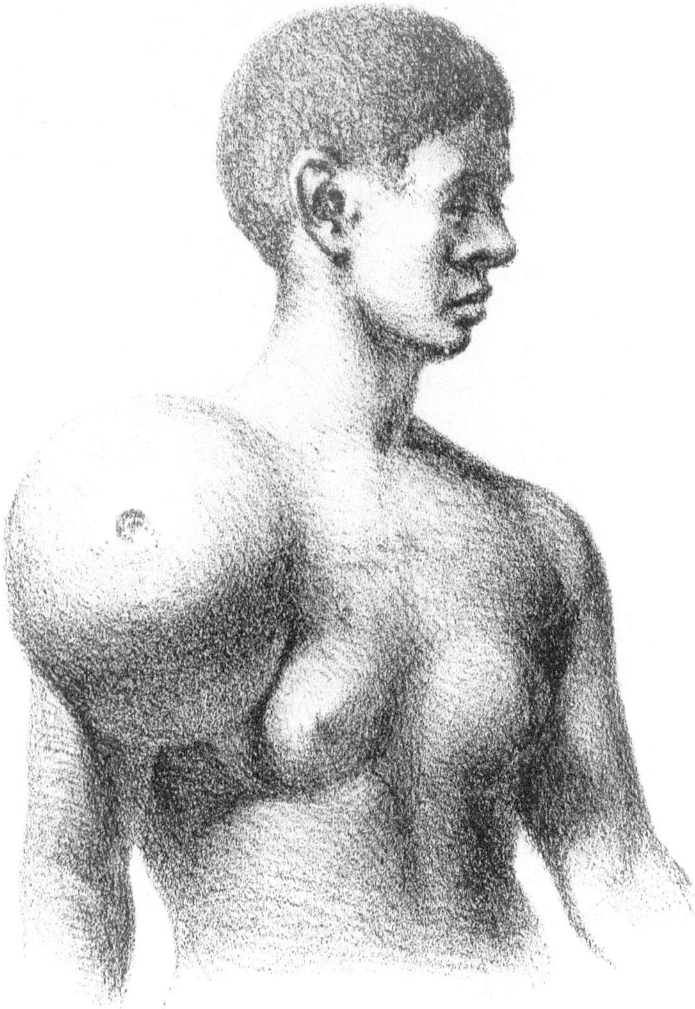

Fig. 4. A twenty-five-year-old Virginia slave with bony tumor at shoulder joint, before surgical excision at Medical College of Virginia Infirmary. She died subsequent to the operation. From A. E. Peticolas, "Case of Osteoid Cancer, With Remarks," *Virginia Medical and Surgical Journal* 2 (1854): facing p. 380.

been considered a personal illness in the isolated, white, rural family dwelling became in a three- or ten- or thirty-home slave community a matter of public health and group concern.

In the slave quarters, sneezing, coughing, or contact with improperly washed eating utensils and personal belongings promoted transmission of disease-causing microorganisms among family members. Poor ventilation, lack of sufficient windows for sunshine, and damp earthen floors merely added to the problem by aiding the growth of fungus and bacteria on food, clothing, floors, and utensils, as well as the development of worm and insect larvae. Improper personal hygiene (infrequent baths, hair brushings, and haircuts; unwashed clothes; unclean beds) led to such nuisances as bedbugs, body lice (which also carried typhus germs), ringworm of skin and scalp, and pinworms. In a household cramped for space, these diseases became family, not individual, problems. And when two or more families shared homes and facilities, the problem of contagion was further aggravated.

Contacts outside the home also facilitated the dissemination of disease. Children who played together all day under the supervision of a few older women and then returned to their cabins in the evening spread their day's accumulation of germs to other family members. Even mere Sunday and evening socializing in an ill neighbor's cabin was enough to "seed" the unsuspecting with disease. Contaminated water, unwashed or poorly cooked food, soil infested with worm larvae, and disease-carrying farm animals and rodents also contributed their share to the unhealthfulness of the quarters.

The two major types of seasonal diseases—respiratory and intestinal—that afflicted Southern blacks reflected living conditions within most slave communities. Respiratory illnesses prevailed during the cold months, when the enslaved were forced to spend much time indoors in intimate contact with their families and friends. Several important contagious diseases were spread through contact with respiratory system secretions: tuberculosis, diphtheria, colds and upper respiratory infections, influenza, pneumonia, and streptococcal infections (including sore throats and scarlet fever). The community life of the slave quarters also provided excellent surroundings for dissemination of several year-round diseases contracted through respiratory secretions. People today tend to regard these illnesses—whooping cough, measles, chicken pox, and mumps—as limited to the younger population, but enslaved adults who had never experienced an outbreak of, say, measles in Africa or the United States were quite susceptible to infection and even death. Measles and whooping cough are still important causes of fatality in developing countries, as they were in the antebellum South.

As warm weather arrived and workers spent more time outdoors, intestinal diseases caused by poor outdoor sanitation and close contact with the earth became common. Respiratory diseases decreased in frequency and insects became important culprits in the spread of disease, particularly maladies of the digestive tract and various "fevers." What more could a mosquito or housefly wish than a large concentration of human beings, decaying leftover food scraps, scattered human feces, or a compost heap? Mosquitoes discharged yellow fever or malarial parasites while they drew fresh blood from their victims. Flies transported bacteria such as *Vibrio* (cholera), *Salmonella* (food poisoning and typhoid), and *Shigella* (bacillary dysentery); the virus that causes infectious hepatitis; and the protozoan *Entameba histolytica* (amebic dysentery) from feces to food. Trichina worms, embedded in the muscles of hogs inhabiting yards often shared with the enslaved, were released into a person's body when the meat was not completely cooked. Finally, there were large parasitic worms, a concomitant of primitive sanitation.

Intestinal disorders were at least as common among antebellum Virginia's blacks as were respiratory diseases. The human alimentary tract is distinguished among all other body systems in that it receives daily large amounts of foreign material, usually in the form of food, which it must sort and assimilate into a usable form. In the Old South, where living conditions were generally unhygienic, seemingly good food and drink often concealed pathogenic organisms ranging from viruses to worm larvae. Hands entering mouths sometimes contained the germs that others had cast off in feces, urine, or contaminated food. It is not surprising to find that dysentery, typhoid fever, food poisoning, and worm diseases afflicted many Southerners, especially those living in the poorest, most crowded circumstances, without sanitary facilities or time to prepare food properly. The enslaved often fit into this category.

Though their major medical problems were communicable diseases, enslaved blacks, in the course of a day, also faced health challenges unrelated to contagion or parasites. Inadequate clothing and food, poor working conditions, harsh physical punishment, pregnancy, and certain bodily disorders also made the enslaved sick or uncomfortable, at times rendering them useless to their owners and burdensome to friends and family.

Even though adequate clothing was important, it did not play as crucial a role in the maintenance of health as did housing. Of course, clothing covered and protected the body from exposure to wind, sun, rain, snow, cold, and insects. It also limited the severity of many minor falls to cuts, scrapes, and bruises and of some accidents to smaller areas of the body. But only a few disorders are spread by contact with infected clothing (smallpox, body lice, impetigo, typhus) or by contact of exposed skin with other objects (tetanus, yaws, hookworm, brucellosis).

Except in cases where the enslaved were truly underclothed in winter and therefore possibly had less resistance to respiratory ailments, the danger of contracting disease through inadequate or dirty apparel was relatively small. Of the articles of clothing that owners provided their bondspeople, shoes were probably the most important in terms of health and disease. Not only did they provide warmth in the winter to feet and toes highly susceptible to frostbite, but they also protected against hookworm penetration, scrapes, scratches, burns, and some puncture wounds that would otherwise have caused tetanus.

Did enslaved people receive a diet adequate to keep them healthy, laboring, and producing vigorous offspring? Opinions vary on this question, for diets differed from individual to individual, and our understanding of nutritional needs has changed often. Based on current dietary standards, the typical daily ration—one quart of whole ground, dry, bolted cornmeal, prepared from white corn (the South's favorite) and a half pound of cured, medium-fat ham with no bone or skin, could not have provided enough essential nutrients to sustain a moderately active twenty-two-year-old male or female, much less a hardworking laborer or a pregnant or lactating woman. Field hands fed this diet alone (with water) would soon have become emaciated and sickly and would have shown symptoms of several nutrient deficiencies. It is highly unlikely that any bondsperson could have survived very long on a diet consisting solely of pork and cornmeal.

Most owners provided supplements to the basic hog meat and cornmeal, a practice most urgently recommended by agricultural writers throughout the South. Vegetables topped the list of required additional foods. Planters could, if they planned ahead, have a ready supply of at least one or two varieties throughout the year. These writers also suggested adding, when available, fish, fresh meat, molasses, milk, and buttermilk to slaves' diets.

Many agricultural authors and slave owners indicated in their writings that blacks often raised vegetables, poultry, and even pigs on their own plots of land near the quarters. The assumption was that extra food from this source would supplement rations supplied by the owner. Surprisingly, however, some of these same writers also pointed out that the enslaved usually sold what they raised to the owner or at the marketplace, thereby defeating the major purpose of the plan. In all likelihood bondspeople did not dispose of all their produce, but saved some for future needs. The fact that there were enslaved people who sold rather than kept food indicates that, other than those saving every available penny to purchase their freedom, some slaves received sufficient nutrition from their regular rations, supplemented by homegrown food, to feel quite comfortable relying on their owners for proper nutrition.

Kenneth F. Kiple and Virginia H. King, in their book *Another Dimension to the Black Diaspora*, assess the adequacy of a slave diet consisting primarily of pork and cornmeal supplemented occasionally with other foods.[17] They conclude that the enslaved received sufficient amounts of carbohydrates and calories but generally lacked some essential amino acids, vitamin C, riboflavin, niacin, thiamine, vitamin D, calcium, and iron. And slave children, who all too often began life with nutritional deficiencies owing to their mothers' poor pre- and postnatal diets, also lacked sufficient magnesium, calories, and protein in their diets. Not surprisingly, Kiple and King assert, enslaved adults and children suffered higher morbidity and mortality than whites because of lower resistance to infection and disrupted basic metabolic pathways. Among the most common resultant black health problems were respiratory and intestinal diseases, skin and eye afflictions, "teething," tetanus, "fits and seizures," and rickets. Diet, controlled to a large degree by the owner, greatly affected enslaved people's health.

In addition to providing food, clothing, and housing, slave owners also directed working conditions, punishments, and care of women and children. Though warm weather helped the crops grow, it did not always have the same effect on the black laborers who tended them. Planters recording the effects of excessive heat on their field hands made it clear that even though blacks originated in tropical Africa, they were not immune to sunstroke. For instance, Hill Carter of Shirley Plantation wrote during the 1825 wheat harvest, "Hotest day ever felt—men gave out & some fainted."[18]

Slave owners also recognized the potential hazards of overexertion and exposure. Some indulged their bondspeople by easing their tasks; others found this impossible, especially at certain times of the year. Hill Carter and no doubt many others worked their slaves in intense heat when it was necessary to harvest a crop. Charles Friend of Prince George County, Virginia, alternatively, had second thoughts when the ditching operation to which he had assigned many bondsmen evolved into a messy and unhealthy job: "We have the ditchers knee deep in water and mud. If I had known how bad it was I should not have put them to work at it but hired labor to do it."[19]

Farm accidents also took their toll. Falls, overturned carts, runaway wagons, drownings, limbs caught in farm machines, kicks from animals, and cuts from axes or scythe blades were the commonest types. Occasionally enslaved people suffered more remarkable mishaps, as when a 260-pound Culpeper County field hand jumped eight feet from a hayloft onto a pile of hay in which a wooden pitchfork lay concealed. The point punctured the man's scrotum and passed into his abdominal cavity, but miraculously pierced no internal organs. Thanks to prompt surgical attention he was doing "light work" around the plantation about three weeks later.[20]

The whip was an integral part of enslaved people's lives in the Old South. Those who had not experienced its sting firsthand were acquainted with persons, usually friends or relatives, who had. Whites held out the threat of whipping as a means of maintaining order. When strong discipline was called for, so, very often, was the lash. Even the mildest and most God-fearing of owners permitted application of this painful instrument in extreme cases, though some insisted that the person's skin not be cut or that a responsible witness be present when punishment was administered.

From a medical point of view, whipping inflicted cruel and often permanent injuries upon its victims. Laying stripes across the bare back or buttocks caused indescribable pain, especially when each stroke dug deeper into previously opened wounds. During the interval between lashes, victims anticipated the next in anguish, wishing for postponement or for all due speed, though neither alternative brought relief. In addition to multiple lacerations of the skin, whipping caused loss of blood, injury to muscles (and internal organs, if the lash reached that deep), and shock. (Rubbing salt into these wounds, often complained of as a further mode of torture, actually cleansed the injured, exposed tissues and helped ward off infection.) Paddling, another form of whipping, jarred every part of the body by the violence of the blow and raised blisters from repeated strokes. In addition to the possibility of death (uncommon), there was the danger that muscle damage inflicted by these instruments might permanently incapacitate or deform a person for life. One Old Dominion bondsman who experienced the sting of the paddle recalled years later: "You be jes' as raw as a piece of beef an' hit eats you up. He loose you an' you go to house no work done dat day."[21] No work done that day or, in many cases, for several days. Ellick, a rebellious member of Charles Friend's White Hill Plantation slave force, was slapped one day "for not being at the stable in time this morning" and "soundly whipped" the next day for running away and for not submitting to a flogging earlier that morning. He spent the next week recovering in bed, only to receive another whipping upon his return to work. This time he ran off for two days before settling back into the plantation routine.[22]

The daily routines of enslaved women and children were often upset by health conditions peculiar to these groups.[23] Enslaved females probably lost more time from work for menstrual pain, discomfort, and disorders than for any other cause. Planters rarely named illnesses in their diaries or daybooks, but the frequency and regularity with which women of childbearing age appeared on sick lists indicates that menstrual conditions were a leading complaint. A Fauquier County, Virginia, physician considered the loss of four to eight workdays per month not unusual for enslaved women.[24] Among the menstrual maladies that afflicted bondswomen most often were amenorrhea (lack of menstrual flow), abnormal bleeding between cycles (sometimes caused by benign or malignant tumors), and abnormal discharges (resulting from such conditions as gonorrhea, tumors, and prolapsed uterus).

Some enslaved women took advantage of their owners by complaining falsely of female indispositions. One unnamed Virginian who owned numerous slaves complained to Frederick Law Olmsted about such malingering women: "The women on a plantation . . . will hardly earn their salt, after they come to the breeding age; they don't come to the field, and you go to the quarters and ask the old nurse what's the matter, and she says, 'oh she's not well, master; she's not fit to work, sir'; and what can you do? You have to take her word for it that something or other is the matter with her, and you dare not set her to work; and so she lays up till she feels like taking the air again, and plays the lady at your expense."[25] Owners found it difficult to separate the sick from the falsely ill; as a result, they often indulged their women of childbearing age rather than risk unknown complications. Thomas Jefferson, for instance, ordered his overseer not to coerce the female workers into exerting themselves because "women are destroyed by exposure to wet at certain periodical indispositions to which nature has subjected them."[26]

If whites treated women's gynecological complaints with a certain delicacy, they regarded pregnancy as almost holy. In addition to receiving time off from work and avoiding whippings, expectant women in Virginia were protected from execution in capital offenses until after parturition.[27] At least three cases arose in the Old Dominion between the Revolutionary War and the Civil War in which enslaved women obtained execution postponements for this reason, though all were presumably put to death following delivery.[28]

Children, like women, were exposed to certain unique disorders that caused illness or death. Though their labor did not usually account for much, young slaves' serious illnesses did mean lost time from work for mothers watching over them at home or distractedly worrying about them while performing daily tasks. Enslaved children suffered more frequently than their white counterparts from most illnesses, especially diarrhea, neonatal tetanus, convulsions, "teething" (not really a disease, but considered a cause of sickness and death prior to the twentieth century), diphtheria, respiratory diseases, and whooping cough, owing to poorer living conditions and diet. And their mortality rate far exceeded that of whites, especially in infancy.[29]

Worms occurred frequently in black children. The poor sanitary conditions at many slave quarters were conducive to the development of these parasites in the soil. Children playing in the dirt inevitably picked up worm larvae as they put fingers in mouths. Failure to use, or lack of, privy facilities only served to spread worm diseases to other residents of the quarters and to white and black visitors, who could then carry these parasites to their own quarters.

Some black children had overt sickle cell disease with irregular hemolytic crises, severe joint pains, chronic leg ulcers, and abdominal pains. The medical records relating to antebellum Virginia do not provide any clear descriptions of the disease, probably because its symptoms resemble so many other conditions and because the sickness was not known until 1910. These children were often the "sickly" ones, useless for fieldwork or heavy household duties, expensive to maintain because of frequent infections, and, if female, often unable to bear children if they survived puberty. Their lot was a poor and painful one.

Enslaved children also developed diseases that no one could identify or treat. John Walker's young bondspeople appeared one day with "head ach swelled faces & belly diseases"; Colonel John Ambler's evidenced swollen feet and faces, and bones cutting through the skin; and Landon Carter's had "swelling of the almonds of . . . [their] ears which burst inward and choaked . . . [them]." The white tutor at Nomini Hall, Phillip Vickers Fithian, noticed that one enslaved mother on this estate in Westmoreland County, Virginia, had lost seven children successively, none of whom had even reached the age of ten: "The Negroes all seem much alarm'd."[30] Childhood was generally the least healthy period of life.

In many ways, then, the state of Southern blacks' health depended on the kind of living and working conditions whites provided. These conditions varied widely from place to place and from individual to individual and were a subject of much comment in both Northern and Southern publications.

Medical Care of Enslaved People

Bondage placed the enslaved in a difficult position with regard to health care. When taken ill, they had a limited range of choices. Owners wished their bondspeople, legally *an article of property*, immediately to inform the person in charge about any sickness so the malady might be arrested before it worsened. But some blacks, as *human beings*, felt reluctant to submit to the often harsh prescriptions and remedies of eighteenth- and nineteenth-century white medical practice. They preferred self-treatment or reliance on cures recommended by friends and older relatives, black herb and root doctors, or influential conjurers among the local black population. This desire to treat oneself, or at least to have the freedom to choose one's mode of care, directly conflicted with the demands and wishes of white owners, whose trust in black medicine was usually slight.

To further compound the problem, unannounced illnesses did not entitle ailing bondspeople to time off from work. To treat their own illnesses, the enslaved had to conceal them or pass them off to the owner as less serious than they actually were. Owners who complained that blacks tended to report sickness only after the disease had progressed to a serious stage often discovered that bondspeople had treated illnesses at home first. The blacks' dilemma, then, was whether to delay reporting illnesses and treat those diseases at home, risking white reprisal, or to submit at once to the medicines of whites and, in a sense, surrender their bodies to their owners. The result was a dual system in which some people received treatment from both whites and blacks.[31]

When illness afflicted an enslaved person, whites responded in several ways. They almost always applied treatments derived from European experience. Most often the master, mistress, or overseer first attempted to treat the ailment with home remedies. If the patient failed to respond to these home ministrations, the family physician was summoned. Some slave owners distrusted "regular" doctors and called instead "irregular" practitioners: Thomsonians, homeopaths, empirics, and eclectics, for example. Owners who hired out their bondspeople to others for a period of time arranged for medical care when signing the hiring bond. Whatever the situation, white Southerners often displayed concern for the health of blacks held in bondage. The reasons were threefold: the enslaved represented a financial investment that required protection; many owners felt a humanitarian commitment toward their bondspeople; and whites realized that certain illnesses could easily spread to their own families if not properly treated and contained.

Those responsible for the care of sick bondspeople made home treatment the first step in the restorative process. They knew that physicians, though they possessed knowledge of the human body and the effects of certain medicines on it, were severely limited in the amount of good they could do. Because no one understood the etiology of most diseases, no one could effectively cure them. Astute nonmedical observers could make diagnoses as well as physicians and could even treat patients just as effectively. Physicians played their most crucial roles in executing certain surgical procedures, assisting mothers at childbirth, and instilling confidence in sick patients through an effective bedside manner. At other times, their excessive use of drugs, overready cups and leeches, and ever-present lancets produced positive harm by depleting the body of blood and nourishment and exhausting the already weakened patient with frequent purges, vomits, sweats, and diuretics. Laypeople often merely followed the same course of treatment that they had observed their physicians using or that they had read about in one of the ubiquitous domestic medical guides. Anyone could practice bloodletting or dosing with a little experience. And a physician's services cost money, even when no treatment or cure resulted from the consultation.

Home care, of course, stemmed from people's natural instincts to relieve their own and their families' illnesses as quickly as possible. The unavailability of physicians, the inaccessibility of many farms to main highways, and the lack of good roads and speedy means of transportation reinforced such thinking among white rural Southerners. Even when a physician was summoned, hours or even a day passed before his arrival, during which time something had to be done to ease the patient's discomfort. People learned to tolerate pain and to cope with death, but the mitigation of suffering was still a primary goal. To that end most people stocked their cabinets with favorite remedies (or the ingredients required for their preparation) in order to be well equipped when relief was demanded. On large plantations with many bondspeople, this was a necessity, as Catherine C. Hopley, tutor at Forest Rill near Tappahannock, Essex County, Virginia, noted: "A capacious medicine chest is an inseparable part of a Southern establishment; and I have seen medicines enough dispensed to furnish good occupation for an assistant, when colds or epidemics have prevailed."[32] Some physicians made a living selling medicine chests and domestic health guides designed specifically for use on Southern plantations. Self-sufficiency in medical care was desirable on farms and even in urban households, especially when financial considerations were important.

An additional feature of home medical care for the enslaved was the plantation hospital or infirmary. Its form varied from farm to farm, and it existed primarily on the larger slaveholdings. It was quicker and more efficient to place ailing bondspeople in one building, where care could be tendered with a minimum amount of wasted movement and where all medicines, special equipment, and other necessary stores could be maintained. Of course, infectious diseases could

INFIRMARY FOR SLAVES.

THE Subscribers beg leave to inform the public that they have rented and fitted up as an INFIRMARY FOR SLAVES, the house in the City of Norfolk, near Calvert's Lane, formerly occupied by Mr. J. Scott. The location is private and central, and the house airy, well arranged and sufficiently commodious. Competent Nurses are engaged; and, in addition to the personal attention of the undersigned, an advanced Medical Student will be constantly in the house to see that the sick are properly ministered to at all times.

The *entire* expense for the treatment of any one case, Medical, Surgical, or Obstetrical, *including* medicines, food and nursing, will be as follows:

Per day..................................$1 00
" week.................................. 5 00
" month..................................18 00

☞ Cases of Small Pox, Measles, and other contagious diseases will not be received.

The advantages of an establishment of this kind, so common in many parts of the South, will be apparent to all who have any experience in hiring out servants. Non-residents, especially, will be saved much trouble and expense by having their servants, when taken sick, sent to the Infirmary, where they will receive the most careful attention and nursing at a comparatively trifling cost. It also recommends itself to those who have servants in the adjacent counties suffering from chronic diseases, where the remoteness of medical aid renders it more expensive and difficult to be procured as often as needed.

All applications must be in writing, and if from a distance, *post paid.*

WM. J. MOORE, M. D., Office 42 E. Main—residence 15 N. Catharine.
GEO. L. UPSHUR, M. D., Office 57 S. Fenchurch—residence 7 Bermuda.
R. W. SYLVESTER, M. D., Office 20 W. Main—residence 7 S. Granby.

Fig. 5. Advertisement for slave infirmary in Norfolk, 1851. From William S. Forrest, *Norfolk Directory for 1851–1852* (Norfolk, Va.: n.p., 1851), 17.

spread quite rapidly through a hospital and subject those with noncontagious conditions to further sickness.

Armed with drugs from the plantation or home dispensary, one person, usually white, had the responsibility of dosing and treating ill bondspeople. The master, mistress, or overseer spent time each day with those claiming bodily disorders and soon developed a certain facility in handling both patients and drugs.[33] The approach was empirical—if a particular medication or combination of drugs succeeded in arresting symptoms, it became the standard treatment for that malady in that household until a better one came along. Overseers and owners inscribed useful medical recipes into their diaries or journals and clipped suggestions from newspapers, almanacs, and books.

An overseer's or owner's incompetence or negligence was the enslaved person's loss. New and inexperienced farm managers, unskilled in the treatment of illness, necessarily used blacks as guinea pigs for their "on-the-job" training. As a consequence of living on the wrong plantation at the wrong time, some enslaved people probably lost their lives or became invalids at the hands of new, poorly trained, or simply inhumane overseers or owners.

Despite the policy of many owners of delaying a call to the physician until late in the course of an enslaved person's disease, there were times when owners desperately wished for the physician's presence. More practitioners should have retained in their files the numerous hastily scrawled notes from frantic slave owners begging for medical assistance or kept a record of each verbal summons to a sick bondsperson at a distant farm or village household. For physicians did play important roles, both physiological and psychological, in the treatment of illness. Dr. Charles Brown of Charlottesville, Virginia, for instance, had a thriving country practice during the early nineteenth century. He handled many types of problems: James Old wanted him to determine whether his enslaved woman, then "in a strange way," was pregnant or not; Bezaleel Brown needed his opinion "if I must bleed her [Jane, who had pain in her side and suppression of urine] either large or small in quantity"; and Jemima Fretwell wished Brown to "cut of[f] the arm" of an enslaved four-month-old who had been "so very badly burnt" that "the [elbow] joint appears like it will drap of[f]."[34] Sometimes physicians made daily visits to dress wounds or to keep track of household epidemics. In emergencies, some owners panicked and fretted away many hours after learning of their physicians' temporary absence.

Between the household remedies and the standard treatments of the physicians stood "irregular" medicine. The impact of alternative movements on the medical care of blacks in Virginia was great. Most slave owners either treated with conventional medicines or called in regular physicians and rejected the new cults as quackery, but a sizable minority, difficult to estimate, became enthusiastic proponents of the system known as Thomsonianism. This movement, which had followers in areas of heavy slave concentrations (64 percent of the Tidewater counties and 66 percent of the Piedmont counties during the 1830s and 1840s), appealed to owners who were fed up with the ineffective and expensive treatments of their regular physicians. One Tidewater resident turned to Thomsonianism after experienced Norfolk physicians had unsuccessfully managed a household scarlet fever outbreak. All twenty cases, the happy slave owner reported to the editors of a Thomsonian journal, had been cured. Another man, in Goochland County, stated that a local Thomsonian practitioner had cured his bondswoman of a disease that one of the most respected regular physicians of the area had found intractable to the usual blister and salivation treatments. And a Prince Edward County Thomsonian doctor claimed to have cured an enslaved ten-year-old who had been suffering from rabies (a misdiagnosis, no doubt). With adherents to the sect so widely diffused throughout the state, the services or success stories of practitioners no doubt reached at least a portion of the slaveholding class and influenced its thinking.[35]

Beyond the masters' and overseers' eyes, back in the slave cabins, some bondspeople took medical matters into their own hands. When under the surveillance of whites, the enslaved usually (but not always) accepted their treatments. Some even administered them in the name of the owner. But others developed or retained from African heritage their own brand of care, complete with special remedies, medical practitioners, and rituals. The result was a dual system of health care, the two parts of which often conflicted with each other.

Owners did not appreciate bondspeople overusing the plantation infirmary, medicines, or the family physician, but they preferred this to black self-care for several reasons. Their quarrel with the enslaved was the same as the physicians' with the slave owners: they waited too long before seeking medical assistance and often misdiagnosed illnesses. Owners permitted blacks a small amount of freedom in treating minor ailments at home, but lost their patience when sickness got out of hand. James L. Hubard, in charge of his father's lands during the latter's vacation at Alleghany Springs, Virginia, reported that Daphny had treated her own son with vermifuges (worm medicines) for several days before realizing that the boy was suffering not from worms but from dysentery. Hubard quickly altered medication and summoned a physician, blaming the entire affair on "the stupidity of Daphny." An enraged Landon Carter found a suckling child with measles at the slave quarters. "The mother," he wrote in his diary, "let nobody know of it until it was almost dead."[36]

Whites often accused the enslaved of negligence or incompetence in the care of their fellow blacks. Dr. G. Lane Corbin of Warwick County, Virginia, for instance, promoted bondspeople's use of collodion, a syrupy dressing, because it required so little attention once applied: "This I consider of moment in regard to our slave population, whose negligence and inattention to such matters [as the proper dressing of wounds] must have attracted the notice of the most superficial observer."[37] Enslaved people frequently were charged with irresponsibility, ignorance, slovenliness, and indifference in the management of other blacks' illnesses. "They will never do right, left to themselves," declared one Franklin County planter.[38]

Furthermore, some whites argued, the enslaved did not even care for their own personal health properly. Recovery was retarded and even reversed, Dr. W. S. Morton of Cumberland County remarked, "by their [the slaves'] own stupid perversity in refusing confinement to bed, and to follow other important directions when in a very dangerous condition."[39] Owners and physicians often confirmed this but were powerless to combat it. It was difficult for whites, unless they were present at all times, to force ailing blacks to take medicines or to remain constantly in bed. A most spectacular instance of death following defiance of medical orders occurred in Portsmouth, Virginia, when a black male patient of Dr. John W. H. Trugien, confined to bed with a stab wound of the heart, sustained a massive effusion of blood from that organ upon exerting himself by rising from his pallet.[40]

To offset the failures and harshness of white remedies or the negligence of owners, or perhaps to exert some control over their lives, some enslaved people treated their own diseases and disorders or turned to other trusted blacks for medical assistance, with or without the owner's knowledge.[41] Black home remedies circulated secretly through the slave quarters and were passed down surreptitiously from generation to generation. Most of these cures were derived from local plants, though some medicines contained ingredients that had magical value only. Occasionally whites would learn of a particularly effective medicine and adopt it, as when Dr. Richard S. Cauthorn announced in the *Monthly Stethoscope* (1857) that an old folk remedy (milkweed or silk weed, *Asclepias syriaca* in the U.S. Dispensatory) that had been used for years by blacks in the counties north of Richmond worked almost as well as quinine for agues and fevers.[42] Otherwise, most whites simply ignored or tolerated the black medical world until something occurred to bring their attention to it—either a great medical discovery or a slave death caused by abuse.

Because blacks practiced medicine in virtually every portion of the Old Dominion and because their methods were based partially on magic, problems occasionally arose. The main source of trouble was usually not the misuse of home remedies, but the "prescriptions" and activities of so-called conjure doctors, whose system existed in the South because the enslaved brought it with them from Africa and the West Indies. These men and women used trickery, violence, persuasion, and medical proficiency to gain their reputations among local black communities. They were viewed as healers of illnesses that white doctors could not touch with their medicines and as perpetrators of sicknesses on any person they wished—all through "spells."[43]

Superstition was a powerful force within the enslaved community, and a difficult one for white nonadherents to understand or overcome. For instance, the older brother of an enslaved patient of Dr. A. D. Galt of Williamsburg observed to the doctor that his medicines were useless because Gabriel "had been tricked" and "must have a Negro Doctor" to reverse the progress of the illness. Galt soon claimed to have cured the man, though he did admit that Gabriel suffered frequent relapses, "probably from intemperance in drink."[44] In another case, an enslaved woman took sick and eventually died on a plantation near Petersburg from what her fellow bondspeople believed were the effects of a conjurer. Some speculated that the young man whom she had refused to marry "poisoned or tricked" her, though the overseer attributed her death to consumption.[45] Virginia Hayes Shepherd, a formerly enslaved woman interviewed at age eighty-three in 1939, described an incident to illustrate how superstitious her stepfather had been: "He believed he had a bunch something like boils. White doctor bathed it. After a few days it burst and live things came out of the boil and crawled on the floor. He though he was conjured. He said an enemy of his put something on the horse's back and he rode it and got it on his buttocks and broke him out."[46]

Whites did permit blacks to fulfill certain medical functions. Some planters assigned "trusted" bondspeople to the task of rendering medical assistance to all ailing blacks on the farm. In most cases, they simply dispensed remedies and performed venesection and cupping as learned from the white owner or overseer. Though not complete black self-care, this activity did represent a transitional stage in which the enslaved had the opportunity to apply some of their own knowledge of herbs and such gained from elders, in addition to white remedies. These nurses, predominantly women, usually won the respect of both blacks and whites for their curative skills. "Uncle" Bacchus White, an eighty-nine-year-old former slave interviewed in Fredericksburg, Virginia, in 1939, attested: "Aunt Judy uster tend us when we uns were sic' and anything Aunt Judy couldn't do 'hit won't worth doin.'"[47] A white lady writing at about the same time provided a similarly romantic view of the black plantation nurse: "One of the house-servants, Amy Green—'Aunt Amy' we children called her—was a skilled nurse. My father kept a store of medicines, his scales, etc. So with Aunt Amy's poultices of horseradish and plattain-leaves and her various cuppings and plasters the ailments of the hundred negroes were well taken in hand."[48] Given such high testimony and devotion from plantation folk, one could hardly dispute the novelist Louise Clarke Pyrnelle's depiction of Aunt Nancy, a fictional antebellum household nurse, who claimed, while dosing several young slaves, "Ef'n hit want fur dat furmifuge [vermifuge—worm disease], den Marster wouldn't hab all dem niggers w'at yer see hyear."[49]

To black women often fell another task: prenatal and obstetrical care of whites and blacks, especially in rural areas.[50] At least one enslaved woman on most large Virginia plantations learned and practiced the art of midwifery, not only at home but also throughout the neighborhood. Owners preferred to employ these skilled accoucheurs in uncomplicated cases rather than pay the relatively high fees of trained physicians. Physicians, remarked one member of the medical profession, attended less than half of all births in the state. He estimated that nine-tenths of all deliveries among the black population (another physician set it at five-sixths) were conducted by midwives, most of whom were also black. He further asserted that midwives attended half the deliveries of white women. Physicians often saw obstetrical cases only when problems arose. As a result of this demand for competent nonprofessional obstetrical services, black midwives flourished in the countryside.

Blacks did play a significant role in the health care system of the South. They assisted whites and blacks in delivering children, letting blood, pulling teeth, administering medicines, and nursing the sick. The techniques and drugs they used were overtly derived from white medical practices. But unknown to masters, overseers, health officers, or physicians, blacks did also resort to their own treatments derived from their own heritage and experience. Occasionally the white and black medical worlds merged or openly clashed, but usually they remained silently separate.

CHAPTER 8

Medical Experimentation and Demonstration on Blacks in the Old South

"An abundance of materials in the southern medical journals reveals that slaves had a fairly significant role in medical education and in experimental and radical medical and surgical practice of the antebellum South," remarked J. Walter Fisher in a 1968 article describing some of the medical uses to which slaves were put in the Old South.[1] Further investigation into this subject indicates that Southern white medical educators and researchers relied greatly on the availability of African American patients for various purposes. Black bodies often found their way to dissecting tables, operating amphitheaters, classroom or bedside demonstrations, and experimental facilities. This is not to deny that white bodies were similarly used.[2] In Northern cities and in Southern port towns such as New Orleans, Louisville, Memphis, Charleston, and Mobile, where poor, transient whites were abundant, seamen, European immigrants, and white indigents undoubtedly joined blacks in fulfilling the "clinical material" needs of the medical profession. But blacks were particularly easy targets, given their positions as voiceless slaves or "free persons of color" in a society sensitive to and separated by race. This open and deliberate use of blacks for medical research and demonstration well illustrates the racial attitudes of antebellum white Southerners.

Interestingly, people generally assumed that information gained from observation of Negro bodies was applicable to Caucasians. Despite the political rhetoric then current in the Old South about a separate medicine for blacks and for whites,[3] the research and teaching reflected, in fact, the opposite. Blacks did not seem to differ enough from whites to exclude them from extensive use in Southern medical schools and in research activities.[4]

Use of blacks for medical experimentation and demonstration was not the result of a conscious organized plan on the part of white Southerners to learn more about the differences between the races or even how better to care for their black charges. The examples related in this chapter reflect the actions of individual researchers and medical institutions. Taken together, however, a pattern emerges. Blacks were considered more available and more accessible in that white-dominated society: they were rendered physically visible by their skin color but were legally invisible because of their slave status.

Throughout history medicine has required bodies for teaching purposes. Students had to learn anatomy, recognize and diagnose diseases, and treat conditions requiring surgery; researchers had to try out their ideas and new techniques; and practitioners had to perform autopsies to confirm their diagnoses and to understand the effects of diseases on the human body. The need for human specimens became more recognized and more emphasized in America during the first half of the nineteenth century as the ideas of the Paris school of hospital medicine reached this country.[5] Bedside experience, clinical-pathological correlations, and statistical studies became increasingly important. And medical schools throughout the United States, including those in the South, attempted to meet the new demands of students for a modern education. Clinics, infirmaries, and hospitals were opened in conjunction with those colleges; patients, however, were not always willing to enter. To fill beds, it became essential to use the poor and the enslaved. Medicine thus capitalized on the need of the indigent and the helpless for medical care. In the South, white attitudes toward blacks ensured the selection of patients of this group as specimens, though some whites were also used.

Competition for students among Southern medical schools was fierce during the thirty years preceding the Civil War, which led each institution to publicize the positive aspects of its program in newspapers, medical journals, circulars, and magazines. One of the major requisites of any school was an abundant supply of clinical material—living patients for medical and surgical demonstrations as well as cadavers for anatomical dissections and pathological examinations. Institutional reputations were made and broken on the basis of the availability of teaching specimens. The Transylvania University Medical Department in Lexington, Kentucky, serves as a case in point. One of the causes for its decline from eminence during the 1830s was its purported difficulty in procuring bodies for clinical teaching. Despite numerous attempts by both faculty and students to dispel rumors about the shortage of specimens and demonstration materials at the medical school, it was impossible to reverse the negative impressions of students. In contrast, a medical school was established in nearby Louisville (Louisville Medical Institute) in 1837, owing in part to the presence of a large black (as well as transient white) population, well suited to the needs of teaching institutions.[6]

To train students in disease management, the better Southern medical schools either established infirmaries or arranged with local authorities to treat patients in poorhouses or city hospitals. In Georgia, Kentucky, Alabama, South Carolina, Virginia, and presumably in other Southern states, the patients used for the education of students were frequently black. Newspaper advertisements by the Atlanta Medical College, for example, encouraged owners to send their sick and injured slaves to the infirmary for treatment. There, "an intelligent nurse and faithful servant will be in constant attendance." No mention of the presence of medical students was necessary. The boarding fee was reasonable (fifteen cents per day), and the doctor's fee was waived if the case turned out to be incurable and the enslaved patient had to be sent home.[7] Probably typical of patient use for demonstrations at the Atlanta Medical College Infirmary was what a professor of materia medica termed "An interesting case of Hepatic Abscess in a negro man" who "was subject to the examination of the Students for several weeks during the course of lectures, and was lectured upon and prescribed for in presence of the Class." Similarly, he wrote that a black woman suffering from tuberculosis "had been under our occasional observation for a year previously."[8]

South Carolina medical institutions were even more explicit in their public requests for black patients. In the late 1830s both Charleston medical schools operated infirmaries during the regular teaching sessions, from November to March, and both catered to the large black population resident in the city and surrounding area. The hospital of the Medical College of the State of South Carolina admitted the enslaved, poor whites, and free blacks. As an inducement to lure patients from the competing medical-school hospital, infirmary officials made slave owners liable for no professional charges, the only account rendered being that for food and nursing. This was so, they explained, because "the sole object of the Faculty . . . [is] to promote the interest of Medical education within their native State and City."[9] The surgery established by the faculty of the other school, the Medical College of South Carolina, admitted the enslaved and free blacks only. An advertisement placed in the *Charleston Courier* requested planters with servants "laboring under Surgical diseases," local physicians with slave patients requiring surgical intervention, and "such [free] persons of color as may not be able to pay for Medical advice" to call at the hospital. "The object of the Faculty," the announcement continued, "is to collect as many interesting cases, as possible, for the benefit and instruction of their pupils."[10]

By 1841 the Medical College of the State of South Carolina had established a permanent year-round hospital with large wards for black and white patients. College officials claimed that they had little trouble filling beds at this new infirmary, because "the slave population of the city, and neighboring plantations, is capable of furnishing ample materials for clinical instruction." Students at the school saw not only "all the common diseases of the climate" but also a variety of operative procedures, owing to the presence of a slave population "peculiarly liable to surgical diseases requiring operations for their relief."[11] The medical college continued to use black patients for surgical demonstrations throughout the antebellum years. During the late 1850s, for instance, surgical cases occurring among blacks while school was in session were admitted to the "Coloured Wards" of a newly constructed public hospital and were reserved for the exclusive use of student doctors.[12]

The use of black patients for medical-school training was not confined to the lower South. The Hampden-Sydney College Medical Department (called the Medical College of Virginia after 1854), located in Richmond, employed many of the same techniques as the South Carolina and Georgia institutions to attract persons of color into its infirmary wards. Faculty physicians announced in an 1853 publication that "the number of negroes employed in our factories will furnish materials for the support of an extensive hospital, and afford to the student that great desideratum—clinical instruction." They placed ads in country editions of Richmond newspapers informing rural slaveholders of the infirmary's facilities, charged lower rates for blacks, and attempted (unsuccessfully) to establish first a slave hospital, then a free hospital for all indigents and enslaved persons.[13] Though none of the infirmary's records are extant, evidence from case histories published in the local medical journals indicates that a majority of the patients were black.[14]

Neither whites nor blacks held hospitals in high esteem during the antebellum period. Not only did patients object to having medical students and doctors touching and poking them and discussing their illnesses and the merits or problems of particular modes of treatment in their presence, but they also feared that experiments might be performed on them and that they would be permitted to die so autopsies could be undertaken.[15] Nor were medical school announcements, circulated to attract students, calculated to encourage the sickly to request hospital admission. A Transylvania University Medical Department advertisement for the 1846–47 session, though perhaps more wishful than accurate, was typical: "Clinical instructions fully equal to the wants of the class, are given at the hospital. Experience during the last session fully attested, that there were always patients sufficiently numerous for all useful purposes. Valuable opportunities are here presented for the study of the physical signs of Thoracic Diseases."[16] Illiterate slaves did not have to read such circulars to learn about medical-school hospitals: their reputations preceded them.

Though fears about mistreatment in Southern hospitals were generally unfounded (doctors and students appeared, usually, to do their best to cure patients on the wards), concerns regarding the use of deceased patients were real. Autopsies and anatomical dissections were (and are) integral and important aspects of a medical education, but people expressed great aversion to the prospect of having their bodies minutely investigated after death. Complained one Georgia physician, "There is a superstitious prejudice existing in reference to them [autopsies], and it is seldom we can secure a case, except where the light of science has made headway."[17] In 1861 a resident physician at Charleston's Roper Hospital made the following entry in his casebook after one of his white patients died: "No autopsy could be held in this case, as his friends by some accident heard of his death immediately on its taking place, and forthwith came for the body."[18] The result was that physicians and students had to resort to grave robbing, hurried dissections before bodies were claimed, and deception to obtain cadavers for autopsy and anatomical investigations.

The attitudes of white Southerners both toward the use of human bodies in medical education and toward blacks were silently but clearly revealed in the medical profession's heavy reliance on cadavers of persons of color. Human anatomical dissection was illegal in many states during the antebellum period,[19] although medical schools continued to teach anatomy. Unless approached by angry relatives or friends of deceased persons, city authorities rarely questioned medical educators regarding the sources of their anatomical specimens. Southern blacks, because of their helpless legal and inconsequential social positions, became prime candidates for medical-school dissections. Physicians usually found it much more convenient to obtain black specimens than white. "In Baltimore," commented Harriet Martineau after an 1834 visit, "the bodies of coloured people exclusively are taken for dissection, 'because the whites do not like it, and the coloured people cannot resist.'"[20] Dr. Henry M. Dowling of Leesburg, Virginia, had little difficulty receiving permission for an autopsy on a twelve-year-old slave girl with a suspected case of worms because the victim's owner was "a gentleman of intelligence, and unaffected by the vulgar prejudices entertained on this subject" by others.[21]

When it came to obtaining Caucasian bodies for postmortem examinations, however, even "gentlemen of intelligence" found ways to refuse physicians. For example, of twenty-four individual autopsies reported by white Southern physicians in the *Transylvania Journal of Medicine and the Associate Sciences* (1828–39) and the *Transylvania Medical Journal* (1849–51), nineteen were performed on blacks and only five on whites, in a state where the white population far exceeded the black. Also indicative of the race differential is an article that appeared in the *Transactions of the Medical Association of the State of Alabama*, describing an 1853 typhoid-fever epidemic in the vicinity of Sumterville. Of the approximately forty-five blacks and twenty whites who contracted the disease, a young white physician and his sister as well as ten other persons of both races died. The three autopsies performed by the reporting physician, however, were all on slaves.[22]

The enslaved were not entirely voiceless in the matter of autopsies. Some masters honored the wishes of deceased slaves' relatives or friends and refused which it would execrate if performed upon their master or other whites."[37] Southern medical schools could and did boast that their cities' large black populations provided ample supplies of clinical and anatomical material. And white physicians trained at these institutions carried with them into their own careers this idea of the medical usefulness of blacks. When new techniques or treatments required experimentation, physicians tested them on readily available and legally silent enslaved or free black patients. There was little fear of retribution, and as long as death or debility attributable to the new technique did not result, the cost was negligible. People of color, therefore, did have reason for fearing misuse at the hands of Southern white physicians.

Generally speaking, in the era prior to acceptance of the germ theory, there was only a fine line between seeking an appropriate treatment and engaging in actual experimentation.[38] A physician confronted with sick patients administered whatever treatments he had found efficacious from previous experience without really understanding their actual operation within the body. If the standard remedy failed, another compound was tried, regardless of its "scientific" merit. Few practitioners attempted to perform controlled experiments to determine the properties and effects of the drugs they used or to establish basic physiological or surgical principles that would serve as guides for the medical profession. Medical practice at this time was basically empirical, as Southern white physicians indicated in their journal articles. And here blacks often served as the test subjects for new remedies. Dr. T. S. Hopkins of Waynesville, Georgia, for instance, prescribed nitric acid solutions in seven cases (five black and two white) of asthma after a medical friend in an adjoining county had had success with an accidental administration of this medicine to a sick child. He "deemed [the] experiment justifiable, particularly when it could result in no harm to the patient."[39] Similarly, a Madison County, Alabama, practitioner, Joseph Evelyn May, faced with a severe case of malaria in an enslaved person, administered as a last resort extremely large doses of quinine combined with calomel. It worked, so May felt justified in having attempted so radical and unorthodox a procedure.[40]

Empirical trials of remedies on patients were not unusual in the practice of medicine anywhere in antebellum America, but outright experimentation upon living humans may have occurred more openly and perhaps more often in the South, owing to the nature of slave society. No studies of human experimentation and use of white medical specimens in the North or South presently exist to substantiate this claim. Comparative statistics of this nature are difficult to obtain. Certainly the indigent and socially voiceless were used by medical people for their own ends in the North and, as Ronald Leslie Numbers has pointed out, in Europe at that time. The social status of Dr. William Beaumont's experimental subject, a poor French-Canadian trapper named Alexis St. Martin, is illustrative of this attitude. Beaumont induced St. Martin by force and by various legal and financial means to submit to some nine years (1824–33) of intermittent experimentation on the physiological activity of his stomach, part of which had been permanently exposed in a gunshot accident. The ethics of human experimentation were not established at this time—people generally accepted the research of Beaumont and others without questioning their ethics or the patients' rights.[41] It did not seem odd or unusual then to use persons of color as a number of physicians in the South did. Some whites took advantage of Southern blacks by testing new techniques or remedies in the name of medical progress. In several instances physicians purchased blacks for the sole purpose of experimentation; in others the physicians used free blacks and enslaved people owned by others. Though white subjects were included in one or two cases of experimentation, blacks always made up the overwhelming majority of patients. A few major medical breakthroughs did result from the research performed upon persons of color, for which the physicians involved received fame and glory. The slaves, identified, if at all, by first name only, are unknown now to their descendants and to the general public.

A tale passed down by residents of the Alabama Black Belt illustrates the inclination of some Southern whites to use blacks for experimental purposes and to discount the worth of slave lives in their society. When the region around Marion was first being settled, people were unsure of its healthfulness. They feared the mists, swamp gases, and miasmata that rose from the low ground. According to tradition, a number of farmers purchased a bondsman, set him up in a hut with tools, supplies, and food, and left him there for a period of time to see if he could survive. Finding him still healthy when they returned, the settlers moved in, and the area grew rapidly.[42] Whether true or not, the story illustrates some Southern whites' attitudes toward using blacks in experiments.

A number of physicians had similar inclinations. Dr. T. Stillman of Charleston, for example, operated a private infirmary in the 1830s that specialized in the treatment of skin diseases, although he also cared for patients with a variety of other disorders. During October 1838, Stillman concluded his usual lengthy advertisement in the *Charleston Mercury* with an offer to purchase from slave owners any chronically diseased slaves they might wish to "dispose of." He would pay "the highest cash price" for fifty blacks "affected with scrofula or king's evil, confirmed hypochondriasm, apoplexy, diseases of the liver, kidneys, spleen, stomach and intestines, bladder and its appendages, diarrhea, dysentery, &c."[43] It was obvious from the wording of the advertisement that Dr. Stillman planned to test newly formulated remedies on these fifty chronically ill persons of color for the benefit of medical science, as well as, no doubt, for personal gain.

In a few instances actual discussions of the kinds of experiments to which the enslaved were subjected are available, from the point of view of both the patients and the physicians. There lived in Clinton, seat of Jones County, Georgia, during the 1820s and early 1830s, a physician-planter who was attempting to discover permission for postmortem examinations. Colonel S. B. Stevens of Quincy, Florida, objected when Dr. Richard Jarrot proposed to perform an autopsy on the body of 102-year-old Moses, dead of what appeared to be acute pleuritis.[23] The master of a large Lowndes County, Alabama, plantation released for postmortem examination the body of only one of eight enslaved children who had died during a violent dysentery outbreak in 1851 despite the request of the attending physicians for other cadavers.[24] And a Virginia slave owner, "unwilling to do violence to his [bondsman's] prejudices and feelings," withheld assent when a physician requested an autopsy on the enslaved man's wife.[25]

Occasionally, the prevailing attitude of whites—that dissection was acceptable when confined to the black population—was expressed in print. A correspondent to the Milledgeville, Georgia, *Statesman and Patriot* in 1828 agreed that it was necessary to dissect corpses to learn anatomy, but opposed the use of whites for such a procedure. He endorsed a proposal then before the state legislature that permitted local authorities to release bodies of executed black felons to medical societies for the purpose of dissection, assuring the safety of white corpses. "The *bodies of colored* persons, whose execution is necessary to public security, may, we think, be with equity appropriated for the benefit of a science on which so many lives depend, while the measure would in a great degree secure the sepulchral repose of those who go down into the grave amidst the lamentations of friends and the reverence of society."[26]

The Kentucky House of Representatives seriously considered a similar proposal. It rejected by the narrow margin of seven votes a bill "to authorize and require the Judges of the different Circuit Courts of this state to adjudge and award the corpses of negroes, executed by sentences of said judges, to the Faculties of the different chartered Colleges in this state, for dissection and experiment."[27] In Virginia the vast majority of cadavers obtained for dissection at the five antebellum medical schools were those of persons of color.[28] The faculty of the Medical College of Georgia (MCG) in Augusta hired, between 1834 and 1852, several bondsmen to act as intermediaries in the purchase of bodies from slave owners in the surrounding plantation country. In 1852, MCG purchased Grandison Harris in Charleston to obtain cadavers and to perform janitorial duties. He robbed graves and also bought black bodies for the next fifty years or so.[29] And the Medical College of South Carolina openly acknowledged in its circular of 1831 that it obtained "subjects . . . for every purpose" from the black rather than the white population of Charleston so as to carry on "proper dissections . . . without offending any individuals."[30] This undisguised use of persons of color for dissection in Charleston continued into the post–Civil War era.[31]

Blacks usually knew full well how the bodies of their friends and relatives were being used, and they were both offended and frightened. The Rev. Robert Wilson of Charleston in 1856 overheard one aged black woman exclaim to her friend as they passed a building housing the city's medical school, "Please Gawd, when I dead, I hope I wi' dead in de summah time."[32] Classes ran only from November to March, the cold months when bodies did not decompose rapidly. A former bondsman, Charlie Grant, recalled many years after the event how, as an adolescent boy near Florence, South Carolina, he was paid two dollars by a local doctor to dig up and carry to his office the body of a one- or two-year-old enslaved child who had just been buried. Though Grant did not let on, he knew what was happening: "Dr. Johnson want to cut dat child open. Dat what he want wid it."[33] Blacks' fear of medical schools and dissection inevitably carried over into the postbellum period, when whites, as a means of maintaining control over former slaves, reinforced the idea of "night-doctors" who stole, killed, and then dissected African Americans.[34] The accuracy of the belief that whites actually killed blacks for use in dissection is hard to verify.[35] But the fear blacks harbored was well known, as illustrated by four of the nine verses of the following poem, probably written by a white in black dialect in the late nineteenth or early twentieth century. It poked fun at these very real concerns of persons of color:

THE DISSECTING HALL
Yuh see dat house? Dat great brick house?
Way yonder down de street?
Dey used to take dead folks een dar
Wrapped een a long white sheet.

An sometimes we'en a nigger'd stop,
A-wondering who was dead,
Dem stujent men would take a club
An' bat 'im on de head.

An' drag dat poor dead nigger chile
Right een dat 'sectin hall
To vestigate 'is liver—lights—
His gizzard an' 'is gall.

Tek off dat nigger's han's an' feet—
His eyes, his head an' all,
An' w'en dem stujent finish
Dey was nothin' left at all.[36]

The abolitionist Theodore Dwight Weld was not exaggerating when he claimed in his 1839 polemical work *American Slavery as It Is*, "'Public opinion' would tolerate surgical experiments, operations, processes, performed upon them [slaves], the best remedies for heatstroke. This man, Dr. Thomas Hamilton, borrowed the slave Fed from a grateful patient in order to test some of his medications on a human subject. He had a hole dug in the ground which he then had heated with fire to a high temperature. Fed sat naked on a stool on a platform placed within this ovenlike pit with only his head above ground level. To retain the heat, Hamilton fastened wet blankets over the hole. Fed took a different medicine each of the five or six times he entered the pit over a period of two or three weeks, so that Hamilton could determine which preparation best enabled this bondsman to withstand high temperatures. Fed fainted each time from the heat and from exhaustion (he had put in a full day's work before each experiment). According to Fed's account of the proceedings the doctor found cayenne pepper to be the most effective preparation. Experimentation did not end here, however. Fed claimed, in a book written in London some years after his escape from slavery, that Hamilton came to his master's farm to perform other experiments on him for nine months, after which time "I had become so weak, that I was no longer able to work in the fields." Dr. Hamilton bled the slave every other day for three weeks and repeatedly blistered him "to ascertain how deep my black skin went." Hamilton never published a description of his experiments, so Fed's account of these events cannot be verified directly. Extant records place both men in the same neighborhood, one as slave, the other as physician, at the same time. Other aspects of Fed's narrative also bear up under historical scrutiny.[44]

Hamilton's crude experiments did little to advance medical knowledge. The same cannot be said for Dr. James Marion Sims's use of slave women to develop a cure for vesico-vaginal fistula. Vesico-vaginal fistula is a break in the wall separating the bladder from the vagina, which allows urine to pass involuntarily to the outside from the vagina rather than from the urethra. Women suffering from this defect, usually the result of trauma during childbirth, are incontinent of urine and continually uncomfortable. The constant flow of urine produces fetid odors, irritated skin, and frequent infections of the reproductive organs. Sims, a South Carolinian practicing in Montgomery, Alabama, during the 1840s and early 1850s, became interested in this condition when three cases among enslaved black women came to his attention within a few months, and a chance occurrence gave him the idea of how to cure it. While treating a white patient for a traumatically malpositioned uterus by placing the woman on her knees and elbows, he suddenly realized that by putting vesico-vaginal fistula patients in the same position he would be able to visualize the fistula and perhaps even repair it. No physician prior to this had developed a consistently successful surgical treatment for the condition owing to difficulties in visualizing the defect, repairing the passage through the bladder wall, and preventing infection during the procedure.

Once Sims had conceived of a way to operate on patients with vesico-vaginal fistula he set about putting his ideas into practice with the cooperation of his enslaved subjects. He never disguised the fact that what he was doing was entirely experimental. The three black women who served as the first patients, Anarcha, Lucy, and Betsey, desperately wished relief from their sufferings. So too did several other patients, all enslaved, who submitted to Sims's attempts at a cure over the next four years, 1845 to 1849. Each woman underwent up to thirty operations in quest of relief. When local physicians lost interest and ceased assisting Sims with the procedure, the persistent doctor trained his enslaved patients to assist him. Finally, in May 1849, Sims succeeded in overcoming all the complications that had been plaguing his procedure for four years. One by one, the black women were cured and sent home.

It is significant that all the subjects in Sims's experiments were black. When he decided to pursue his idea of curing vesico-vaginal fistula he "ransacked the country for [Negro] cases" and found enough to warrant enlarging his eight-bed slave infirmary. Sims agreed with each slave owner to pay all costs of maintenance except taxes and clothing and "to perform no experiment or operation ... to endanger their [slaves'] lives." It was not until after his success with enslaved women became known that white women ventured to submit to the operations. Interestingly, Sims discovered that white patients often failed to persevere as well as black patients during the painful and uncomfortable procedure. Typical of the problem was the woman about whom Sims remarked in his medical notes: "The pain was so terrific that Mrs. H. could not stand it and I was foiled completely." Perhaps it was Sims's recognition of this difference between black enslaved and white patients that prompted him, in a speech several years after his successes, to praise so highly the black women upon whom he experimented. "To the indomitable courage of these long-suffering women, more than to any one other single circumstance is the world indebted for the results of these persevering efforts. Had they faltered, then would woman have continued to suffer from the dreadful injuries produced by protracted parturition, and then should the broad domain of surgery not have known one of the most useful improvements that shall forever hereafter grace its annals."[45]

Sims's reliance on black patients for experimental purposes was continued by Nathan Bozeman, his successor in Montgomery. Bozeman purchased Sims's practice when the latter moved to New York and continued to operate the slave infirmary. In 1855 he perfected a new type of suture for relieving vesico-vaginal fistula with the cooperation of seven new enslaved patients.[46]

Other examples can be offered of the white Southern physician's bias toward the use of black subjects in medical experimentation. Dr. Ephraim McDowell of Danville, Kentucky, revered in American medical history as the first to perform successfully an ovariotomy (removal of an ovary), operated initially upon a white woman, Mrs. Jane Todd Crawford, in 1809. Little known is the fact that McDowell's subsequent four ovariotomies, during which he improved his technique, were all performed on black women—again, this in Kentucky, a state with a relatively small black population.[47] Crawford William Long of Jefferson, Georgia, is often cited as the first to operate on an anesthetized patient. In March and again in June 1842 he removed tumors from the neck of James M. Venable, a white man. Two of Long's next three experiments with ether were on black patients: the amputation of an enslaved boy's toe in July 1842 and of a bondsman's finger in January 1845.[48] John M. B. Harden, a physician in Liberty County, Georgia, removed and measured the circumferences of certain blood vessels from the bodies of one black man and three hogs during the 1830s "to determine the relative areas of the Trunks and Branches of arteries." Harden published his findings, which he considered of significance to anatomical and physiological knowledge, in a regional medical journal.[49]

A final example of the usefulness of persons of color to physicians in a slave society was the performance of cesarean operations on pregnant women. Attempts at delivering children abdominally when they could not pass through the mother's contracted or occluded pelvis had been generally unsuccessful throughout history. Physicians in antebellum America continued to perform this procedure and occasionally met with success. The racial statistics, derived from compilations of the Philadelphia physician Dr. Robert P. Harris in the 1870s and early 1880s, are revealing: of fifteen Northern women whose race was reported, thirteen were white, one black, and one Mexican (California); in the South, twenty-nine of thirty-six women were black.[50] This trend continued throughout the nineteenth century: by 1881, fifty-one of sixty Caesarean procedures performed in Northern states had been on whites, while only twelve of fifty-nine in Southern states had been on whites. Physicians in Louisiana performed the most procedures (twenty) of those in any state, nineteen of which were done on blacks.[51]

It is to be expected in a slave society that the subjugated will be exploited. Such was the case in the American South where blacks acted not only as servants and laborers but also as medical specimens. Some medical scientists living in that society took advantage of the enslaved's helplessness to utilize them in demonstrations, autopsies, dissections, and experiments, situations distasteful to whites and rejected by them. Some whites, usually the poor and the friendless, found themselves in the same position as blacks. But given the racial attitudes of that time and place, persons of color were particularly vulnerable to abuse or mishandling at the hands of researchers, medical teachers, or students.

CHAPTER 9

Slave Life Insurance in Virginia and North Carolina

In late December 1853 an agent of railroad contractor John Buford stopped at the Southampton County, Virginia, farm of Samuel Drewry and solicited the hire of six healthy male slaves to form part of the crew building the Virginia and Tennessee Railroad. Drewry was aware of the dangers of jobs on public-works construction projects of this sort and of the poor treatment hired slaves sometimes received. He therefore replied that in addition to paying $150 per worker for a ten-month contract (March through December) Buford would have to purchase one thousand dollars of life insurance on each hired hand. After a month's delay, during which Drewry informed Buford that the Great Dismal Swamp Land Company (a wood-and-shingle gathering operation in southeastern Virginia) was paying $160 plus insurance, the two men came to terms—Drewry's terms.[1]

This incident illustrates the interest in slave life insurance that slave owners were beginning to demonstrate in the late antebellum period. Enslaved blacks were frequently employed on dangerous jobs in public-works construction, coal mining, iron manufacturing, and railroad and steamboat operations. A number of industrial concerns that owned slave workers protected their large investments by purchasing life insurance. Similarly, owners who hired out their bondspeople to industry bought life insurance or insisted that the lessee do so, and a few slave owners took out policies on valuable or favorite servants not hired out.[2] Whatever the reason, during the late 1840s and 1850s, whites were insuring the lives of their slaves in increasing, but never overwhelming, numbers.[3]

Life insurance did not become popular in the United States until the late antebellum period. Prior to 1800, Americans had purchased marine insurance on goods and occasionally a life insurance policy to protect against a pirate's ransom (an important consideration at the time) or the hazards of a long voyage. But people did not buy insurance to cover everyday risks on their lives. Slowly the concept of term insurance gained acceptance as companies began to offer this kind of protection. In 1794, the Insurance Company of North America inaugurated the sale of life insurance policies, followed by the Pennsylvania Company (1809), the Massachusetts Hospital Insurance Company (1818), and the New York Insurance Trust Company (1830). Still, public response was poor until the Girard Life Insurance and Trust Company introduced, several years after its founding in Philadelphia in 1836, a new plan whereby management shared some of its profits with policyholders. This idea of distributing profits caught on rapidly and spurred the establishment during the 1840s of other mutual life insurance companies. These firms began actively promoting sales to secure their shareholders' investments and ensure solvency. Given this new impetus, the life insurance business grew rapidly during that and the subsequent decade both in number of companies chartered (at least fifty-nine between 1840 and 1860) and total insurance in force (at least $4,690,000 in 1840 and $204,752,000 in 1860).[4]

The burgeoning life insurance industry did not confine its activities to the Northern states, though most business did center in that region. At least sixteen companies were founded in the Southern and border states between 1840 and 1860, but, unfortunately, few records exist for these firms. Most firms did not survive for more than a few years, and only one, St. Louis Mutual, was still in existence in 1937, when a major historical survey of life insurance companies was conducted.[5] Those Southern companies that did sell life insurance often found sales to white customers scarce. For example, a group of Virginia agents stated, in a petition requesting lower taxes for out-of-state insurance companies, that "in towns numbering one, two, or three thousand inhabitants there are seldom more than six or eight persons who have their lives insured."[6] Though comparative regional figures are not available, white Southerners appear to have been less willing to invest in life insurance protection than Northerners. As antebellum Southerners' written opinions on the subject of life insurance are rare, it is only a conjecture that residents of the region adopted this innovation as reluctantly and cautiously as they adopted others. Another reason for the difficulty Southern firms had in selling policies locally was fierce competition from several large Northern firms. Advertisements in most urban newspapers of the South attest to the number of "outside" companies doing business in this relatively small market.

A logical extension of the insuring of white lives was the taking on of slave risks. This form of insurance had existed for some time prior to the 1840s, but mainly as a protection to slave traders transporting blacks from Africa to the Americas or from one domestic slave market to another. Few, if any, Northern or Southern companies insured plantation, industrial, or urban bondspeople on a regular basis until the 1840s, when life insurance began gaining in sales and in the number of new firms.[7] But even after the introduction of slave life insurance, slave owners did not flock to the doors of agents. Had more slave owners purchased such life insurance at the time it might have become, as historian Robert S. Starobin asserted, "significant for the future stability of industrial slavery."[8] White Southerners wrote little on the subject in diaries, letters, and articles. Historians can thus merely suggest reasons why only about 3 percent of all industrial slaves and a substantially smaller number of plantation bondspeople employed during any year in the 1850s were covered by life insurance.[9] The problem of cost was undoubtedly a major factor. Owners were probably reluctant to lay out an extra five to fifteen dollars annually for every laborer, even if the number insured was limited to prime hands, and marginally successful farmers could not afford to buy life insurance for their family slaves.[10] Few white heads of households owned personal policies to protect their surviving spouses and children, much less policies on those they enslaved. Though agents advertised frequently in local newspapers, the concept of slave insurance was still so new that many masters must have simply ignored the publicity or put off inquiries for a future time. Then too there was the confusion in the Old South about the enslaved as people and as property. Farmers had been insuring their horses, barns, and even their crops (during transport to markets) for generations. With the introduction of life insurance, owners may have had difficulty deciding about the desirability of protecting themselves against the loss of their human property. The situation was more clear-cut when owners hired out their enslaved workers or purchased bondspeople for dangerous industrial labor. Then the slave was obviously a piece of property, an investment requiring financial protection.[11] But on large plantations, for instance, bondspeople were still treated ambiguously as both persons and property.

Some white Southerners disapproved of the whole concept of slave life insurance. Dr. Josiah Clark Nott of Mobile, Alabama, was probably the best-known and most vocal opponent. He prepared a lengthy article, published in the widely read *De Bow's Review* in 1847, at the very time that this kind of life insurance was gaining popularity. Nott feared that bondspeople would be the sufferers in the long run, as slave owners succumbed to temptation and permitted the sick or injured to die. Being the working class of the South, Nott argued, blacks "are exposed much to the causes of disease, and are less protected in sickness than the higher classes." Free men and women have an innate love of life; they and their families naturally do everything possible to save themselves and loved ones from death. However, he continued, "if the slave become unsound and there is little prospect of perfect recovery, the [insurance] underwriters cannot expect fair play—the insurance money is worth more than the slave, and the latter is regarded rather in the light of a superannuated horse." Nott believed that the typical slave owner treated his bondspeople kindly and carefully, but that insuring the lives of enslaved workers would change his attitude when serious illness or injury occurred: "Any man who will drive a horse cruelly, will drive a negro or operative to death, if he can gain anything by so doing."[12]

Nott's dire predictions did not prevent the formation of companies to insure the enslaved in Virginia, North Carolina, and other Southern states during the late 1840s and the 1850s. The Richmond Fire Association, the North Carolina Mutual Life Insurance Company, the Asheville Mutual Insurance Company, the Lynchburg Hose and Fire Insurance Company, and the Greensborough Mutual Life Insurance and Trust Company all took risks on bondspeople, but they also heeded Nott's caveats in several ways.[13] They limited the amount for which the enslaved could be insured, required a medical examination before approving a policy, restricted the term of the insurance policy, prohibited the free movement of insured bondspeople from place to place, charged extra premiums for dangerous jobs, and insisted on proof of proper treatment in health and of medical attention in sickness. Each of these means of protecting the company's liability also protected the bondsperson's life.

No insurance company in Virginia or North Carolina insured a slave for full value. The usual maximum was two-thirds or three-fourths of the stated valuation, but not to exceed $800. When John Buford, the railroad contractor, made inquiries regarding the purchase of life insurance on Samuel Drewry's six hired bondsmen, he learned that the Richmond Fire Association would not take slave risks for $1,000 as Drewry had demanded. The highest the company would go on an eighteen- to forty-year-old male railroad hand was $600.[14] The North Carolina Mutual Life Insurance Company of Raleigh (not to be confused with the Durham-based, African American–owned, postbellum company of the same name) advertised slave coverage at two-thirds of the market value and rejected several applications on bondspeople written for $1,000. James F. Jordan Jr., secretary of the company, returned one policy in 1855 to an agent in the field, explaining, "In no case at the present time does our company insure for more than $800: unless the slave to be insured is a first rate mechanic and a number 1 risk. The committee have given the limit in this case as Humphrey is only a laborer."[15] Similarly, the Lynchburg Hose and Fire Insurance Company insured the enslaved "to an amount equal to three fourths of their value provided it does not exceed Eight hundred Dollars the head."[16] By refusing to cover the full worth of a bondsperson, insurance companies were heeding Nott's warning that owners might consider their enslaved workers more valuable dead than alive.

Before accepting a slave policy, insurance companies required certification that the person was healthy. Local physicians in major towns acted as regular medical examiners for the firms. In rural areas reputable doctors received a small fee to perform this service when called upon.[17] Some companies routinely required both the family and company physicians to examine the enslaved. Such was the case with Franklin A. Slaughter, a general insurance broker in Fredericksburg,

Virginia. He instructed Dr. Andrew Glasswell Grinnan of Madison Court House to submit with every application to insure a bondsperson "a certificate from the slave physician and a personal examination to be made by you as the Medical Examiner."[18] For their efforts physicians received between fifty cents and two dollars per examination (the amount was higher for examinations of whites).[19] Not all doctors were satisfied with the amount of the compensation. Petersburg, Virginia, physicians in 1859 balked at what they considered to be insufficient remuneration for their services. They unanimously adopted a resolution setting the fee for insurance examinations at five dollars for white persons and three dollars for blacks, regardless of any company's established rates.[20]

The quality of doctors' examinations and reports was of the utmost importance to a company. Poorly conducted physical examinations meant approval of poor life insurance risks. Insurance firms insisted that local agents employ regular physicians of good standing in the community, not homeopaths, Thomsonians, hydropaths, or other sectarians.[21] One or more physicians at the home office read each examination statement to evaluate medical reports from the field and brought doubtful cases before the company's directorate or policy committee. The discovery of any chronic disease or serious acute illness automatically disqualified an enslaved (or white) person from obtaining insurance. For example, the North Carolina Mutual Life Insurance Company rejected a bondsman suffering from hernia because his occupation was "unfavorable to that disease." Several other bondsmen were rejected by the firm as "unsound," as were two pregnant bondswomen.[22] In Virginia, three of thirteen black railroad workers scheduled for hire to John Buford failed to receive insurance approval.[23]

The medical check on enslaved applicants' health sometimes placed owners in awkward positions. When a physician declared Mrs. Clanton's bondsman Charles "unsound" for life insurance in 1854, Thomas Wrenn, the lady's brother and slave manager, was immediately on the defensive. Had he known that anything had been amiss with Charles, Wrenn explained to his Southampton County, Virginia, neighbor, Samuel Drewry, he would have stated so at the time of application. Yes, Charles had suffered from "a certain disease" last year, but the doctors had cured it, and Charles had been perfectly healthy ever since. Wrenn, therefore, objected strongly to the results of this physical examination.[24] Mr. Drewry himself, having earlier in 1854 driven such a hard bargain with John Buford over the insuring and hiring of his enslaved workers, felt compelled to reaffirm the perfect health of his bondsman Colonel prior to his departure for southwestern Virginia and the railroad. Colonel had died of dropsy and pneumonia a few weeks after his arrival at the work camp, and Drewry apparently feared the insurance company would question Colonel's soundness during the months before he began work and decide not to honor his claim. So Drewry disagreed with the doctor's diagnosis of dropsy (usually a chronic condition) and described in detail Colonel's health record for the previous year. "This is the amount of all the sickness I am aware he [Colonel] ever had," Drewry concluded in a letter to Buford, "so from these circumstances I think they [the doctor] must be mistaken." He convinced the Richmond Fire Association, for almost a year later Drewry received assurance from the company's agent that his claim would be paid.[25]

Insurance companies also protected themselves and their slave risks by limiting the terms of policies to four or five years. Whites could buy insurance for life at a set annual premium based on age at time of purchase, but slave owners had to renegotiate policies on their bondspeople every few years and pay higher rates. This gave insurance companies the power to drop from their rolls any enslaved workers injured or taken chronically ill during the previous few years. The rule was also designed to protect the enslaved from "premature" deaths at the hands of mercenary owners. However, during any contracted multiyear term the company had to renew the policy annually as long as the premium was paid, regardless of health. There was also an upper age limit beyond which the enslaved could not be insured. Franklin Slaughter of Fredericksburg insured bondspeople only up to the age of sixty-two, and the North Carolina Mutual Life Insurance Company to age sixty. Superannuated bondspeople thus could not be subjected to maltreatment or neglect for insurance purposes, as companies would not insure them.[26]

Virginia and North Carolina insurance houses limited the movement of insured slaves to certain regions or states. Franklin Slaughter advertised his rates of slave insurance contingent upon a continued residence within the state of Virginia. He was willing to take risks on enslaved persons of color "to be conveyed to, or to reside in any slaveholding state in the Union," but at a higher premium.[27] Written into most slave insurance policies were the words "in case the said slave shall, without the consent of this Company, . . . pass beyond the limits of the State, . . . this Policy shall be null and void."[28] Though designed to protect the company, this rule also helped enslaved blacks. "Fevers" were the commonest cause of illness and a frequent cause of death in the antebellum South. Medical opinion held, with some truth, that persons who moved from one place to another, especially in the South, required several years' residence to acclimate to the new disease environment, as different forms of fevers usually prevailed. In fact, residents of the lower South paid a higher premium than those of the upper South even when they were acclimated, and much more when they were not. For example, a one-year, $1,000 policy on a twenty-two-year-old slave cost $35 in New Orleans in 1854 and only $16 in North Carolina. But even high premiums did not adequately compensate some companies for their slave losses in the Deep South. One Connecticut firm went into bankruptcy under a heavy barrage of claims on bondspeople, and a New York concern ceased issuing slave policies after a two-year trial period.[29] Hence, it was not surprising to read in a policy on an enslaved (or white) person that the insured could not "go to any locality South of the State, in which he or she now lives" without the company's approval.[30]

Owners did occasionally seek permission to move their enslaved workers to other states. In the minutes of the North Carolina Mutual Life Insurance Company's board of directors meetings are several instances: Alexander Graham of Fayetteville, North Carolina, was permitted to hire out two insured slaves in South Carolina without additional premium, though William Groves of Wilmington, North Carolina, was allowed to move his insured bondspeople to Florida only if he paid a 1 percent additional premium. The company authorized J. Wells of Hillsboro, North Carolina, to send an insured bondsman to Knoxville, Tennessee, by railroad through South Carolina and Georgia at no extra cost but insisted that W. A. Holeman pay an additional half-percent premium to send his bondsman Prince to Alabama.[31] The directors of insurance establishments feared, with justification, that the movement of people through different parts of the South would increase the risk of death.

Slave owners and hirers paid extra premiums not only for transferring bondspeople but also for putting persons of color to work at certain occupations. Franklin Slaughter considered that railroad engineers and firemen were at the greatest risk and so added a 2 percent surcharge for enslaved workers so engaged. Miners were charged an additional 1.5 percent while coal pit, steamboat, fishing boat laborers, and those involved in coasting were charged 1 percent more. Besides adding extra premiums for these occupations, the North Carolina Mutual Life Insurance Company also collected more for enslaved laborers engaged in rice fields, "getting oysters," and hauling seines.[32] The Richmond Fire Association refused to insure enslaved railroad hands over the age of forty and never for an amount exceeding $600.[33] Most conservative of all was the Lynchburg Hose and Fire Insurance Company. It would take no risks on enslaved laborers "employed upon any public improvement, or in any extra hazardous business" and charged an additional 1 percent for carpenters, house joiners, brick or stone masons, and those laboring in "occupation[s] of a like character."[34] Surcharges and severe restrictions on risks protected the insurance firms but did little to deter owners from hiring out their enslaved workers laboring at dangerous occupations or from obtaining slave life insurance.

A clause commonly found in slave life insurance policies, designed to protect the servant as well as the company, usually stated that "in case the said slave shall die for want of proper medical or personal attendance . . . this Policy shall be void."[35] Firms required some sort of certificate from physicians and witnesses as to the circumstances surrounding the actual cause of, and the care tendered prior to, death.[36] A typical witness' statement read, "This is to certify that Bill a slave of J. A. Linn, and a Tanner by trade aged about 17 or 18 years-laboured with me in the Tan yard from 1st of August, 1855, to 1st of November, 1856, that said Boy began to complain sometime before the 1st of Nov., 1856, and continued lingering until the 22nd of Feb. 1857 when he expired. I saw him after death and witnessed his burrial, & know him to be the same boy insured in your company in Policy No. 426."[37]

The available evidence does not substantiate Nott's dire predictions of inhumanity to enslaved blacks whose lives were insured. The proportion of deaths among one North Carolina company's white and black clients remained about equal for the years 1857, 1858, and 1860. Companies in Virginia and North Carolina attempted to safeguard their investments by establishing guidelines and rules and in so doing served to protect the lives of black servants.

The North Carolina Mutual Life Insurance Company of Raleigh was probably the major insurer of enslaved people in the Carolinas. Established in 1849, North Carolina Mutual counted among its directors some of the most prominent business and political figures in the capital city—the mayor of Raleigh (William D. Haywood, vice president of the company); the cashier and the teller of the Branch Bank of Cape Fear (William H. Jones, treasurer, and F. C. Hill); three respected physicians (Charles E. Johnson, president; William H. McKee; and R. B. Haywood); the principal clerk of the state House of Commons (Perrin Busbee, attorney); the U.S. attorney for the Raleigh District (H. W. Husted); the editor of the state Democratic organ, the Raleigh *North Carolina Standard* (William Woods Holden); the principal of the Institution for the Deaf and Dumb (William D. Cooke); and an influential local merchant (Charles B. Root).[38] Agents made great use of these prestigious names in assuring prospective clients of North Carolina Mutual's respectability as an insuring and business institution. With sales representatives and policyholders throughout North and South Carolina and in parts of Virginia, Alabama, and Georgia, North Carolina Mutual was by the eve of the Civil War a well-known and trusted firm.[39]

Though established to provide financial security for survivors of white heads of households (motto: "In Distress We Succor"), North Carolina Mutual rapidly became an insurer of slaves. The company approved its first policy on April 1, 1849. In early July it had issued eighty-three policies on white and forty-five on enslaved people. A year later, 610 policies were in force, the majority of which were probably for bondspeople.[40] By June 1857 (and probably earlier) three times as many enslaved as white people were being insured annually (see Appendix, Table 2).[41] Over the eleven years during which the company grew and prospered (1849–60) the directors constantly modified and adjusted their handling of slave accounts to keep pace with changing internal and external economic conditions and with the increased volume of slave risks.

In their first business prospectus (issued 1849) the directors of North Carolina Mutual included a few remarks on slave life insurance: "The insurance on slaves in this State opens a new field of thought to our Planters, and other slave owners, and proposes to secure them in the possession of that kind of property, which constitutes half of the actual wealth of the State."[42] Despite the fact that insurers of the enslaved could not "participate in the profits of the company" as could holders of regular life policies, applications arrived in unexpected numbers, raising several unanticipated problems. According to the rules, for instance, bondspeople could be insured for up to two-thirds of their market value, but the declarations that agents sent to the home office did not include information on the enslaved person's value. Only late in August 1849, almost five months after the start of operations, did the secretary of the company, James F. Jordan Jr., instruct all agents to rectify this matter. At about this same time, J. Hersman, one of the company's traveling agents, presented the directors with the results of his fact-collecting trip to Baltimore on slave insurance.[43] No record of this report or of the directors' reactions to it is available, but the fact that such a mission was even authorized reflects the board's desire to obtain as much information as possible on the subject and to act cautiously until they understood fully the implications of so large a slave owner response.

During its first fourteen months of operation, North Carolina Mutual paid only two claims on the 610 policies sold, one on an enslaved person and one on a white person. This favorable report, the board realized, did not reflect the experiences of other life insurance companies and could not be taken as indicative of future claims.[44] The board's circumspection proved warranted, as the number of deaths increased more than fivefold the following year, to eleven, while the number of insured persons only doubled, to 1,161 (see Appendix, Table 2). This was the one time in the company's sixteen years of full activity that the amount paid in slave losses ($5,288) exceeded that for whites ($5,000). North Carolina Mutual was still financially sound, having $46,117 on hand at the close of the fiscal year (June 1851), but the directors were understandably concerned. Calling these mortality figures to the attention of "those who hold the opinion that the bills of mortality among slaves are not so great as among whites," the board announced in its annual report for 1850–51 a 15 percent increase in slave premiums. It further justified this increase by pointing out that North Carolina Mutual's rates on bondspeople were 15 to 33 percent lower than those of other companies.[45] A comparison of North Carolina Mutual's premiums in 1849 with those of Franklin Slaughter's for the same year indicates differentials ranging from 7.8 to 20.7 percent lower. The directors made it clear in their annual report that this rate increase was an economic necessity and not a device to discourage slave owners from insuring their enslaved blacks with North Carolina Mutual: "Its [slave life insurance's] utility has thus far been recognized on all hands; and it is confidently predicted that the day is not far distant when this species of property will be almost universally under insurance."[46]

During the 1851–52 fiscal year, the board of directors continued to adjust its regulations regarding slave risks. Up to this point neither the bylaws nor the written insurance policies had included any statements refusing payment on claims for death owing to the slave owner's negligence. Such an oversight could have been very costly to the firm, so on September 6, 1851, the board voted to refuse claims on bondspeople who had died "from want of proper care during sickness, or from neglect in procuring proper medical attendance." Words to this effect were hereafter included in all policies.[47] A few months later the question arose as to whether the company would insure the lives of free blacks. The board voted unanimously to refuse "this class of risks," no doubt because of the reportedly high mortality rate of members of this usually impoverished and often sickly group.[48]

In June 1852 the directors decided to evaluate the success of their slave insurance program. They found that over the previous three years the company had received $18,206 in premiums and paid out $14,713 in claims on bondspeople. Profits, it was decided, were too small compared with the risks incurred, so another 15 percent rise in premiums was voted.[49] Thus, a slave owner who had paid $7.44 per year in 1849 to insure his twenty-year-old bondsman for $600 for one year, or $8.28 annually for five years, now, after two rate increases of approximately 15 percent each, had to pay $10.02 for one year, or $11.28 annually for five years (see Appendix, Table 3). For the remainder of the 1850s, premiums on slave insurance remained at the rates established in 1852. The premiums for whites never changed from 1849 to 1860.

Despite the increased cost of insuring the enslaved, owners and hirers continued to purchase policies in large numbers. In July 1856, the directors acknowledged in their annual report that "insurance on the lives of slaves . . . has become quite an important feature in the transactions of this Company."[50] An analysis of the number of policies issued on whites and enslaved people was not published until the 1856–57 annual report, but the total policies in force each year between 1854 and 1860 averaged about 2,200, and the racial breakdown remained constant for three of these years, at three black risks for each white risk (see Appendix, Table 2). During the same period the company paid claims on between two and four times as many bondspeople as whites, a further indication of the large number of slave policies being issued. Mortality rates, as mentioned earlier, were about equal for both groups. Because North Carolina Mutual took risks only up to two-thirds of a bondsperson's value, the total amount paid out for slave losses annually was smaller than the amount for whites. The average coverage for bondspeople (based on claims paid) rose from about $550 in the early 1850s to approximately $800 ten years later, a reflection of the rising purchase price of the enslaved during the last pre–Civil War decade. Whites usually insured themselves for about four or five times this amount (see Appendix, Table 3).

During the period of rapid company growth in the mid-1850s, as both white and slave claims began to increase, officials became concerned with the quality of medical examinations provided applicants. In 1854 the board discussed this matter at one of its regular meetings and recommended that insurance examinations "be conducted with the utmost care, and circumspection."[51] Death payments continued, however, to increase during the 1854–55 fiscal year (up over $14,500 from 1853–54) despite company warnings to examining physicians. The directors made their point even more explicit in the next annual report, stating "that the examinations of the applicants for insurance by our Examining Physicians are in many cases insufficient; that they suffer much to escape their attention, which a more thorough and searching investigation would reveal."[52] When white claims dropped some $8,200 during the ensuing year but claims on the enslaved rose, another strong statement from the board appeared and so did a change in policy. Referring to the decline in white claims, the directors expressed "their conviction that like benefits and advantages would follow the employment of the same caution and ability in the taking of applications for insurance on the lives of slaves." To encourage such "caution and ability" it was announced that thereafter the company would pay physicians a fee of one dollar for examining slaves. (This had increased to two dollars by 1858.) Prior to this, North Carolina Mutual had paid two dollars for whites but had refused to reimburse slave owners or doctors for medical examinations of bondspeople, a practice that had encouraged imperfect if not outright dishonest medical reports.[53]

The verbal message and financial incentive may have produced the desired effect, as during the next year (1856–57) claims on enslaved persons dropped from thirty-one to seventeen and profits on black policies rose from $2,013 to $8,034. Still, the board suspected duplicity on the part of a few agents and examining physicians in the field. Because some deaths "have been the result of chronic constitutional diseases," company officials believed that "sufficient care has not been taken . . . to exclude all unsound persons from the benefits of Insurance in this Office."[54] The results of this public exposure must have satisfied the directors, for nothing further on the subject appeared in minutes of board meetings or in annual reports.

Though available records do not contain information on the number of industrial bondspeople insured by North Carolina Mutual, they do indicate that this group provided the company with a significant amount of business. For instance, included with the table of premiums on bondspeople at the end of each annual report was a list of "extra rates of insurance on slaves." With experience, company officials learned that the risk on the enslaved employed on boats (steam, canal, fishing, pilot) or coasting was greater than for any other kind of work. Consequently, beginning in July 1854, North Carolina Mutual imposed a

2.5 percent surcharge on bondspeople so employed.[55] It was also discovered that slave laborers engaged in running a railroad incurred more dangers than those who did stationary railroad work such as grading and ditching. By 1855, the insurers of the former were being billed one-fourth percent more than the insurers of the latter, and in 1860 enslaved graders on the railroad from Rocky Mount to Tarboro, North Carolina, were entirely free of any extra premium.[56] Among other industrial slave laborers not subject to surcharges were shingle gatherers and turpentine workers.[57] A number of deaths each year occurred among what appear to be industrial slaves. Causes such as "drowning," "noxious gas in well," "accidents," "falling off embankment," "killed in a well," and "killed on Manchester Railroad" are indicative of the types of employment of some of these workers.[58] Extant insurance policies of enslaved laborers from several industrial concerns[59] and the appearance of business company names, such as James C. Sproull & Co., Boatwright & Miot, Freeman and Houston, and Dickenson, Grant & Gauze, in the list of claimants for slave losses further illustrate the importance of industrial slave insurance to North Carolina Mutual's business.

During the first eleven years of its existence, North Carolina Mutual grew and prospered. By 1860, the company had more than $190,000 on hand, compared with less than $90,000 only five years earlier. A dividend of 20 percent was declared, with the thought that similar dividends could be declared annually in the future.[60] But then civil war and economic chaos disrupted the directors' plan, and within six years, despite several attempts to save it, North Carolina Mutual was forced to cease operations and disband.[61] During its existence the company had insured more than 7,200 lives, half to two-thirds of whom were enslaved people, and had paid to slave owners more than $176,359 in compensation for the deaths of 265 bondspeople.[62] North Carolina Mutual was, until the outbreak of hostilities, part of a growing network of insurance companies that insured enslaved people's lives and thus provided a small measure of financial support for the South's "peculiar institution."

CHAPTER 10

The Georgia Freedmen's Bureau and the Organization of Health Care, 1865–66

> The mortality of the Negroes in and near large towns and cities still continues to be very great. The small-pox still rages among them. One colored carpenter in this city [Macon], who employs four hands, said . . . that it was as much as he and his men could do to make the coffins that were ordered from him.
>
> —*New York Times*, January 22, 1866

> I was sorry to hear that the small-pox had broken out in Athens. . . . [A]s for the Negroes I don't care how many of them have it—so they die. It is a real luxury now to know that they are shuffling off their thieving coils.
>
> —Martin J. Crawford to Mrs. Howell Cobb, November 3, 1865[1]

> For the present I do not regard it my duty to assume the charge of those cases of smallpox that may occur in the city—it is fully able to provide its own sanitary institutions, and support its own poor.
>
> —Dr. J. W. Lawton, surgeon-in-chief, Medical Department, Freedmen's Bureau, Georgia, to Dr. A. T. Augusta, assistant surgeon, Lincoln Hospital, Savannah, November 21, 1865[2]

Of all the functions and activities of the Bureau of Refugees, Freedmen, and Abandoned Lands (Freedmen's Bureau), provision of medical care should have been the least controversial. Bureau physicians did not enforce labor contracts, adjudicate disputes between former slaveholders and freed people, or teach black citizens to read, write, and calculate. They established and manned hospitals, dispensed drugs, and treated smallpox, cholera, and malaria. Their mandate was to facilitate for blacks the transition from free medical care provided by slave owners to self-care and to ease for whites the problems of providing such care to large numbers of indigent freed people during the unsettled immediate postwar period. Unfortunately, these ideals, conceived in Washington, D.C., were difficult to realize at the state and local levels. In organizing its operation, the Medical Department could not avoid entanglement in the bureau's political disputes with civil authorities and local white residents because it was an extension of that federal agency. Its presence and assistance was necessary, even welcomed, but it was also resented for intruding into local affairs. Moreover, some of the Medical Department's actions seemed calculated to advance political points rather than to help the sick and injured. In addition, bureau physicians encountered numerous bureaucratic and financial problems as they attempted to establish and maintain their facilities. The losers in all this disorganization and political manipulation during the bureau's first year of operation were sick freed people. They, at times, received poor medical care and ultimately failed to receive assistance in developing medical independence. This situation existed throughout the South. The following example of Georgia is only one of many.[3]

When Gen. William T. Sherman departed Savannah in January 1865 to commence his march northward, the war in Georgia was unofficially at an end. Gov. Joseph E. Brown remained in office until April, however, presiding over the affairs of state as though military defeat and massive property destruction had not demoralized and disrupted the lives of most Georgians. This dislocation was most apparent in the cities and large towns where former slaves—hundreds and thousands of them who had trailed behind Sherman's forces through the state—now remained in expectation of something, though they knew not what. Blacks also began swelling the populations of towns more remote from the path of the Union invaders, especially in the weeks after the official surrender of Georgia to Gen. James H. Wilson in April. With housing, food, and clothing quite scarce even for whites, newly freed African Americans experienced extreme hardships through the cold winter and wet spring months. During the transitional period, when state and local governments were bankrupt or unwilling to expend their meager resources on "renegade" blacks, and when the Union occupation forces made little provision for the care or governance of camp followers and migrants, the state of health of freed people declined in short order.[4] The Medical Department of the Freedmen's Bureau soon undertook the task of providing necessary care for these people.

On March 3, 1865, Congress passed the Freedmen's Bureau Bill and sent it to the White House for President Lincoln's signature. Gen. O. O. Howard, chosen to organize and administer the new agency, had served under Sherman during his march to the sea and had seen destitution and disease firsthand among the freed people and white refugees.[5] Recognizing the need for a medical department, though not specifically authorized to create one, Howard soon "found it necessary to . . . extend medical aid as far as practicable to refugees and freedmen who became sick and were unprovided for by any local supply from a private source."[6] In the spring, Howard began by appointing surgeon Caleb W. Horner as chief medical officer of the bureau. During the summer, Horner chose military physicians to serve as surgeons-in-chief of the various states under bureau jurisdiction. By late September, the Medical Department was prepared to begin rendering assistance on the local level.

The spring and summer months of 1865 were dismal ones for those black citizens of Georgia who expected that the end of the war and the achievement of freedom would bring happy and prosperous times. Brig. Gen. Rufus Saxton, assistant commissioner of the Freedmen's Bureau for South Carolina, Georgia, and Florida from June to September 1865, betrayed his partiality for the South Carolina Sea Islands by assigning only three agents for the remainder of that state and two agents for all of Georgia.[7] Gen. Edward A. Wild, Saxton's assistant commissioner in Georgia, appeared to be more concerned with abandoned lands than with refugees or the 465,000 freed people. In August, an inspector general of the Department of Georgia discovered Wild near the town of Washington torturing members of the Chenault family to discover where they had hidden large amounts of gold rumored to be in their possession. This sort of neglect and mistreatment did little to relieve the multitudes of freed people and refugees congregated in crude shelters in Macon, Atlanta, Savannah, Augusta, and elsewhere. The congested quarters and unsanitary conditions in those places had caused much sickness and suffering during the warm season, complicated as the summer turned to autumn by an epidemic outbreak of smallpox. General Wild was dismissed from the bureau on September 2, 1865, leaving Georgia with no assistant commissioner until the arrival of Gen. Davis Tillson late in the month.[8]

On the day that General Wild left his office in Augusta, surgeon John W. Lawton reported for duty as surgeon-in-chief of the bureau for the district of Georgia. Lawton, former chief medical officer of the 100th Ohio Volunteers during the Atlanta campaign, had been appointed by Dr. Horner to this new position on July 24, less than a month after his regiment had been mustered out of service.[9] Upon assuming the duties of surgeon-in-chief, Lawton received instructions from Horner to "ascertain the number of persons in the district entitled to the benefit of this bureau requiring medical attendance . . . , recommend the establishment of hospitals . . . and designate . . . medical officers and attendants" in the various parts of the state.[10] In addition to these tasks, Lawton faced such problems as racial prejudice, lack of financial support from those groups receiving medical care, uncooperative local officials, a poor supply system, and a major smallpox epidemic.

Lawton's first task was to hire physicians to care for the sick in the major cities of the state. He found two readily accessible sources of capable medical practitioners with whom he could contract for services—army surgeons recently mustered out of the military or willing to transfer their commissions to the Freedmen's Bureau and established physicians already residing in towns requiring bureau assistance. Upon his arrival in Augusta, Lawton discovered that the contracting of physicians was a joint procedure that required the approval of both the district surgeon-in-chief (himself) and the assistant commissioner. As General Wild was no longer in charge of the bureau, and since his replacement had not yet been designated, Lawton could make no contracts with physicians.[11] On September 17, he wrote a note to Horner in order to "call your immediate attention to the need of med. officers in this Dist." Explaining that he could presently hire no contract physicians, Lawton requested that army doctors be temporarily detailed to the Georgia district, "for I frequently get letters from various points calling attention to the demand for aid for the poor white & colored people, and I cannot help them."[12]

Lawton was not entirely without staff at this time. C. H. Taylor, a black assistant surgeon in the U.S. Army, had been commissioned to serve in the Freedmen's Bureau on August 19 and assigned to duty at the Lincoln Hospital for Freedmen and Refugees in Savannah on September 3.[13] In addition, J. V. DeHanne, assistant surgeon, U.S. Volunteers, had been appointed to serve in Georgia at the same time as John Lawton.[14] Taylor, however, did not report for duty until September 19, nor DeHanne until the end of September, leaving Lawton with only a staff on paper for several weeks. Once the new assistant commissioner finally arrived in late September, staffing of the Medical Department proceeded smoothly. On September 23, General Saxton ordered Alexander T. Augusta, a black physician educated in Canada and serving as surgeon with the First U.S. Colored Troops, to report to Lawton, where he was placed in charge of Lincoln Hospital.[15] On October 1, Dr. DeHanne was ordered to establish a freedmen's hospital in Augusta with a special smallpox ward under the care of Acting Assistant Surgeon M. J. Jones, U.S. Volunteers.[16] The first two Southern civilian physicians to be commissioned with the bureau's Medical Department were L. Carter and Joseph R. Bettison, assigned to operate a freedmen's hospital and smallpox ward in Macon. These and all other full-time commissioned medical officers of the bureau were compensated for their services at the rate of one hundred dollars per month, with the exception of Lawton, who received two hundred dollars monthly.[17]

Though the arrival of Gen. Davis Tillson, the new assistant commissioner, solved Lawton's hiring dilemma, it also raised a new issue that exposed a slight difference in the philosophies of the two men. Shortly after taking charge of the bureau, Tillson inaugurated the policy of designating local persons in the various towns and counties as bureau agents without pay and authorizing them to collect a small fee from the parties with whom they dealt on official business. Lawton, however, was wary of placing white Southerners in the Medical Department. "I want a few good Medical officers to take charge of Hospitals at different points in the state . . . and prefer Northern men," he wrote to a prospective employee in Illinois.[18] The issue appears to have never become critical; a combination of Northern and Georgia medical officers was hired.

Lawton received a number of requests for job information from Northern physicians, predominantly from former army staff surgeons.[19] Their motives for seeking such employment in the destitute and often unfriendly South were not usually revealed in their letters, though the steady income of one hundred dollars per month would presumably have been an inducement. Some who had been mustered out desired to remain in the military and considered the Freedmen's Bureau an acceptable alternative to active duty. Lawton discouraged physicians who applied with this idea in mind: "I do not disguise from you the fact of some unpleasant circumstances accompanying this service as we can not have the discipline and control of men as in the army—but a person of good executive ability can make a good Hospital, pleasing himself and satisfying the demands of the Med Dept of the Bureau."[20] Others wanted to come South for the purpose of nursing black men, women, and children back to health. Dr. Augusta and Dr. Louis Masson, "a French Surgeon who served during the four years of the war in the U.S. Army and who desires now to direct his special studies on the colored populations of the South," were of this mind.[21]

Whether physicians came for altruistic, financial, or other reasons, or merely out of a sense of adventure, they did not seem to be deterred by the dangers of endemic and epidemic diseases in this region. Not all who were offered contracts came to Georgia, presumably because they preferred to practice elsewhere or because of a change of heart. A letter such as the one Lawton sent to Dr. Masson, written as the surgeon-in-chief was attempting to hire a predominantly Northern staff, might have given those applicants second thoughts: "If you come, I would like you to come *at once*, and write me how soon you can come. Don't bring much baggage." (Dr. Masson did not come.)[22]

Southern civilian physicians offered their services to Lawton for many of the same reasons as their Northern counterparts—altruism, financial need, and spirit of adventure. But they also had more to risk, both personally and professionally, than did Northerners. Personally, these men incurred the animus of local residents firmly opposed to the incursion of the Freedmen's Bureau into their communities. Professionally, the health of their towns was at stake: to leave one portion of the population untreated was to risk the spread of disease to white and black residents alike. Some of these physicians may have been Union men during the war and were therefore eager to display their loyalty to those now in command. Caring for people's health problems compelled some to transcend politics and personal prejudice, if for no other reason than lives were in danger. Lawton found several local civilian medical men ready and willing to aid the Freedmen's Bureau in its work.

Of the five hospitals established in Georgia by the Freedmen's Bureau, three were administered initially by local physicians. A French physician, Noel D'Alvigny, who had been a resident of Atlanta for more than twelve years, curator of the Atlanta Medical College museum, and director of a Confederate hospital in Atlanta during the war, was placed in charge of the freedmen's hospital in that city. D'Alvigny had established a reputation for quick thinking and bravery during Sherman's occupation of Atlanta by outwitting the Union troops who had come to burn the Medical College building before departing the city. He had signed a contract with the U.S. government to treat the sick and wounded during the occupation and therefore came to the Freedmen's Bureau highly recommended by Dr. H. H. Buck, the U.S. Army post surgeon in Atlanta.[23] In Columbus, on the Georgia-Alabama border, Dr. T. S. Tuggle, a local resident recommended by subassistant commissioner Capt. P. Slaughter, was commissioned as a medical officer in charge of the freedmen's hospital. He, like D'Alvigny, had been employed by U.S. authorities during the occupation.[24] Drs. Carter and Bettison of Macon have already been mentioned. Bettison, a surgeon in the Confederate army during the war, had been held prisoner in Washington, D.C., for a period of time in 1863 and then released.[25]

All employees of the bureau were required to take an oath stating that they had never borne arms or given aid and counsel to the Confederate cause during the Civil War. Though a few Georgia physicians could sign this oath in all honesty, most could not. Several times during the three years and three months that the Medical Department functioned in Georgia, Washington officials attempted to force the issue and require all physicians to sign the oath. Dr. Carter refused to sign, explaining that he was as loyal to the U.S. government "as any man" but must "respectfully decline to take . . . the oath laid down . . . as I would commit the crime of Perjury were I to take it."[26]

The medical needs of the freed people and white refugees often required the extended and intensive care that only a hospital setting could provide. In addition, such infirmaries could serve as headquarters for whatever dispensary (outpatient) operations the bureau medical officers found time to provide. With these necessities in mind, Lawton and his staff immediately set about the task of acquiring suitable facilities in Augusta, Savannah, Macon, Atlanta, and Columbus.

In Augusta, home office of the bureau Medical Department, the surgeon-in-chief noted that "the buildings used at present for Hospital purposes [by the freedmen are] . . . in a wretched condition, and utterly unfit for the purpose" of providing adequate medical care. The buildings hardly shielded patients from the elements and contained no cooking facilities, forcing the staff to prepare meals outside over open fires. Lawton combed the city after his arrival in early September and soon fixed upon a group of unoccupied buildings known as "Darkie" Hospital, "built . . . by the Rebels."[27] Maj. Gen. James B. Steedman, military commander of Georgia, had previously assigned this property to General Wild for use by the Freedmen's Bureau as a school or hospital, so Lawton now politely demanded and received title to the buildings.[28] Two days later, Drs. DeHanne and Jones arrived in Augusta to assume their duties at the newly opened facility.

The bureau's task in Savannah was simplified by the fact that a freedmen's hospital already existed—a result of government activities during the occupation. Smallpox and other diseases had followed the many freed people who packed into Savannah in the wake of Sherman's army, and authorities had been forced to establish the Lincoln Hospital in town and the Tybee Light Quarantine Vessel off Tybee Island at the mouth of the Savannah River. Dr. Richard Arnold, a physician of national repute and mayor of Savannah, had worked closely with local and military physicians during this period to care for the sick of both races. In late September, the Medical Department inherited the Lincoln Freedmen's Hospital and the responsibility of treating the multitude of unhealthy freed people and refugees still congregated in Savannah. By October 1, Dr. Augusta, the medical officer in charge of Lincoln Hospital, had been transferred into the service of the Freedmen's Bureau.[29]

Drs. Carter and Bettison experienced little difficulty in establishing a freedmen's hospital at Macon, though it was small (fifty beds) and located in a swampy section of town. Prior to the installation of the bureau hospital at Macon, the military district's surgeon-in-chief informed General Wild of "the condition of the poor whites and blacks in Macon & vicinity needing medical care." The city authorities apparently soon undertook the responsibility of caring for many of its white and black citizens, as well as for several U.S. soldiers, all stricken with smallpox, until the freedmen's hospital could be opened in October.[30] This type of cooperation between the town and the bureau was not always so freely given.

In Columbus, Dr. Tuggle was able to acquire and convert a suitable house into a hospital but was delayed until November from opening the facility because of a lack of medical supplies. The Freedmen's Bureau agent, Captain Slaughter, had reported in October that there were many sick and needy refugees and freed people in the area, but no funds or supplies with which to aid them. He had, in fact, "given a poor (col[ored]) woman three very sick persons to care for and have promised to see her paid for her trouble, but as no funds are here and no way to get it I am at a loss to know what to do." The establishment of a hospital and medical branch office in Columbus was a welcome relief to this harried agent.[31]

It was not until December that Dr. D'Alvigny was able to establish in Atlanta any sort of permanent shelter entitled to the name "hospital." A small number of freed people had been fortunate enough to receive medical treatment "in the [military] post hospital by the kindness of Dr. Buck in charge" prior to the opening of the bureau's facility, but the majority of the sick were treated by D'Alvigny "at their shanties, in their tents scattered about town, & . . . [at] the *Contraband Camp*." In late October, he and Colonel Curkendall, the local bureau agent, located a building in which to house a temporary hospital, but the project to convert the structure into a useable infirmary was delayed for more than a month.[32] D'Alvigny fumed in a letter to Lawton, "Col'n Curkendall . . . probably described [to you] the still unfinished shanty called Hospital where my patients are cramped up in the Medical College yard, and also close by my Small Pox Comp[ound] where I ought to have at least three Tents more."[33] Not until late in February 1866 was D'Alvigny even partially mollified by the establishment of a separate smallpox hospital on the outskirts of town for the exclusive use of the freed people.[34] He could finally, on March 9, write to Lawton, "Everything is going Smooth here"—his first letter without a complaint since assuming the position of medical officer in the bureau.[35]

The very heart of Lawton's mission in Georgia was, of course, the treatment of unhealthy freed people and refugees. It was imperative, therefore, that his physicians be well supplied with drugs and medications; his hospitals with sufficient beds, medical implements, and miscellaneous equipment; and his pantries and storage bins with adequate stocks of rations and clothing. This emerged as a most challenging task, for the ways of medical purveyors, quartermasters, and treasury agents were unfathomable. The sick refugees and freed people of Georgia suffered most from the resultant mistakes and delays.

One reason for the confusion was the poor organization of the "centralized" supply system under which the Medical Department was forced to operate. The nearest War Department medical purveyor's office was at Hilton Head, South Carolina, a short distance up the coast from Savannah. This office supplied certain provisions needed by the medical officers in Georgia, but not many of the drugs, medicines, and medical equipment—items that were usually handled by the Nashville, and occasionally, St. Louis offices. Thus, while the purveyor at Hilton Head furnished the general anesthesia ("brandy instead of whiskey will be issued during the coming quarter"), his counterpart in Nashville equipped physicians with lithotomy and optical instruments used to perform the surgery.[36] The paperwork involved was tremendous, as all requisitions had to be made in triplicate and quarterly reports compiled for the chief medical officer of the bureau in Washington. Lawton's office served as a clearinghouse for all requisitions; he had to approve them and then send copies to the correct purveyor's office and to Washington. After six months of complaints from his physicians in the field, Lawton suggested to Dr. Horner in Washington that a depot for medical and hospital supplies be established in each state. Horner tersely replied, "The Commissioner decides that it is inexpedient, *at present*, to modify" the current system.[37]

If the system frustrated and upset Lawton, it positively exasperated and infuriated most of the local medical officers. Dr. Carter, who had ordered provisions for the Macon freedmen's hospital in early or mid-October 1865, finally reported to Lawton on November 24, "Supplies of Medicines have arrived from Nashville and our Hospital is dispensing its favors on all who have applied for admittance to it."[38] Another physician, employed on April 30, 1866, to locate a temporary medical dispensary at St. Marys, near the Georgia-Florida border, ultimately borrowed medicines and drugs from physicians in the area because he had still not received his supplies from the medical purveyor three months after placing the order. On July 27, the quartermaster's office at the military post in Savannah informed Lawton that the supplies intended for St. Marys had been mismarked and sent to Darien, Georgia.[39] Dr. Tuggle, who had postponed the opening of his hospital in Columbus the previous fall in part because the supplies had arrived late, reported to Lawton, in January 1866, that the situation had not improved much: "I must again call your attention to the difficulties experienced by me in procuring the necessary supplies to carry on the hospital successfully. I cannot get even a wash pot though repeatedly applied for. I have been obliged to fell the shade trees around the building to procure fuel, and the rations supplied are insufficient."[40] The nettled and unlucky Dr. D'Alvigny, writing to Lawton from Atlanta on January 8, told an even darker story:

> Many of my patients . . . died from the Want of comfort and clothes: Some of them entirely Naked. Last week the weather was very inclement . . . at which time I was not able to be Supplied with wood and five of my patients died from sudden chills. . . .
>
> I have not been able to give my female patients a change, even of chemise, since they are under me. Some are now laying all the time in Bed from want of covering their Frames. Notwithstanding repeated requisitions [for supplies] made by me.[41]

Tuggle described to Lawton, on January 1, 1866, another reason for his impatience with the purveyor's offices and the supply system: "The smallpox is becoming prevalent in and around the city and the vaccine matter furnished me is totally inert, not one of the patients vaccinated has exhibited symptoms of its taking. This is a serious matter and I therefore beg you to forward me by mail, some reliable matter immediately."[42] And Dr. Carter's graphic description of the overcrowded conditions at his hospital in Macon reinforced the need for a better supply system: "You seem to think that the Report of [111 patients] . . . and only 50 Beds is an error. That report is litterally [*sic*] correct. . . . Some beds are occupied by three persons where they are Small in size[,] Larger [patients] two to a bed[.] Some patients had no bed but had to ly [*sic*] on a pallet or do the best they could[.]"[43] Perhaps Lawton's decentralized supply scheme would also have met with numerous snags had it been adopted, but it might have avoided some of the lamentable situations that directly affected the sick freed people and refugees.

Lawton and his staff were not entirely at the mercy of the cumbersome government supply system, however, and were more than willing to take advantage of any opportunities to bypass it. Within three weeks of his arrival at headquarters in Augusta, Lawton had already requested aid from Henry W. Bellows, president of the U.S. Sanitary Commission in New York. Though Lawton's request arrived too late for Bellows to ship supplies directly to Georgia—"We have already made over to Gen. Howard at Washington, all the Supplies suited to Freedmen's wants, left on our hands at the conclusion of our labors . . . on October 1"—some Sanitary Commission stores did eventually find their way into the state.[44] Such Northern benevolent groups as the Christian Society of Ohio, which several times eased Dr. D'Alvigny's ill humor by furnishing freed people with old clothes, were often of more immediate value to local medical officers than some national aid associations.[45]

The bureau's Medical Department also profited from its close ties to the military occupation forces. When medical provisions were scarce, the medical officers fully exploited the rule fixed by the surgeon general in Washington authorizing transfer of "the surplus Medical Property of Post Hospitals" to the Freedmen's Bureau.[46] In addition to surplus medical supplies, the surgeon general also permitted, as of February 1866, "transfer to the Medical Officers of the Bureau . . . , without charge, [of] all captured Medical Property found in Rebel Hospitals in Georgia." Within a month this material had been distributed to the local medical officers.[47] Another method of bypassing the government system was to grow some of the needed food on the hospital grounds.[48] This program actually originated in Washington with Dr. Horner, probably as an economy measure. All medical officers obtained land suitable for use as gardens,[49] though some later abandoned this project for various reasons.[50]

Immediately upon finding themselves free from the bonds of slavery, some blacks adopted an attitude of extreme independence, summed up in a phrase repeated by the bitter and defensive Dr. Richard Arnold of Savannah in an October 1866 letter: "The mortality [from cholera] is certainly great among the Blacks, but I am satisfied that [that] belongs to their new status of being 'nobody's niggers but their own.'" His cook, Arnold continued, had assumed that philosophy prior to her sudden attack of cholera, and now Arnold took great pleasure in repeating how Mrs. Arnold had "boldly nursed her as if she had been her slave, instead of being 'nobodys nigger but her own.'"[51] African Americans in other parts of the state were willing to go without medical attention as a means of demonstrating their newly gained independence to each other and their former masters. This was a dangerous practice during a smallpox epidemic when the potential victims included entire communities. At Athens, seat of the University of Georgia, the white population was understandably concerned in late January 1866 when some freed people avoided contact with local physicians during a smallpox epidemic. Judge R. S. Taylor of the Cooke County Inferior Court asked Asst. Comm. Davis Tillson to take firm action on the matter: "At Cooke armory the disease has been more fatal, because, they [the freedmen] refused any attention from the Doctor saying they would manage their own affairs. I would suggest that you would compell them through the agent of the Bureau at this place to go to the Hospital. I think by this means that the disease would soon be arrested. We have done our part in attending the wants of these unfortunate and ignorant people."[52] Only a small minority of freed people in Georgia adopted this unrealistic medical "self-help" attitude. Most were more than willing to consult bureau or local physicians when a serious health problem arose.

Black citizens did work with the Freedmen's Bureau on matters of public health through benevolent associations. Even before the Medical Department of the bureau had been extended into Georgia, at the suggestion of the assistant commissioner a group of African Americans in Augusta formed a freedmen's aid society, which provided medical care for the black population of the city. The funds raised supported a hospital, a physician, a black midwife, and a lying-in ward.[53] When the bureau's Medical Department replaced this local medical program in the fall of 1865, the Colored Benevolent Society pledged seventy-five to one hundred dollars per month in support of the Freedmen's Hospital Fund.[54] Though the Medical Department received funds from the War Department, freed people were encouraged to assist by giving what they could to the Freedmen's Hospital Fund in the major cities of Georgia. These funds were used to hire additional attendants and for other expenditures.

When the Colored Benevolent Society of Savannah was unable to raise as much money as its counterparts elsewhere, Dr. Augusta, himself black, was angered by what he interpreted as freed people's apparent lack of interest in their own welfare. He wrote to Lawton of this situation and his plan to remedy it on December 3, 1865:

> We have been doing all we could to get the Colored Churches to contribute towards the support of the Hospital, but it seems impossible to depend on them any longer; in fact, if we had to depend on them alone for the time the Hospital has been under the Bureau, we should have had to stop operations long since.
>
> The whole amount subscribed by them up to the present time is $487.30. . . .
>
> I have suggested to the Pastors of the different Churches to hold a Union meeting of all the Churches, to lay before them the claims of the

Hospital, as well as to make a report to them of all the money they have contributed and the number of Colored people that has been treated in Hospital, during the time.[55]

Apparently Augusta's appeal was successful enough to sustain the hospital through the winter and spring months, as he filed no further complaints about the matter with Lawton.

Dr. D'Alvigny, seemingly always harried, reported on October 28, 1865, that he had "not yet found the Benevolent Society" in Atlanta, and on November 26 that he had located it but had only received about thirty dollars for support of the hospital. By January, these contributions had terminated entirely. After this inauspicious beginning, however, the society undertook to hire and support nine nurses at the freedmen's hospital. Unfortunately, this commitment required more funds than the association's limited resources could contribute over an extended period of time. In April they reduced their obligation to that of merely supplementing the government allowance so that D'Alvigny could "keep a set of nurses who will perform for good wages" at the smallpox hospital. The leaders of the society sent an apologetic note to the doctor explaining their situation and praying for continued aid from the Freedmen's Bureau: "Enny thing that we can do for them [the nurses] here shall be don by us and what the Government will do let it do for we are verry much in nead of healp."[56]

Doctors Tuggle and Carter were unable to raise any funds among the freed people of their communities. In fact, Tuggle reported that he frequently had to pay incidental expenses out of his own pocket: "The colored population of this place evince no disposition to assist us with either money, clothes or delicacies for the sick. All those things are needed to carry on the hospital creditably and advantageously."[57]

The differing responses of African Americans to the medical needs of their communities reflected many factors, including the personalities and public images of the individual medical officers and the leadership within local black societies. In addition, the city of Augusta, relatively wealthy and almost untouched by the invading armies, supported a black population that might have been better able to contribute supplies, funds, and time to the hospital than were the freed people of Atlanta, Savannah, Columbus, or Macon. The fact that Savannah's and Atlanta's black communities accomplished as much as they did is remarkable considering the adverse conditions under which they labored.

One of the most delicate and troublesome issues facing the bureau's medical staff concerned the amount of responsibility city authorities were willing to assume in the health care of freed people. At bottom, the arguments between city and bureau reflected the differing conceptions each had of the ultimate role of the agency in Georgia. Lawton and his successors assumed that the freed people were the South's problem and that the bureau was there only temporarily, to assist during a period of readjustment. His officers rendered medical services to African Americans while civilian physicians and public health authorities recovered from the dislocations caused by the war. Lawton therefore resisted attempts by cities to send all freed people to bureau hospitals for treatment; the cities, he believed, had to accept more and more responsibility for their own infirm, be they black or white. On this matter, he and Assistant Commissioner Tillson shared similar views. Both preferred dispensaries, "where poor colored people can come to be examined gratuitously, and charge[d] a small amount for medicines," to hospitals, which they felt should be run by municipal health officers. Both men anticipated an early "discontinuance of medical aid" to the state of Georgia.[58] The municipal health officers, alternatively, found it impossible to handle the increased patient loads resulting from the migration of rural freed people to the cities. The cost to the cities of caring for the large numbers of newly arrived black citizens was more than their already strained resources could bear.[59] When smallpox erupted in Savannah in November 1865, the medical crisis was soon transformed into a political confrontation.

The rapidly rising incidence of smallpox among the city's freed people during the early part of the month (twenty-five patients in the hospital with two to three new cases arriving each day) caused terrible overcrowding at the temporary smallpox hospital located on a plantation outside of town. Bureau physicians Augusta and Jones soon found it difficult to provide adequate care to patients both at the regular freedmen's hospital in town and at the smallpox facility. Furthermore, in mid-November, the owner of the property upon which the smallpox hospital sat received his pardon from the government and applied for the restoration of his land. Then, on November 21, Dr. Jones's contract was terminated, owing to his failure to take the amnesty oath, leaving Dr. Augusta with no assistant physician, a poorly functioning staff, and two hospitals filled with seriously ill patients.[60]

Augusta appealed to Lawton on November 17 for permission to establish a new and permanent pest house (smallpox isolation hospital) somewhere in or around Savannah and to hire a replacement for Dr. Jones. He also apprised Col. H. F. Sickles, subassistant commissioner of the local bureau office, of the situation. Sickles immediately took up Augusta's cause by echoing his request to Lawton, but in more emphatic terms: "For God sake. If there are any devisable means within your power, or principality, or heighth or depth, or any other means! whereby any additional assistance can be had for our Hospital in the way of contract Surgeons or otherwise, It will be a great and phylanthropic enterprize—If executed!"[61] Instead of agreeing, however, Lawton sent Augusta a lengthy communication defining his understanding of the Medical Department's role in Georgia:

> For the present I do not regard it my duty to assume the charge of those cases of smallpox that may occur in the city—it is fully able to provide its own sanitary institutions, and support its own poor. If the result of the war has been to throw an extra burden upon cities South by the freedom of these millions of slaves, they must meet it. The time *must* come when the United States Government will withdraw from the care of the Freedmen and force their care upon local (Town or County) Authorities. This may as well be done, if possible, now as months or years hence, and the aid of the Bureau is to be rendered only until the [city] authorities can make proper provision. . . . I cannot help thinking that as long as we will do for them, the [city] authorities will be quite willing to allow it. While the Smallpox is limited, the city can provide.

Augusta was to refuse all but a few smallpox patients. The bureau's proper province was "the care of the Aged, infirm and Orphans who have no one to care for them and those *sick*, who have gathered in the city from other places." Lawton believed that with the bureau's refusal to provide assistance, "the city will be forced to provide for these cases, or let the disease run riot in the city—a choice to which they are welcome and the results also." He therefore refused to commission another physician to work with Dr. Augusta: "Let the city hire the physician you mention, to care for the unfortunate ones." To ensure uniformity in the enforcement of these rules, the surgeon-in-chief sent similar letters to his medical officers in other Georgia cities; to inform his superiors of these directives and obtain their approval he sent a copy of the letter to Dr. Horner in Washington.[62]

The result of this confrontation was that on December 28, after much angry negotiation, all smallpox patients who had been citizens of Savannah prior to Sherman's occupation were treated at the city's pest house, while stricken nonresidents were sent to the bureau's new pest house at Thunderbolt, six miles from town. Lawton, discovering that the commissioner in Washington agreed with his philosophy but not with his coercive methods, approved of the Savannah settlement and hired a physician to fill the vacancy at the smallpox pest house.[63]

Lawton's directive stood as the guiding principle of the Georgia Freedmen's Bureau's Medical Department during its three-year existence. Implicit in Lawton's statement was the assumption that white Southerners would attempt to avoid caring for blacks whenever possible. Sometimes that suspicion seems to have been well founded, as when Dr. Carter reported that Macon authorities were sending black smallpox victims from the city hospital to the bureau's pest house and instructing them to say that they were from the country. Carter refused to admit another person until prospective patients provided proof as to residence. A similar incident occurred in Atlanta. Further negotiations regarding jurisdiction and care of freed people's health needs continued to take place in these cities until the bureau's Medical Department curtailed and then ceased operations in late 1868 and early 1869.[64] When bureau physicians enforced rules this strictly, and when city authorities refused to care for freed people as well, black citizens' health took second place to the principles for which each disputant stood.

Political considerations also dictated the Medical Department's response to calls for medical assistance from rural Georgia. One major goal of the Freedmen's Bureau throughout the South was resumption of normal agricultural pursuits, the usual occupation of most African Americans prior to Emancipation. As freed people returned to plantations and farms from the cities, and as they signed labor contracts that sometimes specifically excluded medical care coverage, the needs of rural blacks increased. Those rural freed people who suffered from chronic ailments or who were too old to support themselves also required outside assistance, as they were no longer being cared for by former owners.[65] The centralized urban system of medical care under which the Medical Department was operating could not possibly serve all or even most of Georgia's former slaves.

It is here that confusion of bureau goals becomes most apparent. The Medical Department offered hospital and dispensary care to Georgia's urban blacks, but it offered rural freed people (who were obeying bureau directives by signing labor contracts and engaging in agricultural work) little in the way of regular medical care. Consistent with the policy of self-help, Lawton (and his successors) preferred to supplement local practitioners with material aid rather than establish an official medical post with a hospital and full-time medical officer. The bureau did establish several dispensaries outside the five larger cities, but only for short periods of time and only after local agents, doctors, white residents, and even, in one or two instances, freed people pleaded for help.[66] Chronically ill and aged freed people were transported to one of the five major hospitals. The general response from bureau headquarters to calls for assistance from outlying areas, however, was usually either to send a small supply of medical stores to a local physician or the regular bureau agent (not a medical officer), with the admonition that this should not be expected in the future, or to refuse aid, explaining that this was a matter for county or town authorities.[67] Thus, though the bureau pressed rural public officials to care for their own freed people, rural authorities did not receive as direct, regular, reliable material assistance from the bureau as did urban areas. Officials of the bureau seemed to believe that the paternalistic health care system that had existed in rural Georgia during slavery times still existed. Again, freed people were the losers, owing to unresolved political differences between the Freedmen's Bureau and local authorities.

Politics even affected the physicians who willingly treated blacks in rural Georgia. For example, Dr. Couch of Newton, near Albany, lost much of his regular medical practice after the war because he cared for so many African Americans and favored federal Reconstruction policies.[68] Dr. Head of Americus won such favor among local freed people that they petitioned the bureau for a dispensary with him in charge. The bureau agent in Americus, however, believed that whites were more interested in obtaining the dispensary to reduce their own tax burden than to improve the health of blacks.[69] One final example comes from Albany, where the bureau dispensary's physician, a Northerner named Dalton, reported that freed people were afraid to trust the local physicians but were also afraid to send for him (Dalton) because whites discouraged them from attending his clinic.[70]

The Medical Department of the Freedmen's Bureau came to Georgia expecting to aid newly emancipated blacks until they could help themselves or until local governments were willing and able to provide such assistance. These turned out to be elusive goals. Thousands of formerly enslaved people received medical attention, especially those who were citizens of, or migrants to, the five major cities in the state. Virtually all the freed people of areas served by the Medical Department were entitled to free vaccinations against smallpox, and many actually received them.[71] The medical officers administered diagnostic physical examinations to those who appeared at their dispensaries with complaints. Drugs were made available at nominal fees. People requiring special treatment were placed in bureau hospitals and not asked to pay a fee. Though many freed people received aid, others who should have did not, owing to bureau policies and white Georgians' recalcitrance. Granted, the state of medicine just after the Civil War was not much improved over antebellum practices. The germ theory of disease had not yet been developed, so patient mortality from infections was usually quite high, especially in hospitals. What is being questioned here is not, however, the scientific attitude of bureau physicians toward disease, but the racial attitude consciously or unconsciously exhibited by those directly and indirectly responsible for care of the freed people. Lawton himself is a prime example. His refusal to hire another physician for the Savannah freed people and his order to close all the hospitals to large numbers of smallpox victims simply to force a political issue seem selfish and shortsighted decisions. He allowed an admitted and emotional dislike of Southerners to overrule what should have been a rational decision in a time of crisis. Lawton appears to have lost sight of the fact that he was dealing with people's lives. Had the situation been different, had hundreds of whites been under the care of the bureau, would Lawton have closed the hospitals? This question cannot, of course, be answered with any surety, but the harshness of his actions during the confrontations with city authorities raises doubts about his commitment to the well-being of freed people. It is also curious that Lawton did not apply pressure to the Atlanta city authorities when they refused to aid D'Alvigny in his efforts to build an adequate hospital as winter approached.[72] Furthermore, how could it be expected that one or two physicians in each city could adequately treat hundreds of freed people each week; train unskilled, inexperienced hospital attendants; write innumerable reports and requisitions; raise funds among the local citizenry; and attend to other spontaneous, miscellaneous problems as they arose? The Medical Department developed no basic programs of self-help upon which freed people could build, mounted no health education campaigns among blacks or whites, and trained no black or white physicians or medical assistants. There was no overall plan, no blueprint. The bureau did not attempt to introduce a system that could have ensured permanently adequate medical care for blacks. It simply filled a temporary gap, providing, in some cases, the same direct care for freed people that they had received when enslaved, and, in other cases, offering indirect care by sending supplies. The bureau only sought to continue its health care work until it could coerce or persuade local authorities to take responsibility for the freed people in their areas. These humanitarian activities were admirable and useful but did not go far enough.

The medical system that the Freedmen's Bureau favored encouraged white public officials to care for blacks only in compliance with bureau demands or in their own self-interest when smallpox or cholera threatened the entire population. It taught African Americans in areas where the bureau's Medical Department was active to expect free or low-cost medical care on application. Once the bureau was gone, however, freed people had no system of health care upon which to rely. Hospitals and dispensaries were left in the hands of white officials and white doctors. Freed people remained as dependent on the largess of whites as they had as slaves before the Civil War.[73]

African American Medical Schools

CHAPTER 11

The Rise and Decline of African American Medical Schools

Introduction

Freedom—the emancipation of 4 million enslaved people during and after the Civil War—altered the relationships among Southerners of both races and shifted some responsibilities to a group that had had, ostensibly at least, little experience in coping with such concerns. Medical care became a particularly difficult problem, as African Americans had developed no organized system of dealing with health problems during the era of slavery. Individual farms, plantations, or rural neighborhoods had spawned a few persons of color who gained recognition as skilled midwives, nurses, healers, or root doctors. But the enslaved usually could not turn openly to their own people for medical care with owners and the Euro-American medical world looking over their shoulders. (See Chapter 7.)

Emancipation suddenly released blacks from the necessity of looking to whites for medical care. But freedom also often excluded them from the white medicine to which many had grown accustomed. Physicians had to be paid, and local government authorities frequently took their time in establishing mechanisms whereby public funds could be used to care for sick poor black citizens. As discussed in Chapter 10, this situation prevailed despite efforts of federal agents of the Bureau of Refugees, Freedmen, and Abandoned Lands (the Freedmen's Bureau) both in establishing public hospitals and in encouraging towns and counties to care for all their indigent or helpless citizens. With the departure of the bureau in the late 1860s and early 1870s, blacks again lost any assurance they once had of receiving regular medical assistance from white physicians in time of need. White physicians did take African American patients, often at no charge. But they could not provide extensive free care and remain in practice. Black patients had now to insinuate themselves into a private enterprise medical care system from which they had been previously excluded. Most freed people could not pay for every ailment requiring professional aid. In times of public health emergency, as when smallpox, cholera, or yellow fever threatened whites and blacks, blacks received attention because disease could spread from them to whites. But in normal times they, like poor whites, had to fend for themselves. African Americans needed access to more and better medical care than that provided by the white and black healers of the region.

Emancipation occurred during an era of great medical advances. The introduction of ether and chloroform anesthesia in the 1840s and of Joseph Lister's antiseptic methods in the 1860s portended revolutionary changes in surgical practice. Physicians could make better diagnoses owing to the development of the stethoscope, percussion, and pathological anatomy in early-nineteenth-century France. Louis Pasteur was beginning his work on microbes, and Rudolf Virchow had already published his ideas on cellular pathology. It was an exciting time in medicine, one that, like Emancipation, held great promise for the future.

So, for freed people, a new world of opportunity stood potentially open in 1865. Because they could now openly participate in the free enterprise system, they could serve their people as lawyers, teachers, storekeepers, ministers, skilled artisans, and, of course, physicians. To take advantage of these possibilities, however, required education and money. No group was more aware of these needs than the small groups of conscientious white Northerners who expanded or inaugurated educational and Christian missionary work in the postbellum South. They saw the ignorance and poverty of freed people and the difficulties blacks faced in altering that situation. With few educated leaders and little money, African Americans could not easily establish schools that would provide a chance for individual or race advancement. If, as some said, blacks needed their own professionals, they would have to gain their training somewhere. During the first two decades following Emancipation, white Northern missionary associations and former white abolitionists established a number of freed people's schools across the South to teach literacy, basic knowledge, practical job and housekeeping skills, religion, and sometimes ministerial courses.[1] A few of these institutions (many of which are still in existence, often referred to as "historically black colleges and universities") originally included or later added medical education as part of their mission.

White medical schools in the South refused to accept African Americans into their programs, and a handful of Northern schools irregularly admitted a few freed people into medical classes.[2] Howard University, an institution founded in the District of Columbia by Northerners, with funding assistance from the Freedmen's Bureau, took the first significant step to alleviate the problem. Its trustees established in 1868 a medical school that freely accepted both blacks and whites. The Northern missionary groups that established schools in the South had a few visionary individuals who persisted in their attempts to add medical programs to

CHAPTER 12

Lincoln University Medical Department

Near the village of Oxford, in rural southern Pennsylvania, sits one of the oldest traditionally African American institutions of higher education in the United States. Lincoln University (LU) began educating small numbers of free black students, primarily future teachers, ministers, and African missionaries, in 1856, under the name Ashmun Institute. Conceived of and fostered by white Oxford Presbyterian minister John Miller Dickey, Ashmun grew slowly during its first ten years of existence. Though sanctioned by the Presbyterian Church it received no regular funds from national or local church agencies, but rather relied on Dickey and other donors for financial support. Because black education was never well accepted by antebellum Northerners or Southerners, Ashmun remained an isolated institution until 1865. Only after the Civil War, and the emancipation of the enslaved, did Ashmun come into its own and begin to expand its programs.[1] At that time the school housed the skeleton of a medical college, the second in the country founded specifically to include the training of persons of color. This medical institution gained little repute during its short existence and soon became an all but forgotten chapter in LU's history. Yet this seemingly insignificant episode in the life of a remote but vital black college reflects accurately the spirit and aspirations of postbellum African Americans and their white supporters. As part of that new era of black freedom, the story of LU's medical department, though sketchy in many of its details, deserves recounting.[2] It demonstrates the need both blacks and some whites felt immediately after Emancipation to produce competently trained black medical practitioners.

The story of the LU Medical Department begins in April 1866 when Ashmun Institute amended its charter and changed its name to Lincoln University.

Simultaneously the board of trustees added several nationally known names to the local ones that had previously overseen the school's development. Among the board members now were Gen. Oliver Otis Howard (1830–1909), recently appointed head of the Freedmen's Bureau in Washington, D.C.; Republican senator Edwin Denison Morgan (1811–83) of New York; New York businessman and philanthropist William Earl Dodge (1805–83); Bishop Matthew Simpson (1811–84), a leader in the antebellum sectional split within the Methodist Church; Baltimore abolitionist Andrew B. Cross (1809 or 1810–89); and Rev. Edward Norris Kirk (1802–74), a New England Congregationalist involved in the American Missionary Association's efforts to establish black schools and colleges in the South. Aiding this board in attempting to meet the educational needs of African Americans was a provision in LU's new charter that permitted the school to "confer all such literary degrees and academic honors and titles, as are usually conferred by University Corporations."[3]

The men who sat on LU's postwar board of trustees knew well the conditions under which freed people lived in the war-torn South. Those who had not observed them firsthand had read descriptions in Northern newspapers. Former slaves had left the lands they had tended for so many years and poured into Southern towns, taxing public resources and overloading health facilities. With poor housing, bad weather, lack of good food, and overcrowding came sharp increases in contagious diseases. Local authorities argued with federal officials and with each other about who would pay for black health care. Some hospitals refused or gave poor treatment to blacks, and other facilities admitted so many patients they became seriously overcrowded.[4]

Given such problems, the spirit of the times, the postwar composition of LU's board of trustees, and the school's now broader mandate, it is not surprising that LU began attempting to fill the new needs of black citizens, especially their need for black professionals to help them rise above their immediate difficulties. LU's catalogs soon announced plans to add theological, law, and medical departments to the preparatory and collegiate instruction already offered. The two-year theological program was inaugurated immediately, in 1866; law and medicine, publicized in 1869, were not introduced until 1870.[5]

Little is known about the exact impetus for, or the actual deliberations that resulted in, the formation of a medical department at LU. An 1874 faculty memorial to the trustees aimed at saving the by then moribund medical department provides evidence that college officials were motivated to found a medical school by their knowledge of the terrible plight of Northern and Southern blacks searching for adequate health care and the desires of some freed people to improve their situations by entering the professions:

> [T]he colored population are excluded from most of the existing [medical] institutions. . . . Their sick however respectable and curable are cruelly

> sent to wards occupied by contagious diseases and vicious patients. The skill of educated physicians is not within their reach from prejudice. . . . They are banished from the consulting rooms, lest their presence should alienate more profitable patronage. Their poverty prevents them from creating the instrumentalities which would bring relief. To alleviate that deplorable situation, to improve the economic opportunities of intelligent young blacks, and to develop a powerful force for raising the "standard of Social Morality" within the black community, the trustees saw their new endeavor as worthwhile and even crucial.[6]

That Lincoln was already attempting to foster the improvement of black health through education is revealed by the presence of required collegiate courses in anatomy and physiology taught during the students' junior year by J. Willis Houston, M.D.[7] But clearly the faculty and trustees now had grander plans—the training of black physicians to care for the freed people.

The twelfth annual LU catalog, published in June 1869, contained the first mention of a medical program, and even named courses and faculty:

> Medical Department
> A course of Lectures on the following subjects will be delivered to the Students of the University during the next Collegiate year:
> Chemistry, Materia Medica and Pharmacy.
> S. B. Howell, M.D.
> Anatomy, Physiology and Surgery.
> J. Willis Houston, M.D.
> Principles and Practice of Medicine.
> D. D. Kennedy, M.D.
> Hygiene, Toxicology and Medical Jurisprudence.
> D. W. Hutchison, M.D.[8]

Nowhere in the university's records prior to this date appears any indication that the faculty or trustees had contemplated establishment of such a department,[9] though the move appears a logical extension of the university's larger commitment to serve the educational needs of freed people.

At a meeting sometime before June 1870 (presumably before June 1869, but available documents do not substantiate the date), the LU faculty as a body voted to create departments of law and medicine. President Isaac N. Rendall undoubtedly supported that sentiment,[10] as he caused the previously mentioned announcement to appear in the catalog published in June 1869, and an even more definite statement to run in the following (April 1870) catalog. The latter advertised formation of a medical class beginning September 15, 1870, and included a schedule of expenses and a list of the faculty. The catalog announcement continued, "All medical students will be registered in the offices of practicing physicians, and on completion of the prescribed course, and satisfactory examination, will receive from the Board of Trustees, the degree of M.D."[11] Though the board of trustees must have known and approved of the faculty's and Rendall's actions before June 15, 1870, earlier minutes do not reflect it. Surely the board, given its composition and interest in furthering education for African Americans, played a more active role in promoting LU's interests than merely rubber stamping so important a change as the addition of departments of law and medicine. Yet the earliest minutes, from June 15, 1870, simply read: "On motion of the Reverend Albert Barnes it was resolved that the action of the faculty in creating the law and medical departments, and in appointing the persons named in the catalog to give lectures, be approved." The board also approved purchase of library books to support studies in these professional schools.[12] Despite the lack of hard evidence to support this presumption, all indications suggest that President Rendall, the faculty, and the board had cooperated in this endeavor over a period of time, probably since 1867 or 1868.

True to its word, LU did inaugurate a medical course in September 1870, with three students and four faculty members. Though geographically isolated, this small Pennsylvania college, by expanding programs to fit the needs and desires of its constituents, acted like other contemporary black institutions. One of LU's sister institutions, Howard University, had opened a medical school two years earlier with hopes and aspirations similar to Lincoln's. The spirit of the time encouraged such bold experiments in the higher education of freed people.

Our knowledge of the LU Medical Department's (LUMD) actual operation is severely limited, owing to the paucity of source material. Who directed the program? Why was the curriculum arranged as it was? What motivated students to enroll? Why did the physicians who served on the faculty agree to do so? We cannot answer these questions from the information at hand, but we can paint a rough portrait of LUMD based on available evidence.

The 1870–71 catalog, the first issued during the life of the medical department, failed to include specific details regarding curriculum, length of courses, and the first year program of instruction. What can be gleaned is a sense of the administration's expectations of the department: "The design of the Board of Trustees in establishing the Department of Medicine is to afford the student an opportunity of thorough instruction in the principles of medicine as a science, and in the application of these principles to the treatment and cure of diseases. It is hoped that the measures already adopted, and those in contemplation, will result in securing for the students a complete course of didactic and clinical instruction."[13] The specifics of the curriculum, outlined in the 1871–72 catalog and reprinted in the subsequent (1872–73) edition,[14] seem well designed to accomplish these goals. They were, however, difficult to attain, especially at an isolated, financially disadvantaged institution like LU. In fact, for that period, they were revolutionary. Only Harvard University and Chicago Medical College had similar requirements.[15]

To gain admission into the medical program, a student had to be a graduate of LU's or another institution's collegiate department, no mean task for whites, much less for blacks in those days.[16] The administration quietly modified this rule the following year, allowing prospective students who might not have graduated from college the option simply to "pass a satisfactory examination before the Faculties of Arts and Medicine,"[17] a rule common to many schools of the time. Once matriculated at Lincoln, students faced three years of study in a fully graded (sequential rather than the traditional repetitive) curriculum, as follows:

Studies of the First Year	Studies of the Second Year	Studies of the Third Year
Anatomy	Medical Chemistry	Pathological Anatomy
Physiology	Materia Medica	Physiology
General Chemistry	Pathological Anatomy	Therapeutics
Materia Medica	Physiology	Tokology (Obstetrics)
	Theory and Practice of Medicine	Theory and Practice of Medicine
	Clinical Medicine	Clinical Medicine
	Surgery	Surgery
	Clinical Surgery	Clinical Surgery

Because material presented in the second and third years presumed mastery of information taught earlier, medical students could not advance with their classes or be admitted with advanced standing until they had "passed the required examination in the studies of the year or a majority of them."[18] Presumably to avoid the potential problems of traditional medical school oral examinations (personality conflicts, unfair questions, favoritism, and lack of permanent records), the rules demanded that all examinations contain written portions, though other testing procedures might be used in addition. Furthermore, no student could graduate until he passed examinations in every subject in the curriculum listed earlier, "presented a certificate from the Demonstrator of Anatomy that he had satisfactorily dissected the three parts of the human body," reached the age of twenty-one, studied medicine for three years, spent "one continuous year" at Lincoln, and written a satisfactory thesis.[19]

In an era of keen competition among medical schools and declining entrance and graduation requirements, these stringent regulations seemed unnecessarily tough, out of place, or meaningless (another example of catalog rhetoric so common in these late-nineteenth-century publications).[20] Few schools insisted on evidence of prior liberal arts study or even knowledge of English grammar and literature. Nor did medical colleges in the early 1870s offer a graded curriculum, with the exceptions noted earlier. Medical schools stood to lose students, and therefore profits, if requirements were too difficult. LUMD's faculty and trustees, however, were trying to address, honestly and appropriately, the realities of medical education for African Americans of the 1870s. Few had had the opportunity to obtain a basic education by that time. The black struggle for survival in a hostile and war-torn society worked against the acquisition of even primary schooling. Furthermore, the kind of educational enrichment and encouragement offered as a matter of course in many white middle- and upper-class homes, both Northern and Southern, often did not or could not exist in the lower-class black household. LU officials apparently recognized these problems and took measures to ensure that graduates of the medical program could overcome these circumstantial deficiencies in background and so compare favorably with the products of white medical schools. Though all but one of the students who attended LU did satisfy the admissions requirements, the faculty members who actually taught and the facilities available at the school could not have fulfilled the educational program outlined in the catalog. LU (and Howard, which graduated its first medical class in 1871) had taken on a big responsibility in opting to train black professionals and did not want to risk failure. So the lengthy program and cautious attitudes of LU faculty and trustees in their handling of the new medical program are understandable, if seemingly unreasonable or unattainable. That the curriculum and requirements were advanced for their time is an interesting feature. They were instituted out of necessity.

Innovative, unique, and forward looking as it was, the experiment in black medical education at LU was doomed to failure from the outset. The reasons for its demise had less to do with race than with the realities of conducting a viable medical education program at that time and in that place. To understand the problems in Lincoln's program, it is necessary to look closely at the school's location, faculty, manner of teaching, classroom facilities, teaching apparatus, clinical resources, and financial status.

The biggest difficulty in sustaining a medical school at LU was its location. Dickey built the college on a remote site, adjacent to a small black settlement some four miles from the village of Oxford. As Horace Mann Bond described the location in his history of the school, "It was isolated from the world; the dirt road that bordered its northern limits was only a track leading uncertainly to Oxford. United States Highway 1 was seventy years away in the future. There was no railroad; mail and passengers came by stagecoach on the highway two miles south at Elkdale."[21] Secure from antebellum slave stealers who regularly crossed the Maryland-Pennsylvania border to kidnap unsuspecting blacks and sell them South at the Baltimore market, the college was, by 1870, also secure from benevolent prospective Philadelphia physician-teachers who would have had to make a determined effort to visit the place for regular classes. Even though a rail line had been built by that time, train travel required a trip from Philadelphia's Market Street Station to Wawa Junction and a change to cars bound for Buttonwood Station, near Hinsonville. There one might obtain a horse and buggy for the short remaining ride to LU.[22]

In addition to location, the state of LU's finances hindered development of the medical department. In its early years, Lincoln relied primarily on the funds that founder John Miller Dickey raised or contributed himself, an amount just sufficient to operate the school. Expansion of the university's programs in theology, law, medicine, and precollegiate education after the Civil War strained an already stressed budget. Donations from Northern whites such as trustee William E. Dodge and other benefactors dedicated to improving black educational prospects, and appropriations from Gen. O. O. Howard's Freedmen's Bureau and the Education Department of the Commonwealth of Pennsylvania, helped but could not keep up with the school's rising expenses. LU's indebtedness, $3,660 in 1866, rose to $11,290 just before the medical department first opened in 1869 and doubled in the next three years.[23]

Had the school a greater reputation, better facilities, and larger salaries it might have attracted a residential medical faculty as had rural contemporary schools such as the University of Virginia in Charlottesville. But it was just starting out and so was fortunate to obtain the services of even local physicians willing to travel the four miles from Oxford. At the many proprietary medical schools that mushroomed around the country in the postwar period, physician-teachers collected fees from each student for their courses of lectures on particular subjects. LUMD students, however, paid a flat fee of $26 for the year, and each faculty member in turn received a salary ($300–$500) or taught gratis.[24] Recruiting a teaching corps for the medical department under those circumstances was not easy. And yet the faculty that expressed willingness to or actually did teach at LUMD surprisingly included some prominent Philadelphia physicians, a few even with regional and national reputations.

Like many medical schools of that period, LUMD initially enlisted local or readily available talent to teach its classes. The June 1869 catalog first announcing the school's opening named four instructors. Samuel Bedell Howell (1834–1903) of Philadelphia, an 1858 University of Pennsylvania medical graduate, had already been teaching courses in natural sciences to LU students since 1868 when he was called to the medical department's chair of chemistry, materia medica, and pharmacy. He continued instruction in the natural sciences after LUMD's official closing in 1876, apparently making the strenuous journey from and to Philadelphia on at least a weekly basis. Howell, who had pursued studies in practical geology immediately after graduation while practicing medicine and surgery in the Schuylkill mining region of Pennsylvania, also taught at the Philadelphia Dental College and the University of Pennsylvania.[25] Like Howell, Dr. Joseph Willis Houston of Collamer, Pennsylvania, was lecturing to undergraduate students at LU on anatomy, physiology, and botany before establishment of the medical department. He donated his services from 1868 (perhaps earlier) through 1872 when, the next year's annual catalog announced, "protracted illness" prevented him "from repeating his lectures."[26] Houston's name appeared on the initial roster of medical faculty members in 1869 as teacher of anatomy, physiology, and surgery, and again in the subsequent two catalogs.[27]

The other two men listed in that first catalog—David Dickey Kennedy (1829–81), an 1853 University of Pennsylvania medical alumnus,[28] and D. W. Hutchison—practiced medicine in nearby Oxford. They were named in the 1869–71 catalogs as lecturers on principles and practice of medicine and obstetrics, and hygiene and obstetrics, respectively. Kennedy also provided medical care for ailing students at LU as resident physician during the 1870–71 and 1871–72 school terms, and presumably longer.[29]

During the years that LU offered instruction in medicine (1870–74) the annual catalogs listed a total of twelve faculty. Half, it appears, never had the opportunity to impart their knowledge to interested students: Harrison Allen (1841–97; University of Pennsylvania, M.D., 1861; anatomy), S. J. Clark (anatomy), Henry Hartshorne (1823–97; University of Pennsylvania, M.D., 1845; practice of medicine), F. A. Hassler (materia medica and pharmacy), William F. Jenks (1842–81; University of Pennsylvania, M.D., 1866; obstetrics), and Horatio C. Wood (1841–1920; University of Pennsylvania, M.D., 1862; materia medica and pharmacy) all taught and/or practiced medicine in the Philadelphia area, and all expressed a willingness to teach African American students to become physicians. At least three of these men, Allen, Hartshorne, and Wood, had published extensively and earned national reputations in their respective fields.[30]

Evidence suggests that these men actively supported the school's efforts to raise funds and consulted and advised the trustees on various matters relating to the medical department. But extra salary money simply was not forthcoming, nor was goodwill or a worthy cause sufficient remuneration for these six physicians, whose names and participation would have greatly enhanced LUMD's standing. Fully aware of the benefits of appointing men such as Allen, Wood, and Hartshorne to the teaching staff, the 1871–72 medical department faculty sent a clear message to LU's president and board: "The friends of these gentlemen would probably do something toward the endowment of their chairs; at all events, their names would add dignity to our department and make us more widely known." But these faculty members were also realists. In that same report, they suggested election but postponement of actual teaching assignments of those three illustrious Philadelphia physicians "until their chairs could be endowed, or partially so." After all, their fees for teaching were $500 each per annum plus travel expenses, money the trustees did not have and could not raise. So Allen, Wood, and Hartshorne received faculty appointments but not instructional duties.[31]

Of the remaining two physicians, both from Philadelphia and both actual teachers at LU, little is known. Dr. Houston's generosity in instructing students gratuitously was matched initially by Dr. Theodore H. Seyfert[32] (University of Pennsylvania, M.D., 1867), who gave lectures in physiology beginning in February 1872.[33] (Others may also have donated their services, though the available records are not specific on this matter.) Elmore C. Hine (Yale, M.D., 1861) acted as dean and professor of surgery and obstetrics after joining the faculty in January 1872. He and Howell received an undetermined salary from LU.[34] Howell, Hine, and Seyfert carried most of the teaching load at the tiny medical school during the second half of the 1871–72 school term, throughout the 1872–73, and probably the entire 1873–74 academic years.[35] Between September 1870, when students began medical studies, and January 1872, Howell, Houston, Kennedy, and Hutchison most likely served as instructors.

Had Lincoln been located in or near Philadelphia, it undoubtedly would have been a more visible institution, and so better able to obtain financial support and perhaps more volunteer or nominally paid medical faculty members. As it stood, Hine, Howell, and Seyfert traveled out to the school once a week, at great expense in time and money, to teach a handful of students.[36] Other physicians would have taught—were, as mentioned earlier, even appointed to the faculty—but did not, assumedly because of the distance and lack of salary guarantees. Certainly they sympathized with the little school's plight and wanted to help, just as Dr. Hartshorne, for example, devoted time and service to such causes as the advancement of women physicians and the medical and spiritual needs of the Japanese.[37]

In November 1872, Dean Hine and his small faculty (still smarting from the American Medical Association's refusal to admit Hine as the delegate from Lincoln University to its annual meeting because of the school's precarious situation), including those appointed but not teaching, used these arguments and the lack of adequate clinical teaching facilities (hospital or dispensary) in rural Chester County to convince the board of trustees to reestablish the medical department in Philadelphia. That ruling body needed little prompting to recognize the advantages of such a move, both to the university and to the medically needy black population of Philadelphia. On June 17, 1873, it expressed "confidence" in the medical department but not in the financial strength of LU, which was "in such a condition that we dare not incur any additional expense" for medical instruction. If the three additional needed faculty and the removal to Philadelphia could somehow be accomplished without expense to LU, the board would certainly endorse such changes. Otherwise it could do nothing to assist at present.[38] Attempts to obtain outside funds from potential donors failed.[39] Student tuition the basic college curriculum. In 1873 Joseph W. Healy was able to organize what turned out to be a short-lived medical department at the American Missionary Association's Straight University in New Orleans. Three years later, Dr. George W. Hubbard, with the assistance of a private gift and the Freedmen's Aid Society of the Methodist Episcopal Church, opened a medical department (Meharry) at Central Tennessee College in Nashville, and in 1882, Henry M. Tupper received permission from the American Baptist Home Mission Society to begin training medical students at Leonard Medical School of Shaw University (Raleigh). Two other white-founded missionary schools later followed the lead of Meharry and Leonard (Flint Medical School in 1889 and Knoxville College Medical Department in 1895).[3] Once a generation of black physicians had been trained, a few black doctors founded their own independent medical schools to further increase the number of trained African American healers. These so-called proprietary schools, opened in the last dozen years of the century, were similar to the much larger number of white-owned proprietary medical schools in both the North and South founded during the Gilded Age. No state, North or South, operated or contributed public funds in support of a medical school for African Americans during this period. The first of these independent medical educational institutions was Louisville National Medical College in 1888, followed the next year by Hannibal in Memphis, in 1899 by Chattanooga National Medical College (its founder was a graduate of the Louisville institution), and in 1900 by Knoxville Medical College and the University of West Tennessee College of Medicine and Surgery in Jackson, Tennessee, and later (1907) Memphis (see Appendix, Table 4).[4]

Back in 1876, as the Reconstruction decade drew to a close, a spokesman for the Freedmen's Aid Society (FAS) of the Methodist Episcopal Church, one of the Northern white missionary groups dedicated to improving the lot of formerly enslaved people in the South, explained, in paternalistic language typical of the era, the need for white support of efforts to train black physicians: "In the olden time the master's physician attended the slave in his sickness, and spared no effort to save his valuable life; but now the physician who practices among the freedmen loses caste and business among the whites. Under such circumstances the poor freedmen are neglected, and not infrequently they suffer and die for want of medical attendance. The remedy is, educate colored physicians. The training of good men for physicians is the next great duty that confronts us in the preservation and elevation of this people."[5] In 1910, just thirty-four years later, another white man, Abraham Flexner, speaking for the American Medical Association, an organization also concerned about the training of physicians, urged that most of the black medical schools founded since Reconstruction be closed: "Of the seven medical schools for negroes in the United States, five are at this moment in no position to make any contribution of value to the solution of the [Negro health] problem. . . . They are wasting small sums annually and sending out undisciplined men, whose lack of real training is covered up by the imposing M.D. degree."[6] When he made these recommendations about black medical schools, only seven of the original fourteen remained in operation, and Flexner wanted that number reduced to two. What had happened to the optimism of Reconstruction that such an important spokesperson of the Progressive Era would sound so negative about medical education for African Americans? And what had happened to all those medical schools?

The following chapters will provide case histories of several black medical schools in an attempt to answer these questions. We will look at the circumstances surrounding establishment of the schools, at some of the problems the schools encountered as they struggled to survive in the late nineteenth and early twentieth centuries, and, finally, at explanations for their closing, or, in the cases of Meharry and Howard, for their survival.[7] These chapters will argue that finances underlaid each school's success or failure, that because of poor access to funds, one group of African American medical schools—black-owned proprietary institutions—were doomed to failure from the start, and that the schools founded by Northern white missionary groups had a better chance for survival but could ultimately endure only with the blessing of white organized medicine and the funding of large white philanthropic organizations allied with organized medicine.

fees, at $26 per year, added little to the medical department's coffers.[40] The final recourse, open appeals in the school's catalogs of August 1873 (p. 42) and May 1874 (p. 30), and presumably in other publications, for $6,500 "to develop the Medical Department in Philadelphia" also generated no new funds.

The board's inability to rescue this important educational program from dissolution illustrates dramatically the young school's financial instability. Dependent on private benefactors and state and federal funds, LU's small endowment could hardly begin to pay operating expenses. So the school struggled as Freedmen's Bureau and then state education department payments ceased in the early 1870s. With LU already deeply in debt, the board could do little more than retrench when the financial Panic of 1873 even further reduced the university's income. Challenges by the school's new financial agent, Rev. Edward Webb, to President Rendall's and the board's leadership, and by the school's alumni to the LU administration's refusal to hire black faculty or elect a black board member, created an unsettled situation unfavorable for support and development of programs like the medical department.[41]

After limping through the 1873–74 academic year, the faculty, president, and finally the trustees recognized the futility of the medical school endeavor as it existed. The gloomy annual report from President Rendall spurred a special board committee to recommend on June 17 that "action of radical effect" be taken with regard to the medical and law departments. The trustees responded by reconstituting a committee on the medical department, which was charged with considering the matter. That committee's apparent inaction over the summer caused frustrated and alarmed faculty members to appoint, on the first day of the fall term, September 17, 1874, President Rendall a committee of one "to prepare a Memorial to the Board of Trustees in reference to the Law and Medical Departments." That document, approved by the faculty on September 24, was read to the board the following day.[42] In it the faculty members expressed their desire that the integrity of the university "in all the Departments of instruction" be maintained. They viewed any move to suspend operation of the medical and law departments as a threat to that integrity, especially as these programs had been established to satisfy such worthy and important needs: "The Faculty therefore feel that they would justly incur the censure of the Board, *if they should allow any of these departments* established with so many formalities and with such public demonstrations, *to be disbanded*, and the cherished plans of the Board *to be defeated*. . . . Those jealous of our prosperity will not be slow to use our failure to our injury. We cannot personally escape the discouragement of failure. We cannot prevent the loss of confidence in our wisdom and influence." The memorialists then rehearsed the various reasons for having established a medical department at LU and asserted that, because these conditions still existed, the training program needed to continue. Furthermore, the board could not, in all fairness, abandon the students who had devoted the past few years of their lives to medical study at Lincoln and now lacked, in some cases, but one year of instruction to graduate. In a few instances, the faculty remarked, students had even given up the opportunity to transfer to other institutions in favor of completing study at LU. They too had a stake in the future of LU's medical department. In concluding their memorial, the faculty urged an increase in support to both professional departments (law and medicine) by removing them to Philadelphia and fostering their development there.[43] The trustees, moved by this eloquent statement on behalf of medical and legal education at Lincoln, again referred the matter to a select committee, which included the school's founder and board chairman, John Miller Dickey, and its president, Isaac N. Rendall.[44]

And what of those persons whose careers hung in the balance—the students? Their small number, six between 1870 and 1874, rendered them insignificant as both financial contributors with tuition fees and lobbyists in the effort to keep the medical department alive. But it was their presence that justified the whole enterprise. Who were these students? Unfortunately, as with so much of the history of LU's medical department, not much is known about the young men named in the annual catalogs[45]:

Name	*Home Town*	*Entered Medical Department in*	*Received A.B. in*
William F. Brooks	Philadelphia, Pa.	September 1870	1870
Charles P. Colder	Germantown, Pa. (later Philadelphia)	1872	September 1870
Jesse Gould	Bridgeton, N.J.	September 1870	1870
George Henderson	New York, N.Y.	September 1871	1870
Bayard T. Smith	Wilmington, Del.	January 1872	———
Benjamin James	New York, N.Y.	September 1872	1872

Assuming that information in the catalogs is correct, both Mr. Colder and Mr. Henderson undertook medical studies before actually completing requirements for a bachelor's degree. Bayard Smith may have entered the medical program by satisfactorily passing exams before the arts and medical faculties, as outlined in the catalog and described earlier, or by graduating from another collegiate institution, as he was not an undergraduate at Lincoln. Interestingly, in light of LUMD's tough admission requirements, all students but Smith (whose background is uncertain) earned collegiate degrees, an unusual circumstance for a medical school student in the early 1870s.

The students pursued their medical studies under difficult conditions, given the irregularity and changing nature of the faculty presence on campus over the years, as well as the lack of clinical reinforcement of information read in books or discussed in class. It is difficult to assess the quality of teaching facilities available on campus. Students could, when taking anatomy or surgery, consult one of two disarticulated human skeletons owned by Drs. Howell and Houston or look at a poorly maintained printed set of anatomical plates kept at the school. Mr. Brooks had a chance to go to Philadelphia sometime during the 1871–72 school year for a lesson in dissection, and the medical class as a whole dissected a cadaver on campus in March 1872.[46] The catalogs make mention of chemistry and physiology laboratories, a dissecting room, a medical specimen museum, a collection of medical botanical specimens and pharmaceutical preparations, a "manekin" for learning obstetric and gynecologic operations, and a weekly public clinic, but how much of this material and activity was planned for the future and how much was actually then present at LU is not known.[47] Student textbooks must certainly have been available and central to their studies. The catalog lists several for each subject.[48]

Some students found that even the lengthy nine-month-per-year, three-year program in force at LUMD did not allow them sufficient time to learn the required material. These difficulties in completing the prescribed course on time probably resulted from the less-than-ideal teaching situation and facilities at the university as well as, perhaps, from financial distractions and the presumably deficient educational backgrounds of the students. President Rendall reported in June 1873 that Mr. Gould and Mr. Colder had both lost a half year from their studies during 1871–72, and so would not graduate that year. Brooks, the third student of the initial group, had graduated third in the LU undergraduate class of 1870 and delivered the mathematics oration at his commencement. He served as vocal music and writing instructor at Lincoln during his first two years in the medical class and then left to teach mathematics at the Colored High School in Philadelphia. He intended to resume medical studies after the medical department had progressed further. Clearly he had interests beyond medicine. Of the six students who had enrolled at LUMD, four, Rendall stated in his June 1873 annual report, were far enough along to be ready for graduation the following June.[49]

For some unknown reason no students graduated in June 1874 or at any time thereafter. Though teaching took place during 1873–74, the catalog issued in May 1874 omitted any mention of the medical department, its faculty, or its students. Save for the previously discussed statement of need for a $6,500 endowment to move the school to Philadelphia, this and every subsequent catalog ignored the medical program—acted, in fact, as if it had never existed. The board of trustees' Summary of Operations Book listed six medical students in its June 1874 student head count, but did not even include this category in any of the following years' listings.[50]

If the board's high level select committee created in response to the September 24, 1874, faculty memorial ever reported back to the trustees, that fact never appeared in the minutes. All evidence points to a suspension of medical instruction with the close of the 1873–74 academic year. After September 25, 1874, the board minutes do not refer to the medical department for almost two years, until June 5, 1876. On that date the trustees heard and accepted letters of resignation from Drs. Hine, Seyfert, Allen, and Jenks, all still officially faculty members, though in name only. Next morning the board responded further by recording in the minutes its "high appreciation of the services [these four physicians had] rendered to Lincoln University." After deploring the necessity formally to sever the relationship between Lincoln and these men, the trustees expressed their embarrassment at the university's inability to pay $300 back salary owed Drs. Hine and Seyfert since 1874. They assured the two physicians that Lincoln's debt would be paid "at the earliest possible date."[51]

And that was all. As one recent investigator, aptly applying a medical metaphor, summed up the situation, "No doubt the delinquent sums were paid in good time; so far as I find, however, the record of the Medical Department of Lincoln University terminates with the above-quoted Board minute of 6 June 1876. Clearly it has the effect of an obituary notice on the Department, even though the Department had never been declared dead. The Board seems to have buried the Department without ever having laid it out—not surprising perhaps in view of the fact that the Department had from the start hovered between life and death, with its final years spent, as it were, in an oxygen tent. In any case, buried or not, the Department gives no further twitches of life beyond the faculty resignations of June 1876."[52]

The official demise of Lincoln that June day did not spell the end of medical schools for African Americans in the United States. Howard University, then the only other medical school in the country that regularly admitted blacks, had also gone through a crisis in 1873, but succeeded where LU had failed.[53] Located in a large city, it had better access to faculty of both races, clinical facilities (Freedmen's Hospital, a legacy of Reconstruction), money (the U.S. government and missionary societies), and students. Howard continued to train black physicians throughout the period and survives today, as does Meharry Medical College, founded in Nashville in October 1876, just a few months after the LU Medical Department's closing. Over the next forty-five years, almost a dozen missionary and proprietary black institutions opened their doors with aspirations similar to Lincoln's only to close in short order for want of funds, sufficient facilities, and qualified faculty. LUMD's story was repeated, with some variations, in each instance.

One final question remains: What happened to those six students? Though seemingly abandoned by LU, they all managed to continue their careers apparently without a break. Jesse Gould and Benjamin James transferred to Howard University Medical Department for the 1874–75 and 1875–76 sessions and received M.D. degrees in 1876, the year that LU's medical faculty tendered its official resignation. Gould then opened a practice in Ohio, later moving to his hometown of Bridgeton, New

Jersey, where he practiced medicine and farmed. James followed the advice of his benefactor, William E. Dodge (an LU trustee), and journeyed to Liberia in 1877 as a medical missionary. After his wife and one of his children died there, James sent his other two children to Baltimore, following them later. He subsequently practiced medicine in Beaufort, Sheldon, Jonesville, and finally in Hardeeville, South Carolina.[54] William Brooks may have spent 1874–75 at Lincoln, since he received an A.M. degree in June 1875. He remained a teacher in Philadelphia for some time, but returned to Lincoln for seminary training in the mid-1880s. He then moved to Charlotte, North Carolina, where he served as a Presbyterian minister and teacher at Biddle University. As of 1878, Charles Colder was a teacher at an unnamed school in Maryland. Bayard Smith and George Henderson entered Yale Medical School, earning their degrees in 1875 and 1876, respectively, and then opening practices in their home states of Delaware and New York. Henderson resided in Brooklyn the last eight years of his life. An 1896 obituary notice in the *Journal of the American Medical Association* stated his age as forty-five and called him "a colored practitioner of good position." He died, the notice continued, from "an overdose of morphine accidentally taken, for the relief of pain."[55]

Lincoln University managed to launch four of its six medical students' careers before its experiment in medical education collapsed. The people involved knew how important an endeavor it was and said so in their memorial to the board:

> The Board of Trustees and the Faculty of the University stand before the colored population of the country as champions of their interests in these respects; and as pioneers in the practical organization of the agencies for their protection in them.
>
> We have put our hand to the plough, and it would seem that unless God release us from the duty of sympathy and self-sacrifice for his suffering poor, we cannot look back.[56]

Despite these noble sentiments, those in charge had to look back, assess the realities of the situation, and at least suspend operations in rural Chester County until more money and new facilities became available. None ever materialized.

LU had tried, beginning in 1866, to help African Americans take advantage of their newfound freedom by offering them more than merely basic educational opportunities. Hopefully, confidently, white school authorities developed programs that trained ministers, teachers, lawyers, and physicians. They expected graduates of these curricula to form the basis of a successful black professional group that would serve as a model for others and to lend their services to their brothers and sisters in the South and the North who needed spiritual uplift, a good education, legal aid, or medical services. In some of these goals Lincoln succeeded, but in the realm of medical education LU simply did not have sufficient resources. Other institutions would have to fill that gap.

CHAPTER 13

Straight University Medical Department

Black Medical Education in Reconstruction New Orleans

Three Northern religious groups established colleges in New Orleans during Reconstruction: the American Missionary Association (AMA; loosely associated with the Congregationalist Church) founded Straight University (SU) in 1869, the American Baptist Home Mission Society opened Leland University in 1869, and the Freedmen's Aid Society of the Methodist Episcopal Church chartered New Orleans University in 1873. The charters of Straight University and New Orleans University authorized both schools to establish medical departments, which both did. Straight's medical school began first, but failed because of problems relating to religion, politics, money, personalities, and race. New Orleans University's medical school started years later and graduated a number of physicians of color before closing in 1911 in the wake of the Flexner Report.[1]

SU opened its doors in the fall of 1869. Full of promise, this new institution of higher learning provided a congenial setting in which the region's African Americans could gain not only a college education but also professional training in the fields of theology, law, and medicine. Straight's first catalog announced establishment of a medical department following a $35,000 appropriation from the state legislature and the appointment of a faculty of distinguished local physicians. Six years later, however, in September 1875, a report on the school's activities made no mention of a medical department. What had happened?

Historians' descriptions of Straight's history during the Reconstruction period have characterized the medical school as a successful enterprise until at least 1877, when an arsonist destroyed SU's main campus building, thereby contributing to the university's decline. According to one writer, "From 1870 to 1877 Straight probably had one of the strongest medical departments in the state."[2] Another author echoed those words and extended the life of the medical school beyond the 1877 blaze: "Within a few years [of the fire] the law department became independent and the medical school ceased to exist."[3] In reality, the medical department operated for just one (1873–74) or perhaps two (1872–73, 1873–74) academic years, graduated no physicians, employed a teaching faculty of one, and had quite poor instructional facilities. A major reason for so much confusion in published histories of Straight's medical school is the sparseness of pertinent documentation. Very little remains with which to trace the medical department's brief existence. The following discussion is based on those few extant source materials.

In late 1868, Rev. Joseph W. Healy moved from Chicago to New Orleans to serve as agent of the AMA for the Southwest and as pastor of the First Congregational Church of New Orleans. The AMA tended to the spiritual and educational needs of Louisiana's freed people until 1866, when racial turmoil forced the association to drastically reduce its involvement. Healy, an energetic and enthusiastic worker, intended to revitalize the AMA's efforts. He organized schools and churches for newly freed blacks and cultivated a relationship with the federal government's Freedmen's Bureau, which was also attempting to provide educational opportunities for African Americans. Healy, who wished to establish a university for Louisiana freed people,[4] chose New Orleans as the appropriate location. The AMA, a leader in establishing colleges for African Americans during the early years of Reconstruction,[5] lent its support to Healy, as did the Freedmen's Bureau, which provided financial and other assistance to religious groups in the region interested in establishing schools. As a result of Healy's efforts, including a March 1869 visit to AMA and Freedmen's Bureau officials in Washington, D.C., when he thought his program's progress was being stalled unnecessarily, the AMA purchased land for a university in the heart of New Orleans, near the intersection of Esplanade and Claiborne. The Freedmen's Bureau donated $20,000 to erect school buildings and purchase furniture, and, by the end of June 1869, Healy and his co-organizers had filed the appropriate papers with the state of Louisiana incorporating a university for "the education and training of young men and women, irrespective of color or race." The trustees were empowered "to confer all such degrees and honors, as are conferred by Universities in the United States of America," including a degree in medicine.[6] Healy's plan was moving forward.

Among the people Healy convinced to support this new university was Seymour Straight, an Ohio wholesale grocer and commission merchant who did business in both Cincinnati (Straight, Deming and Company) and New Orleans (McFarland, Straight and Company). Straight, also the owner of four cheese factories in Ohio, lived in New Orleans during the winter and spring months. Though a Baptist, he gave generously of his time and money to the AMA's Louisiana activities on behalf of the freed people, beginning as early as 1863, and served as an AMA vice president from 1864 to 1883.[7] In recognition of Straight's financial donations and labor in helping found the new school, AMA officials agreed with Rev. Healy's suggestion that the university be named for him.[8] Straight continued donating to the school after the enterprise had been launched and served for several years as president of the university's board of trustees.

Rev. Healy was able to secure the support of a number of prominent Louisianans willing to serve on the school's twenty-one-member board of trustees, including ten, as he put it, "carefully selected" "colored" men. Among the African American trustees were popular Lt. Gov. Oscar J. Dunn; Rev. John Turner, chaplain of the state senate; and wealthy and prominent New Orleans citizens Aristide Mary, Fabius Dunn, and John R. Clay. White board members included Gov. Henry Clay Warmoth, Mayor Edward Heath of New Orleans, U.S. Treasury officer Charles Clinton, and real estate speculator and attorney Charles Heath.[9]

The language of the school's charter clearly indicates that Healy had included medical education in the university's master plan. Perhaps his March 1869 meetings in Washington with Freedmen's Bureau officials, including Gen. Oliver Otis Howard, sparked this idea. Howard University in Washington, named for General Howard, its organizer and benefactor, had the year before opened its medical department concurrently with several other academic departments.[10] SU, like Howard, was nonsectarian, biracial, and coeducational in its admissions policies and broad in its program offerings.

Just as classes at Straight's Normal School were beginning in the fall of 1869 in temporary quarters at a local church (the permanent buildings would not be completed until February 1870), Healy saw an opportunity to obtain classroom facilities for his projected medical department. Representatives of the American Baptist Home Mission Society, a Northern missionary group, and a local Baptist missionary society approached Healy about ways to obtain Freedmen's Bureau aid for a theological school. The bureau had refused the Baptists' request (the grounds of the refusal are uncertain in the extant documentation), but Healy proposed a way to satisfy the Baptists and obtain a medical school building in the bargain. He suggested that the Baptists patronize the various departments of "unsectarian" SU, including its theological school, and ask the bureau "for a Building, the lower part of which shall be a chapel, and the upper stories the Medical College of the University." The Baptists would own the new facility. "Thus our work will be cooperative," he explained to AMA officials. "We have facilities for a Normal Col[lege] and Theo[logical] depart[ment]s: and . . . [the Baptists] furnish facilities for the Med[ical] Dept." Both missionary groups would get what they wanted, and recently freed African Americans would gain additional educational facilities.[11] For reasons not explained in extant correspondence, however, Healy's proposal to work with these Baptist groups was not implemented. (The persistent problem of interdenominational rivalry in Reconstruction Louisiana over churches and educational institutions, in which Healy had been involved, could have been a factor.)[12] The incident does demonstrate, however, Healy's sincerity in wishing to offer persons of color in the lower Mississippi Delta the opportunity to become medical practitioners.

Reconstruction politics played a significant role in the medical school's establishment, or rather in the delay of its founding. Title VII ("Public Education") of Louisiana's 1868 Constitution contained three articles bearing on Straight's history: Article 135 allowed the Louisiana General Assembly to establish public schools and other institutions of learning across the state but forbade the state from organizing such schools "exclusively for any race"; Article 140 prohibited the General Assembly from appropriating funds to support private schools; and Article 142 directed the legislature to establish and maintain a university with law, medical, and collegiate departments in New Orleans, stipulating that no rules or regulations be made by the university or the General Assembly "violating the letter or spirit of the articles under this title." The last provision presumably referred to Article 135's prohibition against segregated schools. Whites opposed to racially mixed schools feared that Article 135 would be used to integrate the Louisiana State Seminary (later to become Louisiana State University), which received annual state appropriations. Gov. Henry Clay Warmoth and seminary president David French Boyd opposed mixing races at the school, while State Superintendent of Public Education Thomas Conway, a former chaplain for a black regiment, was a strong integrationist. Conway wished to force the seminary's integration through the state's "beneficiary program" by selecting two students from each parish to attend the school gratis.[13] SU's founding in 1869 coincided with this controversy, and the facility's proposed admissions policy almost brought Healy's medical school the money it needed to open.

Correspondence among AMA officials regarding the founding of SU does not mention any plan to have that school designated as the institution mentioned in Article 142. Funds raised to open Straight came from the Freedmen's Bureau, the AMA, and private individuals such as Seymour Straight. However, opening a reputable medical school required more money than the founders could raise at the time. Additional dollars were needed for erecting or renting a classroom building, purchasing furnishings for classrooms and equipment for laboratories and demonstrations, and paying faculty salaries. Hoping to open the medical school for the 1870–71 term, President Healy urged the school's board of trustees to apply to the state legislature for financial help during the January 1870 legislative session. Sympathetic legislators cooperated, proposing an act with several sections relating to the establishment of a university containing legal and medical departments. Embedded in the penultimate section was a $35,000 appropriation "for the use of the medical department, to construct suitable buildings, and secure illustrations of medical science." The proposed legislation also provided that "the faculty [of the university] shall receive one indigent student from each parish free from charge for tuition, which obligation shall continue for ten years."[14] This effectively established a state beneficiary program for African Americans. By essentially making SU "the state college for negroes," as one historian of Louisiana State University termed it, this compromise satisfied the opposing groups on the racial mixing issue and gave Straight funds to start a medical school.[15]

Rev. Healy had been involved in the behind-the-scenes negotiations,[16] using the integration controversy as a way to gain an appropriation for the medical school. "But for his [Healy's] persisting in urging it," reported board president Seymour Straight to AMA Secretary George Whipple in New York, "the effort [to solicit funds from the legislature] would probably not have been made." Once the board had decided on this strategy to obtain an endowment, three or four trustees "worked hard to get it through."[17] The tactic seemed to work. On February 23, 1870, the state Senate passed the bill; the House of Representatives approved it one week later.[18] In addition to the $35,000 appropriation for construction of a suitable building and the purchase of teaching materials, the bill included directives that the medical department operate with no fewer than seven faculty members and that students be allowed free access to the wards of New Orleans Charity Hospital for the practical study of diseases and their treatments.[19] The bill was signed into law as Act 81 on March 9, 1870.

The establishment of a medical school at SU thus seemed assured, but, almost a month later, on April 5, Seymour Straight, still publicly elated by the prospect of opening a medical school, betrayed his private misgivings in a letter to George Whipple at AMA headquarters: "If we get the $35,000 from the State and a part of this amount from the U.S. Government for a Medical Department, and if distant friends interest themselves for [*sic*] us, as they give us reason to expect, we may hope to make this a leading Institution, and one of the most useful of any in the Southwest."[20] President Straight's uncertainty over funding is partially explained by the sequence of events following enactment of the appropriation bill. In order to complete some unfinished legislative business, Governor Warmoth recalled the General Assembly for an extra session upon the close of the regular session. During that extra session, Sen. C. C. Antoine of Caddo Parish introduced Bill 226, titled "An Act to Aid the Medical Department of Straight University." This bill was quickly adopted by both the Senate and the House.[21] Extant records do not explain why it was necessary for the legislature to approve a new bill supporting the medical school when one had been passed just a few weeks earlier. It is nevertheless significant that, unlike its predecessor, the newly approved bill failed to receive Governor Warmoth's immediate signature.

While the bill sat on the governor's desk, Rev. Healy continued his search for a medical department facility, despite the uncertainty regarding secure funding for the medical school. In May 1870, a church building and adjacent property in New Orleans became available at a low price, and Healy proposed its purchase to the school's trustees and the AMA secretary in New York. "This property is 50 × 200," he explained to his superiors, "and extends between two streets. The lot on one Street, 50 × 150[,] is vacant and would make a good lot on which to build a Med. College. Very near the Charity Hospital."[22] Seymour Straight, however, felt that the property was unsuited for a medical school. "I see not how we could use 50 feet wide in a block . . . for a medical college, 80 being needed to give room light and ventilation. A Corner lot 60 feet wide would do well."[23] Discussions about the procurement and possible use of this property continued through the summer and into the fall. The fact that the debate centered over such details indicates that SU and AMA officials were still confident about the success of their fund-raising efforts.

Such confidence seemed justified when, in late summer, President Healy reported to readers of the *American Missionary*, the AMA's monthly magazine, that the Louisiana legislature had "adopted the Medical department, and made an appropriation of thirty five thousand dollars toward its endowment." He followed that disclosure with an announcement of the commencement of medical lectures "as soon as buildings and cabinets [of teaching and laboratory materials] have been secured."[24] The university's annual catalog also announced faculty members. Healy and Straight enlisted the services of seven local physicians, some quite prominent, including city health board president Charles B. White as dean, along with health board secretary S. C. Russell and well-known surgeon Andrew W. Smythe.[25]

The best laid plans of medical school organizers, however, appear to have been for naught, for the university never received the anticipated legislative appropriation. Though discussions about the acquisition and use of the St. James Church and adjoining property for the medical department continued into September,[26] SU did not operate a medical school during the 1870–71 academic year.[27]

SU's medical department failed to open because of the action of one member of the university's board of trustees, Gov. Henry Clay Warmoth. Warmoth, who had signed Act 81 providing the SU medical department with a $35,000 appropriation during the General Assembly's 1870 regular session, vetoed Bill 226 of the extra session ostensibly because the assistance it provided violated state constitution Article 140 forbidding state funding to private institutions.[28] Furthermore, the state auditor refused, on the same grounds, to issue warrants for payment of the $35,000 to the school. SU's trustees responded by filing suit for the funds through the state court system.[29]

In 1871, with the funding issue working its way through the courts, SU officials became involved with a second medical institution—a dispensary[30]—that brought to New Orleans the eventual dean and leader of the university's short-lived medical department. A Bristol, Rhode Island, businessman, Elisha Hathaway, donated land valued at $20,000 to the AMA. This property was earmarked for the care of indigent freed people in New Orleans.[31] During the 1871 legislative session the General Assembly approved appropriations to a number of benevolent associations around the state, including one for $5,000 requested by the trustees overseeing the new Hathaway Home for the Poor and Friendless, allowing them to open the establishment.[32] University officials hired James T. Newman, an African American physician originally from New Orleans then practicing in Chicago, to staff the home's dispensary, at a salary of $1,000 per year. With the planned medical department in mind, SU president Healy informed the AMA board in New York that Newman, "a colored physician of note," would also "act as medical advisor and instructor of our med. class."[33]

The arrival of a black physician in New Orleans on April 20, 1871, caused sufficient interest to prompt at least one local newspaper to cover the event. According to a reporter for the *Louisianian*, a leading black newspaper founded by prominent New Orleans businessman and politician P. B. S. Pinchback, Newman came to the Crescent City highly recommended by Moses Gunn, the distinguished chairman of the Department of Surgery at Rush Medical College in Chicago. Gunn called him "an able diagnostician and a bold and skillful surgeon, a sound practitioner and a polished gentleman." Another prominent Rush faculty member, J. Adams Allen, soon-to-be-named president of that medical school and current editor of the *Chicago Medical Journal*, indicated that Newman had published a number of articles in the medical literature that "have been generally reproduced throughout this country and Europe." After reporting these warm recommendations, the *Louisianian*, never mentioning Newman's race, extended the newly arrived physician a "welcome to our midst" and the wish that "he will succeed among us."[34]

Despite such high praise, Newman's medical credentials are difficult to verify. As far as can be determined, Newman never graduated from a medical school, though he may have enrolled and taken courses. He never provided clear and unequivocal information to Louisiana officials or medical directory compilers over the approximately fifty-five years he practiced medicine in the state. He could possibly have received his medical training through apprenticeship, for he did once allude, in correspondence with an AMA official, to his "preceptor."[35] His medical apprenticeship does not explain the educational data he submitted for publication in national directories. In these profiles, he variously claimed the University of Toronto and the New Orleans University Medical Department as his medical alma maters, but there are no corroborating records at either institution.[36] What can be documented about Newman's earlier career[37] are the nine articles he published in the *Chicago Medical Journal* between 1867 and 1869, and two in the *Chicago Medical Times*, a professional journal issued by members of the medical sect known as the Eclectics.[38] These articles indicate that he practiced briefly in an unidentified rural area and approximately five years in

Chicago before moving to New Orleans in 1871. Newman spoke French fluently, as evidenced by his translation of an article on the use of aconite in respiratory diseases for the *Chicago Medical Times*.[39] His knowledge of French was likely a legacy of his New Orleans heritage.

Few members of the New Orleans medical community evidently questioned Newman's medical credentials or his skills as a medical practitioner, for he obtained immediate access to the city's medical professional community. From 1871, shortly after his arrival, through at least 1875, he served as visiting surgeon at Charity Hospital, and from April 1873 through 1875 as a state sanitary inspector in New Orleans. His lucid annual reports as sanitary inspector tell of the varied public health problems facing the city at that time.[40] Those public health activities meshed well with Newman's work as medical director of the Hathaway Home for the Poor and Friendless, a post he held for several years. In this latter capacity, he annually provided medical care for hundreds of impoverished people of all colors and national origins, no doubt sending many of them to his surgical and medical wards at Charity Hospital for further treatment.[41]

With Newman's arrival in 1871, Straight officials had on their payroll an employee who could administer and teach at the proposed medical department. Because Newman moved to New Orleans before publication of SU's 1870–71 catalog, university officials were able to insert his name on the medical college faculty roster as an instructor at the school they hoped to open in the coming academic year. But Newman's presence in New Orleans unfortunately did not result in the immediate opening of SU's medical department. A year later, in August 1872, school officials were still promising that "lectures [in the medical department] will commence at an early day."[42] The trustees had taken legal action against the state auditor's refusal to warrant the $35,000 appropriation to the medical department, but the legal system worked slowly. The Eighth District Court of Orleans Parish had agreed with the trustees and ordered the auditor to issue warrants for payment, but the auditor had appealed the decision to the state supreme court.[43] That suit remained unresolved during the 1872–73 academic year.

Newman may have had an opportunity during that 1872–73 academic year to teach medical subjects to an advanced student. James Patrick Hays, a white pharmacy student who had previously studied at Queens College, Dublin, attended SU that year and received a master of pharmacy degree at Straight's June 1873 commencement exercises. SU's new president, Samuel S. Ashley, said of Hays, "Our first medical graduate is a *white man*."[44]

Not only did Hays not fit the SU founders' original conception of medical students, but he also did not receive an M.D. degree. Yet he was the only graduate of the Straight University Medical Department to receive an advanced degree. A second student, Leon Dewitt Stocking, author of a reportedly "well prepared thesis on 'Experimental Physiology,'" received a bachelor of medicine degree. (The degree remains a mystery, for it does not appear in contemporary SU catalogs.) At the closing ceremonies, Dr. Newman presented what one writer called "an able 'defence of the medical profession,' which received the hearty approval of the several disciples of Esculapius who were present."[45]

In May 1873, shortly before these graduation exercises, the trustees learned that the Louisiana Supreme Court had issued a ruling annulling the district court's order to pay the $35,000 appropriation to the medical school. The high court decided that because SU was a private corporation, controlled by a board of trustees responsible only to private individuals and not to the State of Louisiana, it was not a public institution of learning. The medical department, it concluded, was therefore, based on Article 140 of the 1868 Constitution, not eligible for the funds appropriated by the legislature.[46] Despite this seemingly fatal blow to SU's medical program, the medical school opened, and Dr. Newman finally taught medical students in the fall of 1873.

The Supreme Court's negative decision coincided with a dispute over integration at Louisiana State University (LSU). As a result of the state legislature's refusal to appropriate funds to all-white LSU, pursuant to state constitution Article 135, the segregated school's subsidy was diverted to integrated SU.[47]

On Monday evening, October 20, 1873, twenty-six-year-old James T. Newman, now dean of the Straight University Medical Department, and Louis A. Bell, professor of law, assembled their classes at the university buildings for opening exercises.[48] Both addressed the approximately twenty-five students, ten of whom had registered for the medical course. All were males, and some were white.[49] (No list of these first medical students' names has survived.) Newman reminded those present of the importance of the occasion: "It is no ordinary purpose that calls us together this evening. We do not come to debate any of the vexed questions now agitating our country from one end to the other. We do not come to speculate as to the probable character of the next Cabinet. We do not come to celebrate the commencement of an old and established institution. But we do come to inaugurate a new college devoted to the interests of medicine and surgery, the inauguration of which will mark the commencement of a new epoch in the history of the healing art in this city."[50] Newman then offered a long historical discourse on medicine and invention and perseverance that ended with an admonition to the students: They too would have to work hard and persevere to succeed in their chosen profession.

All seemed well that first evening, but there were problems that arose later at the fledgling school, not the least of which was money. Despite the state legislature's appropriation, SU was in a precarious financial situation. The national financial panic that year only compounded the problem. The AMA exerted strict central controls over fiscal matters from its New York headquarters. Payments for expenditures often took months, as Dr. Newman soon discovered. In addition, the

AMA overextended itself nationally by establishing too many schools too quickly and now found it had drastically to reduce funding for SU and other educational institutions.[51] As a result of these problems, new SU president Samuel S. Ashley, reviewing projected costs for the 1873–74 academic year with his superior in New York, wrote that he would try to "diminish somewhat the expenses to the [American Missionary] Assoc. of the Medical and Law Departments."[52] This is a surprising statement, given the medical department's already spare budget, which was composed only of Newman's $1,000 salary. Newman himself paid for such teaching materials as chemicals, books, and instruments.[53] SU's medical department operated not from new or leased facilities tailored and equipped for the needs of a medical school, as had been originally planned, but out of the university's main buildings, which were not ideally suited for medical instruction. The students had access to, and were expected to attend, teaching sessions at the surgical and medical wards that Newman directed at Charity Hospital. They were also expected to participate in anatomical demonstrations, probably at an off-campus site.[54] To all appearances, the school lacked funds for adequate laboratory equipment, facilities, and faculty. This situation did not bode well for the medical department's future.

Hiring appropriate teachers for the current term was a real concern. Newman, according to school records, was the only paid member of the medical faculty.[55] He had the authority to hire more faculty, though the source of funds to pay these teachers is not indicated in available records. In any case, Newman's search for colleagues was unsuccessful. Even with the help of friends in New Orleans and elsewhere, he was unable to hire instructors by the end of November, a month after the start of classes. At that time, Newman told one prospective professor: "There are several chairs vacant."[56] He did not elaborate on the cause of the openings.

Timely payment of salaries may have been a concern of prospective faculty members, for SU's medical department could not have opened at a less propitious time. In the aftermath of the financial Panic of 1873, everyone associated with the university was short of cash, including the students and SU officials who paid faculty salaries. President Ashley's daughter, Mary, described the situation to AMA field secretary E. M. Cravath in New York: "Please write what shall be done here about tuition. Times are very hard; Banks pay nothing—merchants have no money—and employers can not pay their employees—and if the tuition is insisted on many of our scholars must leave. Everything is in a bad condition here especially for the laboring classes."[57] This financial crisis exerted great pressure on SU, while the university tried to entice teachers to serve in the medical department. In November 1873, President Ashley wrote to AMA headquarters in New York that he had "borrowed until my credit is exhausted." He had "received nothing scarcely from Gen[eral Charles H.] Howard," who served as the Chicago district secretary for the AMA, "and yet was expected to pay the salary of Dr.

Newman" and other faculty members.[58] Charity Hospital's treasurer suggested to one potential medical department instructor in early October that he first check with AMA officials about "what you can depend on relative to the prompt payment of your salary" before accepting the position.[59] Local physicians who in previous years had agreed to serve on the faculty if the school opened may have contributed their time to present lectures or teach in the clinics, which would have been a great help to Newman, who had little luck recruiting and who appears to have undertaken much of the classroom and clinical instruction himself.[60] Beyond such minimal assistance, Newman operated the medical school alone.

Even Newman did not receive his pay in a timely manner during these hard times. Shortly after the medical department opened, the dean urgently requested "a prompt remittance" of his salary for the previous two months to "enable me to obtain Books, Chemicals and Instruments, which are absolutely necessary in the prosecution of the work on [*sic*] which I am engaged."[61] He was paid a month later.[62] This pattern of delinquent salary payments continued through the year.[63]

SU's financial situation had not improved by the close of the medical school's inaugural academic term on April 1, 1874. On the day that Newman informed AMA field secretary Erastus M. Cravath of the successful completion of the medical school's first year of instruction,[64] SU president Ashley advised Cravath of a board of trustees' resolution "that the Law and Medical Dep[artmen]ts should be self supporting." This decision meant that "the [American Missionary] Association will not be expected to carry them [the medical and law departments] after the present arrangements close."[65] Professors Bell and Newman were now on their own.[66]

Both instructors rose to the challenge. Students in the law school reacted in a way seemingly calculated to maintain good relations with SU officials. Most of the students, both white and black, Protestant and Catholic, arranged for themselves a scriptural study class for the summer and asked President Ashley to serve as their instructor every sabbath morning. Ashley wrote glowingly to an unidentified correspondent about the prospect of training Christian lawyers: "I therefore feel, that by aiding the Law Dept. the Assoc. is doing a religious, protestant, evangelical work. I think that Prof[.] Bell ardently desires and faithfully endeavors, to make his Department a moral and religious agency." Not so the medical school, according to Ashley. He concluded his remarks about the law department with a backhanded rebuke of Dr. Newman, providing the first hint in available AMA correspondence that the medical department did not enjoy the SU administration's full support: "With a pious man at the head of the Medical Dept. the same work could be done there."[67] Was Dr. Newman's religious commitment an issue?

Newman, apparently not a religious individual, and not backed by a class of religiously inclined medical students, took a straightforward, businesslike approach to the problem of saving his department. Unlike the law program, the medical department required funds to pay for more than simply a classroom, a collection of reference books, and a faculty member. Laboratories, a dissecting room, teaching models, equipment, supplies, and instructors, in addition to classrooms and a library, were necessary. Facilities during the 1873–74 academic year had been inadequate, and Newman was constantly vigilant for a building suitable for the medical school. He finally located one, on the corner of Common and Villeré streets, close to Charity Hospital and the wards that he oversaw there as a state sanitary inspector. Newman proposed its purchase to the trustees. The board, at the same meeting that removed funding from the medical department, granted the medical dean permission to raise money to purchase a medical school building.[68]

Financial and religious difficulties, it turned out, were not the only problems Newman confronted in his crusade to keep the medical department operating for a second year. Several SU trustees and President Samuel S. Ashley also opposed the school's continuance because the recently enacted state Civil Rights Act of 1873 promised equal access to all public institutions, including, they presumed, the state-subsidized medical school. Such access, they felt, eliminated the need for a parallel medical department at SU.[69] Ashley and others thus informed Field Secretary Cravath that they did not wish to extend the medical department's life. They also questioned Newman's suitability as dean. These remarks understandably put the dean on the defensive.[70] In early June, Newman, armed with the trustees' authorization to raise money to purchase a building, informed Cravath that he had "arranged my business that I will be able to start upon my mission on or about the last of this month." Well aware of Ashley's objections to his fund-raising efforts and to his continued service on the faculty, Newman sought reassurance from Cravath that the project "meets the approbation [of the] American Missionary Association" before he expended any time and effort. He addressed directly the negative comments others were making about him, denying their validity without further explanation, saying, "A great many of the objections urged against the medical Dept while you was [*sic*] in this city have been wiped away simply because they did not exist, and especially those against myself." He also asked Cravath for travel funds as a token of the AMA's support. "I am enthusiastic of success & only ask you to give me a trial."[71]

Newman must have been more persuasive than his opponents on the university's board of trustees, for a month later the SU Medical Department dean began his fund-raising mission with a note of thanks to Cravath and a request: "Please have my endorsments [*sic*] made out—Send money at your earliest conveince [*sic*]." In response to the field secretary's reiterated admonition to avoid soliciting money from church groups, Newman replied that he did "not expect to ask a cent of religious bodies." Showing the same enthusiasm and confidence he had displayed in some of his Chicago medical journal articles several years earlier, he stated, "I shall raise the money among medical men. My preceptor says that he will head the list with five thousand dollars." Newman did not elaborate as to the identity or location of this evidently wealthy former teacher. The letter, like others by the SU medical dean that summer, almost defiantly contained the return address of "Medical Department, Straight University, New Orleans."[72]

Unfortunately for Newman, he would not be able to use that return address for much longer. Just three weeks after writing that spirited letter to Cravath, Newman ran into a bigger impediment, one related to larger issues of New Orleans race relations and medical politics. These problems arose when a group of white physicians, intent on starting a medical school to compete with the University of Louisiana Medical Department (the predecessor to Tulane University Medical School), purchased the building Newman had selected at the corner of Villeré and Common streets. Dr. D. Warren Brickell, a well-known figure in antebellum medical circles, and his associates paid $40,000 for the building, frustrating Newman's grand plan and angering him because, as he explained to Cravath, "we could have bought it for ([$]20,000)." Like the medical students at the University of Louisiana Medical Department and SU, students at this newly formed Charity Hospital Medical College had access to Charity Hospital's wards.[73]

Newman saw the loss of the building and the opening of Charity Hospital Medical College as direct threats to African American accessibility to New Orleans' medical schools. "This second school in this city will make more objections than the old school [University of Louisiana Medical Department] did against the colored Medical student," he explained in a letter to Cravath. Though some people had argued, "predicated upon the Justice of the civil rights Bill [of 1873]," that "the colored student would have no difficulty in entering the State University [University of Louisiana Medical Department]," Newman felt these people were either misinformed or jealous of SU's medical program. "They spoke without proper advisement," he told Cravath, "or with an intention of checking the growth of our infant [medical] department."

Taking a cynical position, the Straight University Medical Department dean asserted, "Human ingenuity framed and passed that [civil rights] Bill. Human ingenuity can readily find ways and means to circumvent it." To support his allegation, Newman pointed to what he described as "a tacit understanding" between the white school's faculties "that colored students are not to be admitted." School authorities had inserted a clause in their catalogs barring students from admission until they pass an examination given by the faculty as a means of implementing white-only admissions. Though an examination appeared to be a reasonable requirement, Newman contended it was a ploy. "[I]f I was a member of any faculty and was disposed to be unjust, Sir Astley Cooper might present himself and I could keep him out."[74] "From what I have said you can readily see the necessity of a colored school," insisted Newman, who felt that his situation had become desperate.

Since the loss of the prospective school site, the Straight University Medical

Department's dean had been surveying other properties and now proposed to Cravath his "last resort": the purchase of a "magnificent Hospital" building that well-known New Orleans physician Warren Stone had built "many years ago." Newman reported that the structure, located "only one block from charity Hospital," on the corner of Claiborne and Canal, "could easily be converted into a medical school" if he could raise $5,000 to purchase it. Though "Dr Stones [*sic*] Building is sadly in need of repairs," Newman thought that "three thousand dollars will put it in a splendid condition for our purposes." He now urgently requested the AMA's approval to raise funds for the purchase and refurbishing of this structure: "If the Association will only not withdraw their protectorate from around me I will yet build up a Medical school that we may all feel proud of." Again showing both his verbal flair and his excitement over the prospect of opening a medical school for African Americans, Newman concluded his letter in memorable style: "I am as confident of success as Columbus was of the existence of a new world."[75]

Newman's confidence appears to have won him a second chance at obtaining a permanent home for his medical school, but not enough to win him sufficient funds for completion of his plan. As late as the end of October, Newman still had not collected sufficient funds to purchase Stone's hospital building. The Straight University Medical Department consequently did not open.[76]

Why did so worthy an enterprise fail when there was an obvious need for a medical school to train African American physicians? Two strong personalities, one white, one black—Rev. Joseph Healy and Dr. James T. Newman—both worked hard to establish the school. Their lack of success can be attributed to several factors, but money appears to be the overriding reason. Even before the Panic of 1873 undermined the finances of SU and the AMA, SU's board of trustees could not raise sufficient funds to open the medical department. Like other Northern Christian missionary schools, Straight's primary focus was providing a basic college or normal school education for newly freed slaves, not offering professional training. The trustees consequently channeled most of their resources to the core curricula. SU officials did try to take advantage of Louisiana's Reconstruction political turmoil over school integration to obtain a legislative appropriation for the medical department, but the plan backfired when the governor, the state auditor, and the Supreme Court successfully reversed the General Assembly's action. Then poor money management at AMA headquarters and the consequences of the Panic of 1873 placed the burden of establishing the medical school on Dr. James T. Newman's shoulders.

Newman seemed adequate for the task, but money was not the only issue he faced. In addition to unspecified personality and religious conflicts with some board members, Newman also encountered racism within the New Orleans medical profession and resistance from his own university's trustees regarding the need for an African American medical school. The forces arrayed against the establishment of SU's medical department were overwhelming in the early 1870s. It would be more than a decade before an African American medical school would open in New Orleans, under the auspices of a different religious organization; once again, Dr. Newman was involved.[77]

CHAPTER 14

The Education of Black Physicians at Shaw University, 1882–1918

In the 1912 Leonard Medical School (LMS) catalog, Charles F. Meserve, the institution's president, boasted, "As a proof of the wisdom of the policy and methods of the Leonard Medical School, it can be stated that its graduates rarely fail to win for themselves positions of influence and usefulness in the communities where they settle. They are not obliged to go to States where a license is not required in order to practice medicine."[1] Two years later, in 1914, having trained more than four hundred black physicians in its thirty-two years on the Raleigh, North Carolina, campus of Shaw University, LMS reduced its medical education program from a full four-year to a limited two-year (basic science) curriculum. In 1918, Leonard closed its doors forever. How could LMS's status change so radically in so short a time? Why did it close if its graduates were performing so well on licensing exams and in the communities where they practiced?

As mentioned in Chapter 11, Leonard was not the only black medical school to open and then cease operations during the late nineteenth and early twentieth centuries (see Appendix, Table 4). Of the fourteen founded during this time, all of which began with similar high hopes, only two—Howard and Meharry—endured beyond the early 1920s. One might argue that these schools were not providing medical training equal to that offered at, for example, Johns Hopkins or Harvard. Some in the medical reform establishment of the time saw little value in schools that turned out lesser-trained physicians. Abraham Flexner's famous 1910 report on medical education in the United States spoke for those with such attitudes: "A well-taught negro sanitarian will be immensely useful; an essentially untrained negro wearing an M.D. degree is dangerous."[2]

Were these medical schools really so poor as to deserve the fate they suffered? Did external pressures contribute to their demise? Judgments of quality aside, did LMS and other black medical schools provide for needs in the black population of the United States that would not have been met otherwise? The answers to these questions are important because, after 1923, only Howard and Meharry remained to train the vast majority of African American physicians in the United States. The small number of black physicians in practice during the remainder of the twentieth century can be attributed in part to the closing of schools like Leonard.

Information about the demise of the black medical schools is difficult to obtain. Though the American Medical Association (AMA) published annual education and state licensure exam reports, neither the AMA nor the Association of American Medical Colleges (AAMC) preserved many original papers, letters, and unpublished reports or minutes of meetings of the late nineteenth century. Some important information was exchanged among leaders in medical education at the Carnegie Foundation for the Advancement of Teaching (a cosponsor of the Flexner Report) and the General Education Board (a philanthropic wing of the Rockefeller family fortune that donated large sums to medical education). Those papers have been preserved, but with one notable exception, records of black medical schools are scarce. The small archives department in the Shaw University Library in Raleigh contains invaluable material on some of the operations of LMS. On the Colgate-Rochester Divinity School campus in Rochester, New York, is another small cache of papers on Leonard—part of the American Baptist Historical Society collections. From these documents we can reconstruct a history of Leonard. The problems it encountered in its attempt to provide quality medical education to a generally poor, undereducated racial minority in the late-nineteenth- and early-twentieth-century South were typical of all such schools. Though the details were, of course, different for each school, the basic problems were similar. Leonard can serve as a case study for black medical education at those institutions.

The seeds of failure at Leonard were sown early. Internal problems grew unchecked, making it increasingly difficult to respond to external pressures of the medical reform era. The school never had a chance to be self-sustaining. It could have been saved and improved, but no one was willing to take the necessary steps at any time in its thirty-six-year history.

LMS was an addition to Shaw University, one of those post–Civil War institutions of higher learning established by Northerners to educate freed people.[3] The New York–based American Baptist Home Mission Society (ABHMS), an organization with a long tradition of benevolence and missionary zeal, sponsored and supported Shaw in Raleigh as it grew from a small struggling school for local freed people in 1865 to one of the larger and more highly regarded colleges for African

Americans at the turn of the century. During the period from 1865 to 1920, Shaw offered college preparatory, college-level, and theological courses as well as, for various lengths of time, legal, pharmaceutical, medical, and missionary training programs.[4] With fateful significance, Shaw was maintained as a charity institution, part of the larger mission of Northern Baptists to aid and educate former slaves and their children and grandchildren. Funds came from the outside, for the most part, not from student fees, endowment funds, or local support—a weak system of funding that would plague the institution for much of its history.

The medical school at Shaw had its origins in the dreams of Henry M. Tupper (1811–93), the university's founder and first president. A white native of Massachusetts, Tupper joined the Army of the Potomac shortly after graduating from Newton Theological Seminary in 1862 during the Civil War. Deeply interested in serving the religious needs of African Americans, the young minister decided, upon the cessation of hostilities, to do missionary work among the freed people in Raleigh, North Carolina, under the auspices of the ABHMS. Tupper worked with small groups of blacks and, during the second half of 1865, established a "theological class" that became the basis of a school.[5] Relying on contacts developed with the Freedmen's Bureau, ABHMS, and Baptists in Massachusetts, Tupper gained enough financial support to establish a permanent school to train African Americans for the ministry. In 1870, Elijah Shaw, a woolen manufacturer of Wales, Massachusetts, donated $5,000 to aid in the purchase of land for a permanent home for the "Raleigh Institute." For this gift (and later ones) the school was renamed in his honor.[6]

According to Henry L. Morehouse, a white officer of the ABHMS and well-known champion of black education during the late nineteenth century, Tupper had decided as early as 1866 to add a medical school at Shaw University when it became feasible.[7] The president of Shaw explained this desire in the university catalogs during the 1870s: "The colored people at present are without educated Physicians, and thus are subject to all manner of quackery and imposition, and many suffer and die for want of medical attention."[8] Though the need was there, the wherewithal to undertake so ambitious an enterprise was not. Howard University had started its medical school in 1868 with, in part, federal financial support.[9] Central Tennessee College had just opened its medical department under the auspices of private philanthropists (the Meharry brothers) and the Freedmen's Aid Society of the Methodist Episcopal Church.[10] Tupper had broached the subject of a medical school at Shaw several times with the ABHMS board and wealthy, public-spirited Northerners, but as of 1878 had received only words of encouragement. He reported great interest and enthusiasm among his students for the opening of a medical school.[11]

So anxious was the president to see this project through that he made a proposal to the ABHMS board that would later undermine the maintenance of the institution. At the time, however, the idea seemed logical, applicable, and feasible. Tupper's communication to the board read:

> 1st. I offer to purchase a site for building said department.
> 2nd. I will deliver the brick on the ground free of expense for said building, the building to be about 40 × 60 feet, three stories high.
> 3rd. I estimate that it will cost about $5,000 to erect the building and furnish it.
> 4th. I propose to find five men who will give $1,000 each, and think I can do it with the blessing of the Lord.
> 5th. Form a class next October, and have the building completed one year from next October.
> 6th. Make the tuition pay for the medical instruction.
> 7th. If there be objections to having the Home Mission Society engage in such a department of work, let the trustees operate this department of the school independent of the Home Mission Society. Why not? We are all brethren.
> 8th. There is no medical college for colored people from Washington to New Orleans.[12]

He managed to gain the board's official, conditional, but still only spiritual endorsement in December 1878.[13] Tupper then quickly took action.

He did not find five $1,000 donors; instead he came up with one, his brother-in-law, Judson Wade Leonard of Hampden, Massachusetts, who pledged the whole $5,000 on condition that a matching amount be raised within six months.[14] The Home Mission Board endorsed Leonard's philanthropy and encouraged others to follow suit by publicizing the gift in its new magazine, the *Baptist Home Mission Monthly*.[15] To raise remaining funds, Tupper traveled north after the spring 1880 school term. He returned to Raleigh in July with $3,900 in cash and pledges, enough to feel confident about further pursuit of his proposal.[16]

Shaw students had actually been engaged in digging clay for brickmaking since January 1880. Now the work began in earnest.[17] The thirty-four-room medical dormitory was completed in the spring of 1881.[18] While the dormitory was under construction, Tupper turned his energies to securing land for a medical classroom and laboratory building. An appeal to the North Carolina General Assembly netted Shaw a square acre of land adjacent to the campus—land that had been part of the governor's mansion. The legislature designated this plot specifically for Shaw's medical school.[19] Spurred by this success in March 1881, Tupper turned again to his wife's brother to fund the medical science building, and Leonard again came through. By the fall of 1882, LMS had two new buildings and some extra land.[20] Tupper then secured the services of "some of the

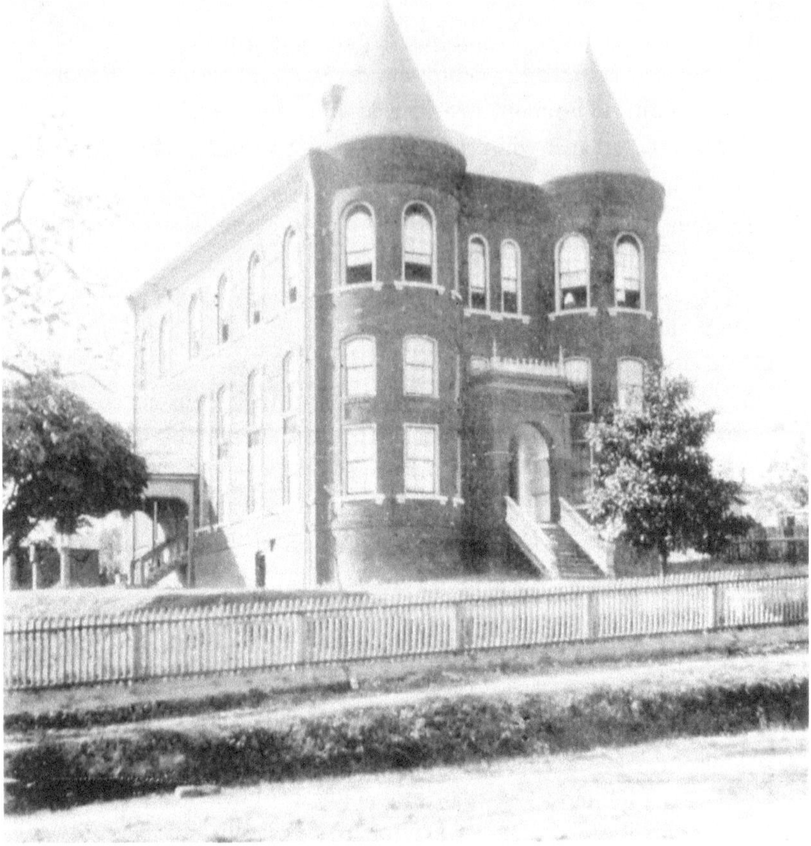

Fig. 6. Leonard Medical School, Shaw University. This building, adjacent to the campus, was constructed in 1882 on an acre of land that the North Carolina legislature designated for Shaw's medical school. From *The 29th Annual Catalog of the Officers and Students of the Leonard Medical School . . . For the Academic Year Ending May 31, 1909* (Raleigh, N.C.: Edwards & Broughton, 1909).

leading white physicians of Raleigh" to teach at the school and obtained partial support from drug manufacturers for establishment of a dispensary (a kind of outpatient clinic) so "that our medical students may have the advantages of clinical instruction."[21] During the previous year, thirteen students had pursued a preliminary medical course in anticipation of matriculation at Leonard. Tupper was pleased with the school's progress. The only hint of future problems was this brief allusion in an enthusiastic report to *Baptist Home Mission Monthly* readers in the summer of 1882: "If we have the ability to furnish our medical building with apparatus and appliances, so as to make it a first-class medical school, we may expect to see it crowded with students."[22]

That was a big "if," especially in view of the sixth and seventh items in Tupper's proposal to the ABHMS board. These portions guaranteed that tuition fees would cover the cost of medical instruction. LMS was to be self-sufficient—not a drain on Shaw's other programs or on the university's main financial support, the ABHMS. The ABHMS board, in fact, had emphasized from the outset that though it approved of Leonard, it also had no financial obligations to the school.[23] Here then was the root of Leonard's biggest problem and the cause of its ultimate failure—money. The problem existed from the school's inception. Tuition fees never paid the medical instruction expenses. The Leonard family's gifts really amounted only to the funding of two buildings, establishment of a small ($5,000) scholarship fund, and occasional small donations to cover shortfalls in operating expenses. A few donations from the Rockefeller family over the years helped ease specific financial problems.[24] But no substantial endowment fund existed. No other Northern philanthropists and no wealthy graduates of the medical school gave large sums to LMS. The state offered no further assistance. Leonard, in fact, soon became a financial drain on Shaw, precisely the situation Tupper and the ABHMS board had sought to avoid. Leonard could not become the first-class institution Tupper had dreamed about until it obtained proper funding. That never happened.

Tupper, of course, understood Leonard's financial needs, but could not have predicted their persistence in November 1882, when the first class of students formally began its studies. He simply proceeded according to plan. The school catalog for 1881–82 listed eight students in the preliminary course and seven in the regular recitation course (though two students were listed in both).[25] The following academic year (1882–83), during which the medical school had its official opening, three young men matriculated as second-year students and eight as first-year students. At the end of that school term, Tupper expressed satisfaction, pronounced the school "a grand success," and praised the students in nineteenth-century white paternalistic terms: "In the medical department, the closing examination was very satisfactory indeed. The students have studied with diligence and more enthusiasm than I have ever witnessed among colored students, and those competent to judge, do not hesitate to give as their opinion, that the class has made as much progress as is usually done by white students. Our medical school is a grand success."[26]

Leonard soon received national recognition from two different sources. First, the newly created John F. Slater Fund, established by a Massachusetts businessman to assist in the education of worthy black students, donated $500 to LMS, half for purchase of medical apparatus, half for student scholarships. Though the amount fluctuated, Slater Fund money aided LMS annually until 1905.[27] Second, *Medical News*, a prestigious Philadelphia medical journal, included a one-column piece on the school based on information contained in the college catalog and Shaw's student newspaper, the *African Expositor*. The story, written by one of Shaw's trustees, Dr. W. W. Keen, extended a warm welcome to LMS and a wish for its success. "[Blacks] need physicians of their own race, and this medical school will not only provide them, but will also open a new avenue of self-support to the black man."[28]

Ironically, Leonard received a very different sort of greeting from home-state physicians. Noting that his information derived from the *Medical News* article rather than directly from authorities at LMS, Thomas F. Wood, editor of the *North Carolina Medical Journal* (Wilmington), remarked, "We have never seen any authoritative account of this Medical College, but we trust that the good sense of the managers of it will prevail, and that they will allow it to cease, before much harm is done."[29] Because, according to his information, the school had shorter terms than at other medical colleges and only a three-year curriculum, Wood felt LMS graduates would be less well trained than their white counterparts. "In fact a much larger course should be prescribed for them, as they have more difficulties to overcome." Blacks, he continued, lacked the "degree of inborn quickness of perception of which the higher races are remarkable, and superadded to this a long training of the senses, and an immense amount of learning is necessary for success in the medical profession."[30] The editor then jabbed at the smallness of Raleigh, the quality of LMS's teaching staff (three white Raleigh physicians), and the poor learning capability blacks had displayed in other educational situations. He predicted the failure of the medical school.[31]

Though black students did have some educational deficiencies owing to poor basic schooling and the constant pressures of poverty, Tupper remained undaunted. At first, he later recalled, "there were few who had pursued their [preliminary] studies a sufficient length of time to commence that of medicine, and it took two years—from 1880 to 1882—to find half a dozen in all our schools who were competent to enter our Medical Department."[32] That problem seemed to have been overcome by the 1885–86 session. Once embarked on the new medical course, Tupper, his white medical faculty, and his black medical students strove for success.

Thanks to the generosity of Northern friends of Shaw University, the lecture rooms and laboratories were soon stocked with supplies and anatomy models.[33] In January 1885 the twenty-five-bed Leonard Hospital opened its doors to the sick and poor of the local black community and to the medical students of Leonard. Clinical instruction, increasingly recognized as an essential component of good medical education, was now provided. (Unfortunately for patients and students, for those months when school was out of session, the hospital was closed.) Again, as with all other aspects of LMS's development, private Northern philanthropy and local black fund-raising through fairs and community appeals financed the school's programs. The ABHMS allocated no money.[34]

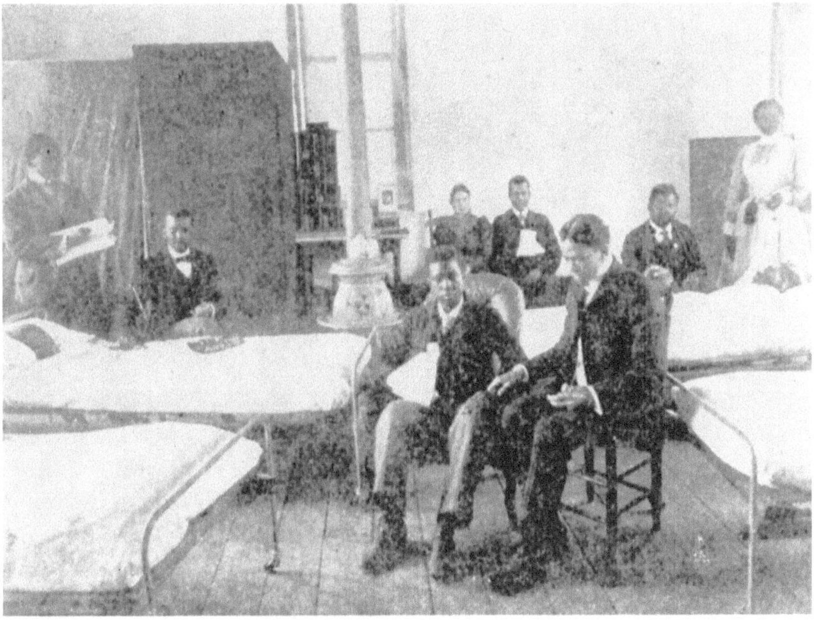

Fig. 7. Male ward in Leonard Hospital. From copy in North Carolina Collection, University of North Carolina Wilson Library, Chapel Hill.

When, in 1886, the first six students had completed their studies and exams and were ready for graduation, Shaw University celebrated. The Reverend Mr. Tupper wrote in the school's newspaper, "Few events connected with the founding of Shaw University have ever awakened so deep an interest as the closing exercises of the Leonard Medical School, on the evening of March 31st."[35] In addition to students and invited guests, a large number of interested black citizens attended the ceremonies. Eugene Grissom, M.D., superintendent of the North Carolina Insane Asylum in Raleigh (later called Dorothea Dix Hospital), who delivered the keynote address, treated the occasion with the same seriousness and earnestness found at a white medical school graduation. Not once did he allude to the uniqueness of this commencement or to the race of the young physicians being honored.[36] It was Lawson A. Scruggs of Liberty, Virginia, the class valedictorian and soon-to-be resident physician at Leonard Hospital, who brought home that message to an audience that did not really need reminding. "The colored man must go forward," he announced in an oration titled "Medical Education as a Factor in the Elevation of the Colored Race." "He must harness himself for the battle, and we who stand before you tonight, are pioneers of the medical profession of our race." He concluded with the hope that physicians of color would increase rapidly in number and so improve black health, both at home and in Africa, and that the race would then be in a position to concern itself with spiritual, moral, and economic elevation.[37]

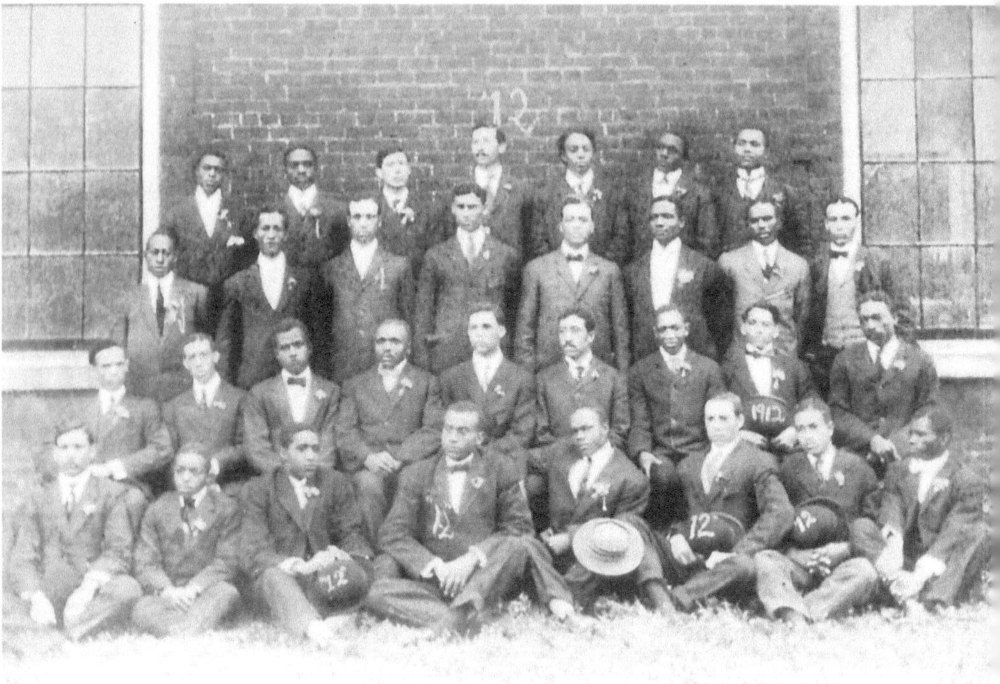

Fig. 8. Class of 1912, Leonard Medical School. From *The 29th Annual Catalog of the Officers and Students of the Leonard Medical School . . . For the Academic Year Ending May 31, 1909* (Raleigh, N.C.: Edwards & Broughton, 1909).

Demonstrating the capabilities of blacks as physicians, Leonard's first graduates succeeded admirably on the state licensure exams. Tupper reported gleefully in 1886 to the school's trustees and to the ABHMS, "The best evidence that the school is doing good work is the fact that those who graduated at the close of last session and recently presented themselves before the State Medical Board passed a creditable examination, much to the surprise of some of the examiners. The scene as described by one of our faculty, also a member of the State Medical Board, was, to say the least, intensely interesting and exceedingly gratifying."[38] During Tupper's remaining seven years as president of Shaw, LMS sources reported that students who graduated continued to perform well on state boards.[39] Meanwhile, regular LMS budgetary deficits seemed to disappear with the annual emergency financial help of Northern friends, medical faculty teaching by local physicians remained stable and satisfactory,[40] and new black doctors found good locations for their practices.[41] Leonard Medical School was, to all outward appearances, succeeding.

On November 12, 1893, Shaw University and LMS marked the end of an era: Rev. Henry M. Tupper died after twenty-eight years of service to the institution he had founded. To succeed him, the ABHMS and the university's trustees selected Charles Francis Meserve, a forty-four-year-old New Englander with twelve years' experience as superintendent of Haskell Institute, a large American Indian industrial training school in Lawrence, Kansas.[42]

Meserve found financial matters at Shaw in an alarming state when he arrived on campus in March 1894: "I found the departments of Law, Medicine and Pharmacy in good condition, but it is these three departments that have caused the financial strain through which the University is passing. . . . I am not prepared to recommend the discontinuance of these departments for the reason that they are of such high order and have done such grand work. . . . It is, however, but true to state that these departments cannot continue unless money is forthcoming from some source."[43]

Meserve thus put the school's trustees and the ABHMS on notice that he would not jeopardize Shaw's existence for the sake of the medical, law, and pharmacy schools. It was not that he opposed training black professionals. On the contrary, in an interview Meserve granted a *Raleigh News and Observer* reporter in September 1895, the president stated, "The colored people need those of their own race in the professions. . . . Why, now, we can't begin to supply the demand for physicians. Not long ago, I had a letter from the private secretary of the Governor of Alabama, asking us to send them physicians, there was a county containing 22,000 colored people, with no physicians among them of their own race."[44] For Meserve, though, Leonard was but part of a greater enterprise—Shaw University. When he acted to close the medical school some twenty years later, he did so to save that larger enterprise.

The institution's financial instability was, of course, an old story. As early as 1886, the year of Leonard's first graduation ceremony, the need for a large endowment fund had been recognized. Using the *African Expositor* and the *Baptist Home Mission Monthly*, Tupper at that time made regular appeals to Northern Baptists for $40,000 or $50,000 and, when that amount was not forthcoming, for $25,000. In an 1886 article titled "The Leonard Medical School, Shaw University—Its Endowment a Necessity," Tupper further explained that the $5,000 endowment fund Leonard then possessed yielded only about $250 per annum, which, combined with the low tuition of $60 per student, barely paid operating expenses such as fuel, repairs, and regular additions to the teaching equipment. Salaries for the instructors alone totaled $2,750, an amount difficult to raise each year. These regular appeals for money from Northern friends consumed much of Tupper's time and energy. "We are sure," he continued, "a moment of reflection will convince any one that the present financial condition of our Medical Department must be a source of anxiety, if not wasted energies."[45] By the spring of 1888, two graduating classes later, the situation had not changed. For the previous six months the *Baptist Home Mission Monthly* had advertised for "a $25,000 Christian philanthropist," but to no avail.[46] Still, Tupper and the

ABHMS "earnestly hoped for" his appearance.[47] An expanded version of Dr. Scruggs's valedictory address on black medical education was published in the Christmas 1888 issue of the *Monthly* in hopes of stimulating interest, but again with no success.[48]

Other Southern black schools found themselves facing similar situations. By the late 1880s and 1890s, the strong sense of mission that had stimulated and sustained Northern interest in the welfare of former slaves was waning. The very term "freedman" now seemed anachronistic. Though missionary organizations like the ABHMS continued to provide evidence of Southern blacks' educational needs, Northern benefactors seemed to be losing the paternalistic spirit that had existed twenty-five and thirty years earlier. Black migration to Northern towns and new interests in caring for the large numbers of European immigrants in the northern United States also contributed to a declining concern for Southern blacks. Furthermore, money had become tighter during the economic turmoil of the 1890s. Not surprisingly, then, ABHMS field secretary Henry L. Morehouse wrote a long article for the *Monthly* in 1894 proclaiming "a great crisis in our educational work for the colored people and the Indians." The ABHMS could not, he maintained, support with present funds all the educational activities for which it was responsible without curtailing its other, equally important missionary work. In explaining the need for a permanent endowment to relieve this crisis, Morehouse pointed to the severe distress at Shaw. "Even now, the very existence of the excellent medical and industrial department of Shaw University is trembling in the balance for the lack of $6,000. Dr. Tupper's death takes away the skillful management which has kept those departments in successful operation. They are not and cannot be maintained by the Society, both for lack of means and because this is not its legitimate work."[49] It was at this inauspicious moment in Leonard's financial history that Meserve assumed the presidency of Shaw.

The situation was grim. Meserve discovered and reported to the Slater Fund agent in a carefully written but frank letter of appeal that for a few years before his death Tupper had borrowed "large sums of money at a high rate of interest to keep the institution alive." He described in detail Tupper's actions to save the medical school.

> My predecessor was enabled to keep the institution going only by devoting all the money he could possibly collect from the students and other sources to paying the salaries of the medical professors. Even this was not sufficient, for year by year he was obliged to transfer funds from other departments to the medical, and, after this was done there was a large deficiency which was met by borrowing from banks. This is not all paid yet. To such an extent was this carried on that he was not able to equip the medical school with the apparatus that is so indispensable in such

> an institution. Furthermore, the buildings in all departments have been neglected, and imperatively demanded repairs were not made, so that all the money possible from all departments might be saved and devoted to paying the salaries in the medical department. To such an extent was this carried on that some of the buildings were endangered, and there is not a building here but what needs extensive repairs both outside and inside in order to prevent decay and destruction.[50]

Not only was LMS in danger of failing, but its problems were threatening Shaw as a whole.

Meserve believed that nonreligious activities such as medical education were not the proper work of missionary associations such as the ABHMS. He felt strongly that Shaw should remain first and foremost a vehicle for teaching Baptist principles to African Americans and for producing good, Christian teachers who would then spread their knowledge and faith to other African Americans. As he explained it to the Slater Fund agent, "It would be impracticable for the Home Mission Society, organized distinctively for the prosecution of Missions and collecting its money from the churches for that purpose, to engage in the general work of educating Negroes of the South especially along the higher professional lines. . . . It does not feel warranted . . . in attempting to carry on a Medical School, a School of Pharmacy, and a Law School, to be paid for out of its Mission fund."[51]

Desperate to eliminate the primary drain on Leonard's fiscal resources—medical faculty salaries—Meserve described the problem in full to Slater Fund agent J. L. M. Curry, and asked for help. The $1,000 that Slater already gave annually paid the salaries of two medical school teachers, both of whom received $100 per month for the five-month term. Meserve now asked Slater also to pick up the six remaining faculty salaries, totaling $2,750, "to save the life of the institution." He minced no words. "The closing of the medical school is staring us in the face on account of inability to meet running expenses." In addition to financial exigencies, Meserve argued, Shaw was a fitting recipient of Slater money because the funds would be used to pay an unusual faculty. "Its Faculty is unique, consisting of seven white Professors, men who were born and bred in the South and who are all practicing physicians in the City. . . . These white physicians [are] doing more to break down any prejudice that may have existed and to build up education for the colored people in the South, than could be done in any other way."[52] For reasons not spelled out in Slater Fund or other records, that organization refused to increase its allowance to Leonard, and, in fact, ten years later ceased funding the medical school entirely.[53]

Somehow, by dint of skimping and sacrificing on the part of faculty and students, Shaw and Leonard made it through the 1895 crisis. The old debts were paid off.[54] But again, the basic problem had not been solved, only patched over. Leonard needed an endowment so that its instructors could be paid, its needy students funded with scholarships, its laboratories and classrooms regularly restocked with supplies, and its hospital enlarged and open year-round. Leonard needed to grow with the times, but it could not.

Outside the walls of LMS times were certainly changing for medicine. Louis Pasteur and Robert Koch had proven that microbes caused disease, ushering in the era of bacteriology. German scientists had moved medicine into the laboratory, from which they were reporting exciting developments in pathology, physiology, immunology, and microbiology. Innovative surgery was being performed. Students studying abroad brought these new techniques and ideas back to the United States, where standards of medical education began to improve. The opening of the Johns Hopkins Medical School in 1893 symbolized that improvement. Furthermore, some medical educators began to feel that the rapid, uncontrolled proliferation of proprietary medical schools, which had been occurring since the Civil War, had to be reversed. The Association of American Medical Colleges, the American Medical Association's Council on Medical Education, and the individual state boards of medical examiners all now strove to increase the standards of medical education.[55]

These changes were occurring just as Leonard Medical School was getting its start. As the AAMC gained more member schools and began setting standards, and as state examining boards incorporated more and more new medical and basic scientific information into their tests, medical colleges like Leonard found themselves in trouble. Longer school terms, better-trained faculty members, improved clinical facilities, modern technological and chemical equipment, new laboratories, and solidly educated students were needed.

Failure rates on state licensure exams became the measure of a school's worth once the AMA began publishing this information in 1904. Leonard did not fare so well, in comparison either with some of the other black schools or with other medical students around the country (see figure 9). In the periodic inspections that the AMA's Council on Medical Education made after 1904, Leonard always received C ratings, compared with Howard's and Meharry's As and Bs.[56] Flexner, in 1910, had little good to say. Of LMS's laboratory facilities, for example, he reported, "These comprise a clean and exceedingly well kept dissecting-room, a slight chemical laboratory, and a still slighter equipment for pathology. There are no library, no museum, and no teaching accessories. It is evident that the policy of paying practitioners [to teach] has absorbed the resources of a school that exists for purely philanthropic objects." The report added that clinical facilities were "normal," consisting of a sixteen-bed hospital with only three patients at the time of the visit, and "no dispensary [outpatient clinic] at all."[57] Flexner's comments underscored the problems facing Leonard.

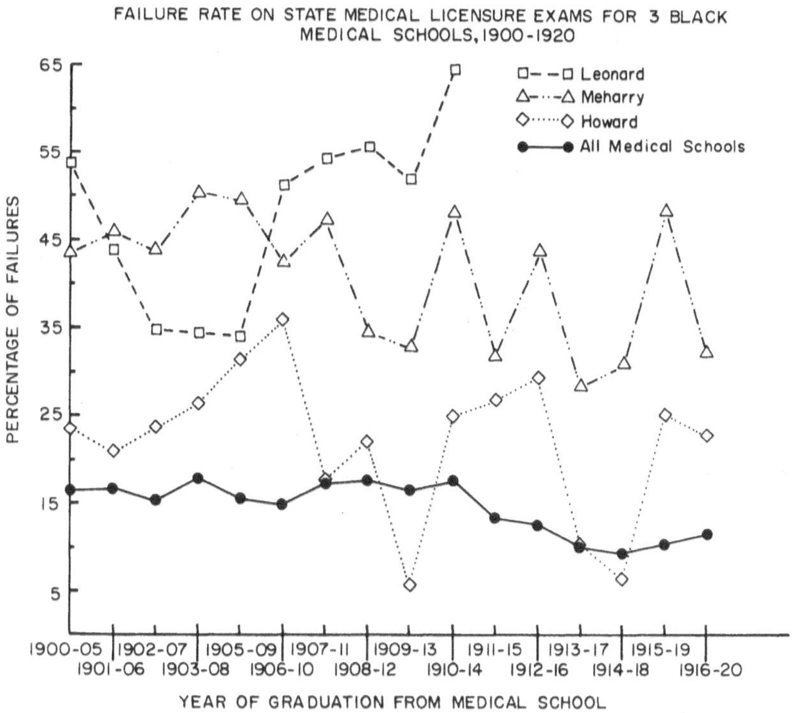

Fig. 9. Failure rate on state medical licensure exams for three black medical schools, 1900–1920.

Spurred on by these negative statements, the school's administration tried desperately to keep up. Terms were lengthened gradually from four to eight months, laboratories were upgraded and new ones built, microscopes were purchased, admissions standards were raised, more faculty and courses were added, and finally in 1911 a new, modern hospital was constructed.[58] But still, the core of the matter was that lack of money wore Leonard down. The local Raleigh physicians who made up the faculty did their best, but many had trained in the pre-bacteriology era with its different approach to medicine. They gave their time at no small cost. LMS could not afford to bring in many of the new breed of scientific physicians or basic science teachers. The school was too far behind to catch up without a large infusion of money to upgrade faculty, students, and facilities. Despite Meserve's optimism in the 1912 catalog, Leonard was doomed. Rockefeller's General Education Board saw Meharry, a bigger, more dynamic black medical school in Nashville, and Howard, more visible in Washington, D.C., and possessing better facilities, as the logical recipients of its largess in the area of black medical education.[59] Leonard did not have the growth potential, the financial strength, or the strong faculty to meet the higher educational standards of a new era.

Unquestionably, more black physicians were needed, and General Education Board money could have been well spent at Leonard. Letters from Leonard graduates in practice indicated that they were faring well, seemingly as well as their counterparts from Howard and Meharry.[60] At the end of the 1914 term, however, LMS closed the newly built Leonard Hospital and reduced its program to a two-year basic science curriculum. In 1918 LMS closed its doors forever. The editors of the black-run *Journal of the National Medical Association* sadly and reluctantly agreed with the trustees' decision:

> Our . . . requiem for the school . . . is fare thee well Old Leonard, your work is done. Honor to you and to the lamented and beloved Dr. Henry M. Tupper who brought you into existence. Honor to those who fostered you and gave you support. Honor to your noble professors. Honor to the many sons whom you sent into the world who are today the only living vestige of your having existed. We love you, Old Leonard, and mourn your loss, but we recognize that this is a new era, a new day has dawned—your work is done. . . . All standards of education, and especially medical education, have been raised. . . . Not being able to meet these exacting conditions, it was necessary that you die, and while it is with great sorrow, we had far rather bid thee farewell than to have you merely to exist.[61]

Leonard closed because of underfinancing, because no individual or organization was willing to step in and support it monetarily. By 1910, when Flexner wrote his negative report, even the promise of a new clinical facility (the expanded Leonard Hospital) could not alter the school's pattern of decline. Leonard needed an endowment and operating capital to pay professors, buy equipment, maintain teaching and clinical laboratories, and provide for the other usual expenses of a modern medical school. Instead, the school drew off funds from the rest of the university, impeding, indeed reversing, the growth of the larger institution. Meserve had to close Leonard to save Shaw. He could hang on no longer. So, having satisfied a need for some thirty-six years, LMS passed quietly from existence.[62]

CHAPTER 15

Training the "Consecrated, Skillful, Christian Physician"

Student Life at Leonard Medical School

In the 1909 catalog of Leonard Medical School (LMS), a black medical college affiliated with Shaw University in Raleigh, North Carolina, the institution's white president, Charles F. Meserve, laid out in no uncertain terms, as he had for the past decade, the philosophy of the school and the conditions under which students worked:

> The race is greatly in need of consecrated, skilled Physicians and Surgeons, and the Leonard Medical School has been established to meet this want. No one can do more to improve the daily life of the masses than the consecrated, skillful, Christian physician. . . . Not *self*, but the *race*, must ever be his motto, and this requires not ability alone but the most rugged and strongest character. . . . Young men of clean, pure lives, honest and reliable, and total abstainers from the use of spirituous and malt liquors, who will refrain from the use of tobacco in any form in the rooms and about the grounds of the institution; such young men as these, and these only, need apply for admission. We want the *best* young men, and only those who will cheerfully comply with our rules and regulations.[1]

Prospective LMS students reading those tough words could mistake neither the moral tone of the statements nor the expectations they represented. Catalogs of the other medical schools that trained most African American students in the late nineteenth and early twentieth centuries (see Appendix, Table 4) rarely contained such an unambiguous articulation of their schools' goals or the character of their students.

LMS was an integral part of Shaw University and as such operated under its same strict rules. The kind of student sought to attend and graduate from Leonard was the same as that sought at Shaw. Many of the African American colleges established during the late nineteenth century by white Northern missionaries and supported by white Northern philanthropists adhered to a similar paternalistic approach to training African American students.[2] Unlike any of the other colleges that established medical schools, however (with the possible exception of Knoxville College),[3] the leadership at Shaw University extended its teaching of strict discipline and Christian values quite deliberately to the medical school.

LMS attracted, for the most part, sincere and serious-minded Christian young men, poor but willing to earn their keep and to use their new skills to help others after graduation. School authorities did what they thought proper to assist those students, both financially and academically. Administrators expected medical students to act with proper decorum on and off campus and to set an example for younger students and for fellow African Americans that would carry over into later professional life. LMS students had many of the same concerns and experiences as their white counterparts regarding medical school admission, financial matters, and academic success,[4] but lived and studied in a stricter campus environment owing to the nature of the school they attended—a Christian missionary institution operated by whites dedicated to training male Christian African American physicians.

Regardless of whether they were established by white Christian missionaries or black physicians, African American medical schools of the late nineteenth and early twentieth centuries varied greatly in atmosphere, academic standards, type of faculty, living accommodations, and facilities. Prospective students could attend a sheltered residential school such as Leonard or a less restrictive but still Christian school such as Howard or Meharry; they could live in a large city such as New Orleans, Louisville, or Washington, or in smaller communities such as Raleigh, Chattanooga, or Knoxville. The white medical establishment viewed none of those schools with favor and ignored them until about the turn of the century. Then the burgeoning educational reform movement collided with inadequate funding, facilities, and faculty at the black schools, and one by one the African American institutions closed, proprietary (independent) and missionary alike.[5] Of the black medical colleges founded during this period, only Meharry and Howard survive today.

Few records are available to document living and learning conditions, grading systems, and the kinds of students, faculty, and administrators that peopled the various African American medical schools. LMS's parent institution, Shaw University, however, preserved such crucial materials as exchanges of letters between the administration and students (prospective, current, and former), faculty grading books, student financial records, faculty meeting minutes, and other official correspondence. Excerpts from the letters and other LMS documents comprise the core of this chapter.

LMS was established as a result of the efforts of Henry M. Tupper, founder and first president of Shaw University. Tupper, a white Baptist minister from Massachusetts, moved to Raleigh just after the cessation of hostilities in 1865 in order to educate freed people under the auspices of the American Baptist Home Mission Society. Money from that organization and from Northern Baptist philanthropists, including Elijah Shaw, a woolen manufacturer for whom the university was named, soon provided financial resources to begin a collegiate institution. Judson Wade Leonard, Tupper's brother-in-law and a Massachusetts manufacturer, contributed money in 1879 to start the medical school. A classroom building and a dormitory building were immediately constructed, and the first class began its studies in the fall of 1882. Despite great financial difficulties, LMS survived, under Tupper's and, after 1894, Meserve's leadership, until 1918, graduating more than four hundred physicians, most of whom went into medical practice in the rural South.[6]

Meserve's statement quoted earlier explains quite clearly the dual mission of the school: to train good African American *physicians* and to train good African American *men*. To do this, the president and his faculty made sure they had knowledge of, and, as much as possible, influence over, their students' lives. From the moment students applied to Shaw, their lives were, in many ways, in the hands of others and always under scrutiny. Their numbers were small, their status on campus high, and their work—whether in laboratory, classroom, or hospital—visible. The school administration invested in them financially, academically, socially, and emotionally, and worked hard to protect that investment. It is instructive, then, to observe students, faculty, and administration during the various stages of an LMS student's career.

A sense of the kind of students who sought admission to LMS and in whom the administration was willing to invest can be gained from their correspondence. The close attention President Meserve paid to all student inquiries about the professional (law, medicine, and pharmacy) schools is indicative of the centralized, paternalistic nature of Shaw University. He personally answered every letter requesting information about, admission to, or financial aid for those schools. For prospective students, ability to pay and ability to master the educational material presented were the two main worries—in that order. Those considerations were also always in Meserve's mind as he sorted through the application correspondence. He assumed responsibility for and oversaw every aspect of the medical school's operation, from admission to graduation and even beyond.

Students from a variety of backgrounds wrote asking for admission and for financial aid. In the post-Emancipation South of the late 1800s and early 1900s, most African Americans had little money to spare and deprived educational backgrounds. School systems provided African Americans with only short academic terms and unqualified or poorly qualified teachers.[7] Finding suitable applicants for medical school, especially at a time when the new scientific medicine was forcing state medical examining boards to increase standards for licenses, was difficult.[8] A typical letter requesting information about admission to LMS reads:

> Will you please send me one of your catalogues and kindly give me full information as to a student entering the medical dept. I finished the junior prep. at Biddle University Charlotte, N.C. but am a little rusty just now. And please state whether or not I can study the Latin over and other languages if required and take the course too in medicine.[9]

These inquiries often contained misspellings and grammatical errors:

> Please send a catalogue of the medical department at Pshaw, and oblige.[10]
>
> I wants to attend your school and with a little assistance I make it all right. Also I would like to enter the medicine department. Will you please give me a scholarship. In reply please send catatogue.[11]
>
> I have a boy wish to to [*sic*] come your school to study medicens you would oblidje me an give me all the infermation in Regards of Rules and Regulations.[12]

Other letters were naïve:

> Pleas forward me a catalog of Leonard school of N.C. Pleas sir state the kind of text books recommended. also how long in your judgment do you think it would take me to complete a medical course (that is to become a practicing physician). I have no knollege of M.D. at present. I am teaching public school. pleas sir write me at once give me all the information you can on the question.[13]

Some inquiries were polished and wise:

> [I] Went out into the world from Hampton [Institute in Virginia] with an idea that I could do well without the Medical profession but I find that the Med. profession is the only profession for the young negro. I should like to enter Oct 1904.[14]
>
> As I have decided to take a medical course in some good school, I thought I would write you for your terms and qualifications that will enable one to be eligible to enter your university. I would like very much to receive the

> course of instruction under your tutorship, as I have met graduates from your school who seemed to be proficient along all lines in connection with their profession.[15]

All inquirers seemed earnest, and most asked frankly for some kind of financial assistance:

> Now sir if you can help me in any way like that I will be ever so much oblige to you for the study of medicine has been on my mind for the past five years so much so till I wrote you in the summer of 94 and you grant me a Schollarship and I could not come on account of my not being able to get the money and I have been doing all that I know to get off and don't see yet where I have the money in fact I know that I haven't got the money. All that I have been doing was teaching Schools and they give such a little for that till there is nothing in it.[16]
>
> I am contemplating entering the Leonard Medical College next term. I have had five years training in hospital work and am a graduate of Tuskegee Institute. My means are very scant, and I am entirely dependent upon myself for my education, with the knowledge I have of hospital work (I can send you testimonials as to my fitness for the study of medicine and hospital experiences) is there any way you could kindly assist me by allowing me to work out a portion of my expenses.[17]
>
> I am a very poor boy and would like to come there after this term closed here (Alcorn College, Mississippi]. Because I would like to study Medicine in short and I think that is the very place for me. . . . If I could get some work there I would be much please in coming there. Have they any printing office up there or any kind of work that I can work at during the summer. If so please let me know.[18]

Meserve responded warmly, sympathetically, and patiently to all letters. His standard reply usually asked for more information about the applicant. For example, in November 1895 he wrote to one potential student: "I have your favor of the 9th inst, and in reply will ask you before I can make a decision to forward me a recommendation from Prof. Blackwell, your last teacher. I would like to know your age and how far you have progressed in your studies. Please forward this at once, because if you enter our medical school you ought to come at the earliest possible moment. Be very particular to let me know your age. Please reply by return mail, if possible and I will at once give you a definite answer."[19] For personal recommendations, he sometimes wrote directly to those who knew the applicants well: "I have a letter from Robert W. Henry of 100 Cohea St [Jackson, Miss.], asking for admission to our Medical Dept. Is he all right? If you say he is I will receive him at once," he wrote to the president of Jackson College in Mississippi in 1903. The reply came back handwritten on Meserve's letter and proclaimed that the applicant was "All right! He is the young man whom you met at my house last spring, and of whom I wrote you a month or more ago. Have you forgotten? He is *able* and willing. Do all you can for him."[20]

Meserve went out of his way to recruit those students with strong academic records or recommendations. "You will find," he proclaimed to one young man in 1897, "that our medical school is especially adapted to the requirements of young men of good ability, but poor in purse. We feel sure that you cannot elsewhere get so much for your money as here at the Leonard Medical school, and when I make this statement, I do not mean to depreciate any one of the other excellent schools. After you have looked the catalogue over carefully please let me hear from you."[21] To another inquirer in 1895 Meserve replied: "I have just received a letter from Rev. C. Ayer, of Clifton Springs, N.Y. in your behalf. . . . I hope that you will read the catalogs, and, if it seems best, that you will enter the Leonard Medical School. We can grant a $60 scholarship to worthy young men, and, as Mr. Ayer speaks highly of you, we would be willing to grant you this favor."[22]

A few who received financial aid from Shaw University wrote letters of thanks to Meserve. In 1905 one grateful recipient informed the president, "I am very much oblige to you and the faculty of Shaw University for granting me a scholarship in the Leonard Medical Department of Shaw University for the session of 1905–06. I have studied very hard during the summer, and it is my endeavor to do my very best during the next school session. I am praying to God to enable me to succeed in meeting the requirements of the faculty and president of Shaw University, and in the main [*sic*] time, I earnestly ask your prayers in my behalf, and I assure you that I shall never bring a disgrace upon Shaw University for having sent me out from its walls."[23]

Some applicants offered to work during the term to defray some of their expenses. Tupper and, at first, Meserve encouraged that approach, though jobs outside the school were difficult to secure. "In reply to your favor of the 22nd inst," answered Meserve to one inquiry in September 1895, "I have to inform you that if a satisfactory recommendation is forwarded by the Principle of your last school, I will grant you a scholarship in the Medical School, as requested, and will also give you an opportunity to work some each month so as to reduce the charges."[24] On another occasion in that same year he responded, "There are so many that desire work that it is well-nigh impossible to obtain it for all and especially for those who wish steady work. There are some of you young men at certain seasons of the year that have an opportunity to work in the up-town barber shops for an hour or two, but there is not much demand for this extra help. Regular help is of course employed, and they do most of the work."[25] As educational standards around the country and at LMS increased, however, Meserve had to insert the following statement in the catalog: "Let no young man think, as many have seemed to intimate in their applications, that they can support themselves by manual labor or other kinds of work and successfully pursue their studies at the same time. Students who enter the Leonard Medical School must be prepared to devote their whole time to study, except what is needed for the rest and recreation necessary to keep themselves in the best physical and mental condition possible."[26]

Some applicants recognized their educational deficiencies and asked about special assistance or preparatory courses. "In receiving your favor of June 1st '96," wrote one dissuaded student, "I noticed that you expressed a doubt as to my preparation for fitness for entering the Medical Dept. As I was only a graduate of the 'Newberry Graded School.' I am very glad you did so, as I don't feel sufficient for the task. Influenced by your doubt I have decided to go in your Literary Dept. for the present and ask that my application be cancelled and you send me another."[27] Another applicant in the previous year had stated, "I thought it would be well to let you know why I prefer going to Shaw University this coming school year. My object is to study medicine and I thought it would be better to enter some University so as to get the proper studies for the medical course. The school which I attended the past term is an Industrial school and I could not get the studies in the Senior Class not all that I should have to enter upon medicine."[28] Still another young man wanted Meserve to send "some information as to any allowance made for candidates who may be a little deficient in passing the required entrance examination."[29] Meserve, whose goal was "to do all we can to assist these young men to get an education fitting them for the duties of life,"[30] guided applicants to what he considered their appropriate academic level.[31]

With the possible exception of a deficient educational background, the chief barrier to medical training for African Americans was lack of money. The total annual cost of attending LMS started out in 1882 at approximately $105 (matriculation fee $5, five months' course of lectures $60, living expenses [room, lights, fuel, and board] $40), plus the cost of books and labs, and had risen but little three decades later ($129 in 1912), about half the cost of most white schools.[32] Despite this relatively low cost, and the $50 or $60 scholarships given liberally, many students simply could not raise the cash. Their letters of withdrawal often explained why they could not attend. "Recent news sent me from home relative money exchange, have greatly affected my [educational] pursuits," lamented an aspiring African American physician.[33] I have had such [financial] reverses that I am unable to enter [Leonard] this session," despaired another.[34] Yet a third complained that "on account of financial embarrassment, I find that I shall not be able to enter this term. If nothing prevents I shall endeavor to enter the term following. P.S. However, I have not given up the desire to pursue a medical course."[35] One student wrote a desperate, poignant letter to Meserve:

> I am very grateful to you for the scholarship granted me in the Leonard Medical School. My purpose sending this letter, is to inform you that I am very sorry that the inadequacy of my means, owing to my want of success and *illness* during the past seven weeks, has disabled me entering school during the forthcoming session. I am willing to do anything so as to obtain my profession.
>
> Please president, couldn't you let me work out my entire way? I would be willing to wait on a private family, whilst taking my lectures, I would also be willing to do out doors work if you have any. I am even ready to come down now & start cleaning up the buildings for the reopening of school.
>
> This is all that I can say Prest. I am earnest & willing to learn & therefore beg to leave my case entirely to your sympathy.[36]

The young man also wrote to one of the school's trustees appealing for help. Meserve, however, firmly but regretfully refused assistance:

> [I]t will be impossible to grant you any further assistance than that stated in my former letters to you. A scholarship of $60 per annum has been granted you, also an opportunity to do some work to reduce your expenses to the minimum. Our charges are made just as low as possible to help poor and worthy young men, and we can not do more than I have stated. All our students are poor and needy, and of course, you understand that we must have money to meet the current expenses of the institution. The income from the students does not half meet the expenses of the institution, the remainder being contributed by self-sacrificing friends in the North. I sincerely trust that some way may open up for you so that you can meet your expenses. . . . I believe there is no other school in the country that offers so many advantages at so small a cost.[37]

That money problem hounded students not just before first year matriculation, but throughout the four years of training. African American students had a difficult time obtaining employment, and the jobs they did find were often menial and low paying. Meserve exerted what influence he could to assist students searching for summer jobs. For example, in 1897, he wrote to a company in Knoxville, Tennessee:

> I was informed by Mr ———, one of our medical students, that there was a possibility of getting employment with you as a porter. [He] has just finished in a very creditable manner his sophomore year in the Leonard Medical School, the medical department of Shaw University. I write to say

> that he is a young man of most excellent character and attainments, and is striving very hard to obtain the means for meeting his expenses in the medical school for the next year. If you can give him employment you may rest assured that you will be helping a very worthy young man. He is one of the worthiest young men of any race whom I have ever known. If you could give him employment at the most liberal wages possible you can rest assured, while it may be a purely commercial transaction on your part, that it will really be in the line of Christian philanthropy and a missionary spirit. He has not been able to meet his expenses this year, but through the kindness of a friend in the North $50 has been allowed him, and were it not for this he could not have made his sophomore year.[38]

In March 1895 the president informed the Pullman Car Company of "a student in the Leonard Medical School connected with Shaw University. He is a young man of integrity, reliability and the best of character and I hope if there is an opening for him, you will give him work for he needs it in order to continue his studies, and I believe will render you faithful service."[39] He wrote to the Wagner-Palace Car Company in 1898 of "a student in the medical department of this institution [who] has been with us since the opening of the year. He is a large, strong man and has shown himself reliable and trustworthy, and he has not, to my knowledge, any bad habits. I believe you will find him in every way faithful and efficient."[40]

Because after 1897 medical students were permitted to work outside the Shaw campus only during vacation periods, unexpected summer sickness or failure to obtain a summer job usually meant the postponement or even termination of a Leonard medical career. The following student letter of December 1896 to Meserve clearly illustrates the problem:

> Your favor of December 9 inst. rec'd. I am sorry to say that I am not expecting to be in this session. My success in the money line is the poorest this year it has been since I have been trying to educate my self. Every [*sic*] since I entered the Leonard School of Medicine, it seems to me that every way I try to make money is almost a failure. I was hired to teach a school this summer for $30 per month. It would have run four months. When I went to take charge, another teacher had taken the school for $25. Then it was to [*sic*] late to get another work. So I have spent most of the summer building a house for my father. I have thought of the school more or less every day since its opening but have not written to any of the boys. I hated to say that I could not come. . . . I read all I have time to spare and hope to be in at the opening of '97. I don't know of any better way than that.[41]

A similar tale of disappointment arrived from Kentucky in the following year: "'Tis my painful duty to say to you, that 'twas impossible for me to reach Leonard this session by any means. After my protracted illness 'twas impossible for me to collect money due me, on account of stringent times. Would you please extend scholarship to Nov. '97? I shall make every effort to be present promptly at the opening of the session."[42] One student who had found summer employment in Pennsylvania in 1896 reported that an injury at work had denied him the necessary means to pay his way at LMS that coming fall:

> I strained my left side by picking up some ice cream freezers. If I had quit work then I might have been O.K. From that day I was not able to do anything; but I continued to work sick. I worked sick two wks. getting worse every day so last Wed. week I began to spit blood which doubtless would have led to a hemorrhage if it had not been for my shrewdness. The following day I went to Philadelphia where I was sent to the Hospital. After I got strong enough Dr. Hirsh of the St. Joseph Hospital told me I could come South and spend some time in the country. But he advised me not to work any more for 3 or 4 mo. I had made all of my school money, but stopping as I did sick and having to pay the Dr. and buy medicine and books with my traveling expenses has almost left me without money and two mo. work I have lost. For five years I have been able to leave Shaw University at the end of the year not owing one cent. Now in my last year sickness compels me to enter school without money. This thought grieves me; but the Lord's will must be done. That I know. Mr. Meserve I am forced to ask you to please be reasonable with me this year. I may be able to pay all of my bills through my father. I have just written to him. I am sure he will help me. I have neither money nor clothes. The Lord will provide.[43]

In the matter of finances, as in so many other aspects of student life at Leonard, the president held great power. Recognizing the severe monetary burdens under which many students labored and the difficulties of attracting, educating, and graduating qualified students, founder Tupper was willing to be lenient when it came to collecting bills. He solicited donations from his Northern friends and borrowed from other Shaw accounts and from local banks to make up the resulting deficits. Meserve, when he took over in 1894, found the university in such desperate straits because of Tupper's policies that he assumed a much stricter stance with medical students whose payments were in arrears.[44] He did, however, allow a few to defer payments to a specified later date. To one student in arrears he wrote, "In view of your past record and the condition in which you find yourself financially, I will allow you to enter at once and shall expect you to pay, with the exception of $20 for which you will give me your note payable to the order of

Shaw University, all the charges for matriculation fee, incidental charge, board, etc., on or before the 20th of March, 1896."[45] At times Meserve refused to become involved when he felt he had done all that was possible or that students needed to learn a financial lesson from life. He informed one student in 1895:

> It surely was unfortunate that you did not send us the money that was due to us, as you promised to send it, instead of keeping it in your trunk, for then surely there would have been no loss. As you have been here some time my heart goes out to tell you to return at the beginning of the year, but the fact is that the $40, or thereabouts, that you are owing Shaw, and similar sums from other students have prevented Shaw University from meeting obligations that should have been met some time ago. I do not see how we can receive you, unless you are able to meet the charges in advance, as all others are required. I think it would be well for you to look around among your friends and have the means provided so that you can return and finish up your medical education.[46]

On the same day, he lectured another student by mail who was also having monetary problems:

> I have looked over your letter carefully and certainly sympathize with you in the illness that you have passed through during the summer and that has deprived you of providing, as you had hoped, means to carry you through next year in your medical course. My hope goes out to allow you to come and pay when you can, but this does not help settle the University bills, and we are in great straits financially.... It is just a hard business situation that requires us to meet our bills, and unless the students meet theirs I cannot meet the University bills as required. I trust that the way will open up so that you can be with us. We shall miss you if you are not here.[47]

Nevertheless, Meserve often made special appeals to Northern whites to support one or another student on an emergency basis:

> I write you with reference to Mr ———, one of our students, a most excellent young man, a graduate of Hampton and now pursuing a course of study in our medical department. He is a faithful and earnest worker and has made above eighty percent in all of his subjects thus far during the year. We find him in every way a most admirable young man. He is hard pressed for funds, and, although I have granted him a scholarship of $60 for this year, he yet needs $15 to meet the necessary expenses for the balance of the year. He told me that you were interested in him, but he was

> too modest to write you and only reluctantly gave me your address. If you could send him, or to me for him, the $15 that he needs to get through, you may rest assured that you are doing an act of charity that is in the highest sense worthy. There are some young men who are eagerly asking for help who are unworthy. I would not recommend [the student] did I not know that he is a young man of a most excellent character and good ability and in every way worthy and deserving.[48]

In keeping with the school's mission of educating young African American men in proper behavior as well as in medicine, President Meserve was not above prompting students as to proper manners when they received financial assistance. He reminded one young man in May 1897: "[Y]ou have been indebted during the past year to Mr. F. W. Hamlin of Milo, Maine. He is the gentleman that has met your expenses and through whose noble Christian spirit and kind liberality you were enabled to pursue your course of study for the year just closed at the Leonard Medical School. I know you will be glad to write him a letter showing him that you appreciate thoroughly his kindness to you."[49] This letter well represents the approach Meserve and other faculty members took in training medical students about appropriate conduct in their private and professional lives. By example, by use of the spoken and written word, by gentle but firm prodding, and by establishment and enforcement of rules, the LMS staff transmitted their ideals and expectations to two generations of future African American practitioners. With financial worries pushed aside (but not forgotten) by the start of the school year, students settled into the routines of academe and of a medical school dedicated to promoting Christian morals.

No diary of daily life at LMS has yet come to light, so conclusions about that aspect of medical students' careers must be drawn from various bits of evidence in several sources. The evidence leaves an impression that, as with other facets of life at the Raleigh school, the administration tried to maintain close control over student living conditions and behavior. Furthermore, because medical students were held in such high regard both on and off campus, President Tupper and, later, President Meserve expected them to act as models for the rest of the university. Early in the history of the school Tupper established that role for medical students. In his annual report for 1885–86 he described making "an appeal . . . to them at the beginning of the session that as they were the oldest and most experienced students so by their example and influence they should be foremost in the moral and religious work of the school."[50] To guide proper behavior, the administration established and published strict rules of conduct. A summary of this code (its details varied over the years but not its tone), appearing in 1910 as part of a pamphlet written by Meserve, titled *The Negro Physician*, is reminiscent of words used in the 1909 LMS catalog: "Another worthy feature of the school is its system of discipline. The medical students are required to reside in the dormitories and are subject to the same regulations as to chapel exercises, strict observance of study hours, abstinence from the use of liquors and tobacco as other students. This is an almost unheard of thing in a medical school. There is no roistering nor midnight carousing at Shaw and men who want that kind of thing do not go there. The ideal of the school is the Christian physician and the University supplies both the teaching and wholesome restraint that such an ideal implies."[51]

To further the goal of training Christian physicians through "teaching and wholesome restraint," Tupper and Meserve made sure that, along with academics, religion was emphasized at Shaw. Meserve even went on record on that point in 1901, announcing to readers of the *Baptist Home Mission Monthly*, "[E]ducational work is not and never has been considered first in the Home Mission schools for the colored people of the South. The idea at the very beginning of these schools, and it is equally true at the present time, was to give moral and religious instruction, and to make this foremost."[52] Though Leonard could not have survived long without a strong emphasis on academics, it did place much value on religion, discipline, and morals. Even the medical faculty—white, well-respected Raleigh physicians and scientists—supported the commitment to Christian education.[53] So medical students, not unexpectedly, took part in the spiritual life of the campus.

The young men at LMS attended weekly worship services at the church on campus. There they were visible to the rest of the college community. (President Tupper did acknowledge and provide for the spiritual needs of non-Baptist medical students by allowing them, according to LMS catalogs, "to worship on Sunday at their own church in the city.")[54] Additional religious requirements included mandatory attendance at chapel on specified days of the week[55] and avoidance of arrival in Raleigh on the Sabbath at the start of the school year.[56]

Many of the medical students went well beyond simple observance of the Sabbath and took on leadership roles in Shaw's Christian community. Tupper boasted to readers of the *Baptist Home Mission Monthly* in 1886 that "all but two or three have made a profession of religion" and that "no class of pupils are more regular in their attendance upon religious services than our medical students."[57] During a religious awakening that swept through campus that year, Tupper wrote elsewhere, LMS students stood out from the rest so that "a higher moral tone pervaded the medical department than at any time since its organization."[58] That religious fervor seems not to have diminished during the thirty-six-year life of the school. Letters from graduates and alumni who visited the campus, all reporting continued involvement in community religious affairs and attesting to the virtues of living by Christian values, reinforced, for those still in school, the spiritual importance of the LMS approach to medical education.[59] By 1906, medical students were not only participating in Shaw's annual "Day of Prayer for Colleges" but had also, for the previous seven years, been sponsoring, organizing, and performing in a yearly "Sacred Concert," which also served as a fund-raiser for the school and Leonard Hospital.[60]

Attending a school like Leonard encouraged students to give of themselves both while in training and after graduation. Not only did the students initiate the Sacred Concert series, but they also, as LMS's needs grew more quickly than its resources, undertook other projects to bring more money to the institution. Leonard Hospital, the small teaching infirmary associated with the medical school, treated primarily indigent patients who could rarely pay for their care. The hospital annually drained a portion of Shaw's budget. Members of Shaw's Medical-Pharmaceutical Association, a student organization, began sponsoring in 1907 a yearly "Pound Party" to help ease that burden. Individuals, churches, and businesses in Raleigh donated money or pounds of supplies to the hospital as their entry fees to the gala. Students gave freely of their time to ensure a successful event.[61] This same fraternity on another occasion solicited contributions from alumni of "not less than $5.00" to aid in the completion of an operating room and convalescent room "here at Old Shaw." "A needy mother appeals to her strong and vigorous sons," they wrote in their circular letter to alumni, adding that "God will smile favorably upon you in responding to this call."[62]

The Christian physician graduates of Leonard continued to put into practice both the spiritual growth and medical knowledge they had gained at their alma mater. A few, like Henry C. Faulkner, class of 1894, became medical missionaries in Africa,[63] while others gave free care to the poor of their communities. One Camden, South Carolina, physician, J. Priestly Pickett, announced in his local newspaper:

> Whereas, God has given me health and strength to accomplish the end I have long sought, namely, to achieve such knowledge of medical science as enables me to render relief to the suffering of my race; and whereas, I desire to return to Him some humble thanks for the same, I, therefore, make the following offer to the aged saints of God's church who have been deprived of their loved ones and who have no one to provide for them in the dark hours of sickness, to-wit: For all members in good standing in their church and who present a certificate of same from their pastor I will give medical advice and write prescriptions without charge. This I do in the name of Him who said "inasmuch as ye have done it unto one of the least of these my brethren, ye have done it unto me."[64]

Annually, senior students who for four years had heard the lessons of Christianity preached to them at Sunday services, weekday chapel gatherings, special convocations, and prayer days, and who had often participated in a variety of religious and charitable activities, listened to one last round of stirring spiritual speeches as they prepared to leave Leonard. Commencement provided the administration and faculty a final opportunity to evaluate the students (they could not be promoted to the next class or be "presented for graduation unless . . . recommended . . . on the basis of good character and habits")[65] and to remind them of the lessons they had learned and the obligations they had now to meet as physicians and committed Christians. Lawson A. Scruggs, class valedictorian, set the tone for graduation orations at the very first commencement exercises in 1886. His speech, titled "Medical Education as a Factor in the Elevation of the Colored Race," included such statements as, "It does not require any unusual foresight to discover that the education of colored men for physicians is in the direct line of Providence . . . and is clearly God's method of uplifting this people. . . . Will it not be the colored Christian missionary, with his Bible in one hand, to enlighten and save the soul, and in his other his medicines to alleviate the suffering and heal the innumerable diseases and afflictions of the body?"[66] Other graduation addresses over the years bore such instructive titles as, "The Temptations of the Medical Profession" (1888), "Work" (1906), and "The Dangers of Success" (1911).[67] From their first day on campus to their last, Leonard students could not help but hear the religious message Shaw faculty and administrators beamed at them.

Though not all aspects of LMS students' lives revolved around religious concerns, the school's emphasis on proper conduct, morals, and respect for authority pervaded the campus. If the students did not always think in those terms, the administration and faculty seemed to. They orchestrated campus life according to what they deemed as the best interests of the students. For example, President Meserve, in November 1906, took advantage of the first anniversary of the abolition of freshman medical student hazing (it was he who had suggested its abolition) by preaching race betterment: "The belief is too general that colored people are rude, noisy and lawless, an opinion that cannot be entertained when we consider that hazing at Shaw University was abolished by the students themselves upon the request of the President of the University, who appealed to them on the score of manliness to take the lead in abolishing a custom that can only be termed a relic of barbarism. We believe it will be difficult to find in any State of the Union a company of over 500 young men and young women courteous, more regardful of the rights of others, and considerate in all their relations with each other than the students of Shaw University."[68]

Students learned that, at least when dealing with school faculty and administration, the rules called for proper procedure, decorum, and respect for authority. One prospective student, having been rejected for admission the previous year because of "circumstances existing at Kittrell College," for which he had been suspended, humbly acknowledged, in his letter of reapplication, Leonard's reputation for strictness. "If you should grant me entrance," he assured President Meserve, "I should be very grateful and try to the best of my ability to conform with your discipline."[69] At the other end of the student hierarchy, the members of the senior class, in January 1897, very politely asserted themselves as they petitioned the president for permission to choose commencement speakers from the working world rather than having Meserve appoint speakers from the graduating class: "We feel that in this way we will be better benefited, because a man who is out amidst the active duties of life, can tell us of the different phases of life and can tell us what to avoid. In short, such a man can give to us needed counsel. In view of this fact, in view of the fact that our studies are hard pressing and in view of the fact that our time is so very limited in which to prepare such pieces as would reflect credit upon us and upon the institution, we therefore, ask the President's liency [*sic*] in this matter."[70] They further requested that the president inform the class ten days before commencement of those who would not graduate. "We ask this for two reasons," they stressed. "First, in order that the men may know as it is very embarrassing to remain here until the verge of commencement and then not to graduate. Second, we ask such a request, so that it will give us more time in making the needed preparations for commencement. We ask these requests not for the mere purpose of asking but we ask them because we have Shaw's interest and her sons['] interest at heart, and because we believe it will be for the benefit of both. The above we respectfully submit to the Pres. for his careful consideration."[71]

On another occasion, in late February 1898, an incident occurred (details are not spelled out in any extant records) for which two members of the sophomore class received immediate punishment. As only one of them had actually caused the trouble, fifteen classmates submitted a petition to set matters straight.[72] Meserve responded first by explaining his philosophy in matters of discipline. Such affairs, he stated, were personal, to be discussed between the parties involved. "Class organizations are not for the purpose at any time, or under any circumstances of considering matters of discipline," he declared.[73] Then, true to his and the school's character, he concluded with a warning and a moral: "There are this year a few members of the class that have failed to attain the quiet dignity of conduct and recognition of the rights of others, that should always characterize the true student. The true student should never forget that he is a man among men, not a boy among men, nor a boy among boys."[74]

That paternalistic and moralistic approach toward the Leonard medical students extended well beyond the classroom. Medical students, though generally older than others at Shaw, could not choose to live off campus, away from the watchful eye of school authorities. "The welfare of the student," Meserve stated without elaboration in the 1896–97 college catalog, "demands that . . . all students . . . live and board at the institution."[75] It is significant that the first structure Tupper had built for the new medical school in 1881 was a dormitory, not a classroom or laboratory building. (As befitted the character-molding thinking of the administration, students made the brick for those and other Shaw University edifices.) Parents could then rest assured that their aspiring physician sons who had left the nest lived in the protective confines of the college. School authorities could also feel comfortable in the knowledge that the newest additions to the Shaw community were safely under their control.

Apparently not all medical students liked the paternalism of Shaw's administration. Some must have covertly attempted to room or board in town, for LMS catalog statements of the on-campus housing-and-eating rule grew stronger over the years. Meserve finally stressed the regulations as bluntly as possible in 1908 and added that students were expected to report to the dining room "as promptly and regularly as they do at their classrooms." "Any who are not willing to comply with the . . . regulations," he concluded, "should not make application for admission."[76] Furthermore, to assure the proper behavior of at least a solid core of students, or perhaps to correct a growing problem among medical students, Meserve began in 1897 to warn scholarship recipients to avoid discipline problems or lose their awards. The following year he had them sign pledges agreeing to obey the school's rules.[77]

Perhaps discipline problems at LMS were growing in the late 1890s, forcing Meserve to publish those warnings and take harsh actions in the face of growing student assertiveness. In the Shaw University Archives, an anonymous typewritten fragment filed with Meserve's unpublished "History of Shaw University" even claims that "there were probably some runners for whiskey houses among the students" and that a number of medical students indulged in drinking. Despite the rules and the lectures and the prayers and exhortations, some Leonard medical students failed to live up to the school's high ideals.[78]

Of all breaches of conduct, the least tolerated and most severely punished occurred in the classroom—cheating. Faculty minutes, grade books, and annual composite grade sheets provide ample evidence of the faculty's assiduousness in evaluating each student's academic performance. Students earned promotion to the next class level by maintaining a prescribed average in all subjects.[79] In order to ensure success, some students took to cheating, and faculty members recorded such illegal activity when it was detected. James M. Pickel, professor of chemistry between 1896 and 1917, wrote, for example, in his 1910 roll book, "There are strong (almost conclusive) indications of cheating in the 3d examination (3/12/10); hence an oral examination was held (3/26/10); this last was optional."[80] To prevent cheating, Pickel had his students take a pledge at each exam, but, as he warned in his "Plan of Teaching Chemistry to the Leonard Medical Students" in 1900, a few years after assuming his position at the school, even that approach did not always solve the problem: "See to it that pledges are, not merely written, but signed. There is a frequent disposition to slight this." To document this observation Pickel noted in his roll book each instance of student failure to write or sign the pledge. He concluded his roll book statement on pledges with an accusation: "There is evidently considerable cheating." He then described how students accomplished cheating and explained the further precautions he took to ensure honesty in tests:

- Don't permit books of any description in examination rooms.
- Don't permit the use of any writing tablets except those to be given out after the students have assembled in examination room.
- Don't permit examination papers to be copied under pretext of making corrections, but insist on the papers being handed in as first written.
- Don't permit the use of extra sheets of paper on the pretext that the rough or first answers are being copied from these sheets. These sheets are doubtless often smuggled in.[81]

Those students caught cheating in any course usually received a failing grade in that subject, but some had to repeat the entire year's work, and at least one was expelled.[82] Leonard, however, was not alone in this problem. Student cheating occurred at other medical schools during the late nineteenth and early twentieth centuries.[83]

Student grades and academic standing were, of course, matters of great moment to the entire medical school community. Those underclassmen who rushed off to summer jobs immediately after finals wrote back anxious letters asking, "How am I standing in my studies. And [tell] whether you or the Medical Faculty think that I am progressing or not? I would like to know before I go too far."[84] The faculty and administration tried as much as possible to identify poor or potential problem students and to inform those students of their deficiencies. Professors' grade books, grade sheets, and faculty meeting minutes contain frank assessments of students' performances and abilities. The comments of the teachers included such remarks as , "Bad English and spelling"; "Ought to quit, poor [preliminary] education"; "Works hard, can't take [it] in"; "Poor education—no foundation"; "Poor education, no ability"; "Failed completely, awful in every way, should drop out." Such assessments reflect the problems African Americans faced in white America a relatively few years after Emancipation, though one can find similar comments written about students at white medical schools of the time as well. Some LMS students had deficient preliminary educations while others, in the faculty's opinion, simply did not possess the capacity for medical-school-level learning. Professor Pickel wrote of one first year student: "Not prepared to be in a medical school." Three years later his assessment of this now senior student had not changed: "Too ignorant of grammar, spelling, pronunciation to have a diploma."[85]

There were other reasons why students performed poorly, such as illness, financial or social concerns, and immaturity. Statements in each annual catalog, remarks in personal correspondence, and comments on faculty grade sheets indicate that a common problem that hurt student grades was poor class attendance. Summer jobs and family obligations, including spring planting and fall harvest, caused some students to arrive on campus days or even weeks after the start of classes or to leave before the end of school. Family crises (financial or social) also took their toll at odd times during the academic year. And those who had to miss an entire session or two to earn money or fulfill responsibilities at home undoubtedly took time to readjust to academic life and to review forgotten material.[86]

Whatever the reason for low grades, once the faculty had identified problem students, they informed them of their low standing and gave them opportunities to improve. Pickel, for instance, often allowed students to retake exams, especially finals, in hopes they would achieve a passing score. He even raised the grades of some whose final exam or average of monthly tests fell just below the needed minimum score.[87]

A few students each year just could not make it. Of one the faculty wrote, "3rd time for exams—still deficient. Should be advised to leave."[88] When that stage was reached, it was President Meserve who informed the student. He described his procedure to the brother of one failed candidate:

> The matter was canvassed very thoroughly by the faculty, and it was the unanimous opinion that your brother could not pass the examination at the board of medical examiners of this or any other state. In order to show their fairness the faculty voted that if your brother should succeed in passing the examination of any state board of medical examiners, they would, upon receipt of this information, grant your brother a diploma signifying that he had graduated from the Leonard Medical School. I talked very frankly with your brother and told him that it was the opinion of the medical faculty that Nature had not intended him for a physician. He was informed as soon as the examinations had taken place that he had not passed.[89]

Some students received a slightly more encouraging letter. "I have to inform you," the president wrote one failed student in March 1895, "that your work in the Leonard Medical School has been of an unsatisfactory nature and that you are not this year received for graduation. I am instructed by the faculty to inform you that it is their opinion that by taking another year in the Leonard Medical School you will be able to do the work successfully and be received for graduation."[90] Throughout his efforts to address the aspirations and problems of students—including letters regarding disappointing grades—Meserve's deep-felt sense of the school's dual mission of training good physicians and good men is apparent. "Your brother," he wrote to the sibling of one of his charges who had not been a successful student, "throughout the whole has conducted himself in a most admirable spirit. He has shown himself under all circumstances a Christian gentleman and he has gone away standing, so far as Christian character is concerned, very high in the estimation of each member of the faculty."[91] Such kind words may have eased the pain and disappointment but could not alter the reality for students who, having completed one to four years of study, suddenly learned that they would not become physicians.

Those who did well in their studies received recognition and rewards, but in those instances, too, the tight, ostensibly beneficent control that the LMS administration exerted over students manifested itself. For example, in March 1895 Meserve wrote to one senior, "In confirmation of my recent oral announcement, I hereby inform you that you have been selected as Salutatorian of your class. The salutatory will be given in the chapel on the evening of Wednesday, the 27th inst. As I orally informed you, you will report . . . for instructions in regard to the writing of the salutatory and also for whatever training may be necessary."[92] To a student in that same year who had done well during the school year and was now working at a summer job to earn expenses for the coming term, Meserve wrote, "I am pleased to learn that you are spending your leisure time in medical reading and trust all the spare time you can find you will devote to improving your mind along these lines that will be of most benefit to you in your future studies."[93]

This paternalistic and moralistic manner characterized LMS from the day it opened to the day it closed. Never during its thirty-six years did administration or faculty try to disguise their approach to training African Americans as physicians. President Meserve expressed himself clearly on the subject in actions and words. Most students accepted those attitudes and the rules that accompanied them. They believed in the ideals for which Leonard stood and did what they could to uphold them both while in school and, as far as can be discovered, after graduation. Judging from these few examples, Meserve's efforts to train consecrated, committed, Christian physicians at LMS succeeded. Meserve bragged to the home office of the American Baptist Home Mission Society in New York in 1895 that advisors at Hampton Institute "have recommended their students who wish to take up a professional course to come here rather than go elsewhere on account of the clean moral atmosphere and the absence of temptations that are found in a large city."[94] And a former Leonard student, continuing his medical training in Chicago, wrote, "Although I am in a large wicked city I have not forgot the good Christian training I received at Shaw and I am putting it to use. I expect with the help of God to be a good Christian Physician."[95] Many of LMS's four hundred graduates appear to have become just that.

CHAPTER 16

Four African American Proprietary Medical Colleges, 1888–1923

The majority of black physicians who graduated from medical school during the late nineteenth and early twentieth centuries attended institutions founded for African Americans. After the Civil War, only a few Northern schools accepted African American candidates for medical degrees, so most aspiring African American physicians studied medicine at predominantly black schools in the South.[1] These schools can be roughly divided into two categories: those with missionary roots and those created as proprietary institutions. (See Chapter 11 and Appendix, Table 4) Among the most successful missionary medical schools were Howard University in Washington, D.C., Meharry Medical College in Nashville, and Leonard Medical School of Shaw University in Raleigh, North Carolina.

By the late 1880s, a generation of African American physicians, trained primarily at missionary schools, had matured professionally. They practiced around the country, but most remained in the South, where the majority of blacks still lived. Several of these physicians of color, following a trend in the white medical world, established independent (proprietary) medical colleges. The first of these institutions was Louisville National Medical College in 1888, followed by Hannibal Medical College (Memphis, 1889), Chattanooga National Medical College (1899), and in 1900 by Knoxville Medical College, the University of West Tennessee College of Medicine and Surgery (Jackson), and the Medico-Chirurgical and Theological College of Christ's Institution (Baltimore). Black medical schools confronted problems related to race not encountered by their white counterparts; black proprietary schools faced additional problems that made their survival in the late nineteenth and early twentieth centuries even more difficult than the black missionary schools.

Though both missionary and proprietary school officials had equal opportunities to cultivate good relations and raise funds among local blacks and whites sympathetic to the institution, the missionary schools, like some of the white schools affiliated with universities, had distinct advantages over proprietary medical schools in almost every other regard. Each was a medical department of a larger university, not a freestanding, unaffiliated institution, and could thus reap the benefits of that association. Even where the home office of the missionary society required separate funding and accounting of supposedly self-sufficient medical departments, these missionary medical schools were able to reduce costs simply by being part of a university. Buildings, for example, already stood or could be built on an existing campus. Libraries, ancillary faculty, and other campus resources were more readily available. Medical department catalogs, announcements, and publicity could be included in general university catalogs, announcements, and publicity. Students were able to live and study in the controlled setting of a college environment, a feature that parents, especially those from rural areas who were distrustful of the supposed bad influences of cities and concerned about their children's safety, liked. Parents also appreciated the fact that missionary schools integrated moral and religious training with education even at the medical school level.[2] Missionary medical schools possessed the further advantage of association with nationally known and respected church organizations dedicated to improving the lot of African Americans. Name recognition, opportunities for fund-raising among sympathetic white Northerners, organizational networks, and other intangibles gave these medical departments an advantage over proprietary schools in building educational programs.

Proprietary colleges run by African Americans were not only independent but also isolated. No missionary magazines reported regularly on their triumphs and their needs or gave them free or low-cost advertising. They had no organized constituency to whom to make financial appeals and few wealthy alumni able to contribute the large sums necessary for capital campaigns supporting improved classroom, hospital, clinic, or dormitory facilities. Philanthropic organizations such as the Slater Fund, the General Education Board, and the Carnegie Foundation bypassed black proprietary schools in favor of missionary schools. African American proprietary schools of the late nineteenth and early twentieth centuries did not have the fiscal strength to go it alone. By 1923, even the toughest of the medical school proprietors, Miles Vandahurst Lynk of West Tennessee, had to surrender and close the doors to his institution.

The worst of American proprietary schools were purely commercial enterprises. Their faculties seemed to care more about collecting student fees than educating future physicians responsibly. Some were simply diploma mills that held few or no classes at all. Legitimate black-owned and white-owned proprietary schools suffered because of the reputation the less rigorous of their number had established. Evidence suggests that some African American proprietary medical colleges fit into this less desirable category.[3] I will present the histories of four late-nineteenth- and early-twentieth-century black proprietary medical schools whose course can be particularly well documented. Only one gained a measure of acceptance from the white and black medical establishments, while the others earned poor reputations. The lack of connection to a larger university or missionary society contributed to the financial problems all four schools encountered and to their inability to improve as national medical education standards rose, but the way each was run also greatly affected that institution's reputation and fate.[4]

Louisville National Medical College (1888–1912)

Arguably the best of the unaffiliated African American medical schools was Louisville National Medical College (LNMC). It grew out of the efforts of three black physicians in the Louisville area in the 1880s who were training African American medical students in their offices. William Henry Fitzbutler was the organizer and prime mover.[5] In July 1872, Fitzbutler, a twenty-nine-year-old newly minted black physician who had lived most of his life in Canada, arrived in Louisville with his wife and children. The first black student at Detroit Medical College (1871) and the first black graduate of the University of Michigan College of Medicine (1872), Fitzbutler was also the first African American to obtain a Kentucky medical license and open a practice in Louisville (1872). He was involved in local and state politics as spokesperson for groups advocating equal educational opportunities for blacks (Kentucky, like all Southern states, provided no opportunities for blacks to obtain medical degrees at state-supported colleges) and as an outspoken critic of governmental racial policies. Fitzbutler not only gave public speeches, worked through legal and legislative channels, and took actions to support these causes but also used the columns of the *Louisville Weekly Planet* (1870s) and the *Ohio Falls Express* (1879–1901), the latter owned and edited by him, to express his views.[6]

Fitzbutler's medical teaching career started within two years of his arrival in Louisville when he began acting as preceptor to a small group of young men. By the mid-1880s, he had learned of two other local black physicians who were also providing medical instruction to students: Rufus Conrad, a homeopath,[7] and William A. Burney, an 1877 graduate of the Long Island College Hospital who lived across the Ohio River in New Albany, Indiana.[8] Fitzbutler, Conrad, and Burney decided in 1886 to open a medical school. With Fitzbutler heading the institution's organization and drive for incorporation, LNMC was chartered by the state legislature and opened for instruction in 1888. The act of incorporation

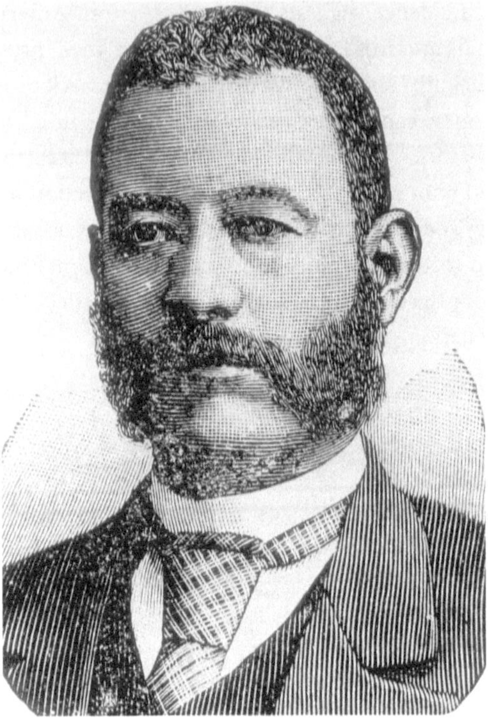

Fig. 10. William Henry Fitzbutler, M.D. From *The Journal of the National Medical Association* (September 1952), cover page.

made no mention of race. LNMC faculty could teach medicine and surgery "to all that may desire to avail themselves of the facilities." As with Kentucky's other medical schools, those earning diplomas at LNMC were entitled to practice medicine in the state. The charter appointed Fitzbutler, Burney, and Conrad as the board of trustees.[9]

An early priority of the school was finding classroom space. The United Brothers of Friendship, a large national black benevolent organization located in Louisville, allowed LNMC the use of its hall for teaching that first year. The following term the trustees were able to purchase a large two-and-a-half-story brick building that had previously housed the Louisville School of Pharmacy.[10] This building, modified for medical instruction, served LNMC for twenty-three years. The school had no campus, no dormitories for many years, no study rooms, and no large library.

Another need was faculty. Fitzbutler, Burney, and Conrad served as the core instructors of the school. During their years at LNMC they taught many subjects, depending on the expertise of their always changing faculty. They also regularly hired LNMC's recent graduates, giving former students a chance to earn money and prestige, as well as to polish techniques, improve knowledge, and gain clini-

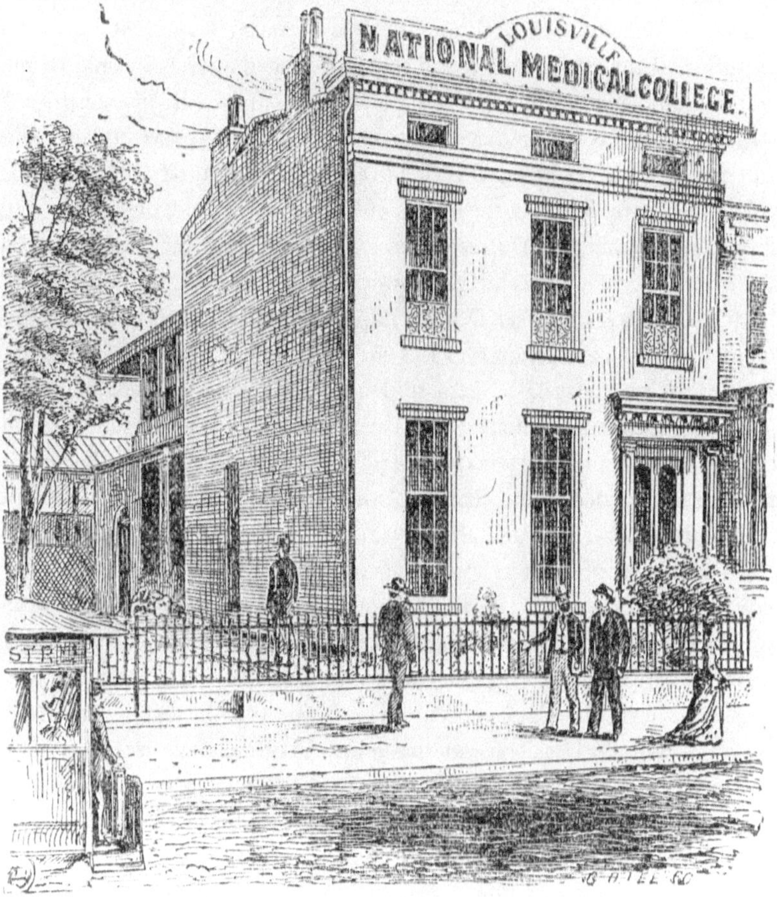

Fig. 11. Louisville National Medical College building (114 West Green Street), from the *Catalogue of the Louisville National Medical College, 1891–92. Fourth Annual Announcement.* Photograph from the National Library of Medicine, Negative No. 82-16.

cal experience as faculty members. Of fourteen faculty rosters extant only two, 1889–90 and 1891–92, contain fewer than 70 percent LNMC graduates. On average, about three-fourths of the teachers in any given year received their medical training at LNMC. Forty-one (71 percent) of the fifty-eight faculty members listed on those fourteen rosters were graduates of LNMC.[11]

Though no discussions of the LNMC faculty's racial composition or of the trustees' hiring policies ever appeared in print, the bias toward black physicians was obvious. Few white physicians ever taught at the school. Of fifty-eight physician faculty members listed in the fourteen available LNMC catalogs, only four were white, the longest employed remaining on staff for three years.[12] These statistics reflected Fitzbutler's commitment to racial uplift. So devoted to the self-help ideal was LNMC that, upon Fitzbutler's death in 1901, LNMC administrators inserted a statement to that effect in the 1902–3 catalog: "It [LNMC] is the only institution of the kind in the world that is managed entirely by colored men, and it is a crucial test of his ability to direct successfully such an enterprise."[13]

In April 1889, LNMC graduated its first class, consisting of six students whose prior training had included attendance at other medical schools and clinical experience as preceptees in the offices of Fitzbutler, Conrad, or Burney. In the school's next catalog the trustees thanked "the public for the good will shown their [the faculty's] efforts, and the patronage which this Institute has received" as LNMC began its second year. During those early years students paid forty-eight dollars for tuition and laboratory fees and received free tickets of admission to the wards of local hospitals. Needy students could purchase "scholarships" that reduced the lecture fees (thirty dollars) by 20 percent and waived the four-dollar matriculation fee. Anyone who possessed "a practical knowledge of the English language, and a good moral character" was eligible for admission. Graduation requirements, other than a fifteen-dollar diploma fee and a stipulation that the third (final) year of medical study be taken at the school, were not discussed. Because LNMC owned no dormitory building, persons needing accommodations had to obtain room and board either in a private residence or in a public house, for between $2.50 and $5.00 per week.[14]

Over the next years, changes occurred in all aspects of the school's basic operations in response primarily to external pressures of national medical education reforms. Of all the black proprietary schools, LNMC most openly acknowledged these reforms in its annual catalogs and reported on how it was addressing the new requirements, always keeping a cautious eye on the school's finances. Though it never joined the Association of American Medical Colleges (AAMC), LNMC quickly moved beyond the very low basic requirements listed in the 1889–90 catalog and attempted to adhere to the guidelines that the newly re-formed (1890) organization regularly publicized. The college, for example, during the 1890–91 session, expanded from a five-month to a six-month/three-year graded curriculum.[15] By the start of the 1891–92 term, LNMC was also asking prospective students for "proof of mental and educational qualifications by examination conducted under management of the Faculty before matriculation." To graduate, applicants had to have reached the age of twenty-one, studied medicine for three years, spent at least the final school year at LNMC, "dissected the parts of the human body, using not less than two cadavers in the operation," and passed final examinations.[16]

Printing requirements in a catalog did not, of course, ensure their fulfillment or enforcement.[17] The catalog shows quite clearly that Fitzbutler, Burney, and Conrad did not adhere strictly (nor did they have to) to AAMC guidelines. For example, students could reduce the three-year curriculum to two if they had "improved the previous time [by study] with regular preceptors" and could enter upon their studies without Latin or physics. They were encouraged rather than required to possess "a good understanding of the elements of Latin and German" as part of their "classified scientific English education" and "a special knowledge of anatomy, physics, and Latin, in addition to what is generally taught in the common schools."[18]

To assist those lacking in certain skills, LNMC offered a short preparatory course during the month before school opened. Instructors reviewed Latin, taught medical etymology and orthography, and gave introductory lectures to the general medical school program. Students could further develop their basic skills by taking courses at State University, a black Baptist collegiate institution in Louisville. Recognizing the need for clinical instruction, LNMC established a free dispensary that provided medical and surgical care and furnished medicines to the public free of charge. The trustees appear to have been scrupulous in their adherence to the rules of the school charter, even insisting that one prospective 1890 graduate, who had passed all his examinations but had not completed a three-year program, continue his studies for an additional year.[19]

Kentucky authorities began tightening medical school regulations in the early 1890s. Among the first activities of the state's newly appointed (1893) board of health was an investigation of medical educational institutions in order to determine each school's quality and, by extension, the competence and certifiability of its graduates. LNMC passed. All its graduates received regular certificates from the state board of health.[20] Fitzbutler and Burney (Conrad died in 1893)[21] used this endorsement, with embellishments, in several subsequent catalogs:

> The Sixth Annual Commencement, or the conclusion of the Sixth Regular Winter Term, marked an era in the establishment of this School. As in all progressive public enterprises, THE LOUISVILLE NATIONAL MEDICAL COLLEGE was under the surveillance of the superstitious, the envious, and the malicious, and the eyes of the public were not opened to the success and practical utility of this Institution, until the State Board of Health, after the most strict inquiry and rigid examination of the Faculty and facilities, placed the School upon equality with the other medical schools in the state, and declared that such a school was necessary in the State of Kentucky, and entitled to the moral support of the Board. The exercises, April 10, 1894, were witnessed by more than a thousand people, who expressed their friendship and admiration.[22]

Additional praise and support for LNMC came, in the early 1890s, from both whites and blacks. Some fifty white medical students from other Louisville colleges accepted an invitation to attend LNMC's third commencement in April

1891. They sat in the front rows of the auditorium "to lend the encouragement of their presence" to the four black graduates about to read their theses and receive their degrees. Fitzbutler used this opportunity to explain to whites the necessity for a black medical school in a town that otherwise denied his race the chance for such an education. Newspaper coverage of this and other LNMC commencements was full and favorable.[23] From the first black medical journal published in the United States came similar praise. Miles V. Lynk, M.D., editor of the *Medical and Surgical Observer* and future founder and proprietor of the University of West Tennessee College of Medicine and Surgery, wrote in 1893, "*The Louisville National Medical [College] Catalogue* has made its appearance on our desk. It will be remembered that this school of medicine was projected solely by colored physicians some six years ago. It will also be remembered that it [was] begun under very discouraging circumstances—everybody hooted at the movement. But we are truly proud to say . . . it has passed the probationary stage and now its diplomas are recognized by the leading state boards of medical examiners. It has turned out twenty-two graduates, among whom are two ladies. All praise to the manly efforts of Professors Fizbutler, Burney and Conrad."[24]

Over the next fifteen years (1894–1908), as entrance, course, and graduation requirements continued to rise nationally, LNMC adjusted its standards as well. The college's catalogs regularly contained both LNMC's requirements and, as they changed, statements of AAMC and other medical organizations' standards.[25] The LNMC regulations usually closely matched these others, especially after Kentucky adopted as part of its medical practice laws the AAMC standards of preliminary and medical school education. When, for example, the AAMC in 1894 voted to require four years of medical study, beginning with candidates intending to receive degrees in 1899, LNMC officials announced a change in requirements to four years of study in its next catalog.[26] Later catalogs stated that LNMC "was the first in Kentucky to require a three years' course, and when four years of medical instruction was generally commended as a requirement for graduation, the Louisville National Medical College endorsed the action of the medical schools that made four years of medical and surgical instruction requisite as one of the conditions of graduation."[27]

LNMC offered clinical instruction to its students from the beginning, through limited access to the hospitals of Louisville, including the Marine Hospital. The free dispensary that LNMC faculty members had established in 1891 also provided some regular exposure to patients, but not the sustained, long-term care experience available in regular hospital facilities. Impetus to improve clinical teaching came not only from the 1894 AAMC change of rules but also from the Kentucky Board of Health a year later when, again responding to national trends in medical education, the board required the state's medical colleges to provide hospital privileges for students if their graduates expected to obtain licenses without examination. The trustees responded by establishing, during 1896, Auxiliary Hospital, located a few blocks from the medical school. It served the city's black community with a lying-in department and treatment facilities for forty patients (acute noncontagious diseases only), all free of charge. Auxiliary Hospital remained open throughout the year, regardless of school sessions.[28]

With a hospital and dispensary to satisfy clinical education needs, a faculty of local black practitioners and recent graduates to teach clinical medicine, a lengthened course of study, and a new set of tougher entrance, attendance, and graduation requirements,[29] LNMC by the late 1890s seemed equal to any other medical school in the country. Fitzbutler and his colleagues felt that this was the case, especially because their institution had continually conformed to nationally accepted standards. As LNMC began its second decade, they explained:

> The establishment of the Louisville National Medical College is the result of a continued effort of more than twenty years to secure for colored medical students the educational privileges from which they have been barred in this and many other States of this country, and while the same prejudices that exclude colored men from the professional schools militate against the rapid advancement of schools opened regardless of nationality, yet by earnest and systematic work this school has made a steady and honorable progress. The number of graduates might have been greater if we had paid less regard to time and qualifications, but by our plan of adhering to regular requirements we have sent out a representative class of doctors that have in no instance disgraced the profession by empiricism or malpractice.[30]

LNMC seemed to be succeeding. The size of the student body fluctuated but averaged between twenty-five and thirty-five students annually. About five doctors graduated each April. Large, elaborate, well-attended commencement exercises received notice in the black and white press.[31] In mid-1899, the administration reported that of fifty-eight graduates, "nearly all of that number are now practicing the profession—many of them with great success—where their services are much needed." By 1908 that number had increased to more than one hundred.[32] The majority of students came from Louisville or other communities in Kentucky, but other students hailed from various Southern and a few Northern states as well.

Another sign of the school's success was Auxiliary Hospital. Not only did it provide students and graduates still living in the Louisville area with opportunities for increased clinical exposure, but it also publicized LNMC's name and spread its favorable reputation. Supported entirely from school funds, private donations, and fees collected from the few private patients admitted, Auxiliary Hospital quickly became a part of Louisville's black community. Its staff included practitioners from LNMC and town, and its board of visitors comprised some of black Louisville's prominent men and women.[33] The public ambulance service took patients to Auxiliary Hospital just as it did to other hospitals in town. The hospital's five-year report, published in 1901, described the institution's modern facilities and equipment. By 1902, LNMC's catalog writer could describe the hospital as "comfortably crowded during the fall and winter months."[34]

The death of William Henry Fizbutler on December 28, 1901, did not slow the growth of LNMC.[35] During Fitzbutler's final year, the trustees authorized remodeling of the classroom building to improve the laboratories and the addition of a library and dormitory rooms. The school also purchased from London a lantern slide projector, which allowed classroom visualization of microscopic images.[36] By 1905, Citizens' National Hospital had opened its doors in a building adjoining and connected with LNMC. The new modern hospital replaced Auxiliary Hospital and provided students even easier access to patients. With new laboratories, a free dispensary, free hospital, and free clinics, the LNMC catalog could state: "It will be impossible for a student to take the course we offer and not to be well grounded in both practice and theory [of medicine]."[37] This and other declarations about the excellent facilities and education offered at LNMC appeared in the school's catalogs at least through 1907–08.[38] Yet four years later, in 1912, LNMC closed.

No detailed information is available to trace the final four years of LNMC's existence and help explain why a seemingly flourishing school would suddenly close. Catalog statements aside, in all probability, LNMC was not flourishing. Given the rising costs of laboratories, equipment, library books and journals, and faculty during this new era of scientific medicine and education reform, LNMC trustees must have had difficulty raising necessary funds. Training suffered. School authorities stated as late as 1907 that "the thoroughness of our instruction is evidenced by the fact that all our students successfully pass the State Boards" and that LNMC "is recognized by all State Boards."[39] But then six of the ten LNMC graduates who took state licensure exams between 1907 and 1911 failed, and state boards of medical examiners (including Kentucky's) placed LNMC on lists of unacceptable schools between 1907 and 1912.[40] Abraham Flexner, hired by the American Medical Association's (AMA) Council on Medical Education and the Carnegie Foundation for the Advancement of Teaching to visit and evaluate every medical school in the country as well as to evaluate the overall state of American medical education, dismissed LNMC (along with four other black medical schools) in his famous report as "ineffectual" and "in no position to make any contribution of value" because of the poor education it imparted to its students. He specifically commented on LNMC's low entrance requirements ("less than high school education") and the eight-bed hospital ("small and scrupulously clean").[41] The combination of a high failure rate for its graduates as state boards increased standards to include the new scientific medicine, loss of recognition by state examining boards, bad publicity from Flexner's report, and an inability to raise adequate sums of money for improving facilities and faculty likely caused LNMC's demise. However, this school appears not to have been a static institution ignoring developments in medical science, practice, or education. Available evidence indicates that the administration, faculty, and students took medical education seriously and worked conscientiously to elevate standards and maintain the comprehensiveness of its program. LNMC's history contrasts significantly with three of Tennessee's black proprietary schools of that period.

Hannibal Medical College, 1889–96

Between 1889 and 1909, the state of Tennessee chartered four unaffiliated medical schools owned and operated *by* African Americans, *for* African Americans: Hannibal Medical College (1889), Chattanooga National Medical College (1899), Knoxville Medical College (1900), and the University of West Tennessee College of Medicine and Surgery (1900). In contrast to LNMC, none of the Tennessee proprietary schools earned favorable reputations in black or white medical circles. All but one (the University of West Tennessee) failed within ten years. (Few of the seven white Tennessee schools in existence in 1900 provided sound education for their students either, prompting Abraham Flexner to comment in his 1910 report that "Tennessee protects at this date more low-grade medical schools than any other southern state.")[42]

The liberal nature and poor enforcement of Tennessee's medical licensure laws, as well as the ease and low cost of obtaining charters, made the state attractive to enterprising individuals, both white and black, wishing to enter the field of medical education.[43] C. C. Fite, secretary of the Medical Society of the State of Tennessee, crudely characterized Tennessee's medical licensure situation in words that were repeated in a nationally distributed medical directory in 1886: "We have no laws bearing upon the practice of medicine. . . . Indians, negroes, confidence men and all that ilk ply their 'trade' with no restriction whatever. A farmer boy too lazy to plow reads an old work on [medical] practice, or 'Every Man his own Doctor,' invests $6 in drugs and is a physician."[44] Fite made these remarks as the state medical society was leading a movement to control through legislation the growing number of itinerants and self-proclaimed healers practicing in the state.[45] After being defeated several times in the legislature, An Act to Regulate the Practice of Medicine and Surgery in the State of Tennessee became law on April 4, 1889. It required each current practitioner to present to the newly established State Board of Medical Examiners a valid diploma from an acceptable medical college or to sit before the board for an examination in the various fields of medicine. Practitioners wishing to enter the state had to submit their educational credentials or pass an examination offered by the board. The board determined the acceptability of diplomas from various medical schools, using the standing of those colleges with the AMA as its guide.[46]

It was just as the State Board of Medical Examiners was organizing itself, preparing to refine and strengthen the new licensing law and beginning to consider the admission and graduation standards of Tennessee's medical educational institutions, that Hannibal Medical College (HMC) in Memphis opened its doors. The school commenced operations on October 7, 1889. During its short existence, HMC failed to build a solid reputation, achieve acceptance either locally or nationally, or attract many students. Finances may have played a role in HMC's failure, but the school's main problems were manner of operation and, as a corollary, quality of instruction. In the early 1890s Hannibal even lost recognition from the Tennessee State Board of Medical Examiners at a time when that body was unwilling to establish firm standards of medical education for the rest of the state's black and white medical schools.

The person guiding HMC's activities and policies was Memphis physician Tarleton C. Cottrell. He founded the institution and served as dean and board member. Born in 1861 during the waning days of slavery, Cottrell grew up on a rural northern Mississippi farm with his parents and seven siblings near Hudsonville and Holly Springs. Little information is available about his early life or his education, though an obituary notice indicated that he held "several diplomas."[47] Despite statements published in an 1888 history of Memphis and in a paid 1890 listing in *Polk's Medical Directory*, Cottrell did not earn any of those several diplomas at Meharry Medical College. He did enroll in Meharry's first-year medical class on two separate occasions, 1880–81 and again two years later, but never progressed beyond the first-year course.[48] He also claimed, in an 1890 medical directory, to have earned a medical degree from Bethel Medical Department of Southwestern University, Little Rock, Arkansas, in 1887.[49] Bethel Institute (now Shorter College), established by the African Methodist Episcopal Church in 1886, had no medical department, nor was there a school in Little Rock called Southwestern University.[50] That Cottrell graduated from this (or any) medical school is doubtful. Those two years at Meharry appear to constitute the entirety of his medical training.

Tennessee's lax medical practice laws allowed Cottrell, despite his scanty medical education, legally to open a medical practice in Memphis in 1883 or 1884. He advertised his presence in both 1885 city directories, paying an extra fee to have one of those listings appear in large type and in boldface.[51] A few years later, on May 29, 1889, Cottrell and four colleagues appeared before P. J. Quigley, clerk of the Shelby County Court, with the three-dollar fee required to obtain a charter in Tennessee and a petition to form a corporation named "Hannibal Medical College, Memphis Tennessee." The school's charge was clearly stated: "To encourage education in the science of medicine, surgery and pharmacy among the young men of the South and South West which shall be equal to any medical college in the South and [upon] the completion of the prescribed course of study laid down by the Board of Directors, together with certificates of good moral character, the Directors shall confer the degree of Doctor of Medicine, Surgery, or Pharmacy."[52]

The five founders included two physicians and two ministers. George M. Anderson, a member of Meharry Medical College's third graduating class (1879), moved to Memphis in 1882.[53] He studied medicine at the same time Cottrell's older brother, Elias, a future bishop and leading figure in the Colored (now Christian) Methodist Episcopal (CME) Church, studied theology at Central Tennessee College, Meharry's parent institution at the time.[54] HMC founder and board member Charles L. Fields was a minister in the CME Church who appears to have lived in Memphis only intermittently.[55] The other clergyman on the board, Alonzo L. Hall, obtained his education at Roger Williams University in Nashville, began his ministry in 1880, and was serving Memphis' First Baptist Church by 1888. In his later years Hall owned a newspaper and a publishing house and wrote at least two books.[56] The college's fifth founder, Henry H. Humes, arrived in Memphis as a schoolteacher in 1883 and held positions between 1884 and 1897 as a laborer, nurse, U.S. Customs House worker, bailiff, and crier of the U.S. District Count.[57]

The name Hannibal, invoking an image of the legendary North African (Carthaginian) general of Roman days who marched across the Alps with his army and won victory against all odds, was well known to and highly regarded by founder Alonzo Hall, whose 1907 book *The Ancient, Mediaeval and Modern Greatness of the Negro* included a section on Carthage and Hannibal.[58] HMC, however, did not live up to its powerful name. Evidence indicates that HMC never became a regularly functioning medical school.

HMC had no single location until its final few years. Between 1889 and 1893, the school moved to a different address each term. During four of HMC's seven official years, Tarleton C. Cottrell's office address, and sometimes also his home address, as well as the business and residence addresses of several other Memphis African Americans, were identical with HMC's.[59] During the academic year 1891–92, for example, HMC operated from a building at 130 Beale Street that also contained the offices of a jewelry agent, an African American newspaper, two dentists, and a physician (Cottrell). A laborer resided there as well.[60] Frequent moves and the use of shared quarters with a practicing physician and others suggest that HMC could not have offered students decent laboratory, dissecting, and classroom facilities or learning materials such as models, charts, laboratory equipment, cadavers, and library books.

Though HMC does not appear to have provided adequate instructional facilities for students, a picture displayed in the 1894 Memphis city directory conveys a very different image of the school's physical plant.[61] The full-page advertisement announcing HMC's faculty and board of directors for the coming academic

Figure 12. Hannibal Medical College Faculty

Name	Race	School Attended	Year of Grad.	Years Taught at Hannibal
Anderson, George M.	black	Meharry Medical College	1879	[1889–91]–96
Chiles, Benjamin F.	white	Physio-Medical College of Indiana	1884	1893–94 [–96?]
Cottrell, Tarleton C.	black	Bethel Med. Dept. Southwestern U.	1887	1889–96
Hall, Alonzo L.	black	Hannibal Medical College	1889	1889–96
Hickman, Clifford J.	black	Eclectic Medical Inst. of Cincinnati	1889	1891–94 [–96?]
Jackson, George Richard	black	U. Michigan College of Pharmacy	1892	1893–96
Jay, Jacob Palmer	black	unknown	unknown	1891–93
Jeter, James Troy	black	Hannibal Medical College	1891	1891–94 [–96?]
Morgan, William F. H.	black	Hannibal Medical College	1891	1891–96
Settle, Josiah T.	black	Howard Law School	1875	1893–96

year, 1893–94 (annual city directories were usually published during the fall of the preceding year), contains a large uncaptioned drawing depicting, a reader would have assumed, Hannibal's building and grounds. Contemporary Sanborn Fire Insurance maps of Memphis indicate, however, that those well-landscaped grounds and the imposing New Orleans–style, three-story rectangular building containing many large windows could not have been at the 121 Beale Street address given elsewhere in the directory as HMC's home base.[62] The HMC advertisement did not represent an existing building.

In addition to lacking a permanent home and adequate teaching facilities and equipment, Hannibal employed an instructional staff of questionable quality and credentials who seemingly could not have been in Memphis during the teaching term. When HMC opened in 1889, Dr. John H. Rauch from the Illinois State Department of Health noted in a report surveying the state of medical education in the United States that only three of HMC's five instructors "claim to have degrees of M.D."[63] One of those three was Tarleton C. Cottrell, holder of an M.D. degree from the nonexistent Bethel Medical Department; another was the regularly trained George M. Anderson.[64] Rauch's 1890 and 1891 reports also stated that "the faculty embraces five professors, two white and three colored men." Neither the third black physician-instructor nor the two white faculty members can be identified from available evidence. It is possible, however, to identify the person Rauch describes as "a minister, who has charge of classes in chemistry and physiology."[65] He was probably founder and board member Alonzo L. Hall.[66]

If Hall was the non-M.D. faculty member who taught chemistry and physiology at HMC, he was in an unusual situation. Medical directories of the time list him as an 1889 graduate of Hannibal, though the school's first term of instruction did not end until the spring of 1890. Yet he must have obtained his degree in 1889, for he also received a Tennessee medical license in 1889 (the year licensure was first required in the state) and so needed to have graduated from a recognized medical school or passed a medical examination. For the first few years of its existence, the Tennessee Board of Medical Examiners recognized all Tennessee medical schools.[67] It is possible that Hall had made special arrangements with his colleagues on the HMC board to receive a medical degree before the end of the regular school and calendar years, or that the HMC board used the powers granted in its charter to issue Hall a diploma, though he may not have attended classes and thus not really "earned" his degree. Regardless of how he obtained that diploma, Hall was simultaneously a medical student, faculty member, and board member at HMC during the 1889–90 academic year. His background provides few clues as to how he could have gained the knowledge and qualifications to teach medical or scientific subjects during the 1889–90 school year. A medical directory of the Southern states published in 1891 reports that Alonzo L. Hall, professor of the theory and practice of materia medica at HMC, was an 1883 graduate of Bethel Medical College, the nonexistent school from which Cottrell claimed to have received his medical degree, and an 1890 graduate of Hannibal. Hall continued to teach at HMC until the school closed.[68] Thus, of the three original HMC faculty members who can be identified, two had questionable credentials: Tarleton C. Cottrell and Alonzo L. Hall.

Of the several faculty members HMC hired over the next few years, at least two (in addition to Hall) were recently graduated HMC students. James Troy Jeter graduated from Hannibal in 1891, opened a medical practice in Memphis that same year, and immediately joined the faculty.[69] Though listed as an instructor at HMC between 1891 and 1896 and as a resident of Memphis in the 1892 and 1894 city directories, Jeter also established residency in Guthrie, Oklahoma Territory, during late 1892 and obtained his Oklahoma Territory medical license in 1893.[70] He later became a leader among Oklahoma's African American health professionals, serving in 1908 as the first president of the Oklahoma Medical, Dental, and Pharmaceutical Society, an African American professional association.[71] Jeter's HMC classmate William F. H. Morgan, a dentist, taught at Hannibal from the fall immediately following graduation (1891) until the end of the 1895–96 term. In the fall of 1891, and possibly earlier, he was treasurer of HMC's board of directors, a position he held until the school closed.[72] As recent graduates, Hall, Jeter, and Morgan had only limited experience with patients and little opportunity to keep abreast of changing ideas and practices in medicine when they assumed their teaching responsibilities. Yet they were now expected to teach science and clinical medicine to students only a year or two behind them.

Two or perhaps three instructors at Hannibal were members of medical sects, rivals of regular (allopathic) physicians during the nineteenth century.[73] Benjamin F. Chiles, the only identifiable white member of the HMC faculty, graduated from the Physio-Medical College of Indiana in 1884, moved to Memphis about 1890, and is listed on faculty rosters from 1893–94 to 1895–96.[74] Clifford J. Hickman, who received his medical degree from the Eclectic Medical Institute of Cincinnati in 1889 and moved to Memphis in late 1890 or 1891,[75] was included on faculty lists for 1891–92 through 1895–96. Interestingly, Memphis city directories indicate that both Chiles and Hickman had left Memphis by late 1894, putting into question their listings as faculty members for the 1895–96 school year. Another faculty member, Jacob Palmer Jay, held an HMC appointment for the 1891–92 and 1892–93 terms, though he lived and practiced in Evansville, Indiana, from at least late 1892 until late 1895. Jay never provided medical directory compilers with the basic information other physicians supplied, such as school and year of graduation. Possibly he was an eclectic physician like Hickman, as an article he wrote for an eclectic medical journal suggests.[76]

Hannibal did include on its faculty, from 1893–94 to 1895–96, two instructors of known reputation and ability, though neither was a physician. George Robert Jackson earned his bachelor's degree from Oberlin College and, in 1892, his graduate in pharmacy (Ph.G.) degree from the University of Michigan, one of only two students in his graduating class of thirty-five to have received a prior college degree. Jackson took courses from two leaders in the fields of pharmacy and pharmacology, John Jacob Abel, who taught the combined medical, dental, and pharmacy classes at the University of Michigan during the academic year 1891–92, and Albert Prescott, the school's first dean. Moving to Memphis in 1893, Jackson first managed, then owned and managed Beale Street's New Era Pharmacy and continued to operate drugstores in Memphis until his death in 1935.[77]

Medical jurisprudence and forensic medicine at HMC were the provinces of Josiah T. Settle, a well-known African American lawyer of Memphis. Settle also attended Oberlin College, though only for a year, then graduated in Howard University's first collegiate class (1872) and later completed studies at Howard's law department. He practiced law and served in the Mississippi State Legislature for a term, then moved to Memphis in 1885, where he was appointed assistant attorney general of the Shelby County Criminal Court and rose to prominence both as a lawyer and as a member of the black elite of the city. So nationally recognized was Settle that he was included in William J. Simmons's 1887 compilation of important African Americans.[78]

Given the educational backgrounds and varied levels of experience of Hannibal's staff, as well as their comings and goings from Memphis at times when they were listed as faculty members, the quality of teaching at the school was uneven at best. Regular instruction was, according to advertisements, occasionally augmented by presentations and demonstrations from local Memphis physicians who were not on the HMC faculty.[79] The number, names, and stature of these volunteer teachers is not known.

Admissions standards at HMC were minimal. Typical of lower-tier medical schools of the late nineteenth century, the school, in its early years and presumably until it closed in 1896, asked only that students seeking admission (1) possess "good moral character," (2) "give evidence of at least a good English education," (3) be at least eighteen years old, and (4) "believe in a Supreme Being."[80] Those enrolled then paid a one-time matriculation fee of five dollars and an annual tuition of twenty-five dollars. Room, board, and books were extra. By the start of the 1892 term, the school had added a twenty-five-dollar graduation fee to the list of charges, providing "materials for practical anatomy and chemistry . . . at cost."[81]

Hannibal's graduation requirements, like those of its contemporaries, looked strict in print, but were probably not rigorously enforced, also a typical practice of lower-tier schools. To receive the M.D. degree, students had to be twenty-one years old, possess "good moral character," have studied medicine for three years, have attended two years of lectures at HMC, have completed a "satisfactory examination in the required branches" of medicine, have "dissected during two courses," and have written a thesis.[82] There is at least one indicator and other hints that HMC officials did not adhere to these printed requirements: Rev. Alonzo Hall, who graduated in 1889, could not have attended Hannibal for two years or dissected during two terms or studied medicine for three years (unless he studied elsewhere previously). Similarly, the two 1891 graduates James T. Jeter and William F. H. Morgan could not have studied medicine for three years at Hannibal, and there is no evidence available that they studied medicine elsewhere before enrolling at HMC.

Even if Hannibal granted M.D. degrees less strictly than the college's written rules allowed, that policy seems not to have enticed many students to enroll. In addition to Hall, Jeter, and Morgan, the only known HMC graduates were Samuel Hutchinson (1892) and John J. Pullen (1892).[83] The only actual extant student number count derives from the 1891 Illinois State Board of Health survey of medical education across the United States.[84] It listed four matriculates at HMC for 1889–90, the school's first session.

Hannibal produced no more physicians after 1892.[85] The exact year in which HMC closed cannot be determined from available sources, but it may not have operated from 1893 to its official closing in 1896. The Memphis city directory lists Hannibal in the collegiate section of both its 1895 and 1896 editions, along with the names of HMC's faculty and board of directors. But the school is not mentioned in the alphabetical or street listings of these volumes, which were compiled during the fall of 1894 and 1895, respectively, nor does it list three faculty members, Chiles, Hickman, and Jeter. Cottrell is shown at 121 Beale, the last known address of the school, but he is listed only as a physician, not as dean or other official at HMC, the way previous listings had recognized him.[86]

Based on its annual moves to new locations, its inadequate facilities and equipment, its use of some undereducated and perhaps unqualified faculty, and its presumably small income from small enrollments, HMC appears never to have been a credible or respected institution. Such actions as granting an M.D. degree to a faculty/board member before the conclusion of the first academic year, awarding an M.D. degree to a faculty/board member two years later, using nonphysicians/nonscientists to teach scientific and medical subjects, continuing to list faculty members on the roster after they no longer resided in Memphis, employing recent graduates to teach, and including "irregular" physicians on the faculty could not have enhanced Hannibal's reputation or its enrollment. It appears that HMC faculty rarely taught their classes and that students obtained their degrees without seeing much of faculty, laboratories, or patients.

For a school trying to lure students to its doors, HMC officials chose to advertise the school in an unusual and limited place—Memphis city directories.[87] Placing ads in the city newspapers during the weeks preceding the opening of the school each year, as other medical schools did, would probably have reached a wider audience. Nor did the HMC board advertise in the *Indianapolis Freeman*, a leading regional African American newspaper of the day, or in Miles V. Lynk's newly established journal, the *Medical and Surgical Observer*, published in nearby Jackson, Tennessee, from 1892 to 1894, and aimed at African Americans in the profession. Every other black medical school then operating (Howard, Meharry, Leonard, New Orleans, and Louisville National) either advertised in the *Observer* or received news coverage in it. About Hannibal, the journal remained almost silent, a telling omission for a publication that invited and included any information thought important to the small black medical community of the time. Lynk's only reference to the school less than one hundred miles from Jackson seemed embarrassed and distancing. He mentioned Hannibal in passing as a foil in order to praise the other independent black medical school then operating, Louisville National Medical College: "We are truly proud to say, not like the Hannibal Medical Institute, of Memphis, it [Louisville National] has passed the probationary stage and now its diplomas are recognized by the leading state boards of medical examiners."[88]

Hannibal had, it appears, not "passed the probationary stage" or earned the respect of the medical profession, black or white. Members of Tennessee's State Board of Medical Examiners and the state medical society held low opinions of the school. Dr. T. J. Happel, secretary of the state board and prominent member of the medical society, commented, in reference to the need for a revision of the medical practice act in 1900, "The Hannibal Medical College, in Memphis, and two other colleges in the State, have already procured charters. Some individuals have procured diplomas by enrolling at colleges without attending the lectures. . . . And if a man gets a diploma, no difference how, from a Tennessee college, he can legally practice upon presenting that diploma to the examiners."[89] Schools like Hannibal, Happel implied, gave the state a bad medical reputation and needed to be regulated. The State Board of Medical Examiners did, at some point not recorded in its published annual reports (its unpublished papers appear to have been lost or destroyed), take action against HMC. It refused to recognize diplomas from the school.[90]

Tarleton C. Cottrell died at age thirty-eight of phthisis, on October 27, 1899, just a few years after his school closed. An obituary notice answers some of the questions about the nature of Cottrell's institution and leaves others unanswered. Interestingly, the obituary refers to Hannibal as "Bethel Medical College," further confusing the issue of where Cottrell and Alonzo Hall actually studied medicine and opening the possibility that the Memphis school was known by two different names, despite its chartered name of Hannibal. It also calls HMC "a projected school for colored men" and explains that "while this school never was built, several young men finished their courses under its name." These statements make it clear that Hannibal had no physical plant of its own and tend to corroborate the harsh assessments of HMC given by respected white and black physicians such as T. J. Happel and Miles V. Lynk. Yet Hannibal did graduate a few physicians who, as the obituary notice stated, "are doing much to relieve humanity."[91]

Cottrell, like black medical school founders William Henry Fitzbutler, Thomas W. Haigler (Chattanooga National Medical College) and Miles V. Lynk (University of West Tennessee College of Medicine and Surgery), was a "doer." In his short life, he, according to the obituary, "was editor of the Crusade Banner, a weekly paper and did much to prove the colored man's ability to edit a paper, . . . was professor in penmanship and drawing," and was a medical school organizer and a physician with "quite a lucrative practice." So involved was Cottrell with Memphis' secret societies for African Americans, especially the Masons and the Odd Fellows, the obituary continued, that "many times he has closed his office to chat with his friends and brethren along these secret lines."[92] Another obituary stated that Cottrell "was generally respected by the white residents of the community and was a man of influence among members of his own race."[93] His medical school, HMC, never earned that respect or influence.

Chattanooga National Medical College, 1899–1904

On May 20, 1899, five African American citizens of Chattanooga filed papers with the clerk of Hamilton County, Tennessee, permitting them to establish and operate a medical school in that city.[94] A few months later, the second independent and third medical college in Tennessee in a decade dedicated to training African Americans opened its doors. (Chattanooga had a white medical school between 1889 and 1910 affiliated, primarily in name, with Grant University of Athens, Tennessee. There appears to have been little interaction between the black and white medical schools that coexisted in Chattanooga for a few years at the turn of the century.) Like HMC, Chattanooga National Medical College (CNMC) failed to establish a sound and credible education program and, like its predecessor at the opposite end of the state, failed to earn a favorable reputation either within or outside Tennessee. It survived for just five years but did graduate a number of physicians who went on to practice in various parts of the country.

Chattanooga in the late 1890s did not want for physicians. Approximately one hundred practiced in that city of 30,000–35,000 persons during the years around the turn of the twentieth century. Only a few of these physicians were persons of color.[95] Of the five men who founded the school and composed its first board of directors, one, Thomas William Haigler, was a physician. Haigler was the central figure at CNMC, the force that kept it alive, and, when he gave up his leadership position, that caused its demise.

As a physician, Haigler had more formal grounding in medicine than did his counterpart at Hannibal, Tarleton Cottrell. Born enslaved in Orangeburg County, South Carolina, in 1856 or 1857,[96] Haigler, according to a 1904 directory of prominent black Chattanoogans "studied the classics at Claflin University, Orangeburg, S.C.; the Business College course, at Clark University, Atlanta, Ga.; Theology, at Gammon School of Theology, Atlanta, Ga.; Philosophy, at Chicago; Pharmacy at the North-Western Medical College University, Toledo, O.; Stenography in the best Short-Hand college, Toledo, O.; He matriculated in the North Western Medical College and the Toledo Medical College, Toledo, O., and in the MaHarry [*sic*] Medical College, Nashville, Tenn. Finally, he matriculated and graduated from the Louisville National Medical College with high honors as Doctor of Medicine and Surgery."[97] The sketch listed his degrees as B.C.S., A.M., Ph.G., Psy.D., M.D., and D.D. Catalogs of the health-related schools he attended corroborate this information.[98]

At the time he opened CNMC (presumably named after his Louisville alma mater) in 1899, Haigler also operated a drugstore (opened in 1890), preached (he had held ministerial positions in South Carolina, Georgia, Tennessee, and Ohio since 1877) at the Temple African Methodist Episcopal Church (soon renamed Haigler's Temple A.M.E. Church), served as surgeon for the Immaculate and

Figure 13. Chattanooga National Medical College Faculty

Name	Graduated from	Race	Residence[1]	Taught[2]
Abby, John Nelson (M.D.)	Louisville National, 1891	black	Memphis, Tenn.	1899–1900
Byrom, Henry M. S. (M.D.)	Meharry, 1894	black	Whiteside, Marion Co., Tenn.	1899–1900
Cain, Commodore I. (M.D.)	Meharry, 1891	black	Rome, Ga.	1899–1900
Councill, William L. (M.D.)	Meharry, 1899	black	Nashville, Tenn.	1899–1900
Haigler, Thomas William (M.D.)	Louisville National, 1889	black	Chattanooga, Tenn.	1899–1900
Maples, William L. (M.D.)	Howard, 1892	black	Knoxville, Tenn.[3]	1899–1904
Murdock, John (M.D.)	Chattanooga National, 1902[4]	black?	Skylight, Oldham Co., Ky.	1899–1900
Parden, Noah W. (LL.B.)	Central Tenn. Coll., Law Dept	black	Chattanooga, Tenn.	1903–04

Compiled from Young and Company's *Business Directory of the Principal Cities of Tennessee and Northern Alabama, for 1900*, 29; and from medical and city directories of the period.

1. Town of residence during year(s) on CNMC faculty.

2. Documented years at CNMC. May have taught at CNMC additional years as well.

3. According to Samuel Joseph Platt and Mary Louise Ogden, *Medical Men and Institutions of Knox County Tennessee, 1789–1957* (Knoxville, Tenn.: Knoxville Academy of Medicine, 1969), 306, Maples died in 1897. Daniel Smith Lamb, comp., *Howard University Medical Department, Washington, D.C.: A Historical, Biographical and Statistical Souvenir* (Washington, D.C.: R. Beresford, 1900), 197, writing in 1900, did not have a report that Maples had died but indicated that he "is said to have recently removed elsewhere" from his last known address in South Pittsburg. He is not listed in medical directories after 1896.

4. Claimed, in medical directories of the time, to have also received M.D. degrees from Kentucky School of Medicine, Louisville, 1900; University of Edinburgh, Scotland, 1891; Michigan Medical College, Lansing, 1873; Michigan Homeopathic Medical College, Lansing, 1873.

Masonic Orders, as president of the Chattanooga Association of Medicine and Surgery, as medical examiner for the Metropolitan and the Mutual life insurance companies, and as treasurer and fund-raiser for a local Masonic lodge. Haigler clearly obeyed his personal motto of "keep a moving." He now added the duties of medical school faculty member, dean, and college president, though by late 1902 he had given up his pastorate.[99]

The four African American men who joined Haigler in organizing CNMC on October 3, 1898, raising $400 in capital stock, obtaining the charter the following spring, and overseeing, as a board of directors, the school's activities, came from nonmedical backgrounds.[100] Noah W. Parden, a graduate of the law department of Nashville's Central Tennessee College (home institution for Meharry Medical College), had practiced law in Chattanooga since the early 1890s. James T. Ross was a local justice of the peace, and J. A. Jones served as pastor at Warren's Chapel in town.[101] No information could be located about the remaining director, A. W. Throne.

Haigler and his board included language in the school's charter that allowed for growth and for attracting students interested in a variety of health-related professions. For example, CNMC could, according to the charter, hire faculty to "instruct and demonstrate in all of the branches of medicine," including pharmacy, dentistry, and "modern hypnotism." Each program, it was stipulated, would require four years of study except hypnotism, which would require six months. The board was also empowered to establish a library, a hospital, and a nurse-training program to provide professional nurses for the hospital.[102]

The board never expanded CNMC's activities beyond medical student education. A picture of the outside of the school's building at 602 East 8th Street appeared in J. Bliss White's 1904 booklet about black Chattanooga and provides the only evidence that the school had a physical plant.[103] That picture tells little about where classes were held or what sort of lecture or laboratory facilities the building actually contained. Space for the medical school must have been limited; city directories indicate that Haigler's residence, drugstore, and medical office shared the same address as the college.[104]

The nature of faculty instruction was as suspect as the quality of the facilities. Only one staff roster for CNMC survives, and that derives from an advertisement in Young and Company's *Business Directory of the Principal Cities of Tennessee and Northern Alabama, for 1900*.[105] That advertisement lists instructors for the school's first year of operation, 1899–1900. Several of the teachers would have had to make enormous efforts to meet their classes on a regular basis. Though three or four African American physicians practiced medicine in Chattanooga during the years the school was in operation, of the six physicians listed on the original faculty, only one (Haigler) lived in Chattanooga, one in a nearby town, and the others in the distant cities of Memphis, Nashville, and Knoxville, Tennessee, and Rome, Georgia.

Figure 14. Chattanooga National Medical College Students and Graduates

Name[1]	Year Graduated or Attended		Source of Information		
	Graduated	Attended	1904–05 Catalog[2]	Medical Directories[3]	Smith[4]
Avery, Robert C.			x	no	x
Boggs, A. A.	1904	1903–04	x	no	no
Bruce, A. K. (Ph.G.)	1902		x	no	no
Buckner, R. J. (B.D.)	1902		x	no	no
Caswell, William		1903–04	x	no	no
Clayburne, Joseph		1903–04	x	no	no
Coleman, James W.	1903[5]		no	x	x
Conyers, S. B.		1903–04	x	no	no
Crawford, Daniel W.	1901		x	x	x
Douglas, William L.	1907[6]	1903–04	x	x	x
Farrier, James A.	1902		x	no	no
Greene, Gene W. L.	1902		x	no	no
Greenlee, J. W.		1903–04	x	no	no
Henderson, William		1903–04	x	no	no
Hurt, Ella		1903–04	x	no	no
Johnson, Calvert P., Jr.	1902		x	no	no
Miller, Isaac Henry	1903		x[7]	no	no
Moses, Stephen Edward (A.B.)	1904	x	no	no	
Murdock, John (B.A.)	1902		x	x	no
Murray, T. T.	1901		x	no	no
Reynolds, Charles H.	1903		x	no	no
Ridout, Johnson		1903–04	x	no	no
Sanson, David H.		1903–04	x	no	no
Scheffield, Henry		1903–04	x	no	no
Sudduth, William Ewart	1904[5]		x	x	x
Thompson, Garfield		1903–04	x	no	no
Turner, James H.	1902		x	no	no

1. Degrees earned other than M.D. are in parentheses after person's name.

2. Information obtained from a list of students copied by AMA officials from "Announcement of the Chattanooga National Medical College, 7th Annual Session from September 2, 1904–April 27, 1905" lent to them in 1916 by a CNMC graduate. This list is housed at the AMA Archives, "Medical Schools Alumni," vol. 44, Chattanooga National Medical College.

3. Polk's and AMA medical directories, 1886–1912. Very few of the graduates of CNMC are listed in these directories, and those who are listed almost never identify CNMC as their medical alma mater.

4. William L. Smith and Dan J. Smith, "The Extinct Black Medical Colleges of the United States: A History" (unpublished manuscript; Los Angeles, Calif.: 1977), 22.

5. Not listed as a graduate in CNMC 1904–05 catalog, but AMA 1916 directory lists him as such.

6. Listed as a freshman in 1904–05 catalog, and as 1907 graduate of CNMC in 1916 AMA Directory (p. 1439), though CNMC appears to have closed in 1904.

7. Miller lent his copy of the 1904–05 CNMC catalog to the AMA in 1916 for list of graduates. Note at AMA Archives says he was then practicing in Nicholasville, Kentucky.

It is improbable that students at CNMC could have heard many lectures from that group of faculty members. The one other known M.D. faculty member from later years, John Murdock, graduated from CNMC in 1902 and moved to Kentucky, yet he announced in a national medical directory that he held the title of "Associate Professor of Materia Medica, Bacteriology and Microscopy" at the Chattanooga school.[106] Haigler did increase the size of the faculty after the school's first year, though the names and hometowns of faculty members could not be located.[107]

CNMC does not appear to have lacked for students. At least twenty-seven African American women and men attended one or more terms; at least sixteen may have graduated.[108] Though the school advertised a "four years' graded course" and fees of fifty dollars per term, it is doubtful that most CNMC students experienced a true four-year graded curriculum.[109] A list of students and graduates compiled by the AMA in 1916 from a CNMC 1904–5 catalog includes only three categories of students: seniors, freshmen, and special. A medical school entering its sixth year of operating a four-year curriculum would be expected to have at least a few students in each of the four classes. Furthermore, Isaac Henry Miller, the man who lent his 1904–5 CNMC catalog to the AMA in 1916, attended, at most, three academic years of classes, but still received his M.D. degree in 1903.[110] Based on the small amount of evidence available, CNMC's academic program, facilities, equipment, and teaching staff appear inadequate.

CNMC enjoyed only a short life. It closed abruptly in 1904 for unexplained reasons. The college seemed to be thriving up to that time, or at least succeeding. Its catalog had already been published announcing the seventh annual session (really the sixth) for 1904–5.[111] School may already have been in session when it closed. Haigler's name disappears from city directories after that year, and by late 1905, his building at 602 East 8th Street was occupied by a grocer, followed, a year later, by an undertaker and a shoemaker. The church with which he was closely associated and which was named for him ceased operations at this time as well. He must have been a sustaining and driving force within that church just as he had been at CNMC. Haigler is not listed in national medical directories from 1906 until 1912, when his name appears, now in Nashville, Tennessee. No information is available to explain why he left Chattanooga and took up practice in Nashville. He died in 1913.[112]

The University of West Tennessee College of Medicine and Surgery, 1900–1923

The University of West Tennessee College of Medicine and Surgery (UWT) graduated at least 155 physicians as well as a number of pharmacists, nurses, dentists, and, through its law school, attorneys during its twenty-three years of operation.[113]

Despite this seemingly impressive record, UWT, like its sister Tennessee proprietary schools Hannibal Medical College and Chattanooga National Medical College, earned little respect from the medical community at large, white or black. For much of the school's history, an M.D. degree from UWT was not recognized by boards of medical examiners in most states. The school's twenty-three-year survival was owed to the strength of personality and character of its founder and president, Miles Vandahurst Lynk (1871–1956). Like Hannibal and Chattanooga National, West Tennessee's history is deeply intertwined with its founder's.

Lynk was in many ways a self-made man. Born of former slaves on June 3, 1871, he grew up on a farm in western Tennessee near Brownsville.[114] The basic education he obtained at rural black schools and through home study enabled him to pass Haywood County's teacher's exam and to obtain a teaching certificate at age thirteen, too young to use it. Wanting to become a physician, Lynk continued his education by studying more advanced subjects such as algebra, biology, geometry, Latin, and physics with a private tutor. To earn money for medical school tuition, he secured another teacher's certificate in 1888 and taught at a rural black summer school. During the next year, Jacob C. Hairston, a newly graduated Meharry physician,[115] who had opened a practice in Brownsville, became Lynk's preceptor. Lynk enrolled at Meharry Medical College in Nashville in the fall of 1889, passing the entrance examinations at a high enough level to begin with the second-year class, and, in the spring of 1891, at the age of nineteen, graduated second in a class of thirteen.[116] He then moved back to western Tennessee, becoming the first African American physician in Jackson, Madison County's seat of government, with a population of approximately ten thousand. To help ease his entry into the community and the profession, Lynk introduced himself to local white physicians and druggists and, according to his autobiography, "gave each my card with the statement that I shall endeavor to practice scientific and ethical medicine."[117] The strategy seemed to work. One of the white physicians in town acquainted his own black patients with the new African American physician. Lynk encountered few problems from his white professional brethren. With time he also won the trust of skeptical African American patients unaccustomed to the presence of a black physician.[118] In the September 26, 1891, issue of the CME Church newspaper, *The Christian Index*, published in Jackson, its editor wrote, "Dr. M.V. Lynk, our Colored physician in this city, has built up such a large practice that it became very necessary that he have a horse and buggy to meet his calls. He now has a splendid outfit and is doing well. Our prediction last winter that a colored doctor would do well here has proven to be true. We are quite glad to see our people giving him their patronage. This is nothing more than right."[119]

As he progressed in his career, Lynk combined self-confidence with boldness and a willingness to take risks in promoting African Americans and their causes both locally and nationally. Between 1891 and 1915, he founded or cofounded a national medical journal—the *Medical and Surgical Observer*—that focused on blacks; a national black physicians' organization—the National Medical Association—that celebrated its one hundredth anniversary in 1995; and a medical school that trained primarily African American physicians.[120] He wrote books and edited a magazine for African Americans on black history, literature, and culture; established a publishing house to print and sell those books and magazines; provided employment to a dozen or more of Jackson's black citizens at the publishing company; earned a law degree; and opened a law school so other blacks could also become lawyers, all from his base in Jackson.[121] Lynk, who bore names similar to those of the CME Church's first two bishops, William Henry Miles and Richard H. Vanderhorst, and who lived in the town that was home to the CME's mother church, Liberty Church, earned further respect for his involvement in that denomination's activities.[122]

In 1900, Lynk undertook an ambitious enterprise to promote the cause of African Americans: the founding of a university to train professionals in medicine and law. It began when he sought to study law in Jackson. Lane College, a local CME Church–sponsored institution, had no law school, and no lawyer in town was available to read law with Lynk (an apprenticeship).[123] Lynk located an African American attorney in Memphis, H. R. Sadler, willing to teach, a small group (including two Lane College instructors, a public school teacher, a public school principal, a letter carrier, an industrialist, and two pastors) willing to enroll as law students, and Lane College board president Bishop Isaac Lane, who was willing to establish a law department. Lynk purchased a set of textbooks and the library of a deceased white lawyer, which served as the basis of a library for the school. Classes were held daily at either Lynk's office or in a room at Lane College. Within nine months, by mid-February 1901, Lynk had earned his law degree, passed the state bar exam, and been accepted to practice law in Madison County, Tennessee. Lynk now applied this model of creating educational opportunities for people of color where none had existed before to establish what he called a "college for the professional training of ambitious Negroes," the University of West Tennessee.[124]

According to its founder, UWT was organized in 1900 "for the purpose of furnishing thorough courses in the professions, regardless of race and color" and "for the purpose of furnishing facilities for the higher education of Afro-American youth."[125] Lynk joined four other African American Jacksonians to form a board of trustees for the new school: Rev. R. E. Hart, pastor of Jackson's Liberty CME Church; postman J. H. Trimble; and two physicians, Samuel Henry Broome (Meharry class of 1897) and John Lucian Light (Meharry class of 1898).[126] The majority of funds came from Lynk and his wife, Beebe Steven Lynk.[127]

Some of the funds went toward housing the school. Lynk located a four-room house with a concrete basement on a 90-by-65-foot lot in the heart of Jackson (southeast corner of Sycamore and Liberty streets). In February 1901 he and his wife contracted to purchase it for $1,800 plus interest, paying $30 per month after an initial down payment of $230.[128] The building still required an additional investment of funds for renovation before UWT staff could begin teaching. Classrooms, laboratories, and an auditorium were fitted to accommodate instruction in medicine, dentistry, pharmacy, law, and nursing. Still more money was spent on desks, supplies, teaching materials, and technical and scientific apparatus for laboratories. To cover the costs of constructing and equipping the school the Lynks mortgaged their home.[129]

Announcements were printed and sent out publicizing the opening of a new professional school for African Americans on September 15, 1901.[130] Thirty or so medical, dental, pharmaceutical, and law students from six states responded to the call, enrolled, and assembled for an opening convocation on the appointed day. A crowd of well-wishers and the curious filled an improvised auditorium (two rooms and the hallway of the newly renovated house) at the refurbished building to see the new students and hear Rev. N. B. Smith, an elder in the CME Church, present a sermon.[131] Classes began.

Available evidence clearly documents that classes at UWT were actually held, unlike the questionable educational activities at HMC and CNMC. An extant 1901 photograph contains pictures of faculty and students, the seemingly well-equipped and well-stocked chemical and pharmaceutical laboratories, a "moot court scene" from the law department, and a "class in dissecting," including cadaver.[132] An article in the *Indianapolis Freeman* described a correspondent's visit to the school and published a photo of the school's building.[133]

The medical faculty at UWT included both blacks and whites. Samuel Henry Broome, a Jackson resident, 1897 Meharry graduate, and cofounder and trustee of the school, taught and served as secretary of the faculty. Walter Fenner Rochelle had graduated from Vanderbilt University's medical department in 1882 and practiced in Jackson for many years. His white colleague on the UWT faculty John T. Herron, an 1884 graduate of Jefferson Medical College in Philadelphia, specialized in and taught diseases of the eye, ear, nose, and throat. As was true at other African American schools in Tennessee, UWT's faculty contained several out-of-town instructors who would have had to travel long distances numerous times during each term to teach their classes regularly, including Meharry graduates Robert G. Martin, Ernest W. Irving, and Jacob C. Hairston (Lynk's former mentor), all from Memphis, some eighty miles away.[134] Lynk himself appears to have done the bulk of the teaching, assuming professorships of obstetrics, materia medica, surgery, clinical medicine, and electrotherapeutics. He was also president of the faculty and dean of the school. His wife, Beebe Steven Lynk, taught medical Latin and botany. She may have assumed instructional duties in materia medica after receiving her Ph.C. (certificate of pharmacy) from the

UWT School of Pharmacy in 1903. *Polk's Medical Directory* listed UWT's 1901–2 faculty at fourteen and its 1902–3 faculty at ten.[135]

Despite its location in rural western Tennessee, UWT School of Medicine did manage to attract students. Lynk reported a student body of seventeen during the 1902–3 academic year, and forty for 1905–6.[136] Matriculates for the 1903–4 term, which lasted six months, paid tuition and fees of forty dollars. They had to attend four years of classes to graduate, though those with a bachelor's degree could attain advanced standing and shorten their stay. There is no way to determine how strictly authorities at the school enforced attendance rules in Jackson, as no listing of students there is available. UWT did not graduate its first medical class until 1904, three years after the school opened, unlike HMC and CNMC, which graduated students during the first year of operation. In 1903, UWT's trustees increased the length of the school term from six months to seven months and the entrance requirements to a four-year high school program or its equivalent.[137] University of West Tennessee administrators and faculty preserved a nonsectarian but religious tone at the school by requiring daily attendance at "morning devotion" and weekly attendance at "some Christian Church on the Sabbath." Rev. W. H. Wilson, D.D., was the school's chaplain. As at Leonard Medical School, the goal was to instill Christian values into students so that their "ethical and religious nature . . . may be fully developed along with their intellectual faculties."[138] Medical students could also participate in the M. V. Lynk Medical Society (which met every Saturday afternoon), the Alpha Literary Society, Young Men's Christian Association, Athletic Association, and Vandahurst Musical Quartette.[139]

By August 1903, and probably earlier, UWT was operating University Hospital, providing students with access to patients. Little information is available about this facility other than what a newspaper reporter stated: "[I]t furnishes abundant clinical material for the medical department, and at the same time is of incalculable help to the poor people of Jackson and surrounding country. Its wards, including good board, nursing, medicine and medical and surgical attention, are free to the poor."[140] The hospital also offered a nurse-training program. A ladies auxiliary committee assisted in running the hospital.

By 1907, UWT had graduated sixteen physicians, one dentist, four pharmacists, and five lawyers.[141] That year, Lynk and his board decided to move the school to a larger city—Memphis—explaining in the 1906–7 catalog: "The rapid growth of the school has made it necessary that we move to a more metropolitan center where clinical facilities will be second to none in the United States." Memphis, it continued, "is a city of nearly 200,000 inhabitants, about half of whom are thrifty Afro-Americans." The many industries there "give rise to numerous accidents and injuries, furnishing to the free clinics and hospitals connected with our school rich material for surgical and clinical work."[142] So, a decade after one

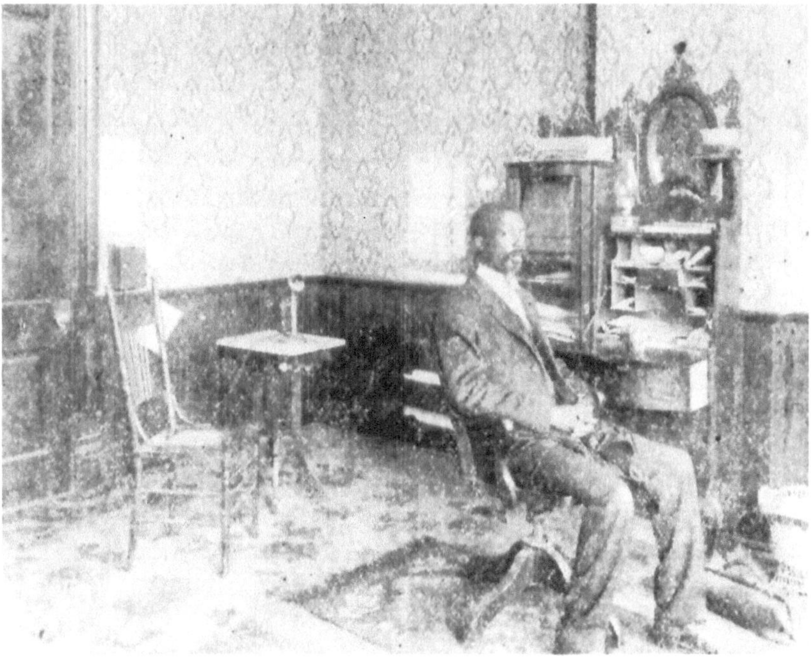

Fig. 15. M. V. Lynk in his office. Photograph from G. P. Hamilton, *The Bright Side of Memphis: A Compendium of Information Concerning the Colored People of Memphis, Tennessee* (Memphis, Tenn.: n.p., 1908), 257.

black independent medical school (Hannibal) had closed in Memphis, another, larger and stronger than its predecessor, prepared to open.

Lynk disposed of his Jackson properties, including the UWT lot and building, which brought $1,500 cash, and purchased, during the summer of 1907, a one-and-one-fourth acre lot in Memphis.[143] The lot was not on or near Beale Street, the heart of black Memphis at the time, but rather in the developing southeastern black suburbs close to good downtown streetcar connections. Two vacant buildings stood on the property at 1190 South Phillips Place, only recently the home of Grace School, a white public school.[144] Laboratories were installed in North Hall, and two large lecture rooms (separated by folding doors) that could accommodate as many as three hundred students were built in South Hall.[145] Clinical instruction was available at three locations. UWT faculty operated a free dispensary (outpatient clinic) at the college building. Several blocks away, Lynk's mentor and UWT faculty member Jacob C. Hairston had recently established a hospital providing black physicians a place to perform surgery on their patients. Slightly farther away, Dr. Cleveland A. Terrell and his nephew Lawrence G. Patterson, both Meharry graduates, operated the Terrell-Patterson Infirmary, also available for UWT teaching purposes.[146]

Memphis had a large African American medical community (more than forty physicians in 1908) from which UWT could draw faculty, the majority of whom had graduated from, and felt a loyalty to, Lynk's medical alma mater, Meharry.[147] Though local white physicians lectured occasionally at the school, UWT trustees recruited an all–African American faculty, not only in the medical school but in every department (including dentistry, pharmacy, and law), throughout the remainder of the university's existence.[148]

Opening ceremonies and lectures began at the new Memphis campus of UWT on September 18, 1907.[149] As with Tennessee's other African American independent medical schools, promise outstripped performance. If UWT provided a superior, or even an adequate education for its students during its sixteen years in Memphis, few people in the medical world, either white or black, other than its graduates, acknowledged that fact. The university encountered difficulties almost from the start, and by the time it closed at the end of the 1922–23 term, medical licensing boards in forty-six states plus Tennessee refused to recognize its diplomates.[150] Furthermore, though UWT was a cut above schools like Hannibal and CNMC in the quality of education provided, it began slipping not long after moving to Memphis.

The three UWT catalogs extant, for 1906–7, 1907–8, and 1909–10, with announcements in each for the subsequent academic year, show that Lynk had full knowledge of the rising criteria in medical education occurring nationally. In 1907, UWT explicitly "adopted the requirements for admission, to the Freshman class, as laid down by the Association of American Medical Colleges" and published them in the catalog for students to see. Stated graduation requirements also adhered to AAMC standards. By 1910, the catalog no longer invoked the AAMC, but that group's influence was clearly present in the requirements listed.[151] Catalogs also described the school's "methods of teaching" major courses, mentioning, for example, daily recitations in the classroom, experiments in the laboratory, dissections, lectures, microscopes, manikins, stereopticon, drug preparations, "outdoor" (outpatient) clinic and hospital patients, bandaging classes, preventive medicine, electrotherapy, and staining techniques—modern medicine for a modern school. Tough-sounding grading, attendance, and tuition-payment policies further gave the impression to prospective students that UWT was a well-managed school where one could obtain a good professional education.[152]

One indication that UWT was failing to keep up with the medical education reforms of the early twentieth century was the result of Abraham Flexner's visit to Memphis in November 1909. Flexner had gone to Tennessee's other medical-school cities—Nashville, Knoxville, and Chattanooga—almost a year earlier, in January. He now inspected UWT and the city's two white schools, Memphis Hospital Medical College, founded in 1880, and the College of Physicians and Surgeons, established just a year before UWT moved to town. Both white schools were housed in excellent, modern facilities, but, Flexner felt, still did not provide an acceptable education to students. Of UWT he thought even less, essentially contradicting all that the school's catalog for that year claimed about programs and facilities.[153] The difference between what Lynk and Flexner reported about UWT's facilities was glaring. UWT's 1909–10 catalog stated:

> About 120 experiments [are] performed in the chemical laboratory. . . . [A] thorough course in qualitative analysis will be given in the laboratory. . . . [S]tudents will be given an opportunity to examine a great number of both crude and prepared drugs from our collection in the pharmaceutical laboratory. . . . Our microscopical laboratory is equipped with Bausch and Lomb microscopes, fitted with Abbe condensers, iris diaphragms 2.3, 1.6 and 1/2 inch oil immersion objectives. Hemocyptometers [*sic*], microtomes, incubators, urinometers and other instruments and appliances are used. In bacteriology most of the important pathogenic bacteria are cultivated, stained and examined.[154]

Flexner saw UWT's laboratory facilities and tersely commented, "There is meager equipment for chemistry, pharmacy, and microscopy. Otherwise the rooms are bare."[155] Similarly, whereas Lynk's catalog pointed to the modern clinical facilities at the nearby forty-patient Negro Baptist Hospital (formerly the Terrell-Patterson Infirmary) and at the fifteen-patient Hairston Hospital, both "directly under the control of our Faculty," Flexner remarked about these same facilities, "The students have access to eight or ten beds, twice weekly, in a small hospital close by." Concerning the UWT "free dispensary in the College Building . . . operated by our Faculty, furnishing abundant clinical material for our students," Flexner stated, "There is a dispensary, without records, in the school building." For Flexner, the medical school at UWT was "without merit."[156] In just a few sentences, Flexner, representing the national medical establishment, publicly cast doubt on the quality of Lynk's medical education program. By reporting equipment and facilities differently from the school's catalog, he also, without saying as much, raised questions about UWT's integrity, just as he did about numerous other medical schools of the period, both white and black.[157] Lynk kept his school open, however, unlike operators of many other schools that received strong criticism in the Flexner Report.

Another national figure, who visited UWT in 1915, six years after Flexner, corroborated his predecessor's assessment, but provided more descriptive evidence to support his negative evaluation. Thomas Jesse Jones of the U.S. Bureau of Education did a survey of all institutions of higher education for African Americans and published a two-volume report of his findings in 1917. The University of West Tennessee, Jones began, "claims to teach courses in medicine, pharmacy,

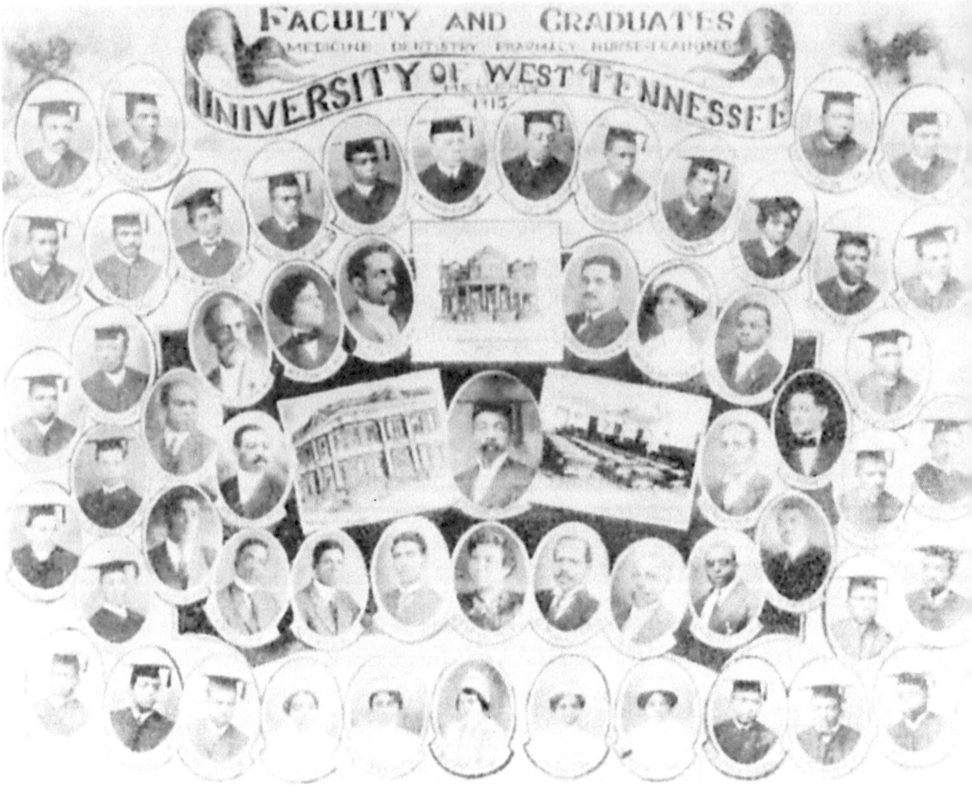

Fig. 16. University of West Tennessee, Faculty and Graduates, Class of 1915. Photograph from M. V. Lynk, *Sixty Years of Medicine, or the Life and Times of Dr. Miles V. Lynk, An Autobiography* (Memphis, Tenn.: Twentieth Century Press, 1951), 50.

dentistry, and automobile engineering." (Lynk did not mention this last program in his autobiography or in other published materials.) On the approximately one acre of land encompassing the school's property, Jones found "four frame buildings, and one brick veneer building." The teaching force consisted of three men, though "some of the Memphis colored physicians lecture irregularly."[158] He went on to report, "The buildings were very dirty and the equipment and teaching force inadequate. . . . All the class instruction was given in one room. The laboratory work occupied two small rooms. There were only one or two charts and four microscopes, of which two were out of commission. One filthy room with four chairs constituted the dental department. The dissecting room was the attic of a small barn or out-building. The so-called 'automobile engineering' [department] consisted of tinkering with two old automobiles."[159] Though Jones, like Flexner, was not a medical person, he had visited numerous institutions of higher learning with which he could compare UWT's facilities, equipment, and faculty size. UWT did not measure up.

Another appraisal of UWT came from an African American dentist who graduated from Meharry Dental College in 1918. Though George W. West, born in Memphis in 1894, did not attend UWT, he knew about its existence and its reputation. In a 1976 interview, West recalled two reasons he and others he knew chose to attend Meharry and not UWT. One reason related to the mistrust African Americans still felt, fifty years after the end of slavery, about the abilities of black professionals: "Well, my mother didn't have to tell me this but, you know, it's a certain idea that we have about things that are operated by colored people because that's something we've been brainwashed from slavery up to now. And I just felt we could get a better education coming to Meharry because the University of West Tennessee was operated solely by colored."[160] His primary reason for not attending UWT, however, related to what he perceived as the school's low educational standards: "The ones that were the heads of the school were accepting some fellows . . . in the school that didn't have the literary foundation. . . . I knew their educational preparation wasn't up to par." West speculated that Lynk accepted them "to fill up the school. And he had no right to accept some of them that didn't have a literary foundation. And that's why I come to Meharry." Lynk, according to West, "was more of a theorist" than a practitioner, which was, in West's judgment, a liability when teaching practical skills in dentistry. "He was everything. He had a degree in engineering, he was a lawyer, and he was a physician, and he was supposed to be a dentist. He . . . was too smart." The school was often short on funds, West knew, because some of the local practitioners helped teach at UWT, but they "got tired of giving their time" when "in fact they [UWT officials] were supposed to pay them."[161] If West is typical of others who knew UWT, the school did not enjoy a good reputation.

Another outside measure of medical schools at that time was results of state licensing exams, published annually in the *Journal of the American Medical Association (JAMA)*. Graduates of UWT never fared well in comparison to either all board candidates or to graduates of other African American medical colleges. Lynk read those reports in *JAMA* and received communications from the Tennessee licensing authorities about his school's performance: "I was in the thickest of the fight and kept close tab of our development," he wrote in his 1951 autobiography. He agreed that there were too many low-grade commercial schools for whites and that some needed to be closed, but he argued that there was a "need for more and better equipped medical schools for our group." Lynk argued that the AMA and others in the medical establishment should have recognized the "need for sympathetic construction rather than indiscriminate destruction," and not have forced the closing of African American medical schools because they lacked large enough endowments to provide better facilities and faculty.[162]

The AMA, AAMC, and state licensing boards continued their relentless push for improving educational and licensing standards throughout the decade following 1910. Even Tennessee, long lax in establishing standards for medical education, in 1915 became the last Southern state to require that prospective medical students pass a preliminary education exam or show evidence of having attained a sufficient basic education to study medicine before being allowed to obtain a license to practice medicine in the state.[163] Now feeling the pressure even more, Lynk, along with a number of administrators from other medical schools, announced in the summer of 1915 that they would require at least one year of college and four years of high school preparation for admission to their schools. Evidence that UWT did not fulfill its promise about raising admissions requirements comes not only from West in 1976. Confirming West's recollections of UWT, the education editors of *JAMA* reported in 1916, and annually thereafter until UWT closed, that the school along with a handful of others "have not announced the higher entrance requirements or evidence has not been received to show they are in effect for all students enrolled."[164] UWT authorities continued to admit less qualified applicants to its classes, prompting prospective students such as West to select Meharry over UWT.

Lynk, in spite of these adversities, showed the same determination and single-mindedness he had demonstrated in his earlier years by not surrendering to the AMA's rating system for a long time. Many years after other African American medical schools, including Leonard, one of the academically strongest, closed, UWT, typical of its founder, dean, and president, determinedly continued to turn out physicians. Between 1900 and 1922, the last year the school produced M.D. graduates, some 155 men and women received medical degrees from UWT (see Appendix, Table 5). Those graduates could not practice in many states, as more and more licensing boards refused to recognize diplomas from the school.[165]

In 1914, UWT got a boost in enrollment when Lynk accepted at least thirty-two third- and fourth-year students from Leonard Medical School who had had to transfer in the wake of a campus crisis at the Raleigh, North Carolina, institution when Leonard ceased training junior and senior medical students. Neither Howard nor Meharry medical schools would accept these transfer students.[166] By 1916, all of this group had graduated, and enrollment at UWT declined drastically. By 1923 it was impossible to hold on any longer, and Lynk closed the school, a decision he did not discuss in his autobiography.[167]

In most ways the UWT College of Medicine and Surgery *was* Miles Vandahurst Lynk. The two names were inextricably linked from the school's founding in 1900. He made UWT what it was. Many who wrote or spoke about him described his willingness to fight and sacrifice for a cause; to apply his mental, spiritual, and financial resources to help other people; and to do what he could to improve the status of African Americans.[168] In 1955, more than thirty years after UWT closed, those associated with UWT held a testimonial reception for Lynk. One alumnus summed up most people's feelings about their mentor: "Undoubtedly, Dr. M. V.

Lynk represented a master mind with a keen mental perception as an educator and as a man of medical science. It was most fortunate for any student to have had the opportunity to have studied under Dr. Lynk for he had an unusual way of getting over information that would be indelibly stamped on their minds."[169]

The four African American proprietary medical schools examined here differed greatly from one another. Hannibal appears to have provided the least substantial education. Its founder and principal teacher, Tarleton Cottrell, probably never earned a medical degree; some of its other teachers also held questionable credentials. Students had little opportunity to do laboratory work or dissections, as HMC had no physical plant other than rented rooms that changed location annually. Chattanooga National had a single, stable location for its few years of existence, but much of its faculty practiced in distant towns, and its primary teacher, founder Thomas William Haigler, was involved in a number of activities other than medical education, raising questions about the frequency of classes and the quality of instruction. Both Cottrell and Haigler had an entrepreneurial spirit that spilled over into the operation of their educational enterprises, seemingly placing profit over learning. Miles Lynk too was something of an entrepreneur, but he channeled that spirit primarily into promoting the advancement of African Americans as a group by founding law and medical schools, establishing a black medical journal and a publishing house, and helping to found a national medical society for African Americans. His proprietary medical school started off strongly, with adequate faculty and facilities, and maintained its momentum both in Jackson and for several years after moving to Memphis before falling behind as medical education changed rapidly and grew too expensive for an independent enterprise. Louisville National Medical College also began strongly and, of all the colleges discussed here, tried the hardest and most honestly to keep up with medical educational reforms. It and the other black proprietary medical colleges enjoyed little breathing space, however, between the time of their founding and the first significant stirrings of educational reform.

With segregation in the South tightening in the late nineteenth and early twentieth centuries and the opportunities for African Americans wishing to pursue medical careers small, the closing of these schools hurt. Medical colleges with outside support, such as Howard, Meharry, and Leonard, held an advantage over the independent schools, though even the black missionary medical colleges struggled to survive. Louisville National, Hannibal, Chattanooga National, and West Tennessee met the same fate as many white proprietary schools of the period that engaged in similar, sometimes questionable, educational activities. The additional factor of race during an era of obvious and often brutal racism, though not discussed in this chapter's recounting of four black schools' histories, cannot be dismissed in accounting for their demise. The need to establish separate medical schools because African Americans were barred from publicly supported professional schools in the states where they lived and paid taxes was part of a larger need black health professionals faced in segregated America. African American physicians, dentists, nurses, and pharmacists had to build a set of medical institutions parallel to the white institutions from which they were excluded—medical schools, nurse-training schools, pharmacy schools, medical journals, medical societies, hospitals, and drugstores—institutions that survived until the race barriers began to fall much later in the century.

CHAPTER 17

Money versus Mission at Knoxville College Medical Department, 1895–1900

In 1895, Knoxville College (KC), a small institution founded twenty years earlier for African Americans in the eastern Tennessee mountains and run by the Board of Freedmen's Missions (BFM) of the United Presbyterian Church of North America, joined the ranks of post-Emancipation missionary schools operating medical colleges. The newly established Knoxville College Medical Department (KCMD) was, by all appearances, a church-run school whose mission was to train black Christian physicians to serve a growing African American population in need of medical care. In reality, KCMD was a proprietary school, nominally overseen by an absentee board (the BFM in Pittsburgh) that allowed the school to exist as long as it cost KC and the BFM nothing and operated by a predominantly white faculty more interested in making money for itself than in educating black Christian physicians. KCMD was thus an anomaly among its sister African American medical education institutions: it was neither a white-run missionary school nor a black-run proprietary school (see Appendix, Table 4). It had a short and, by some standards, insignificant life, lasting just five years and graduating only two physicians. Its history, however, illustrates late-nineteenth-century attitudes and trends in medical education, business, and race relations. Specifically, it shows how, against the backdrop of growing racial tensions among post-Reconstruction Tennesseeans, the school's religious and charitable mission to educate African Americans came into conflict with entrepreneurship and the desire for institutional prestige. The KC administration's intention to train black Christians in medicine collided with the desire of a group of white physicians to run a for-profit (proprietary) medical education business at the college.

President John S. McCulloch, D.D. (1829–1910), a white Presbyterian minister originally from Cumberland County in central Pennsylvania, arrived at two-year-old KC in 1877 with plans to promote basic education among young black Tennesseeans. Typical of such post–Emancipation era denominational missionary institutions, KC offered a normal school curriculum and programs in industrial/mechanical education and domestic sciences, reflecting then current job opportunities and racial attitudes. No official discussions at KC about establishing a medical program appear to have occurred until a sudden convergence of events in the spring of 1895 prompted McCulloch and the BFM hastily to do so. As reported in the annual minutes of the United Presbyterian Church of North America's General Assembly, "Very unexpectedly a desire was found to exist among the [Knoxville College] students for a medical department, and quite as unexpectedly the way was opened up for the organization of such a department. A faculty of seven was secured to give their services without pecuniary compensation until the income from fees should justify it."[1] The minutes provide no further explanation. Following is a more complete description of those precipitating events and of this proprietary medical school's subsequent five-year history and an attempt to understand why KC became involved in such an enterprise, and why it ended it.

The Impetus: A "Wild" Proposition

One day in late April 1895, Robert M. C. Hill, M.D.—professor of materia medica, general therapeutics, and clinical medicine at the Tennessee Medical College (TMC) in Knoxville—rode to the KC campus on the western outskirts of town to pay a visit to President McCulloch. Hill was one of ten local white physicians who, in 1889, had founded TMC under the lenient chartering laws of the state of Tennessee; he served as secretary of the new school and of the Knox County Medical Society.[2] TMC's proprietors had built an impressive new building just a year or so after opening the school, containing a medical museum, laboratories, an amphitheater, and an auditorium.[3] President McCulloch, describing Dr. Hill's visit to the KC campus in his monthly report to BFM secretary J. W. Witherspoon in Pittsburgh, called Hill "the Father of the [Tennessee] Medical College," an institution with a "$12,000 building" that was "an ornament to the city & a very conspicuous building."[4] The purpose of Dr. Hill's visit—to open and operate a medical school for African American students on the KC campus—caught McCulloch by surprise: "He astonished me by volunteering to say, that if the Board [of Freedmen's Missions] will furnish rooms [at the college]—two at least—he will become responsible & have a good working faculty ready for opening in October, & run the school, & equip it with not a cent of cost further to the Board."[5]

McCulloch at first viewed the entire proposition as "wild" and "unworthy of serious thought."[6] Hill pressed the point, however, answering concerns about establishing a potentially costly department at financially poor KC, with outsiders as faculty. Ultimately his arguments persuaded the president at least to entertain the possibility that such an enterprise could work: "When he [Hill] showed me that neither he [n]or any other professor or officer of the Tenn. Med. Coll. had ever received a 'nickel' for their services, when he pointed out how every professor had to be on time, or be marked tardy or absent, I began to think the move less chimerical."[7]

The proposal to start a school was not as outrageous as McCulloch might have thought, given the ease with which late-nineteenth-century Tennessee officials chartered such institutions. In a period of proliferating proprietary medical schools, Tennessee stood out as a haven for these enterprises. By 1895, white residents of the state had seven medical schools to choose from, including three that had formed since 1889 (Tennessee Medical College in Knoxville, Grant University Medical Department in Chattanooga, and Sewanee Medical College in Sewanee) and two that opened in 1895 from a previously merged school (University of Nashville Medical Department and Vanderbilt University Medical Department). For African Americans in Tennessee, Meharry Medical College was thriving, and tiny Hannibal Medical College, founded in 1889, was still operating in Memphis (though only barely surviving). Despite the large number of medical schools in the Volunteer State, however, observers judged few as educationally sound.[8]

The TMC financial arrangement that McCulloch reported to his board was unusual for a proprietary school, as profits from student fees were typically distributed among faculty. In general during that era, faculty members also benefited financially from their association with medical schools because they gained access to clinic patients and earned prestige by linking their names with the institution.[9] Quite possibly Hill meant that TMC faculty members received no salary as such from the school for their services, but shared in the profits, and that KCMD faculty would make a similar arrangement with McCulloch. This issue of money was a continuing source of concern and contention between KC administrators and KCMD faculty.

McCulloch weighed the proposition over the next few days, then included a description of his meeting with Hill in his monthly letter to Witherspoon and the BFM. He was interested in pursuing Hill's offer: "I ask you in all seriousness to consider it," he wrote.[10] Hill, McCulloch explained, was no newcomer either to establishing a medical school or to medical school teaching: he had "made a decided success of the [Tennessee] Medical College, & it was so from the start, including the Dental Dept."[11] Furthermore, McCulloch suggested, finding adequate space for the school would not be difficult: "We could probably make the upper rooms of the Industrial building answer for a while until it could be known whether or not a special building may be required."[12]

McCulloch's receptiveness to Hill's unexpected proposal stemmed at least in part from conversations the president had been having during the previous few months with several of the older undergraduate students regarding their aspirations for obtaining a medical education: "The boys have been talking about it [their desire for a medical school at KC] for some months, & they are considerably excited [now] in view of the possibility of such a department. . . . 'Cato' [C. H. Wilson], the big bass of the Glee Club, is enthusiastic. He intends to go to a medical school next year & he has corresponded with such schools enough to make him more anxious to stay here, if he can have the medical training."[13] The medical school issue was thus on Rev. McCulloch's mind when he wrote his monthly report for the BFM, not only because of Dr. Hill's recent visit but also because Cato Wilson, and perhaps other students, had been pressing him on the subject. Wilson, he reported to Witherspoon, "was in before prayer meeting, *& bored* me about it. There is no time I am so impatient with callers as before preaching or prayer meeting."[14]

As McCulloch indicated to the BFM, Cato Wilson and other African American students wishing to become physicians had several choices in 1895. A handful of Northern medical schools irregularly accepted one or two black students,[15] and of the eight medical colleges founded after the Civil War that catered to black students, six remained in operation (though, as mentioned previously, Hannibal was struggling) (see Appendix, Table 4). There seemed to be room for another black medical school as more and more African Americans chose careers in medicine.

In addition to wishing to accommodate Cato Wilson's and other KC students' desire to remain in a familiar setting and in a small city while attending medical school, McCulloch saw another reason for establishing a medical department at KC: if Cato Wilson was correct in his prediction that "ten students at least, tuition $40, could be had to begin with," then the school could operate without cost to KC and yet reap the prestige associated with having an affiliated medical department as at Howard or Shaw universities.[16]

McCulloch expected the operation of the new department to comport with the moral and disciplinary atmosphere governing the rest of the institution. Like administrators and teachers at other Tennessee black educational institutions, McCulloch (and his successor, Ralph McGranahan) believed that a crucial component of schooling for African Americans in these early years after slavery was the teaching of discipline and religion. KC imposed strict rules of behavior on students, including required religious instruction and chapel attendance.[17] (One historian of African American higher education in the Volunteer State characterized this nonacademic objective of missionary colleges as an "obsession with the moral uplift and character development of the blacks who passed through" such institutions.)[18] "The aim" of KCMD, McCulloch wrote in 1897, "is to provide physicians of high moral & religious character for the people. The great need is apparent."[19] Thus medical students were expected to obey the same religious and behavioral rules as other KC students. Just as at Leonard Medical School in Raleigh, graduates of KCMD would be Christian physicians.[20] Ironically, this mission of moral uplift and character development later became a major factor in the decision to discontinue the medical department.

The BFM expressed an interest in Hill's proposal. McCulloch's letter to Witherspoon was dated May 1, 1895. On May 6, the BFM met and authorized McCulloch "to arrange for a Medical Department at Knoxville"; it gave no explanation as to why it had agreed to establish the medical school, but clearly stated that "there should be no expense to the Board."[21] Thus, just a few weeks after Dr. Hill's unanticipated and unsolicited offer, Knoxville College had a medical department, though with only a weak commitment from its governing board and clear instructions to expect no outside financial support.

Organizational Challenges

The work of building a medical program began. Faculty had to be hired, students located and enrolled, classroom and laboratory space prepared, equipment and books purchased, admission and graduation standards established, and other details recognized and attended to. Unfortunately for KCMD, the school opened just as medical education reform was gaining momentum in America. The Association of American Medical Colleges (AAMC) had recently re-formed and, in order to keep pace with advances in bacteriology, pathology, physiology, and other medical sciences, was annually increasing curricular and graduation standards for its growing membership. Many states (including Tennessee) were implementing licensing examinations and regulating medical education more closely, thereby forcing medical colleges to hire faculty with better and more scientific training and to develop courses in these new subjects that included laboratory work and clinical experiences. Such improvements cost money for, among other items, higher salaries, building renovation and construction, microscopes, libraries, and laboratory equipment and supplies. Dr. Hill's TMC had opened with many of the necessities for this new era of medical education in place, or with funds to develop them. KCMD had no such budgetary support (other than student fees), no well-equipped laboratories, medical library, medical museum, dissecting room, or hospital—it had only Dr. Hill's word that he would take care of organizing the school.

The BFM appointed Hill as dean, with instructions to recruit faculty members who would then be formally nominated to the board for its approval.[22] President McCulloch reiterated to the board his understanding of the agreement he and Hill had made: BFM confirmation of a physician as a medical department faculty

Figure 17. Knoxville College Medical Department Faculty

Name	Race	School	Graduated	Taught[1]
Clark, Benjamin M.	white	Tennessee Medical College	1894	1895–96
Clear, John	white	Kentucky School of Medicine (Louisville)	1885	1896–1900
Derrick, William W.	black	Meharry	1892	1896–1900
Edwards, Augustus G.	black	Meharry	1895	1895–1900
Ford, J. C. (lawyer)	white	unknown	——	1895–1900
Hill, Robert M. C.	white	Toledo Medical College	1886	1895–96
Moore, William H.	white	Tennessee Medical College	1893	1896–1900
Morton, John H.	white	University of Tennessee Medical Department	1888	1899–1900
Price, Levi Jones	white	Hosp. College of Medicine (Louisville)	1877	1895–96
Randall, Edwin L.	white	Missouri Medical College	1869	1895–1900
Yarborough, Charles C.	white	Tennessee Medical College	1893	1895–96

1. School did not operate during 1897–98 term.

member was "to involve no expense for the present in the way of salary, & each professor understands that it is in his own interest to work up his departments, without money compensation, until the income from lecture fees shall have equipped the school, and justified such compensations."[23] Under this arrangement, the school was required to be self-sustaining from the start and to never become a financial drain on the rest of the college or on the BFM.

By late July, Hill had filled four of six vacant faculty positions.[24] Typical of medical school instructors during that era, the KCMD appointees were local practitioners with no special training in medical education or in the courses they were assigned to teach.[25] Atypical of that period's medical faculties was this one's racial composition: one black and three white physicians. At no white Southern medical school did a physician of color hold a regular teaching position. Howard University, founded as a multiracial, coeducational institution in 1868, had a mixed-race medical staff and student body (predominantly white for a number of years) from the start. Of the other African American missionary schools operating at the time, Meharry and Flint had integrated faculties, while Leonard employed only white instructors. Black proprietary schools used black physicians almost exclusively.[26]

KCMD's mix of white and black professors did not come about without some disagreement and tension, however. In the late 1880s and early 1890s, relations between whites and blacks in Tennessee and the rest of the South were becoming increasingly tense, and even rancorous. Writes one historian of Tennessee race relations in the 1880s: "By the end of the decade flexibility had largely given way to rigidity in interracial contacts, white attitudes had become more fixed, blacks more bitter, and the margin for variety in interracial associations narrower. As blacks and whites came into impersonal contact in railroad cars, theaters, hotels, parks, and other public facilities, racial tensions mounted."[27] The Jim Crow era was dawning. These tensions manifested themselves in the selection of teachers at the newly forming African American medical college in Knoxville.

From the start, KCMD's faculty racial composition was a matter of open discussion between the dean and the president. Both agreed that a mixed-race teaching corps was appropriate. According to McCulloch, Hill at first "made some effort to have the Negro represented in the Faculty. He [Hill] thought two or three might be found."[28] In fact, only one African American physician was hired: Augustus G. Edwards of Selma, Alabama, who had graduated from Meharry just a few months earlier.[29] McCulloch provided an enigmatically worded explanation to his superiors in Pittsburgh as to why Hill selected only Dr. Edwards from among the city's black practitioners. He hinted at racial bias, but left open the possibility that poor credentials were the cause: "It was soon apparent that only one of the four or more colored medical graduates of the city would be accepted."[30] Did McCulloch mean that only Edwards of all the local black physicians was considered sufficiently qualified to teach at the medical school (qualifications for these positions are not stated in the available records), or that the white faculty members already chosen would not teach if more than one African American were appointed? Though the chairs in obstetrics, physiology, and principles and practice of medicine remained vacant as classes approached, Hill chose to double the teaching assignments of his current faculty and wait for suitable white physicians.[31] When one of the white instructors resigned at the last minute, he found a white replacement.[32] McCulloch appears not to have intervened as Hill took these actions, despite his approval of Hill's initially stated intention to bring together a well-integrated faculty. The BFM also remained silent.

That racial bias was the motivating factor in the failure to appoint more black professors became quite clear the following year, 1896. This time a chemistry instructor was needed at the start of the school term in early November. The faculty delayed selecting anyone for almost two months, until the end of December, opting again to double their own teaching loads to cover this course because, as McCulloch explained to Witherspoon, a majority was reluctant to hire another black teacher: "Some of the doctors tried hard to find a satisfactory white man [for the chemistry post], but they did not succeed."[33] The man whose name the faculty ultimately sent forward for BFM approval, William W. Derrick, was an 1892 Meharry graduate from Bell Factory, Alabama, who had been practicing in Knoxville since 1892 and had been passed over the previous year for a teaching position owing to his race. McCulloch, who again appears to have avoided intervening in a faculty appointment decision that had been based on skin color, recommended Derrick highly as "a man of unblemished character."[34] Whether the open bias of white medical staff against hiring and working with black members of the profession caused workplace or classroom problems is not revealed in the available records. As will be shown, however, though Edwards and Derrick attended faculty meetings and seemed to cooperate with their white colleagues as appropriate, they also conducted themselves differently from the white physicians in several ways (e.g., they did not focus on money issues, and they led observant religious lives)—thereby winning the admiration of both KC presidents under whom they worked.

Hill and McCulloch had other matters to deal with besides faculty appointments from the end of July to the end of October 1895, as they prepared to open the new school. They had to establish entrance requirements, a curriculum, an academic calendar, and a fee structure, as well as to begin to distribute publicity, admit a class of students, prepare the physical space where teaching would occur, and obtain necessary instructional materials. Available records provide little information as to how these matters were decided, though on most issues the administration appears to have followed the lead of other comparable medical schools, including TMC. McCulloch informed the Pittsburgh board that classes would begin on November 1, 1895, and continue for six months[35] and that applicants would have to meet certain minimal entrance requirements: "a diploma or certificate of graduation from some recognized college, academy, or high school, or a certificate from some County Superintendent of Public Education, attesting that the candidate is possessed of at least the attainments required of second-grade teachers of public schools."[36] They also had to be "of good moral character."[37] Comparable with other African American medical schools, KCMD students would pay $30 for the six-month course of lectures ($25 for "Professors' Tickets," and a $5 matriculation fee) plus $5 in other charges (laboratory and anatomy fees). Room and board cost an additional $6.50 per month. Conforming to AAMC guidelines, KCMD offered a four-year graded curriculum.[38]

Arranging for facilities and teaching materials turned out to be more complex, more disruptive to the rest of the college, and probably more expensive than McCulloch had anticipated when first exploring the possibility of opening a medical school. Clearly KC administrators had not previously considered the basic space and equipment requirements of such an institution; they thus had to scramble at the last minute for classrooms, laboratories, examining rooms, and teaching materials. In late August, for example, just two months before the school's opening, McCulloch alerted the BFM that "there may be call for a dissecting room, but if so it will not be a very heavy item."[39] The clear necessity for such a room and for a teaching laboratory at the medical school soon compelled McCulloch to put into effect his earlier plan to "make the upper rooms of the Industrial building answer for a while."[40] Not only did he have to order the installation of partitions in the Industrial Building for dissecting and laboratory space, apparently at the college's expense ($11.10), he also had to co-opt and partition (for $16.23) "one of the best lecture rooms in the college" for a medical school classroom.[41] That second-floor classroom served for what McCulloch called didactic lectures and also for "meeting patients and treating them in the presence of the class."[42] The medical school possessed no hospital or dispensary space other than this college building classroom. Patients had to pass through the building's halls, among nonmedical students, in order to get to the medical school classroom. In addition, McCulloch informed the BFM, "the giving up of this room may render the use of the library necessary for a class-room [for the college students displaced from the other room], or else Prof. Millin will [have to] take his classes to a large room in McCulloch Hall," some distance from the college building.[43] KC staff and students were shifting and adjusting to accommodate the new medical program.

Publicizing the opening of a medical school to prospective students became a challenge because KCMD had been established so late that the KC catalog for the new academic year had already gone to press. Publicity to attract a medical class appeared only about a month before the first day of classes.[44] In addition to sending out individual circulars designed and produced by the college print shop, school officials inserted a copy of that announcement in Knoxville College's school newspaper, the *Aurora*. The description of the medical program ("Ample facilities for dissecting and laboratory instruction will be provided each student. Laboratory instruction in Chemistry, Operative Surgery, Physiology, Histology, Pathology and Bacteriology required for graduation. . . . Clinical teaching will form an important part of the work. Clinics ample in every department")[45] offered little hint of the hurriedness with which the medical department had been organized; the makeshift nature of classroom, laboratory, dissecting room, and outpatient clinic arrangements; the scrambling to produce a full faculty in time for KCMD's opening; or the inexperience of the "professors" who had basically been (and remained) local medical practitioners until the day Hill asked them to join him in this enterprise.

The First Year

Few responded to the publicity. Two days before classes were scheduled to begin, only two students were registered, Cato Wilson and Cora Rutherford. Wilson, McCulloch reported, "is the first to pay his fees . . . and he paid for the entire year, $35"; two others were expected to arrive "very soon after the opening."[46] The president attended opening-day events and commented, "I like the way they started off."[47] About three weeks later, R. H. Adams arrived; McCulloch

Figure 18. Medical Students Enrolled at Knoxville College Medical Department, 1895–1900*

Name	Hometown	Sessions Attended				Year M.D. Earned
Adams, R. H.	Millen, Ga.	1895–96				
Crenshaw, N. B.	Oakwood, Tex.[4]			1898–99[2]	1899–1900	1900[5]
Fish, W. L.	Altamont, Ky.				1899–1900	
Flack, Pindar M.	Alexander, N.C.	1898–99		1899–1900	1902[6]	
Green, Henry M.	Jellico, Tenn.				1899–1900[1]	1901[6]
Hatcher, Frances	Coal Creek, Tenn.	1895–96				
King, J. G.	Clinton, Tenn.				1899–1900[3]	1900[5]
Knott, A. B. S.	Heiskell, Tenn.			1898–99	1899–1900	
Love, Hugh	Canton, Miss.				1899–1900	1903[6]
Raines, Claude W.	Greenville, Mo.			1898–99	1899–1900	1901[6]
Rowan, Henry E.	Cape Girardeau, Mo.		1896–97			1901[7]
Rutherford, Cora	Baldwin, Ill.	1895–96				
Sheppard, James H.	Bristol, Tenn.	1895–96	1896–97			1899[7]
Taylor, H. P.	Maysville, Ky.			1898–99	1899–1900	1903[7]
Turner, Edwin J.	Atlanta, Ga.		1896–97[1]			1902[8]
Walker, Tillman	New Market, Tenn.		1896–97	1898–99		
Walker, W. H.	New Market, Tenn.	1895–96				
Watson, W. E.	Newton, Miss.				1899–1900	1902[6]
Willis, J. W.	Woodbury, Ga.				1899–1900	1903[7]
Wilson, Cato H.	Darien, Ga.	1895–96	1896–97			1899[7]

*The medical school did not operate during the 1897–98 academic year.

1. listed as second-year student
2. listed as third-year student
3. listed as fourth-year student
4. listed as Butler, Tex., in 1899–1900
5. graduated from Knoxville College Medical Department
6. graduated from Knoxville Medical College
7. graduated from Meharry Medical College
8. graduated from Flint Medical College

Source: Compiled from KC Catalogs, 1895–1901, unpublished monthly reports of KC presidents, 1895–1900, issues of the *Aurora*, 1895–1900, all in KC Archives, and from Polk's and AMA medical directories, 1900–1916.

joked with Witherspoon that "the Medical school has increased fifty per cent."[48] Eventually, six students made their way to Knoxville to attend the first year of medical lectures.[49] Numbers, of course, mattered to McCulloch, since the medical department was to be self-supporting; but they also mattered to Hill, because, as will be shown shortly, he and his colleagues intended to earn money from this undertaking. For the faculty (at least for the white instructors), KCMD was a proprietary medical school.

Though the small student enrollment was a worry, faculty behavior was an even larger one. Faculty issues at first involved missed or late appearances for scheduled classes and staff meetings. Later, the crucial and sensitive matter of financial greed divided faculty from administrators. By the school's fifth year, concern over the faculty's competence and disregard of KC's religious mission, in addition to the instructors' avarice, convinced administration and board members to close the medical department.

Faculty difficulties began almost immediately. McCulloch noted in his November report to Witherspoon that "some of the doctors have not been very regular" in their attendance at lectures.[50] Though instructors were required to register when they arrived for class and to provide an explanation for tardiness or absence, and though the matter was raised at monthly faculty meetings, the problem festered for months. By the end of February, it had reached crisis proportions. Faculty members were missing many classes, arranging make-up classes on very short notice, and in general creating a poor educational atmosphere for the students. Laboratory coursework suffered the most.

Ironically, a modern tool of technology, the telephone, contributed to this problem of faculty attendance. Just before the start of classes in November, the physicians insisted on installing a telephone at KC. "After long hesitation," wrote McCulloch to the BFM, "we have a *telephone*. The doctors said they could not get along without it. It costs $35 the first year and $30 a year afterwards. I hope it will prove a great convenience, & not a nuisance in the office."[51] The phone did become a nuisance: medical faculty made great use of it in reporting that they would have to miss, arrive late for, or reschedule classes.

McCulloch, frustrated, annoyed, and concerned about both the students and the future of the school, expressed his feelings regarding faculty reliability to both Dr. Hill and Rev. Witherspoon: "I fear that the impression is gaining ground that the Medical Department is not going to be a success," he wrote Hill.[52] The students, he explained to Witherspoon, complain "that they often do not know when to expect a lecture. They are well satisfied with the lectures generally, but so often the lecturer does not come. Sometimes he telephones that an urgent [medical] call prevents him, & he names another hour [to do his teaching], but too often, class is disappointed."[53] McCulloch felt that the department's growing negative reputation could "be counteracted," and urged Dean Hill to do something "at once to reassure the students. Can we not have a meeting, & possibly a more definite understanding about punctuality?"[54] The fact that Hill had his own practice and teaching responsibilities at TMC meant that, as at many other medical schools, the dean was usually not on campus to deal with situations like this, or to oversee the day-to-day operation of the medical department; those responsibilities, by default, fell to the president.

McCulloch did exempt one faculty member from his general condemnation of the teaching staff that first year: "Dr. Edwards (colored)," the president informed Rev. Witherspoon, "has been the most faithful" in fulfilling his teaching responsibilities.[55] Here was the first hint that African American instructors might have been more committed to the enterprise than their white colleagues and that members of the college staff noticed.

A showdown faculty meeting finally took place on March 20, 1896. Instructors presented reports and "apologies for failure to come on time"; McCulloch seemed satisfied and told the BFM, "The medical department is doing better."[56] He did not complain about faculty attendance or tardiness again in his remaining reports for the academic term, and only sporadically afterward.[57] Instead, he discovered a new problem concerning the faculty—money.

When Cato Wilson paid his $35 in fees in October 1895, the faculty asked McCulloch to serve as their treasurer.[58] By the end of February 1896, the six students in attendance had paid a total of $140; medical department expenses to that point had amounted to $66.95, leaving $73.05 in the treasury.[59] During the meeting on March 20, at which faculty members apologized for their failings in classroom attendance, they (much to McCulloch's surprise) unanimously "voted themselves $10 each out of the money on hand. . . . I expected," McCulloch told Witherspoon after describing the incident, "that the services [of the instructors] would be gratuitous at least for a year or two."[60] This action went against the understanding that Hill had given McCulloch the previous May when the medical school enterprise had first been broached, and what the president had written to the BFM at the end of July: the faculty was to receive no pay until the school was on a secure financial footing. Apparently McCulloch said nothing at that March 20 meeting and nothing more of a public nature about this misunderstanding for the remainder of the term—quite the opposite, in fact. On April 18, the president penned his annual report to the BFM for presentation at the yearly meeting of the United Presbyterian Church of North America's General Assembly and for publication in the proceedings of that body. His paragraph about the medical department (quoted earlier, near the start of this chapter) actually misrepresented the situation: "A faculty of seven was secured to give their services without pecuniary compensation until the income from fees should justify it."[61] The reason for McCulloch's silence on the matter, both to the faculty and to the General Assembly, is not explained in extant sources, but it raises questions about the potential conflicts that both KC administrators and faculty faced between money and mission.

KCMD instructors gained the prestige of faculty status and the gratification that came with helping to train a new generation of physicians. They may also have found satisfaction in knowing that they were doing their share to improve the lot of African American citizens—both the students and the students' future patients. Teaching at KCMD, however, meant a sacrifice of time and effort: physicians had to arrange home visits and office practices around class schedules, losing patient income. Because they received no set compensation for teaching at KCMD unless fee collections outstripped expenses, they ran the risk of deriving no financial benefit from their service to the college. Alternatively, they did not run the risk run by faculty members at other proprietary schools who invested money in starting up and operating a medical institution that might fail. They paid little if anything, for example, for instructional facilities, catalogs, telephone service, and administrative staff. Those and other expenses would mount up at a de novo proprietary school, but KC had the infrastructure already in place to support these needs. If KCMD failed to attract sufficient students to earn extra money for each teacher, the faculty lost some time and some patient fees but not much of their own money.

As with the faculty, KC and the BFM also derived prestige from their connection with a medical department. For a small college, hosting a successful medical school whose graduates opened practices around the region or even the country could bring fame if not fortune. Because the chartering and licensing laws of Tennessee had not yet tightened up the requirements for medical schools, and medical education reform was just reaching the state, the college needed to invest very little money in the enterprise to derive that fame. It could develop a medical school by simply dividing up rooms in an already existing building, using its print shop to publicize the department's existence, and relying on an unpaid teaching corps of physicians whose only requirement was the receipt of compensation once the school made a profit. It was not until the school was in operation that the negative side of this undertaking manifested itself: the need to oversee matters relating to students, faculty, classrooms, equipment, publicity, grading, licensure, patient visits, record keeping, and finances. Nor did the KC administration or the BFM take into account the impact a medical school would have on the life of the campus. For example, would medical students, older than most KC students, be required to adhere to the same strict disciplinary regulations on such matters as dress, deportment, chapel attendance, living arrangements, and religion? Would medical faculty, who were not paid employees of the college, be subject to the same supervision and rules as other faculty? In the rush to establish a medical department in the spring of 1895, areas of potential friction were not well considered, and conflict arose between the mission of the school and the goals of those who had agreed to teach.

During the first school year some unanticipated expenses arose that the college covered for the medical department and that provide insight into the human side of running a medical school. McCulloch approved the construction of a shed behind the Industrial Building to shelter the physicians' horses, after receiving several complaints about "the seeming cruelty of letting" them "stand out to shiver in the snow and rain" during lectures; the president rationalized his action (the cost was less than ten dollars) to the BFM as "not a work of absolute necessity" but "one of mercy."[62] Another expense related to the anatomy course. McCulloch had to order the college shop to make "two good dissecting tables," but in so doing, he told Witherspoon, he inadvertently alerted KC students and other residents in the area that human dissection was occurring in the Industrial Building: "The dissecting caused a little ripple soon after the first cadaver (stiff) was reported, but curiosity quieted down, and I have heard nothing lately on the subject from outside."[63]

At the end of the first school term in late April 1896, the faculty met "in the medical room for a quiet talk with the students." Earlier that month, the instructors had "expressed very great satisfaction with the progress and diligence of the students," and they now assured them that "the laboratory work which . . . [they] complained of missing is usually not required in the first year."[64] This may have been a self-serving, face-saving rationalization, but McCulloch reported the incident without comment to the BFM. In this manner, KCMD concluded its first year of operation.

The Second Year

The following year started inauspiciously. Though a new physician joined the faculty over the summer, two key instructors left in July, including the school's founder and dean, Robert Hill, who moved to Ohio to care for a sick relative of his wife. At the start of classes, two more faculty left, and a new person was hastily appointed.[65] Despite these losses, the four remaining faculty and President McCulloch agreed to continue operating the medical program and to do so with no changes in fiscal arrangements or physical plant. At a full faculty meeting in July 1896, McCulloch attempted a clarification of monetary policies. When the instructors insisted that he had misunderstood Hill about compensation, McCulloch relented; without Hill to back him up, there was little else he felt he could do: "I found that all the doctors understood that after necessary expenses were paid, the balance [of the student's fees] was to be paid pro rata to them. I read to them what I had written to the Board when the matter was first mentioned, May 1st, 95. I understood Dr. Hill to say that instruction would be given without compensation until a suitable equipment could be secured. It seems that they understood him differently, and that I was mistaken. I found they all expected something out of the money paid by students for lecture fees. They have received nearly $20 each and the treasury is now empty, but not in debt. Thirty dollars are yet due from students."[66] From all appearances, both McCulloch and the faculty wished to keep KCMD operating and to reap the most benefits from its existence at the least cost to themselves. They maintained the status quo rather than attempting to improve the very minimal facilities and equipment used to teach future African American physicians at the school. The disagreements and problems were not great enough to cause either side to threaten KCMD's existence.

Classes began on Monday, November 3, 1896, with two groups of students now being taught—a new entering class and a returning second-year class. Attracting and retaining students was, of course, important to the financial well-being of the medical school and the faculty. Small numbers jeopardized KCMD's existence. Money was a problem not just for the administration and faculty but also for students. McCulloch had hoped for an enrollment increase during KCMD's second year. Instead, it dropped. The October 1896 issue of the school newspaper, the *Aurora*, announced that "all of last year's class [of six] will return except Misses Cora B. Rutherford and Frances L. Hatcher" and tried to encourage prospective students to apply by emphasizing the small number of black physicians in America and the large number of potential patients: "The field for colored physicians will not be crowded for fifty years because there is but one [physician] now to every 40,000 of the colored population."[67] The article also mentioned a reduced cost of $5.50 per month for board, but even reducing fees did not help boost attendance. The 1890s was a period of national economic turmoil that took its toll on many citizens. KC medical students, like African American medical students at other schools, generally had a difficult time earning enough money to pay for their education, and it was even tougher in times of financial disorder.[68] "The money requirement is the greater hindrance," President McCulloch explained to Witherspoon: even dedicated students like Cato Wilson, who had invested time and money taking the first-year course, were having trouble coming up with sufficient funds from summer work to pay for tuition and fees.[69] Ultimately, only Wilson and one of his classmates returned for the second year of courses, along with three new first-year students.[70]

The school year began with, as mentioned earlier, one important course still lacking an instructor: chemistry. Though the faculty was sanguine about filling in until a teacher was found, McCulloch was concerned about the missed instruction. He did not want a repeat of the first year: "I am anxious about the Medical lectures," he told Witherspoon a few days before classes started. "They *must* be given more regularly and promptly than last year."[71] They were: irregular faculty attendance occurred much less often than the previous term.[72] The tiny faculty, teaching both first- and second-year students and covering the chemistry lectures as well, seemed to have come together. A month after classes began, McCulloch cautiously reported to Witherspoon: "The four professors seem to be doing their best, & I have not heard much growling [from the students]."[73] Nearly one month later, the situation remained positive: "The Medical Department has kept up well and I hear no complaints."[74] Dr. Derrick's appointment in chemistry, which began in January, seemed also to work out well for the students: in his January report to Pittsburgh, McCulloch allowed that "the *Medical boys*, still 5 in number, are now doing laboratory work under Dr. Derrick, & seem satisfied. They are dissecting too under Dr. Edwards."[75] The two second-year students, who had missed out on laboratory experiences the previous year, now had the opportunity to make up that material.

The laboratory experience, however, also rekindled issues between McCulloch and the faculty about money. With Derrick teaching chemistry, the laboratories now began to be used more extensively. It soon became clear that the existing materials were inadequate. The faculty, McCulloch reported to Witherspoon, "hinted that a laboratory outfit was essential & that I might get something from the Board to start."[76] McCulloch believed that the cost of laboratory improvements ought to come from student fees (and thus from the faculty's pool of money), not from the BFM. He encouraged the faculty to order the equipment, but then decided to pay for it out of college funds: "I thought rather than have grumbling & complaint I could become responsible for that amount [$15]. The bills have not come in, but I do not think the Board should pay them. I do not wish to let the faculty get into the easy ways of getting money by simply asking the Board for things which they imagine they need."[77] Laboratory work was becoming an essential part of medical education by the 1890s, so the faculty had a legitimate concern about properly equipping the facilities at KC. The larger issue, though, was financial responsibility for such improvements, and it remained unresolved. McCulloch again decided not to invite confrontation with the faculty but rather to allow the institution to absorb the costs. The students did get their materials, as McCulloch informed the BFM in February: "The outfit of the Medical laboratory makes a very respectable show for as small an outlay as $15.00. They [the students] have performed the required . . . experiments."[78]

Despite continued uneasiness over financial matters, the medical department completed its second year smoothly. According to McCulloch, who seemed greatly concerned about harmony on campus and the success of his medical school, "the satisfaction expressed all round is a pleasant contrast from last year. We are hopeful for next year."[79] In his annual report, he used phrases such as "hearty satisfaction" and "regular lectures," emphasized the fact that of five professors "two of them [are] colored," and anticipated "increased attendance" the following year.[80]

This matter of the cost of the medical department versus the benefits deriving from such a program must have concerned BFM members, for, though McCulloch had made no allusion to the nagging and unresolved issue of financing the medical school at KC, the BFM felt it necessary to add a parenthetic statement to the published version of the president's annual report that year, reiterating that the medical department was "carried on without expense to the Board other than providing two rooms in the College for lectures."[81] Though willing to accept compliments for educating much-needed black physicians, the BFM was not willing to spend its money on medical school faculty salaries, physical plant, or educational materials. As a wave of rising standards in medical education and medical licensure spread across the country in the late 1890s, with states (including Tennessee) establishing boards of medical examiners to test prospective practitioners' knowledge,[82] the lack of commitment by the BFM, the college, and the faculty sentenced KCMD to a stagnant program and its graduates to poor showings on licensure exams.

The Final Years: Mission over Money

KCMD did not operate at all during the 1897–98 academic year, owing, once again, to finances and another disagreement between the faculty and the administration. Because of a poor economy and a yellow fever scare, according to McCulloch, many fewer students than usual enrolled in all departments of the college. The start of medical classes was postponed by a month, to November 1, 1897, but still only a few students appeared.[83] When the faculty refused to teach so small a number, saying, according to McCulloch, that "it would not pay to begin with less than seven," the president complained to the BFM that he "had been led to believe they would start with three if no more could be had."[84] Though the fees collected from three or four matriculates would not have contributed much toward improving the facilities and equipment at the school, or toward compensating professors for their teaching time and efforts, the failure to offer classes meant a break in educational continuity for returning students. As a result of KCMD's 1897–98 closure, two third-year students—including Cato Wilson, the early and leading student advocate for establishing a medical department at KC—transferred to Meharry, where they completed their medical training.[85]

The school continued for the next two academic years, enrolling, in 1898, five new students and one who had earlier completed his first year at KCMD, and in 1899, six freshman plus five returning students. A sixth physician joined the faculty to teach surgery in 1899.[86] Though entering student numbers were increasing, problems with money, faculty, facilities, and educational quality persisted. A change of leadership at KC in 1899, however, brought these problems before a new president who confronted them directly.

In July 1899, Rev. John S. McCulloch retired as president of KC after almost twenty-two years of service. He had founded the medical department in 1895 and nurtured it for four years. What had begun as a "wild" idea, "unworthy of serious consideration," had become for McCulloch a kind of pet project that he kept alive despite an accumulation of obstacles that others might have judged fatal to the enterprise. Like his counterpart at Shaw University, Henry M. Tupper, who had been given permission from his superiors at the Baptist Home Mission Society to open and operate Leonard Medical School as long as it was self-sustaining, McCulloch became so attached to the medical school that he could not retrench when maintaining it began to affect the well-being of the rest of the college. McCulloch, however, went even further than Tupper in protecting the life of his medical department: whereas Tupper secretly borrowed large sums of money for Leonard Medical School's fiscal needs and thus placed the entire university in financial jeopardy, McCulloch not only failed to raise funds himself or press the BFM for funds to improve the medical department's educational quality in response to mounting outside pressures for reform from the state and organized medicine but also tolerated faculty and student behaviors that undermined the moral and religious mission of the college. The new presidents at both colleges (Shaw and Knoxville) were surprised at the state of affairs they inherited at their respective medical schools and at the negative impact these medical departments were having on their institutions. At Leonard, Tupper's successor, Charles F. Meserve, viewed the situation dispassionately and implemented an austerity program that included the threat of closing the medical school if certain practices were not corrected. McCulloch's successor, Rev. Ralph W. McGranahan, a Presbyterian minister from Pennsylvania,[87] looked at KC's medical department with a fresh eye, did not like what he saw, and made radical changes that, in short order, closed the school. For McGranahan, the financial and moral costs of maintaining the school were greater than the benefits KCMD brought—a conclusion that McCulloch was apparently unable or unwilling to draw.

After observing and participating in KCMD's operation for a full academic term and presiding over the medical school's first graduation (two students received M.D. degrees),[88] McGranahan recommended to the BFM that the program be discontinued: "I have been trying to shape things up for the best results in all departments," he wrote in his September 1900 monthly report, "and in the Medical department we have a problem."[89] There were really two sets of problems: one relating to the BFM's operation of a medical school at KC, and the other relating to the people who were managing that school and the way they managed it. These were the same issues that had existed since 1895, many of which McCulloch had raised in his reports to the BFM but never resolved, and some of which he had kept silent about and were now revealed for the first time. McGranahan intended to take firm action on them.

McGranahan felt that a medical school should not be conducted at KC for a number of reasons. He had investigated the state of medical education and medical licensure in Tennessee and the rest of the country and found KCMD severely wanting. Medicine was changing rapidly, and KCMD was far behind. The college was not equipped, he explained to the board in Pittsburgh, to house or support a modern medical department that could adequately train future physicians. A proper medical school needed its own separate facilities for classes, laboratory instruction, dissection, dispensary (outpatient) care, and surgical procedures, designed especially for those purposes. The makeshift nature of the KCMD facilities could not suffice for a permanent, respected medical school. Ailing patients and their families, as well as the medical students, deserved privacy and separation from the general public and other students. "A dissecting room should not be on the same hall with the [mechanical] students. A dispensary or operating room is a necessity. We [in the college and mechanical buildings] could hardly tolerate the persons who come to receive such treatment coming on the hall among our students."[90]

Furthermore, emphasized McGranahan, KC needed "ONE MAN EMPLOYED ALL THE TIME IN CHARGE of that department."[91] No one truly oversaw the medical school's operations under the current decentralized faculty arrangement. A faculty member resident on the campus to deal with student affairs, faculty matters, and the medical facilities was necessary in order to organize and unify the department and run it in accord with the rules of the rest of the college.[92] Medical students, McGranahan found, undermined the discipline and routines of the college. They should not, he felt, "mingle with," take classes near, study with, or share dormitory rooms with students at the college or lower levels, as was the case at KC. "You know how inevitably a class feeling rises between students in two departments as distinct as the regular school and the medical department. We have been able to manage that in the small number we have had, but suppose it were increased to 100 or more in the medical department. . . . [W]e would be in great danger of serious and uncontrolled conflict. Students in the medical department do not accept our [school] regulations at all as our other students do."[93] As an example of the problem, he revealed to the board that the medical students had given trouble the previous year "out of all proportion to their numbers. They insist on being called 'doctor' by the other students. You see the effect. A big headed fellow can enter the medical department from 8th. grade and then pose as a superior."[94] In addition, townspeople feared the grave robbing that occurred to obtain cadavers for student dissections: "I had a good deal of anxiety last winter over the stealing of bodies for the dissecting room. It will never do to allow bodies for that purpose to be brought on the same grounds where a promiscuous body of students reside."[95] These were issues McCulloch had not revealed or raised with his superiors in Pittsburgh. The presence of a medical college on campus was upsetting the harmony and discipline of the rest of the institution.

For KCMD to make the changes McGranahan was suggesting and thereby to provide its medical students with an adequate education would require a large outlay of funds well beyond the sums raised through student fees. Neither the college nor the medical faculty could supply those funds. McGranahan, with the approval of the medical professors, turned to the BFM for guidance and financial assistance. He had been surprised to discover, he wrote to the board, that the original arrangements establishing the medical school absolved the BFM of any financial responsibility: "It seems very strange to expect a department" to build itself up "without money, but the letters so state. . . . It seems to me absurd to expect such a thing."[96] The KCMD staff, he continued, were willing to carry on as in the past, "if you can give assurance that in the future you can make provision for . . . securing such funds as would erect the building etc. anywhere"—but if the prospects looked dim for funding the medical school in this way, "I would rather discontinue now than to cripple along and be compelled to stop later."[97] Clearly challenging the BFM, the new president stated, "We . . . await your answer as to whether you can stand back of the [medical] department."[98]

McGranahan did not end this September 1900 monthly report to Witherspoon and the Pittsburgh board here, however, but added another long section in which he explained the second set of problems he saw with the medical department—those related to the people who ran the program. He had originally decided not to mention these matters, but reconsidered before sending off the report. McGranahan felt it right and necessary to tell all so that the board could understand the true nature of the problem and "act intelligently" when it made its decision about the future of the medical department.[99]

For several reasons, McGranahan related, soon after his arrival in Knoxville he "was not satisfied that we had a proper faculty to teach medicine."[100] For one thing, whenever an illness occurred at the college, physicians other than the medical faculty were always called. "The idea of calling one of them [a medical instructor]," McGranahan explained, "only brought a smile." Upon inquiry, he learned that these men had "rather limited . . . practices."[101] Furthermore, most people believed "that the money returned was their only consideration in the work." The president himself soon found "a thousand reasons to believe that they are in it 'for revenue only.'" (He carefully excluded "the two colored men" from this assessment of the medical faculty.)[102] At the very first faculty meeting over which McGranahan presided, the professors voted to divide the six dollars remaining in the treasury "among the five of them, figuring it out to the cent." Such behavior occurred at every meeting, "till I have been disgusted with their hunger for the money."[103] Rather than bother the BFM with petty requests for small amounts of money "to do little things with," McGranahan "quenched it."[104]

Concerned about the character and abilities of the white faculty who were teaching KC's medical students, McGranahan had, a few months after his arrival at KC, turned for more information and guidance to his retired predecessor, Rev. McCulloch. The former president "set forth much of the same doubt that I felt" and told of yet another disturbing issue: the current dean, Edwin L. Randall, was "an unbeliever."[105] Further inquiry, McGranahan continued in his report to the BFM, revealed that Randall was not just an unbeliever but "a blaspheming Ingersolite" who is "very profane as he meets with men" and "makes a boast of his unbelief."[106] At KCMD's graduation exercises the previous June, Randall had made sarcastic remarks about the Bible, and on another occasion had engaged in "a tirade of cursing Jesus Christ" when asked if he was a believer.[107]

Understandably unsettled by what he had learned about the religious views of the dean of this Presbyterian medical school, McGranahan had decided to discuss religion privately with each of the other faculty members. The four white instructors, he found, "don't work at their religion much if they have any to work." The two African American physicians were different: "Dr. Edwards (colored) is a professing Christian and stands well in his profession. Dr. Derrick (colored) is a pronounced Christian and good physician."[108] Based on his own experiences, the information he had gained about the faculty from discreet inquiries and direct interviews, and the opinions of trusted coworkers at KC who thought the medical department "a disgrace, as it is," McGranahan now felt that it was time to either "reconstruct our faculty" or, more likely, "discontinue the department."[109]

When (McGranahan continued in his report to the BFM), true to form, the faculty "asked for a meeting on Sept. 14 for the purpose of dividing the spoils that might have come in during the summer," the president saw his chance.[110] He presided over their partition of the twenty-five dollars in the treasury, then raised the financial questions about space, a full-time faculty member, new equipment,[111] and the future of the medical department already described. The professors agreed to form a committee to request action from the BFM on these matters, but then decided at the next meeting to "continue the department just as it had been." McGranahan would not relent this time, however, telling them that "it rested between their making the statement and my making it."[112] This outraged Dr. Randall, who also accused the president of dragging religion into medicine and of trying to restrict his freedom in the classroom. The dean threatened to "step out and the department can go on" without him.[113] McGranahan welcomed Randall's comments about religion and medicine in the classroom because they addressed the president's concern about the way a Christian medical school should be conducted; he told Randall that those issues would be discussed immediately "if the department went on."[114]

But McGranahan did not want the department to go on. Though he could find other physicians to replace the unbelievers, the president, in his September 1900 report (written after these confrontations with the faculty), recommended taking "the short way out. We have enough here [at Knoxville College] without it [the medical school]. We weaken [the rest of the college] by including this department." He recommended that the BFM close the school and explain that "everything at K.C. must be first class and in the absence of money provision for this department it cannot be first class."[115] McGranahan's major arguments were that the mission of Knoxville College—to educate moral young men and women—was more important than maintaining a potentially prestigious medical school, and that the cost of building and maintaining a modern medical department at KC was too great. The president concluded his report with a plea to the board to act discreetly and "without any reference to these things that I mentioned in this part of my letter." He feared retribution if the medical faculty discovered he had revealed so much about them: "Protect me from a personal attack by these men who will be rob[b]ed of a little income."[116]

The BFM accepted McGranahan's advice and requests within a week, agreeing to suspend the medical department.[117] KCMD, scheduled to begin classes on December 5, 1900, did not reopen then or ever.[118] McGranahan moved swiftly. He immediately sent letters to all prospective KCMD applicants announcing the closing of the school and published a copy of that letter in the October 15 issue of the *Aurora*. Appearing under the headline "Knoxville College Medical Department Discontinued," the letter briefly summarized some of the arguments McGranahan had made to the BFM in his September report. Financial considerations were the primary reason for the school's closing, the open letter explained. Modern medical education required large sums of money for buildings and equipment, money that KCMD did not have and could not raise. The letter continued, "The Medical Department of the college was begun under the mistaken impression that it could maintain itself without any appropriation from outside. This of course would be impossible."[119] Rather than provide a lesser education for its students, the college's board of control had decided to discontinue the department: "Everything connected with . . . [Knoxville College] must be first-class." The board commended "most highly the service of the medical faculty . . . which services were rendered almost gratuitously" and apologized to the students for disappointing them.[120]

Knoxville College had grafted a medical department onto its educational programs in 1895, lured by the low apparent cost and the potential for bringing the college prestige. But KC's president and governing board were not prepared for the undertaking. Rather than furthering the school's mission of educating, both morally and intellectually, former slaves and their descendants, the medical department had proved to be a drag on the college—attracting few students, producing few physicians, costing money and time, undermining the college's moral tone, and upsetting the college's operations. KCMD's two founders, a minister and a physician, had had different goals. Rev. McCulloch viewed the medical school as another way to fulfill the school's mission by training Christian physicians for the nation's needy African American population; Dr. Hill viewed it as a way for him and his faculty to earn extra money. Both thought the financial costs would be low and resisted investing in improved facilities to keep up with rising licensure and educational requirements in the state and nation. KC's overseers, the BFM, had also failed to commit to the undertaking, allowing it to proceed as long as it cost them nothing. Ironically, at a school dedicated to African American medical education, increasingly open racial bias in the larger Knoxville community, as the Jim Crow era began, spilled over into the hiring of faculty. White medical instructors barred most black physicians from teaching at KCMD. Interestingly, the two African American physicians allowed to join the faculty were the teachers most respected by KC staff and students. Not until a change in college leadership occurred did the parties involved—the college administration, the medical faculty, and the BFM—confront the problems that existed in the medical department. It took a new president with a different leadership style to recognize and demonstrate to the BFM the conflicting goals of faculty and administration, and to show how these conflicting goals were undermining the mission of the college.

Knoxville Medical College

Though KC and the BFM chose to discontinue KCMD in 1900, medical education opportunities in Knoxville for African Americans did not immediately disappear. The former medical faculty decided to move operations to another location in town. According to Rev. McGranahan's October 31, 1900, monthly report to the BFM in Pittsburgh, those former instructors asked the president "not to send out any notices that the department was discontinued for it was not, but would be continued."[121] McGranahan responded firmly: "I answered that the department was discontinued and that the notices would be sent to all who applied [for admission to KCMD], and that if they [the former faculty members] started up [a medical school] it would not be as a Department of K.C." He agreed to provide them with a list of people who had written for information about KCMD, but when the faculty "demanded the chemicals and tables of the medical laboratory," he refused to give over what he viewed as school property without the board's permission. He did offer the dissecting tables, but the faculty, considering all the equipment as rightfully theirs, threatened "to take the things by law."[122] McGranahan promptly rescinded his offer to hand over the dissecting tables and letters of inquiry from prospective students.

The outcome of this battle cannot be determined from remaining records, but the faculty did find a new location for their institution and, with or without equipment and supplies from the old school, did begin instruction using KCMD's fall schedule. The new school was named Knoxville Medical College (KMC).[123] New students could start their studies, and former KCMD students could continue them without a break, under the same instructors who had taught at

KCMD. Despite McGranahan's unpleasant parting with the medical faculty, the KC president did forward to Dr. William W. Derrick, treasurer of the new school and one of only two former KCMD faculty members whom he respected,[124] the final tuition payments from two previous medical students and an additional twenty-eight cents that still remained in the department's treasury.[125] Antagonism between the two schools apparently lingered for several years, illustrated by the seemingly spiteful statement included in a half-page advertisement in a 1902 national medical directory proclaiming KMC as "Formerly [the] Medical Department of Knoxville College."[126]

Barred from KC's campus, the new school opened in a building just a few blocks away, down Clinton Road on one of the main streetcar lines to and from the center of town.[127] Even when it moved again in 1904, KMC stayed in the neighborhood, in the former Industrial School for Negroes just four buildings distant from its previous location. The faculty used only the upper floor of the building, sharing quarters below first with a grocer and then, from about 1906 on, with Hamilton and Lillison, an African American undertaker's establishment.[128]

Whether it was the more accessible location, the lack of association with a religious institution, the freer environment away from the watchful eyes of KC administrators and staff, or some other factor, KMC attracted much larger numbers of students than had ever attended KCMD. According to KMC statistics submitted to medical directories and the American Medical Association's Council on Medical Education, thirty-four students attended the independent medical college during its first year of courses, 1900–1901, compared with eleven in KCMD's peak enrollment year, 1899–1900. Most students came from the middle South, though a few lived as far away as Massachusetts, Utah, and Washington State.[129] Registration reached a high of forty-seven in 1904–5, never slipped below twenty-two, and averaged almost thirty-two during the school's ten-year lifespan.[130]

With tuition and fees averaging $40 per annual session until 1907 or 1908 and about $45 thereafter, KMC's faculty could potentially have collected a minimum of $880 each year from students to either reinvest or distribute among themselves. Now that the school was independent, however, it had to pay for items previously obtained at no cost, such as the use of a building, office supplies, classroom furniture, laboratory equipment and supplies, cadavers, advertising, catalogs, and postage. KC had previously covered all or part of these expenses.

KMC's professional staff usually numbered five or six physicians.[131] For the first few years of the school's existence, not much faculty turnover occurred,[132] but by 1905 the only professor remaining from the old KCMD was, ironically, Dr. W. W. Derrick—the man whom, in December 1896, white faculty members had been reluctant to hire because he was African American.[133] Derrick served as KMC's dean at least in 1907, and probably from 1905 until 1910.[134] He also earned the distinction of having taught at the medical school longer than any other instruc-

Figure 19. Knoxville Medical College Faculty

Name	Race	Medical School Attended	Year Graduated	Years Taught at KMC
Blankenship, John P.	white	Vanderbilt Medical College	1874	[1901–02?] –1903
Bryant, William H.	black	Leonard Medical School	1905	unknown
Clear, John	white	Kentucky School of Medicine (Louisville)	1885	1900–1905
Crawford, Daniel W.	black	Chattanooga National Medical College	1901	[?–] 1909–1910
Derrick, William W.	black	Meharry Medical College	1892	1900–1910
Edwards, Augustus G.	black	Meharry Medical College	1895	[1900–1901?]
Ezidore, Ernest N.	black	Meharry Medical College	1907	[?] 1908–1909 [–?]
Green, Henry M.	black	Knoxville Medical College	1901	1902–1910
Moore, William H.	white	Tennessee Medical College	1893	1900–1904
Randall, Edwin L.	white	Missouri Medical College	1869	1900–1903
Watkins, E. L.	black	Knoxville Medical College	1905	[?] 1908–1909 [–?]
Wood, Charles R.	black	Knoxville Medical College	1895	[?] 1908–1909 [–?]

tor, remaining with KMC until it closed in 1910.[135] After 1905, KMC became, like Louisville National Medical College and the University of West Tennessee College of Medicine and Surgery, a medical school operated *by* African Americans *for* African Americans.[136]

The person who became the driving force behind KMC during most of its ten-year lifetime was Henry Morgan Green (1877–1939) of Jellico, Tennessee. Green entered KCMD as a second-year student (information about any prior medical training is not available) during that school's final session, 1899–1900. He concluded his studies at the new KMC the following year and received his M.D. degree after only two years of formal study, in 1901—one of two students to form KMC's first graduating class. After doing postgraduate work at Northwestern University Medical School in Illinois and practicing in Jellico for a short time, Green returned to Knoxville. A 1902 KMC advertisement listed him as the school's secretary as well as professor of bacteriology, histology, pathology, and anatomy. He rose rapidly to prominence in Knoxville's African American medical community, practicing from his downtown office on the second floor of the Famous Building, near the intersection of Vine and Central. When KC developed a nurse-training program and opened a hospital and infirmary at 1825 Clinton Road, between the college and the medical school, he became the Wallace Memorial Hospital's most important medical figure. Though all the black physicians of

Figure 20. Known Graduates of Knoxville Medical College (arranged chronologically)

1901	Green, Henry M.
	Raines, Claude W.
1902	Flack, Pindar M.
	Watson, William E.
1903	Love, Hugh
	Phenix, W. E.
1904	Craig, Thomas E.
	Ezell, G. W.
	Hamilton, C. A.
	Lloyd, Reuben A.
	McCoy, A. G.[1]
	Robinson, John M.[2]
1905	Dantzler, J. J.
	Hampton, W. H.
	Watkins, E. L.
	Woods, Charles R.
1906	Prater, William T.[3]
1907	Stephens, Perry A.
1908	Durham, William A.
	Russell, Samuel M.
1909	Coffey, Alfred V.
	Jones, Benton H.
	McCoy, Elizabeth[4]
	Sims, Otis A.
1910	Flack, William F.
	Perkins, Noah E.

1. Short biographical sketch in G. P. Hamilton, *The Bright Side of Memphis* (Memphis, Tenn.: n.p., 1908), 42. He attended Meharry for three years before transferring to KMC.

2. Obituary in *Journal of the National Medical Association* 62 (1970): 481.

3. Brief biographical sketch in Hamilton, *Bright Side of Memphis*, 48.

4. Mentioned in sketch of her husband, A. G. McCoy, in Hamilton, *Bright Side of Memphis*, 42. Picture of Elizabeth McCoy in Bate, "*It's Been a Long Time*" (Muskogee, Okla.: Hoffmann, 1986), 192.

Knoxville admitted patients to the hospital, it was Green (according to an agent for a major outside agency funding the nurse-training school) who performed "nearly all of the surgical work," including all the major surgery.[137] Green became a great promoter of black hospitals and later founded the National Hospital Association. He remained a visible part of the KMC administration as the school's secretary and, along with Derrick, taught there throughout the decade. On the national level, Green served the National Medical Association as its president and chair of its Pellagra Commission. He was KMC's most prominent graduate and among its staunchest supporters.

KMC did not have a strong reputation, despite Dr. Green's and a few other graduates' respected positions in black medical circles. Members of the National Medical Association's Committee on Medical Education and Negro Medical Schools pointed out in 1909 that graduates of all the schools for African Americans, including KMC, did not fare very well on state licensing board examinations. KMC had one of the poorest records; available statistics show that five of the twelve graduates who took state licensing exams the same year they graduated from KMC failed their exams. Not once between 1904 and 1910 did more than half of KMC's graduates who took licensing exams, regardless of when they graduated, pass them.[138] Some states, such as Alabama, refused even to examine graduates of KMC (and those of a few of the other black schools).[139]

The most telling assessment of KMC came in January 1909 when Abraham Flexner visited Knoxville as part of his survey for the American Medical Association's Committee on Medical Education and the Carnegie Foundation for the Advancement of Teaching. His report, published a year later, revealed just how poor an education the KMC faculty was providing its more than twenty aspiring African American physicians. The school, Flexner stated, had nominal entrance requirements and no laboratory, clinical, or dispensary facilities on site. It supported itself entirely from student fees and rarely afforded students the opportunity to work with patients. Despite the fact that Henry M. Green did most of the surgery at the Knoxville College Hospital, just a few blocks away, and that all the black practitioners in Knoxville, including KMC's faculty, admitted and cared for patients at that same hospital, "It was stated [to Flexner] by a student that twice between October 1 and January 28 'a few students were taken to the Knoxville College Hospital.'"[140] Flexner concluded his account with a most devastating comment: "The catalogue of this school is a tissue of misrepresentations from cover to cover."[141]

Such an assessment indicated that, though the names and faces of the school's faculty had, with the exception of W. W. Derrick, changed over the years, the school's low educational standards apparently had not. Within the African American medical community nationwide, KMC earned for itself a reputation of mediocrity. The school became an embarrassment to other black physicians. Dr. H. F. Gamble, chairman of the National Medical Association's Committee on Medical Education and Negro Medical Schools, stated of KMC in August 1909, without naming the school directly, that "special agents or committees who have investigated Negro medical schools" found "one medical school . . . unworthy of the name of medical school, poor teachers, cheap graduates, cheap schools, and in short, they fail in every respect to measure up to the standard of efficiency" expected of schools of the time.[142] KMC closed its doors after the 1910 term, unable to escape the legacy of its predecessor.

CHAPTER 18

Abraham Flexner and the Black Medical Schools

In 1900 a black student wishing to pursue a career in medicine could choose from ten schools in a variety of locations and settings (see Appendix, Table 4). By 1920 a black student had only three choices and little assurance that any one of these schools would survive until graduation day four years hence. What had happened? The "Flexner Report," containing devastating comments about all but two of the black schools and demeaning statements about black physicians, appeared in 1910, directly affecting the fate of these schools. By 1923, only the two institutions he said deserved to exist, Meharry Medical College and Howard University Medical Department, remained. Those two schools, too, almost closed their doors as organized medicine and medical philanthropies pushed the educational reforms promoted by Flexner beyond the capacities of the black institutions to change. Between 1905 and 1920, black medical education passed through two crisis periods: 1905–12 and 1917–18. Flexner was involved in both.

The Condition of Black Medical Schools in the Early Twentieth Century

As mentioned in Chapter 11, contemporaries classified black medical schools according to their origins as either missionary or proprietary. The precarious nature of these schools' financial arrangements, whether overseen by white missionary groups or by enterprising independent black physician proprietors, put all the African American medical colleges in a vulnerable position from the start. Most of the schools collapsed with the increased pressure for reform in the first decades of the twentieth century. Meharry, Howard, Leonard, Flint, Knoxville, and Louisville National were still struggling to survive and improve when American medicine "discovered" bacteriology, laboratories, public health, and the German education system. With the revitalization of the American Medical Association (AMA) and the Association of American Medical Colleges (AAMC) at the turn of the century and these organizations' relentless application of pressure to improve medical education based on the new ideas in science and education, African American medical schools found themselves caught in a paradoxical situation. On the one hand, they saw the demand for their product—the M.D. degree—growing to the point at which some of them could not accommodate all applicants. In 1907, for example, President Charles F. Meserve of Leonard Medical School told Wallace Buttrick of the General Education Board (GEB), a Rockefeller family philanthropy, that his school had more applicants than places in each class, and more requests from towns for black physicians than graduates each year.[1] On the other hand, every black medical school faced mounting financial pressures as the demand for better trained professors, a longer school year, well-equipped laboratories, and clinical facilities drained limited resources.

The proprietary schools had no sources of income other than student fees and perhaps a small investor or two. Theoretically, the missionary schools could raise funds from other parts of their universities, their home mission societies, or religious sect donors in the North. In actuality, black colleges raised little excess funding to shunt into medical education, and Northern mission societies and individual donors were at this time shifting priorities to such newer, more immediate problems as helping the large numbers of eastern and southern European immigrants who were moving into their cities. Moreover, black students generally came from poor families that could barely pay even the low tuition, fees, and living expenses of medical college, so the schools could expect little extra cash from that source. Few black physicians had succeeded well enough by the early twentieth century to support their alma maters, nor were black philanthropists able to do so.[2] State universities offered little for black students desiring a medical education. The rising demand for black physicians and limited fund-raising opportunities caused problems for black medical schools at a time when they wished to encourage growth and modernization.

Pressures for Change before Flexner

As historians have shown, Abraham Flexner did not inaugurate American medical education reform with his 1910 report;[3] he stepped into the middle of such an era, put his imprint on it, and through his work with the GEB after 1912, influenced the way reforms were implemented. When Flexner began working for the Carnegie Foundation for the Advancement of Teaching in 1908, the AMA's Council on Medical Education (CME) had already evaluated the nation's medical schools three times, twice using state medical licensing board results and once through personal visits. Dr. Arthur Dean Bevan (chair) and Dr. N. P. Colwell (secretary) had published in the *Journal of the American Medical Association* (*JAMA*) the failure rates of individual schools on state licensure board examinations and even a listing of acceptable medical colleges based on a classification scheme they implemented.[4] Though they did not publicize the reports stemming from their site visits, Bevan and Colwell sent these reports to the schools and to the state medical examining boards hoping to spur improvements at the poorer-rated institutions. The African American schools fared badly in these evaluations. Their board failure rates in 1904 and 1905 all greatly exceeded 20 percent, the worst category,[5] and when the two years' scores were combined, each of the six schools with sufficient available data appeared in the bottom 30 percent of the 135 studied.[6]

After its establishment in 1904, well before Flexner's arrival, the CME promoted both higher entrance requirements and higher educational standards, making its appeals both to schools and to state regulatory boards.[7] Most black schools responded by lengthening their terms, improving hospital and laboratory facilities, and, at least in written documents, toughening entrance and graduation requirements.[8]

The CME had also noted, before Flexner, the cost to medical schools of needed changes and the necessity of obtaining outside funding for these reforms. A *JAMA* editorial in May 1907 announced that modern medical education now required two or three times the amount received in fees from each medical student. Proprietary schools, the editorial continued, simply did not possess the ability to raise and pay out such amounts; a large endowment from private sources or state support was needed to sustain a school. Medical education was changing for the better, it concluded, but too many schools lagged behind, unable to keep up with the rising standards.[9] At annual conferences on medical education, the CME began doing more than simply publicizing poor board scores and urging schools to improve; it proposed guidelines for an acceptable education program and wrote a model state medical practice act.[10]

So the CME's efforts before Flexner, though not directed specifically at black medical schools, in effect put them on notice. Administrators at African American institutions understood the message and realized that the expense of change as well as the changes themselves threatened each school's existence. In June 1906, the CME sent a letter to every American medical school, urging adoption of its proposal that all students take at least one year of college-level work in biology, chemistry, physics, and a foreign language before admission.[11] Acceptance of this plan would have immediately reduced the number of students at black medical schools, because few young African Americans went to college before starting their professional education. Furthermore, only a few African American colleges offered such advanced courses, and only a handful of white colleges admitted black students. Reduced enrollments at black medical schools would have meant reduced income, a situation these schools had to avoid, for both missionary and proprietary schools relied on student fees as the major source of funds. Not surprisingly, then, none of the African American medical colleges responded positively to the AMA's request, though each year the number of white schools implementing the plan grew, as did the pressure for black schools to follow suit.[12]

The CME presented other reform ideas during these pre-Flexner years that threatened the black schools in particular. Arthur Dean Bevan, for instance, must have upset authorities at black schools with his comments about instructors, made at the April 1907 annual CME conference in Chicago. He alluded to some medical schools conducted by people respected in the profession, but imparting information and teaching the techniques of a former era. These institutions offered students little practical experience in the laboratory, the hospital ward, or the clinic, instead lecturing and quizzing them in the classroom.[13] Though catalogs of African American medical schools claimed to train modern physicians using modern techniques, other available information belies those statements. Leonard's faculty at this time, for instance, differed little from the faculty twenty-five years earlier, shortly after its opening. These local white practitioners, some highly respected in Raleigh and around the state, had trained early in the modern medical period. Some had not kept up with the new scientific ideas and educational innovations. With a tiny hospital open only during the school year and few laboratory facilities, Leonard could not really offer the best medical education to its students.[14] At Flint and Meharry, both supported in part by the Freedmen's Aid Society, many members of the predominantly black faculty were either recent medical graduates (usually of Meharry) with little practical experience or graduates of many years ago who, because of race restrictions, had not attended postgraduate courses. Faculty at the black proprietary schools consisted primarily of their own graduates, some just a year or two out of school.[15]

Chairman Bevan also attacked "medical schools conducted solely for profit" in his April 1907 address, calling them "a menace" and advocating their nonrecognition. Though the black proprietary schools had their failings, they seem not to have existed "solely for profit" and did turn out needed black practitioners. But the CME pressed hard to eliminate all proprietary schools and thereby put pressure on those run by and for blacks in this pre-Flexner period.[16]

Finally, Bevan spoke quite critically of schools offering courses after four o'clock in the afternoon, when students with full-time jobs were no doubt tired from a day's work and had insufficient time to fit in full-length courses with laboratory and ward work. The AMA House of Delegates instructed the CME just two months after Bevan's address not to rate higher than Class C any medical college that offered evening courses.[17] Howard University Medical Department was then still offering night courses in Washington, D.C., where a strong demand for such a program existed.

So a year before Flexner even began his medical school survey, officials, faculty, and perhaps even students at African American medical schools felt pressure to change their institutions' educational program. They could relate to their own colleges what Leonard president Meserve said of his: "A crisis has come in the life of Leonard Medical School." The school, he felt, had no future if he could not find sufficient financial aid to upgrade it to meet the new educational demands.[18]

By December 1908, when Flexner began his study of medical education in the United States, three of the weakest (both financially and academically) black schools had closed their doors: the Medico-Chirurgical and Theological College of Christ's Institution in Baltimore, State University Medical Department in Louisville (merged with Louisville National Medical College), and Chattanooga National Medical College. Little is known about the first school; it apparently had no strong academic or financial basis and few graduates. The actual date of its closing is not clear, though it is not mentioned in AMA or AAMC records after 1908.[19] State University, despite its name, had no affiliation with the Commonwealth of Kentucky, but received its support from the state's black Baptist organizations. The university continued to train undergraduates and ministers after joining with Louisville National Medical College in 1903, eventually becoming Simmons College.[20] Chattanooga National Medical College (CNMC), named by its founder after his alma mater, Louisville National Medical College, graduated perhaps sixteen students before closing during its sixth year, in 1904. Based on the small amount of evidence available, CNMC's academic program, facilities, equipment, and teaching staff appear inadequate.[21] Three of the seven remaining black schools, the University of West Tennessee and Knoxville Medical College (both proprietary) and Leonard Medical School (Baptist), received ratings of less than 50 percent from the CME in June 1908.[22] The CME also recommended that state examining boards withdraw recognition from these institutions.[23]

Flexner's Evaluation of Black Medical Education

Thus African Americans seeking a medical education already faced challenges when Flexner completed and published his report in 1910.[24] The report (1) announced the existence of black medical schools that turned out practicing black physicians, (2) described the good and bad points of these schools and advocated improvements or closings just as with the white schools, (3) reflected an outlook about black medical education that the AMA readily accepted and applied in its formulation of education policy, and (4) revealed negative white attitudes toward black physicians during an era of increasing racial tension.

Until the Flexner Report, organized medicine had said little directly to or about the black medical schools. Though the CME, almost from its establishment in 1904, had issued annual reports, articles, and commentaries on medical education in *JAMA*, never in the fifteen years of major medical education reform did *JAMA* ever openly discuss the issue of medical education for blacks. Women's medical education received a passing reference in each annual education issue and an occasional article. Black schools received no notice other than the word *colored* posted next to their names in tables, and one-sentence statements when one of them received a gift, completed a building, or closed. Even state medical journals of the period rarely acknowledged the presence of African American schools within their state's borders.[25] The Flexner Report, describing each of the seven existing black institutions and spending fewer than two pages on black medical education problems, at least documented the almost invisible presence of African American medical schools.

But the Flexner Report also harmed the black cause by portraying African American medical education as deficient in general and five of the seven black medical schools as particularly wanting. It said little good about the three proprietary schools—West Tennessee, Louisville National, and Knoxville—or two of the missionary schools affiliated with universities—Flint and Leonard. It did praise the "small and scrupulously clean hospital of 8 beds" at Louisville National.[26] But it also noted the "meager equipment for chemistry, pharmacy, and microscopy" and the "bare . . . rooms" at West Tennessee,[27] the absence of laboratory or clinical facilities at Knoxville,[28] and the paucity of laboratory materials at Leonard[29] and Flint.[30] Flexner's criticisms were harsh ("The catalogue of this school [Knoxville] is a tissue of misrepresentations from cover to cover"),[31] frank ("Of the three negro schools in the state [Tennessee], two are without merit"),[32] chiding ("The school [Knoxville] occupies a floor above an undertaker's establishment"),[33] sarcastic ("It was stated by a student that twice between October 1 and January 28 'a few students were taken to the Knoxville College Hospital'"),[34] and biting ("Laboratory facilities [at Leonard] . . . comprise . . . a slight chemical laboratory, and a still slighter equipment for pathology").[35] Sometimes he allowed the mere statement of facts without comment to convey his message: "The school [Flint] controls a hospital of 20 beds, with an average of 17 patients monthly, and a dispensary with an average daily attendance of one or two";[36] and "There is a dispensary [at West Tennessee], without records, in the school building."[37] Flexner's reports on these five schools told readers that black students, and by implication, current black practitioners who had graduated from these schools, did not receive an adequate medical education. He even stated at one point, "Of the seven medical schools for negroes in the United States, five are at this moment in no position to make any contribution of value to the solution of the [Negro health] problem above pointed out. They are wasting small sums annually and sending out undisciplined men, whose lack of real training is covered up by the imposing M.D. degree."[38]

The report did more than describe poor conditions at black medical schools; it prescribed a limited role for black physicians in their practices and hinted that black physicians possessed less potential and ability than their white counterparts. The tone of Chapter 14, "The Medical Education of the Negro,"[39] illustrated well how, in the world of medicine as in so many other aspects of American life at the time, whites attempted to discount, dominate, and disvalue blacks. It began with a provocative statement: "The medical care of the negro race will never be wholly left to negro physicians." His second sentence explained this assertion by claiming that whites had to teach the black physician "to feel a sharp responsibility for the physical integrity of his people." Black doctors, according to Flexner, lacked responsibility enough to take over full care of their own people, but white doctors possessed that sense. Furthermore, "The practice of the negro doctor will be limited to his own race." Flexner's reasoning for such comments became clearer as he next explained how educating black physicians would also serve white interests in preventing the spread of diseases from blacks to whites. He was clearly writing for a white audience when he concluded, "The negro must be educated not only for his sake, but for ours." To protect the nation's overall health, the responsibility of "educating the [black] race to know and to practice fundamental hygienic principles" fell naturally to the black doctor. Thus, "a well-taught negro sanitarian will be immensely useful." So Flexner not only limited the role of African American physicians to caring for other African Americans but further restricted it to matters of public health.

Where did black medical schools fit in Flexner's scheme? They had two missions: first, to offer "the more promising of the race . . . a substantial education in which hygiene rather than surgery . . . is strongly accentuated"; second, to "imbue these men with the missionary spirit so that they will look upon the diploma as a commission to serve their people humbly and devotedly, away from large cities [in] the village and [on] the plantation, upon which light has hardly as yet begun to break." If Flexner spelled out in more detail how to implement a program to accomplish these goals for black medical education, so different in many ways from the more research- and practice-oriented program for whites described in the rest of his report, he must have done so orally. None of his extant letters to the black medical schools or his published writing discussed these matters.

The two medical schools that Flexner believed to be suited for training black physicians were Meharry and Howard. He admired Meharry founder George W. Hubbard's skill at marshalling slender resources and building his school into a credible institution with good laboratory facilities and a small but well-managed endowment. Meharry lacked only a larger hospital and dispensary. Howard, with its ties to the federal government through a small annual appropriation and the use of Freedmen's Hospital, had its future "assured." Both schools, Flexner knew, needed "developing," and both were "unequal to the need and the opportunity" as they then existed. He urged religious and philanthropic organizations as well as individuals to concentrate their efforts on these two institutions and not to waste separate small amounts of money on the other five schools.[40] Flexner's recommendation on medical education for African Americans in 1910 was to close the five "ineffectual" schools and encourage their supporters to donate time and money toward building Howard's and Meharry's programs.

The Influence of the Flexner Report

In the end, Flexner's black medical school plan prevailed. Only Howard and Meharry survived the reform era, though both continued to train a full range of medical practitioners rather than "sanitarians" for rural African Americans. Of the five other institutions, three closed within two years of the report, one fought on doggedly for another eight years, and one proprietary school defiantly remained open until 1923, though its graduates were unrecognized by most state licensing boards. Knoxville Medical College, criticized severely by Flexner, closed the same year the report was published. The following year, Flint Medical College, sponsored by the same Freedmen's Aid Society of the Methodist Episcopal Church that was supporting Meharry, shut down after twenty years. Flint's president explained that the CME's increasingly intense campaign for improved standards, and the school's lack of money to make the necessary changes, forced its closing.[41] Louisville National Medical College lost its accreditation from the Kentucky State Board of Health and closed in 1912.[42] The influence of the Flexner Report can be seen in the demise of each of these schools.

Few if any African Americans responded directly to the report in writing, though physicians and educators must have discussed it. The Committee on Medical Education of the National Medical Association (NMA)—black counterpart to the AMA—had considered the problems of black medical schools in 1908 and 1909 after the publication of state board scores in *JAMA*, but remained silent (at least in writing) on the Flexner Report and medical education in general after 1910. This committee had no power to implement education policy at black medical schools; it simply advised NMA officers and members of medical education matters and made recommendations for improvements. The committee had recognized the weaknesses of the several black colleges even before Flexner and wished to avoid public embarrassment over them. That, unfortunately, was no longer possible.[43]

In 1912, the end of this first crisis period, only four black schools remained. One of these, the University of West Tennessee, was isolated from the others until it closed in 1923, its president taking an independent course.[44] Howard and Meharry, the two schools of which Flexner spoke positively, seemed to have bright futures, leaving only Leonard to prove itself worthy and secure a firmer position.

The Flexner Report did not conclude an era of medical reform; it appeared in the midst of one. Medical education standards continued to change, to improve, pushed along by the schools themselves, the AMA, the AAMC, state licensing boards, and two major funding agencies, the Carnegie Foundation for the Advancement of Teaching and the GEB. The remaining African American schools still faced difficult times. Howard and Meharry had received A ratings from the AMA in the second round of visits (the Flexner visits of 1909 to 1910), though in a special category called "Medical Schools for the Colored Race."[45] They had to keep up with the latest innovations to retain their positions. Leonard, rated C, had to catch up.

The Flexner Report had brought attention to seven black medical schools: their presence, their needs, their shortcomings, and their potential. Three could not change sufficiently and closed. The remaining schools had to prove themselves. But no one in the white medical establishment, not even Flexner, who wanted Howard and Meharry to endure, helped the schools through this next crisis period until one more had closed and the other two were about to follow suit.

The Search for Funding

On February 21, 1910, Howard University president Wilbur P. Thirkield acknowledged receipt of an advance copy of Flexner's assessment of his medical school: "We are deeply gratified by this favorable representation of the equipment and work of the school." He told Henry S. Pritchett, president of the Carnegie Foundation, that Howard would immediately require of all its freshmen applicants one year of college-level science.[46] Three months later Edward A. Balloch, medical dean, submitted his annual report to President Thirkield, telling him of the faculty's acceptance of the new admissions requirements but concern at the anticipated decline in enrollment and loss of revenue from student tuition. Because Howard relied on fees for most of its income, plus a small allowance from the federal government, Balloch knew that trouble lay ahead. Only by the extraordinary efforts of the school's secretary-treasurer, the underpayment of faculty salaries, and strict economy of educational expenditures did the medical department break even each year. Student fees just covered costs. But, Balloch continued, it was not fair to pay the faculty so little or to provide them with so few supplies and so little equipment. The medical department needed at least

$10,000 over tuition and fees the following year to pay for the cost of education. What Howard really needed was a half-million-dollar endowment. Securing one "should be given precedence over everything else."[47]

Within months Thirkield wrote a letter to Andrew Carnegie, reminding him of his expression of interest in Howard University Medical Department at the recent Carnegie Library dedication on campus.[48] Undeterred by Carnegie's quick response that Howard was worthy, but that he had given them $50,000 for the library the previous year and the government already provided annual financial support,[49] Thirkield held further discussions with Carnegie's personal secretary. In May 1911 he submitted an ambitious proposal for $200,000 to erect and equip a new building for the medical school. This time he enclosed references from Dr. William Henry Welch of Johns Hopkins, Pritchett of the Carnegie Foundation, President William Howard Taft, and Dr. Woodward of the Carnegie Institution, attesting to the value and importance of this investment. He included a fact sheet illustrating the school's need for buildings, salaries for full-time professors, and other budget items. Then, as President Meserve of Leonard Medical School had stated just a few years earlier in an appeal for funds, Thirkield explained that the Howard University Medical Department "has reached a crisis in its affairs." "On the one hand, it is confronted with the necessity of providing medical education for colored students which shall comply with modern standards; on the other hand is the absolute impossibility of providing such education when the income is derived from fees alone." Taking his cue from Flexner's report, Thirkield informed Carnegie that Howard "trains men of science, especially versed in the problems of sanitation and preventive medicine." The work of its graduates would improve white health as well as black because many diseases are transmitted from one race to the other.[50] Despite these appeals and others over the next few years, no dollars from the Carnegie fortune found their way to Howard's medical school.[51]

Dr. Hubbard of Meharry also appealed to Carnegie, for $20,000 to build a hospital. Flexner had urged its construction in 1910 to make Meharry a first-rate medical school. Carnegie agreed and donated $10,000 on the condition that Hubbard raise the rest. This he did, and in 1913 the G. W. Hubbard Hospital was dedicated.[52] But Meharry's further appeals, like Howard's, for larger sums or for an endowment, elicited similarly negative responses. Andrew Carnegie finally told Pritchett, who had urged funding, "If we start helping medical colleges for colored people we cannot discontinue." Their needs, he felt, were too great, and their allies who might help in the funding too few.[53]

The needs of black schools *were* great—too great for individual philanthropists or religious outreach boards such as the Freedmen's Aid Society (supporting Meharry) or the American Baptist Home Mission Society (supporting Leonard) to manage. Yet the Carnegie Foundation, the philanthropic organization associated with Flexner's investigation that ultimately encouraged continuation of Meharry and Howard, refused financial assistance to these schools. In 1912, Flexner himself moved to the other large, education-oriented philanthropic organization in the United States, the GEB. Black medical school officials wrote to both Flexner and Pritchett, hoping that the personnel change signaled a policy change as well, but both the GEB and the Carnegie Foundation turned them down or delayed action for several years.[54]

A Second Crisis Period

Between 1912 and 1918, the situation worsened for the black schools. Leonard could not get the ear of any funding agency after the GEB gave it a tiny amount toward a new hospital in 1910.[55] In 1914, the school, despite its high admission standards and reasonably good laboratory facilities, of necessity dropped its clinical program in exchange for a B ranking from the CME.[56] Earlier that same year, Meharry lost its A rating and received a reprimand from the CME representative who visited the school. A number of problems had been identified: the faculty consisted of only three full-time and twenty-four part-time instructors for 354 medical students; the school's enforcement of student entrance standards could not be verified from existing records; medical, dental, and pharmacy students took classes together; the new hospital, with fifty-eight beds, had only twenty-three occupants at the time of the visit and averaged only thirty; the outpatient department served only six to eight patients per day; no medical library, medical museum, or modern teaching tools such as reflectoscopes or stereopticons were available for student instruction; laboratories were poorly equipped; no course was offered in pharmacology; the curriculum was only partially graded—first- and second-year students took classes together, as did third- and fourth-year students. To that time, the inspector stated in his report, Meharry had retained a class A rating because it was a black school. After each previous inspection, investigators had told school authorities of existing problems and how to correct them. Many of the deficiencies could have been corrected at little expense. Because Howard University upheld proper entrance requirements (it had just begun insisting on two years of college courses) and offered a strong education program, the CME need not keep Meharry "in a classification where it clearly does not belong." So the CME voted to reduce Meharry to a B ranking.[57] Medical education for African Americans seemed to be deteriorating.

The CME, in addition to rating schools, campaigned to tighten state licensure requirements. More and more states began insisting on basic college science courses,[58] or even two years of college, as entrance standards for their medical schools or as prerequisites to taking licensure exams. Some states even refused licenses to graduates of both white and black class B and C schools.[59]

The black schools continued to appeal for help from Pritchett at the Carnegie Foundation and Flexner at the GEB. Neither man ignored the problem, but both found their efforts thwarted or delayed by their own or other agencies. They tried to convince their respective boards to fund African American medical education between 1912 and 1916, but neither foundation would be pushed too quickly.[60] Not until December of 1916 did the two agencies combine forces and offer Meharry, as a stopgap measure, $15,000 a year so that it could remain open, but still without an endowment.[61] As Flexner observed Howard's and Meharry's struggles to maintain their programs, he worried that they (and all other medical schools in the South) ought not be pushed into radical changes too quickly lest they be forced to close unnecessarily. They should not, he believed, be compared to white Northern schools, but rather should be permitted to make improvements based on a less compressed timetable. Flexner strongly disapproved of the CME's constant pressure on Meharry to improve. In late 1914, he feared that Meharry would "be choked" if the CME forced too many changes too quickly on the black schools. But the CME persisted in spite of Flexner's protests.[62]

In fact, the black schools *were* being choked. They were caught in a power squeeze between, on the one hand, two large foundations that put white medical education needs above black, and on the other, a powerful medical organization that refused to recognize the special needs of African American medical schools and African American physicians. The crisis peaked in the fall of 1917. None of the three missionary black medical schools was healthy, and Leonard was about to collapse. Hubbard presented the problems of African American medical schools to the annual meeting of the Southern Medical Association, which passed a resolution urging the AMA to take action to save the schools.[63] Dr. Aaron McDuffie Moore, a Leonard graduate and respected Durham, North Carolina, physician, headed a committee of the NMA that drew up and sent an eloquent and desperate "Appeal for Medical Education for Negroes" to the AMA, the GEB, and the Carnegie Foundation.[64] Meharry and Leonard officials asked the CME for "re-inspections" and A ratings, lest they lose recognition with the licensure boards of several Southern states. The CME responded that it would happily reevaluate the schools, but that without endowments Leonard and Meharry could not improve their education programs in any meaningful and permanent way. Nor could the CME compromise its standards for some schools without jeopardizing its own credibility. The problem was really out of its hands. State licensing boards and medical colleges themselves were increasing the pressure to raise standards.[65] Dr. N. P. Colwell, secretary of the CME, did personally appeal to Flexner and Pritchett to give endowments to the black schools, asserting that the GEB and the Carnegie Foundation were doing these colleges "a grave injustice" by withholding funds.[66] He had, on February 4, 1918, already made these statements publicly in an address to the CME conference of 1918, which was later published.[67] Flexner and Pritchett responded hotly and frankly, asking Colwell to consider "how far this injustice is due to the action of the Council." They felt the black schools were making "good progress under the normal pressure of improvement" and did not need CME's harsh prodding.[68]

By May 1918 Dr. Moore and others were desperate. Leonard faced imminent closing, and black doctors attending recent state association conventions were "very much depressed" over the situation there and at Meharry. Using words that illustrate the stature Flexner had achieved in medical education circles, Moore wrote to him, "We are making our final appeal to you as the most potent representative of the medical profession in America and also as the Financial Agent whose word is final on such matters. We regard your Board [GEB] as an equalizing agency," because tax money in the South was spent on educating white physicians and none was spent on black medical education.[69] Flexner, however, deflected the arrow of blame back at the CME and Colwell. Accusations and denials again flew back and forth. Colwell labeled the situation a "so-called crisis," claiming that recent actions by Florida, North Carolina, and Virginia to deny recognition to class B institutions had "suddenly awakened Meharry and Leonard to the importance of seeking a Class A rating—a rating which they have been content to do without for several years."[70] Interestingly, in the midst of these battles over the fate of black medical schools, fought between organized white medicine and organized white philanthropy, the principal leaders on both sides found one point on which they agreed: that "high-grade white schools such as Columbia and the University of Pennsylvania" needed funding on a large scale before the black schools.[71]

In the end, no agency acted to save Leonard, which closed before the 1918–19 school year began.[72] The annual $15,000 joint Carnegie Foundation/GEB appropriation kept Meharry alive for another year until the two foundations could finally agree on a $300,000 grant, contingent on Meharry's raising $200,000 more.[73] Howard, the school with the most promise in 1910, staggered along without significant philanthropic funding until the early 1920s, as Pritchett and Flexner favored Meharry.[74] The first two decades of the twentieth century ended with three black medical schools still open: the University of West Tennessee existing precariously as an unrecognized proprietary institution, Meharry and Howard with small endowments, and none with an assured future.

Abraham Flexner worked closely on the problems of medical education for blacks from 1908, when he began his study for the Carnegie Foundation for the Advancement of Teaching and the AMA, through the next decade. He believed only Howard and Meharry possessed the potential for success in the medical education system he envisioned and argued for their survival at the expense of the other five. Those five did close, three, it appears, as a direct result of his 1910 report, one (Leonard) despite his attempts to ease the CME's pressure on it, and one (West Tennessee) for other reasons. His strong efforts to provide funding for Meharry helped save that school from closing.

Black Medical Education to Midcentury

From 1920 to 1950, the two remaining black medical schools continued their struggle for existence in the white medical world, one emerging stronger than the other. A black student entering either school during these years might still have wondered, as had students in 1900, whether the school would survive until graduation day. By the 1930s, though, Howard was in a less precarious position than Meharry. Organized medicine and large philanthropies continued to exert influence over the schools.

For Meharry in 1921, the first priority was obtaining an A rating from the CME. Flexner convinced a reluctant CME in 1922 to raise Meharry's ranking after it had twice in two years refused to do so. But Meharry was still not, in the opinion of many, an A school. As one recent historian has characterized Meharry during this period, "laboratory facilities were grossly inadequate; instructors were overworked, poorly paid, and undertrained; library resources were virtually non-existent; and students were indiscriminately admitted."[75] Meharry's president, John J. Mullowney, Hubbard's successor, mismanaged the institution and generated much ill will among faculty and staff and within Nashville's black community. The GEB, under Flexner's influence, poured millions of dollars into the school's budget (about $8 million between 1916 and 1949) and became involved between 1933 and 1938 in the movement to remove Mullowney as president and appoint Edward Turner of Chicago. Turner did much to improve the school in a short time, saving Meharry's A rating in 1938. Money problems continued to plague the school throughout the 1940s. Announcements by the GEB and other philanthropists during that decade that they would soon cease making contributions to Meharry plunged the institution into another financial crisis at the dawn of the civil rights era.[76]

Howard also faced financial problems between 1920 and 1950, but of a different sort. Because the U.S. Department of the Interior provided funds for Howard's operating budget and allowed free teaching use of Freedmen's Hospital, adjacent to campus, large philanthropic organizations such as the Carnegie Foundation and the GEB saw Howard's maintenance as a government responsibility. In 1920 Howard desperately needed help, not with clinical education (Freedmen's Hospital served that aspect well), but in the basic sciences. As Flexner characterized

Howard's wants in a 1920 memorandum to the GEB, "The laboratory branches are starved for support and equipment."[77] He urged the GEB to contribute $250,000 toward a $500,000 endowment and to make funds immediately available for hiring basic science faculty and for laboratory equipment. This time the GEB agreed and donated about $700,000 over the next twenty-one years. This amount, joined with increased government appropriations, a gift from the Julius Rosenwald Foundation, and donations from black and white citizens across the country, provided Howard by the 1940s with an improved physical plant and faculty and a small but solid endowment fund. Leadership during this period from President Mordecai Johnson, and from Numa P. G. Adams, the first African American dean of the medical school, placed Howard in a strong position to face the new problems of the civil rights era.[78]

By 1950, Howard and Meharry together were graduating about one hundred black physicians annually, and white medical schools were graduating a total of about ten to twenty more. The Great Depression had taken its toll on potential black physicians who could not afford to attend medical school. The number of black practitioners in the United States dropped 5 percent between 1932 and 1942, while the number of white physicians increased 12 percent. The strong need for more black physicians continued, but the capabilities of the two medical schools that trained black students remained limited. The many applicants rejected from Howard and Meharry in the late 1940s had few options for attendance at other medical schools.[79] Flexner, in the early 1920s, had saved the two schools he thought worth saving. But the demise of the other black medical schools had created problems Americans were just beginning to face in the 1950s.

The Black Medical Profession

CHAPTER 19

Entering a "White" Profession, 1880–1920

In the late 1890s a young Kentucky physician wrote optimistically to the black sociologist W. E. B. Du Bois: "I am located in a town of 12,000 inhabitants, one-third of whom are colored, and am thoroughly convinced that there is a great field here in the South for the educated colored man. As a physician I am well received by my white professional brother. We ride in the same buggy, consult together, and read each other's books. I have a few white patients, but most of them are colored. I have purchased property on one of our best residence streets and also a business house on the main street of our town."[1] A few years later, in a national monthly medical journal, sandwiched between correspondence on treatments for hysteria and the prevention of dog bites, was the following letter, written, the editor announced, by a Southerner, and printed exactly as received, though without the writer's name:

> WANTS TO KEEP NEGRO PHYSICIANS DOWN!
> *Dr. C. F. Taylor, Ed. of the Med. World.*
> Dear Sir:—What is the negro physician doing as a whole through out the country as a physician and surgeon? What are they doing financialy? How do they compare with the white aplicants in State examinations through out the country? I notice in some places they seams to be makeing more money then the white physicians. What is the best thing we can do to keep them down? Please let me here from you in the nex No. of the *World*.[2]

These two letters, contradictory in one regard, do agree that black physicians in the highly race-conscious New South were gaining recognition and achieving a measure of success according to the standards of the time. They also point to two major concerns of the first generation of post–Civil War black practitioners: reputation and rewards.

Like other physicians, black practitioners faced the problems of gaining their patients' confidence and establishing collegial relationships with other local doctors. They had to *earn* their status among patients and practitioners. Measures of achievement included the number, social standing, financial position, and loyalty of patients; the willingness of already established practitioners to share knowledge, books, and instruments and to call or be called for consultation; and finally, the acquisition of such material displays of wealth as home, office, and "rig" (horse and buggy) or automobile.

These were important matters to black physicians, but, they soon learned, competence, patient acceptance, and material gain were not enough. They also needed to develop group allegiance in order to surmount barriers that the local, state, and national white medical profession had erected to keep them out. African American doctors had to build their own parallel professional structures by establishing hospitals, medical societies, pharmacies, medical journals, postgraduate educational institutions, and clinics as a means of maintaining their standards in medical practice.

In concentrating their efforts on individual career growth and on improving collegial relations, black physicians of this period subordinated another concern: the overall improvement of black health and health conditions. As African American doctors they expected, and were expected by others, to improve the health of fellow blacks both by providing medical care and educating the ignorant regarding good health practices. Though it was an important force, one that inspired African American physicians of the late nineteenth and early twentieth centuries to enter medicine, this broad ideal of racial betterment did not receive as much attention as other goals once doctors actually entered practice.[3]

In addition to these concerns, black practitioners in the turn-of-the-century South lived always with another issue that affected their careers and personal lives—race. For example, they had to overcome black patients' reluctance to use their services, low remuneration from a generally poorer, predominantly black clientele, and an unfriendly reception and professional exclusion from many white physicians. Furthermore, having gained a level of education superior to that of most other African Americans, these doctors became representatives of their race to the white world, and community leaders in the black world. They therefore found it difficult to escape matters of race in their daily lives. The sorts of situations Southern black physicians encountered and the ways they coped with them in their dealings with black patients, white physicians, white patients, and fellow black doctors as they entered the previously white medical profession are the subjects of this chapter.

As Table 6 in the appendix indicates, the number of black physicians in the United States increased markedly between 1890 and 1920 as medical schools devoted to educating African Americans opened their doors.[4] Most graduates remained in the South, where they had grown up and learned medicine (there were no black medical schools in the North), but as the rest of the African American population began to migrate northward in the early decades of the twentieth century, so did black physicians. Though their ranks grew in all parts of the country, black doctors generally constituted only a tiny proportion of the medical profession between 1890 and 1920. Similarly, the proportion of black citizens to black doctors in each state and in the nation as a whole improved greatly during that time period, but, with a few exceptions in cities with black medical schools, the ratio remained much poorer for blacks than for whites (see Appendix, Table 7).

Most black physicians in practice before 1920 had attended one of the dozen missionary or proprietary medical schools established in the South for former slaves after Emancipation (see Appendix, Table 4 and Chapter 11 of this volume). Through every phase of their educational career, beginning with the reading of medical college catalogs and ending with commencement addresses at degree-granting ceremonies, black medical students were told how African Americans needed them, how they could help raise up the race, and how personally rewarding the profession of medicine was. Never did they hear complaints—increasingly common in the white medical community before 1920—about an overcrowded medical field.[5] Black physicians were in demand.

The New Orleans University Department of Medicine and Surgery (later named Flint Medical College), for instance, announced in its 1895–96 catalog, "The school supplies a wide felt need in the far South."[6] That need, a graduating student at Leonard Medical School in Raleigh, North Carolina, explained to his classmates in 1886, extended beyond the mere provision of medical care to educating the ignorant about proper health practices. Lawson A. Scruggs, caught up in the excitement of Leonard's first graduation in 1886, enthusiastically titled his valedictory address, "Medical Education as a Factor in the Elevation of the Colored Race." Discussing the need of black citizens to hear about recent advances in disease prevention, sanitation, and hygiene, Scruggs asserted, "No one can better teach them these practical and important truths than the educated colored physician who is one of their number." The challenges of medicine, he continued, would spur black physicians to help their fellow citizens "with the same self-sacrifice, courage and devotion as has ever characterized the profession. . . . We who stand before you tonight, are pioneers of the medical profession of our race."[7] Booker T. Washington told eager Howard University medical students on the opening day of classes in October 1909: "There is great demand for negro doctors. I think we have about 3,500 negro physicians in America. We need at least 7,000 in America. The white doctor has to seek [his] location, then hang out his shingle, but the location seeks the negro doctor. Everybody knows him. So our apparent disadvantages become our advantages."[8]

President Charles F. Meserve of Leonard Medical School had made similar claims in his 1906 commencement address: "This institution and others of similar character cannot begin to meet the calls that are coming constantly for trained physicians and pharmacists."[9] Letters in his files demonstrated this point. Citizens of one South Carolina town had communicated with Meserve several times over two years and even offered to send a representative to Leonard's commencement exercises in hopes of convincing one of the young graduates to set up practice there.[10] Meserve had to inform a citizen of this town that he thought all graduating seniors had "decided upon where they [would] locate."[11] At black medical schools across the South, prominent residents of large cities such as Montgomery, Alabama, and small ones such as Hertford, North Carolina, courted new graduates.[12] Competition was keen to win the services of these young men and women.

For the young black doctor, all of this attention[13] meant instant prestige and status in the black community. The biographer of the early-twentieth-century Memphis physician Joseph E. Walker described the situation (in exaggerated terms):

> In that age and time a Negro doctor was as popular in Negro life as money is in business. With Dr. before a man's name, he immediately became the community leader, the outstanding figure that received the honor, respect and admiration of the entire populace. Everybody looked up to him and felt complimented to pay homage to him. Negro men accepted the ideas and thoughts of the colored doctor in all things as right and final, and Negro women worshiped them. In another field it would take time to build up—in medicine it was seemingly an over-night affair. The doctor lived in the best home, wore the best clothes, rode the best horse and was the unrivaled suitor of the fairest of the community's fair sex.[14]

But instant status did not mean a problem- and struggle-free transition from poor medical student to well-heeled local physician. Black doctors often encountered a disparity between the status accorded them as educated leaders in the community and the level of acceptance given them as professional healers. Just after graduation, however, with applause and words of praise still echoing in their minds, with confidence in their abilities and success on state licensing exams buoying their egos, and with expectations of developing a thriving practice and of helping their people urging them on, newly minted black physicians knew little of these other matters as they set out into the world. Deep within, though, some must have wondered, as did John Edward Perry on his graduation day in Nashville in 1895, "What does the future hold in store?"[15]

These black citizens, many just one, two, or three generations removed from bondage, had reached this position because of their drive and determination to succeed. They became some of the first African Americans to gain not just literacy or even basic learning but a higher education and a profession. Their letters of application to medical schools; their correspondence with school authorities about scholarships, summer jobs, and money matters; and the writings of contemporary observers about their situations indicate that few came from "monied" backgrounds. Most had limited funds and outstanding debts until several years after opening practices. They (and their families) had struggled and sacrificed to get through medical school and continued doing so as they entered medical practice.[16]

Most, then, arrived in their new hometowns poor, with no horse and buggy or automobile, no office or home, and few material possessions other than some medical books and instruments. They were on their own now to prove themselves capable of earning a living practicing medicine. Courtship with towns anxious for a physician was over, letters of reference from former professors were useless.[17] Black physicians now faced the realities of an impoverished patient population, competition with local established white practitioners, and black patients wary, not just of a new physician but of a black physician. Success was not guaranteed. These new African American physicians hopefully hung their shingles outside their rented offices, arranged their medical books on a shelf, readied their few instruments, and waited for patients to call.

It could be a lonely and trying time. A few months after graduating from Leonard Medical School, Dr. William E. Atkins wrote to his former advisor, "I am now in Hampton, Virginia, my future home. I like Hampton very much and consider the outlook very fair but of course it will take time and patience. I can do both if I just don't get too hungry."[18] Another recent Leonard graduate, John H. G. Williams, moved to Columbus, Georgia, in the spring of 1904 and wrote a more confident letter to President Meserve, though financial prospects also dominated his thoughts: "I have arranged about my license and now have my office opened and also have my horse and buggy. I started last Sat. P.M. . . . got my turnout [buggy] then. I had my first call Sunday P.M. and several since. I am getting along nicely to be at an entirely new place. I think my chances are good here, anyway I am satisfied so far."[19] Frederick Douglass Sessoms, Leonard class of 1906, had little spare cash upon his arrival in Hertford, North Carolina, shortly after graduation. The Reverend G. D. Griffin had invited Sessoms to practice there well before commencement exercises. The young physician had visited the town, talked to its residents, and decided to settle in Hertford. He used some of his limited funds to rent a one-room office, but he did not have enough for a horse. So Sessoms visited his local patients on foot and asked plantation owners to provide him rides to and from their land.[20] And J. Edward Perry recalled years later his actions and feelings shortly after arriving in Mexico, Missouri, in 1893: "With no funds with which to purchase office equipment or the payment for [office] space, the idea suggested itself to begin practice from my residence [rented rooms]. A sign was secured and tacked against the outside wall, cards were printed and I was ready for the first call. . . . There were only three lonely days before a request was made for me to see a [patient]. . . . [That first Sunday] a shadow of gloom hovered over me as I thought of friends, mother and father far away, while I struggled among strangers."[21] Under such circumstances, pursuit of humanitarian ideals of racial health improvement and patient education must have seemed remote and easy to postpone.

Sometimes the local church provided comfort for lonely black physicians in new towns, and also some needed publicity to help start a practice. Upon arriving in Frankfort, Kentucky, for example, Edward Ellsworth Underwood, an 1891 graduate of Western Reserve Medical School, received from the townspeople "a rousing and hearty public welcome at the Corinthian Baptist Church."[22] And even Perry, on that first solitary Sunday in Mexico, Missouri, ultimately found warmth and company at the Methodist Church:

> At the conclusion of the services the presiding elder said, "For many years we have been planting an orchard in Nashville, Tennessee, that has been bearing fruit. All of these years I have not seen until the other day a single apple in this section from our orchard. If you were to spend money and time in growing an orchard, surely you would not be so silly as to say I will not use the fruit from my own trees. I have something to show you this morning that you have never seen before, a colored doctor, an apple from your own orchard."
>
> Those were the words of the solemn minister in the way of introduction. To me this was all a surprise, but I perchanced to have a bountiful supply of [business] cards, which were generously distributed as the crowd surged forth to shake my hand at the conclusion of my remarks.[23]

Any new physician, white or black, arriving in a town would have experienced the same variety of feelings as those described here, their intensity depending on previous training, knowledge of the town, state of personal finances, and personality. But race added an extra measure of uncertainty to the arrival of a black practitioner. As the Mexico, Missouri, minister indicated, in the late nineteenth and early twentieth centuries few black and even fewer white laypeople or physicians had ever met and dealt with, personally or professionally, an African American with an M.D. So the same black citizens who accorded black physicians high status in the community because of educational superiority, professional position, and earning potential also treated warily someone so different from themselves who took on a role ("doctoring") usually reserved for whites.

Biographical and autobiographical sketches of black physicians during this period indicate that they assumed high posts in their churches, service organizations, and social clubs and acted as liaisons with white community and civil authorities.[24] Blacks, wrote one graduate of Leonard Medical School practicing in Maxton, North Carolina, "generally seem to appreciate their people and yet the [black] doctor is such a strange man to a great many, they have to hesitate and 'look him up and down.'"[25] That is exactly what J. Edward Perry encountered after Mexico's daily newspaper announced his presence. For "the first few days," he wrote in his autobiography, "as I passed on the streets, one person would call another and the two, a third one and say, 'He's him.'"[26] Though they appreciated the attention, new black physicians also wanted the chance to prove themselves able practitioners, a sentiment well articulated by John H. Tompkins, newly arrived in Cumberland, Maryland, in a letter to President Meserve back at his alma mater: "In every avenue possible I am striving to do my best, and feel that if I get a start here and have a fair trial for a start I'll do well."[27]

But black citizens did not always find it easy to give their professional brothers and sisters a fair trial. They were distrustful of African American physicians after years of conditioning with white practitioners. Dr. Robert F. Boyd, an 1882 Meharry graduate, reported to 1890 readers of the *Christian Educator*, a magazine of the Freedmen's Aid Society of the Methodist Episcopal Church, that as of three years earlier "very few good [black Nashville] families had ever given colored doctors their practice" because "they did not believe them competent."[28] Worse still was the attitude Dr. Thaddeus A. Walker, another Meharry graduate, encountered upon his arrival in 1887 in Baton Rouge, Louisiana: "I started my practice here with considerable opposition from my own people."[29] Other physicians reported similar problems.[30]

Two sociological studies performed in the early twentieth century confirmed the validity of these physicians' claims. Thomas Jackson Woofter Jr. used a Phelps-Stokes Fund fellowship at the University of Georgia in 1913 to investigate various aspects of black life in Athens, seat of the university. He noted the same disparity between status and attitude that black physicians had observed in their speeches and letters: "All negroes in professions occupy a high position in the negro community. The negro preacher is possibly the most influential. [But] the negro doctors of Athens [Woofter counted five] [still] meet with some little prejudice and suspicion among the masses of the negroes."[31] James W. Martin, a graduate student at the George Peabody College in Nashville, applied his Phelps-Stokes fellowship particularly to observe the practices of black physicians in central and western Tennessee in 1920. He found a number of African Americans who "were personally friendly [with African American physicians], but of the opinion that a physician should be a white man."[32] Commenting on this seemingly contradictory attitude of black patients, a *Washington Post* reporter wrote in 1909, "Now, nobody disputes the right of a Negro to practice medicine. . . . However, there is room for doubt that . . . [additional] Negro doctors would find the demand and reward for their labors considerable enough to pay expenses to keep themselves alive. An indefinable something resides in the breed that disinclines the Negro to give countenance and patronage to members of his own race."[33]

That "indefinable something" keeping black patients from using black physicians' services resulted in part from a reluctance to give up traditional reliance on white doctors and from a sense of uncertainty about black physicians' abilities. For years the enslaved had heard white racist assumptions about black incompetence and seen only white healers when sick, leaving many former bondspeople and their descendents presuming that only whites were capable of learning and practicing regular medicine. In addition, self-dosing in times of sickness was common among blacks. For rural dwellers without ready access to physicians' services, self-reliance in medical matters was a necessity. Such independence from professionals, born of necessity, became habit except in severe situations. And medical intervention, even in the early twentieth century, did not mean certain cure. Medical knowledge was increasing, but primarily in the area of diagnosis rather than treatment. Blacks, even in slavery times when they were supposed to report ailments to owners or overseers, often first used treatments they had brought with them from Africa and the West Indies or had developed in the American South and had shared with others in the slave quarters.[34] They continued to apply these remedies and try out others after the Civil War, especially now that freedom had turned the watchful eyes of their former owners to other matters.

Freedom also allowed the more open practice and flourishing of another activity that interfered with African Americans' acceptance and use of regularly trained black practitioners—rootwork. Based on a belief in the supernatural and on the magical powers of "conjurers" to control events in people's lives, this system, brought from Africa to the West Indies and then to the United States, had a large following among late-nineteenth-century Southern blacks. Conjurers, adherents believed, could, through hexes and voodoo, bring on or relieve people of diseases and physical disorders at will, when asked (and paid) to do so.[35] Regular physicians and lay observers, black and white alike, denounced these beliefs as superstition. One white writer in the *Christian Educator* worried mightily about the problem and tied its solution to the future of African Americans. "So great and so common is superstition among the Negroes, especially in the South, that fears, doubts, and follies embarrass any effort to make him self-reliant." He believed that "the cultured Christian [black] physician, more than any other man" might, through his influence in the black community, "scatter these oppressive superstitions."[36] But even African American physicians could not completely wrest voodoo from the popular place it held in the black mind. Rootwork successfully competed with allopathic medicine and kept some blacks (the number is difficult to determine) from gaining regular medical attention.[37]

Midwifery, common in the rural South through the early twentieth century, also kept black households from employing trained physicians of color. Tradition and cost made the midwife's presence at deliveries a more attractive though not necessarily safer alternative to the physician's.[38]

Cost, of course, played a major role in discouraging African Americans from calling on a physician in time of illness. But that reluctance would presumably have worked equally against physicians of both races, or even have encouraged black patients to try first the local black doctor, who might not charge as much or press for payment as quickly or firmly as the white practitioner. The problem of obtaining payment for services loomed large for the African American physician.

Some black healers, professionally trained or not, created, by their actions, distrust for African American physicians among local residents. A white visitor to Beaufort, South Carolina, shortly after the Civil War learned, for example, of a "Northern colored man" who had opened a medical practice there but soon left because fellow blacks found him "extortionate" and not to be trusted.[39] Incidents such as this one created difficulties not just for the practitioner involved but also for colleagues in the area and for his successors. J. Edward Perry encountered such a situation in 1895 on the Mexico, Missouri, train platform where he had just disembarked to begin his medical career. When the man whom he had asked for directions to the Baptist minister's house learned Perry was a physician, he responded: "A doctor! Lawd! Man, you curtanly made a mistake even stoppen in dis town; de folks here are fighten mad at nigger doctors and I know dey will run you out o' town soon as dey know you are heer." Perry discovered that a black "corn doctor" had recently spent a few days in town selling a patent or homemade remedy, the efficacy of which he had guaranteed, and then skipped out with his "wild promises" unfulfilled.[40]

Less obvious but more insidious than the disliked or lying black healer who came and went in a short time was the well-entrenched but incompetent physician who undermined the standing of fellow doctors. Walter F. White, executive secretary of the National Association for the Advancement of Colored People (NAACP) from 1931 to 1955, described such a man in his 1924 novel, *Fire in the Flint*, about the return of Dr. Kenneth B. Harper, trained in the North, to practice in his hometown of Central City, Georgia:

> Perhaps the greatest factor contributing to the coloured folks' lack of confidence in physicians of their own race was the inefficiency of Dr. Williams, the only coloured doctor in Central City prior to Kenneth's return.

> Dr. Williams belonged to the old school and moved on the theory that when he graduated [from medical school] some eighteen years before . . . the development of medical knowledge had stopped. He fondly pictured himself as being the most prominent personage of Central City's Negro colony, was pompous, bulbous-eyed, and exceedingly fond of long words, especially of Latin derivation. . . . Through his fraternal [society] and church connections and lack of competition, he had made a little money, much of it through his position as medical examiner for the lodges to which he belonged. As long as he treated minor ailments—cuts, colic, childbirths, and the like—he had little trouble. But when more serious maladies attacked them, the coloured population sent for the old white physician, Dr. Bennett, instead of for Dr. Williams.[41]

White makes it clear that Bennett was only somewhat more competent than Williams but that even so, it took young Dr. Harper some time to overcome the prejudice against black physicians that Williams had engendered in Central City's "Negro colony." Only perseverance and successful medical outcomes could win over blacks who had had bad experiences with other black practitioners. White physicians as a group did not encounter this type of problem because its basis was racial; black doctors had a harder time proving themselves to their potential patients because they were black and doctors. A mistaken diagnosis or treatment, a high charge or perceived insult, a charlatan or unqualified physician, cost black physicians a much higher price than they did white physicians.

Drumming up business among reluctant black patients was only one difficulty the African American physician faced upon moving to a new town. His or her presence did more than cause some black patients to consider using a physician of their own race; it often stirred up racial tensions between blacks and whites. Exclaimed one African American woman when, in May 1906, Joseph E. Walker announced himself as the new doctor in town (Indianola, Mississippi): "My God, what is dis here town coming to—dese white folks just now getting ober habing 'er nigger Postmaster and now here comes 'er nigger Doctor—Did Ros'velt send 'm 'ere too?"[42]

Black patients did not worry alone about the effect African American physicians might have on local race relations; the physicians themselves had similar concerns. Sometimes they shied away from a particular state or region, as Leonard Medical School's President Meserve explained to the citizens of a South Carolina town: "I appreciate what you say about the need of a Colored physician in your locality. The fact is, Colored physicians do not desire to settle in South Carolina. You, of course, understand why without my saying anything further. I wish it were not so."[43] (See the state-by-state citizen-to-physician ratios in Table 7.) And generally, African American physicians knew that their arrival would upset the balance of patients and income that had previously existed among practitioners. Though some whites may have extended a helping hand to their black medical brethren, others had underlying or overt negative feelings as well.

The letter to the *Medical World* quoted earlier in the chapter illustrates the nature of the problem black physicians faced. Dr. Taylor's editorial response, printed immediately beneath the letter, ventured "the opinion that [the letter] does not voice the sentiment of southern medical men" and remarked critically on its "literary attainments." Taylor also commented favorably on the good work he knew African American physicians were performing in the South and invited their reactions to the letter.[44] Over the next two months Taylor published replies from black and a few white physicians, all attacking the provocative letter's author, denying the existence of his negative, racist attitude among the general population of Southern white doctors, and supporting the efforts of black practitioners.[45] But racism did exist, as this excerpt from a Clifton Forge, Virginia, physician's response inadvertently demonstrates: "The Southern doctor in question represents a very small minority of the Southern white physicians. . . . Simply regard [the letter] as one of the many obstacles which are constantly being thrown in the way of the man of color when he attempts to rise."[46]

For away from the limelight, in offices and patients' homes, incidents did occur that revealed some of these other beliefs and feelings of white physicians. A white Southern doctor could write an open letter to the *Medical World* looking for ways to limit competition from his black colleagues and receive open rebuffs for his views and denials of their representativeness from members of the medical profession; but back home this same man (and others like him) could (and did) act "to keep Negro physicians down." Dr. J. Edward Perry, for example, met with a less than cordial response from a white Columbia, Missouri, physician to his proposed move to that town in 1895. In reply to the young black doctor's request for "the acquaintance, goodwill and assistance of the [local] representatives of the profession," this man informed Perry that "the practice among your people is done by white brethren in the profession and it would be a mighty hard thing for a man of your age and most especially your color to wring it from their hands."[47] Corroboration of that competitive concern comes from James Martin's 1920 Tennessee physicians study. He found it "generally . . . [though] not uniformly the case" that white physicians "regarded the negro physician as an economic competitor,"[48] so much so in a portion of west Tennessee that "negroes are forced [by their white colleagues] to charge the same as whites do."[49] Similarly, an Oklahoma physician in 1914 described white Southern doctors as "wont" to be "craving for [patients of] the opposite race as an [economic] asset to their practice."[50]

Some of these fears about competition from black doctors can be explained by the state of medicine and the national economy in the late nineteenth and early twentieth centuries. Black physicians were attempting to enter medicine at a time of professional overcrowding, when even in small towns too many physicians were competing for too few patients, and when economic conditions were at best only fair. But in addition to these professional and economic issues in the South were racial ones. White doctors in Tennessee could still say frankly to a white sociologist in 1920, "Mr. Martin, you will find that the negro mind is incapable of any considerable development, and Dr. A., being a colored man, is not to be seriously regarded as a real physician. He is a good negro, but still a negro."[51] And the NAACP executive secretary, Walter F. White, well acquainted with black physicians and their experiences, could, in *Fire in the Flint*, accurately reflect reality by having an inept white Georgia practitioner say of a black practitioner who had corrected his diagnosis and successfully treated his former patient that he "wa'n't goin' to let no young nigger doctor tell him his bus'ness."[52] Black physicians in the South, despite glowing reports to medical journals, alumni and religious missionary magazines, and former teachers, did encounter racial problems in their practices.

A severe one was white physician refusal to consult with or assist black colleagues in the treatment of patients in extremis. Written descriptions of such incidents are rare, but their very occurrence indicates the depth of white antagonism and strength of tradition that some black physicians had to overcome. One encounter took place in the vicinity of Washington, Georgia, in about 1908. Frederick Douglass Sessoms, recently relocated from Hertford, North Carolina, raced his horse and buggy eighteen miles to Barnett, where one of his patients had an abdominal wall abscess that urgently required surgery. Sessoms needed another physician to assist during the operation. The family had seen a white physician pass by shortly before, so Sessoms had the patient's son, Claude Davis, flag Dr. Beasley down on his return from visiting a patient. Dr. Beasley entered the Davis home, examined the patient, and agreed surgery was needed. Neither physician had the necessary instruments on hand, so they agreed to postpone surgery until seven the next morning, assuming the patient survived the night. Sessoms went home and returned at the appointed hour, this time by train, only to find that Beasley had informed the family he could not perform the surgery with a Negro doctor. After determining that an operation might still help his patient, Sessoms acquired a horse and buggy, hurried four miles to the nearest telephone, and called Dr. Thomas J. Wills, an elderly white physician of Sessoms's acquaintance who lived twenty miles away. Wills's initial response to the black physician's request was, "I am very busy," to which Sessoms replied, "But I am no longer urging you, Dr. Wills, I am now begging and beseeching that you help me to save a life—a life that will otherwise be lost." "How can I get there?" answered Wills. He caught a train twenty minutes later and arrived at the depot in an hour, where Sessoms and Claude Davis met him. They performed the procedure and saved the patient.[53]

Not surprisingly, Walter White's stereotypical fictional white Georgia doctor behaved just like the real-life Dr. Beasley. When the young black physician in Central City sought out a colleague to help perform an emergency appendectomy, "he realized his absolute dependence on Dr. Williams [the old black physician in town], for he knew no white doctor would assist a Negro surgeon or even operate with a coloured assistant."[54]

Such openly racist behavior not only endangered patients' lives but also undercut the position of African American physicians before their patients. If African American physicians could not obtain assistance from white colleagues when urgently needed, how could African American doctors be relied upon to treat their patients' medical and surgical problems? Black physician Luther T. Burbridge, in his 1895 Emancipation Day speech, "The Colored Man in Medicine," in New Iberia, Louisiana, cited just this type of situation to exemplify the difficulties facing him and his colleagues: "A surgical operation of importance is to be performed, and the case falls into the hands of the colored doctor. He knows that there is little hope of any professional assistance from the neighboring physicians and his future reputation and success depend, perhaps, upon the issue of the case."[55] Burbridge described those circumstances to illustrate the loneliness of Southern black medical practice and the way these physicians were forced to rely on their own skills. Southern white doctors took advantage of black practitioners' vulnerable positions to isolate them professionally. For, in addition to refusing to consult with or assist physicians of color, they barred their black colleagues from local and state medical societies, refused them admitting privileges to local hospitals, and overtly and subtly tried to reduce their competitiveness for patients who could afford to pay.[56]

As physicians accepted and incorporated more and more of the scientific discoveries and diagnostic methodologies of the late nineteenth and early twentieth centuries into their medical practices, communication of new ideas and approaches to patient problems became increasingly important. To practice good medicine, physicians had to keep up with the latest developments and learn how to apply them to patient care situations. Regularly reading medical journals and occasionally attending postgraduate courses at large medical centers helped practitioners keep abreast of current work in the field. Black physicians, if their response to the 1914 *Medical World* letter is any indication, did the former, and some, based on contemporary and later biographical sketches, also the latter, when time, money, and the lowering of racial barriers in the North permitted.[57]

Collegial face-to-face discussions and demonstrations of newly learned techniques and treatments or exchanges of opinion about difficult cases also taught physicians and improved their skills. Such communication occurred not only informally, at chance encounters or social occasions, but also at more formal county and state medical society meetings. From any of these potentially important and useful learning situations the black physician was usually, and in some areas always, excluded solely on the basis of race and social custom. J. Edward Perry, reflecting on his early career in small-town Missouri in the 1890s, considered that this professional, racially motivated isolation was most detrimental to young black physicians like himself: "There is scarcely a day that the busy doctor is not confronted with some clinical enigma that taxes his scientific resources to the utmost. This is more true of the novice or inexperienced physician than of the one more seasoned in the dispensation of the healing art. At this period, it was my misfortune possibly to be meeting daily more and more cases that produced an anxious mind and sleepless nights. There were three reasons for these restless moments and disturbed emotions. First, a deficiency of knowledge, second, a lack of contact and clinical advice, third, destitute facilities."[58] As Luther Burbridge eloquently described it, "Isolated, as many of them are, from intercourse with colored men of their own profession and despairing of any assistance from the opposite race, often their only recourse is their books and journals. Under such circumstances the Negro physician sometimes finds himself confronted with a deep and seemingly impassable gulf over which it seems impossible to leap and around which he can see no way."[59]

This gulf of isolation based on race appeared almost immediately after blacks entered the medical profession in the 1860s. Alexander T. Augusta encountered it during and just after the Civil War in Alexandria, Virginia, and Savannah, Georgia, in his dealings with white physicians,[60] and then again in 1869 and 1870, when he and two other black physicians applied for admission to the all-white Medical Society of the District of Columbia, and in 1870 to the American Medical Association.[61] It continued into 1882, when Dr. Whitfield Winsey, a Harvard-trained black physician, received seven blackballs from members of the Baltimore Medical and Surgical Society (five were needed for rejection from membership). All voted negatively on account of Winsey's race, one member stating "that his Southern birth prevented him from recognizing a negro practitioner."[62] The exclusionary policies extended to all other Southern medical societies through the 1940s.[63]

The gulf that kept African American physicians from professional intercourse with white colleagues and medical societies also extended to hospitals. White physicians simply denied admitting privileges to physicians of color, forcing them to leave patients who required hospitalization (usually for surgery) at the entrance door, entrusted to the care of these same white doctors. This was a particularly difficult problem because it affected black physicians' earnings, professional competency, and standing with patients. John W. Walker of Asheville, North Carolina, speaking for his state's African American physicians at the 1910 National Medical Association (NMA) annual meeting, described the situation to a group already quite familiar with the problem: "We realize that we are put to a great disadvantage when we have cases to operate upon and have no hospital.

We are obliged to turn [patients] over to white physicians and when we do this it is hard for our people to have the proper interest and confidence in us."[64] Dr. Albert W. Dumas of Natchez, Mississippi, echoed Walker's sentiments, adding, "[White surgeons] carry the patient[s] to the hospital and often you never see [the patients] again until they die or recover."[65] African Americans thus had little opportunity to learn and refine surgical techniques once out of medical school or to provide continuity of care for their patients. Few blacks became surgical specialists, and many lost income because of their actual or presumed inability to perform surgery or because they could not provide needed hospital medical care.[66] In several ways, then, white physicians in the South isolated black practitioners and so reduced blacks' effectiveness as doctors.

Income was another matter that caused tension between black and white physicians in this era of economic stagnation (especially in the rural South). At times, the entry of African American physicians into an already crowded profession worsened existing racial stress. White practitioners appear generally to have surrendered their nonpaying and indigent black and white patients to the new black physicians without strong protest. But African American physicians, like white physicians, had to feed their families. And some, perhaps most, had ambitions besides healing and teaching better health practices to the poor. They were professionals who wanted to make names for themselves and at least live in comfortable homes like those their white colleagues inhabited. This meant competing for patients with white physicians. Walter White's fictional (though representative) Kenneth Harper explained one day to his brother why he returned to Georgia after completing training at Bellevue in New York City:

> "Why did I come back? That's easy. I came back because I can make more money here than anywhere else. . . . I came back here where the bulk of coloured people live and where they make money off their crops and where there won't be much trouble for me to build up a big practice. . . . Oh, I suppose I could've made money [in the North] . . . , but I wanted to come back home. I can do more good here, both for myself and for the coloured people, than I could up there. And I don't think I'll have any trouble down here. Papa got along all right here in this town for more than fifty years, and I reckon I can do it too. . . . Why, I'll have a cinch around this part of Georgia! There aren't more than half a dozen coloured doctors in all this part of the country who've had a decent medical education and training. . . . In a few years I'll be able to give up general practicing and give all my time to major surgery. I'll handle pretty nearly everything in this part of the State"[67]

Harper may have been more naïve than most about the ease with which he would succeed in practice, but his attitude probably reflected that of many young black physicians setting out. They may have meant no harm to their white and black colleagues already in practice, but to earn a living they had to step on a few toes.

John H. Tompkins discovered this when he moved to Cumberland, Maryland, in 1896. He introduced himself to "many of the prominent whites" in town, "including several of the medical profession" and "got their general views of things personally, in regard to having a colored Dr. settle here." "Few of the latter," he reported to Shaw University's President Charles Meserve, "were incourging [*sic*]."[68] That response might have been expected from physicians concerned about losing patients to competitors. In general, ailing whites who patronized black physicians came from the poorer classes, but some white paying patients also turned to African American physicians for their medical care, thereby confirming the fears of certain white doctors. The author of a 1903 study of "The Negroes of St. Louis" found, for instance, that one of the fourteen black practitioners in the city, "who has been here ten years and has an excellent reputation, has a few white patients. They came to him at first by accident, but then continued to patronize him. Two others, whose offices are in districts inhabited by poor whites as well as Negroes, report that they have both white and colored patients."[69] Luther Burbridge noted a similar trend in Louisiana and described it in more political terms: "We feel proud to state that the practice of the colored doctor is by no means confined solely to his own race. For even here in the historic old State of Louisiana, whose fertile vales have often echoed to the cry of the oppressed, the negro physician enjoys in many instances a small, but growing white patronage. This in itself is a confession of a recognition of skill and ability, wrung as it were from the lips of the oppressor."[70]

A number of African American physicians pointedly mentioned in letters about their success the racial mixture of their patients. Wrote a Columbia, South Carolina, man, " I have an extensive and paying practice among my own people and a considerable practice among the poorer classes of the white people." And a Macon, Mississippi, physician bragged to W. E. B. Du Bois, "My practice here is very large among both colored and white. . . . I have had white people come here from a distance and board here to get my treatment." The impact of such success on collegial relations, an Arkansas physician of color admitted, was not always positive: "I have experienced some prejudice among my white friends. We do not have much to do with each other as physicians."[71]

Evidence indicates that, though black physicians attracted some of their white clientele because of professional reputations, they also won white patronage for two less glamorous reasons. Perhaps in recognition of the generally low incomes of their patients, or perhaps in order to draw patients to their practices, some black physicians charged less than the usual fees for medical services. These doctors do not appear to have written to their colleagues, former classmates, or instructors about the practice, nor did newspaper, medical journal, or popular magazine accounts mention it. But James W. Martin, studying Tennessee black physicians in 1920, discussed its silent but pervasive presence in two very different regions of that state and documented its persistence, even when forbidden by white practitioners. Martin reported that the case charges of fourteen black physicians in five middle Tennessee counties (Lincoln, Giles, Marshall, Maury, and Williamson) and eleven in two western Tennessee counties (Haywood and Fayette) were "from 25 percent to 60 percent less than [what] white doctors receive[d] for the same kind of work."[72] Several of the black practitioners told Martin they had "built up a considerable general practice among white people," a practice Martin discovered upon further investigation "to be for the poorer white people, who called [on] the colored physician because his fees were lower."[73] Their clientele among white professional and business classes he found to be "very limited," with the exception noted later.[74]

Concerned about losing patients to black physicians, the white physicians of Tennessee's economically poor and predominantly agricultural "black belt" counties tried actively to compete for African American patients. Martin described the situation and black physicians' answer to it: "The general custom in the Western counties seems to be that the white physicians give directions as to those matters [of fees charged] which the colored [physicians] must obey. As a matter of course, these are often evaded, but secretly."[75] The experience of white and black practitioners in seven Tennessee counties does not necessarily represent a situation that prevailed in the South. But the poverty of most late-nineteenth- and early-twentieth-century Southern blacks—the group that constituted the majority of African American physicians' patients in the region—surely dictated that physicians of color establish a lower fee schedule than that of their white colleagues.[76] And these cheaper prices must have induced some poorer whites to call on black doctors when sick. Whether these practitioners were also more lenient in their collection schedules is not well documented. Lower fees, however, if they cut into the practice of local white physicians, would understandably have upset the white physicians.

If a difference in fee scales between physicians of the two races is difficult to document, another reason some whites preferred black physicians to those of their own racial group is even more difficult to document because of its delicacy. This aspect of Southern African American physicians' practice white doctors could not control, as it took place secretly. One fictional account of black medical practice in the South does confront the subject of sexually transmitted disease treatment directly. The author Walter White describes how Dr. Kenneth Harper began treating certain affluent, respected white males of Central City, Georgia, in the early 1920s:

> A new source of practice and revenue began gradually to grow. The main entrance to his office was on Lee Street. This door was some fifty feet back

> from Lee Street, and the overhanging branches of the elms cut off completely the light from the street lamp at the corner. One night, as he sat reading in his office, there came a knock at his door. Opening it, he found standing there Roy Ewing. Ewing had inherited the general merchandise store bearing his name from his father, was a deacon in the largest Baptist Church in Central City, was president of the Central City Chamber of Commerce, and was regarded as a leading citizen.
>
> Kenneth gazed at his caller in some surprise.
>
> "Hello, Ken. Anybody around?"
>
> On being assured that he was alone, Ewing entered, brushing by Kenneth to get out of the glare of the light. Kenneth followed him into the office, meanwhile asking his caller what he could do for him.
>
> "Ken, I've got a little job I want you to do for me. I'm in a little trouble. Went up to Macon last month with Bill Jackson, and we had a little fun. I guess I took too much liquor. We went by a place Bill knew about where there were some girls. I took a fancy to a little girl from Atlanta who told me she had slipped away from home and her folks thought she was visiting her cousins at Forsyth. Anyhow, I thought everything was all right, but I'm in a bad way and I want you to treat me. I can't go to Dr. Bennett 'cause I don't want him to know about it. I'll take care of you all right, and if you get me fixed up I'll pay you well.[77]

"That," concludes the narrator, "was Kenneth's introduction to one part of the work of a coloured physician in the South."[78]

James Martin found evidence of this work in Tennessee. One pharmacist he interviewed said, "When a young fellow of the aristocratic class, and this is an aristocratic town, gets syphilis or gonorrhea, he usually goes to this negro [physician] and so avoids the embarrassment of submitting such a case to a friend of the family."[79] A few African American physicians there developed a reputation for curing sexually transmitted diseases and attracted a large black and white clientele.[80] Thus black physicians did, in certain instances and for various reasons, compete successfully with their white counterparts for patients of both races.

But success in gaining patients did not necessarily mean financial ease. As a Thomasville, Georgia, physician wrote to President Meserve in 1904: "My practice is as good as I could wish. Collections keeps [*sic*] off the wolf."[81] Smaller fees and a generally poorer clientele must have taken their toll on African American physicians' incomes, though actual numbers are not readily available, making comparisons with white physicians' incomes impossible.[82] Collection of fees for all physicians naturally varied, depending on clientele, physician personality, local financial conditions, and other variables. An Oklahoma physician summed up the situation in his state in a 1914 letter to the editor of the *Medical World*:

"In the state of Oklahoma there are over 100 Negro physicians, some doing well; others are not. They average from $600 to over $3,000 per annum."[83] Turn-of-the-century black medical graduates, often in debt for their education and fiscally overextended in order to open their practices, expressed concern when payments for services did not arrive in a timely fashion. J. Edward Ashburn, a Bowers Hill, Virginia, physician, contrasted for President Meserve of Leonard Medical School the number of patients he saw and the amount actually collected: "In my practice I am doing very well; my field is very large.... [Actual income] is a little scarce, yet I am pushing perseveringly to the front."[84] Jeremiah M. Lloyd of Elizabethtown, North Carolina, echoed Ashburn's story: "I have a large practice in this town and surroundings. But I have not collected much money as the people are poor having lost all of their crops by a large freshet."[85]

So black physicians faced all of the problems any doctor encountered in opening a medical practice and also met with difficulties due to their race as they entered this formerly white-dominated profession. Yet some of them succeeded quite well in the South. In 1890, for example, Dr. Albert L. Thompson, a Meharry graduate, offered readers of the *Christian Educator* a capsule account of his rise to local prominence and fortune: "I began active work in this city [Dennison, Texas] two years ago, and for a while the way appeared dark. I was treated kindly by the [medical] fraternity, and assured that the time would come when I would meet with the success hoped for. So the time moved on, and my practice became larger, and my collections better, until I have been enabled to secure a passable office outfit, a good buggy and horse, and real estate valued at fifteen hundred dollars in a fine portion of the city, within four blocks of Main Street, the business center of the city."[86]

Several available reports announce strikingly positive white physician responses to black practitioners' arrivals, responses that conveyed the promise of friendship and collegiality among potential rivals. Thaddeus A. Walker of Baton Rouge told readers of the *Christian Educator* in January 1887, "I was given the hand of fellowship by a leading white physician, Dr. J. W. Dupree, who welcomed me in these words: 'You are my colored medical brother, and I will go with you at any time.'"[87] And Robert F. Boyd of Nashville, a graduate and future faculty member of Meharry, wrote, "All the physicians of the city treat me white."[88] "I have, when needed," wrote Green J. Starnes from San Antonio at this time, "counsel from the leading physicians of the city."[89] Another African American physician in Texas had "the respect of all the physicians of this city, one of whom made me a present of one hundred dollars' worth of good medical books."[90] President Meserve, who received numerous letters from graduates in practice, most living in the South, boasted in his 1903–4 annual report to a philanthropic fund that his school's alumni "are respected by the white physicians wherever they go, and have no difficulty in getting the white physicians to consult with them when critical cases demand it."[91] Such was the skill and reputation of a Columbia, South Carolina, practitioner that he reported to W. E. B. Du Bois of being often "called upon by white physicians to consult with them in medical cases and assist in surgical cases in their practice."[92] Race seemed not to interfere with professional matters for these physicians.[93] One North Carolina doctor summed it up by stating: "My intercourse with the white members of my profession is cordial along professional lines. I seek no others."[94]

Acceptance by white colleagues represented one measure of success for the black physician. Patronage by patients and the financial rewards that accompanied it represented another. Young African American physicians happily reported their progress, though, as Du Bois cautioned readers of his study of "the college-bred Negro," there were many failures. But people tended to discuss the good and ignore the bad. So letters to Du Bois, Meserve, George W. Hubbard (dean of Meharry Medical College), and others emphasized accomplishments. "I have a fine practice, went in over 500 different families last year and I am doing [even] better this year. I drive my own turn out, and have purchased a home, and married," wrote (on letterhead stationery) a recent Leonard graduate practicing in Portsmouth, Virginia, to Charles Meserve.[95] J. Benton Dickson, an earlier Leonard alumnus, told Meserve that he was "succeeding splendidly" in Jackson, Tennessee, and could now afford to purchase his printed diploma. "I should have sent for my diploma earlier," he explained, "but had a large number of debts to pay off and could not take money to pay for things I could do without awhile, when my other bills were past due." (Dickson's letterhead no doubt helped Meserve understand the source of Dickson's new financial status. In addition to giving his telephone number and morning, afternoon, and evening office hours, it also proclaimed that the young doctor was "in office all night.")[96] "When I came here I was owing three hundred and fifty dollars, all of which is now paid," a Gulf States practitioner wrote to Meharry's Hubbard. "I have supported my family; equipped a fine office, which compares favorably with the best in the city; bought and paid for a horse, buggy, and road-cart, and household furniture amounting to two hundred dollars."[97] And so they wrote about the size of their practices, the mixture of white and black patients, and the financial rewards.[98]

Clearly, the major concern of these new black doctors was survival. They may have wished to fulfill the ideals of race betterment set out by and for them in medical school, for a few mentioned improvement of black health in their reports and letters (e.g., "I am doing all the good I can to all the people I can in every way possible").[99] But these pioneering black physicians believed they first had to establish themselves professionally in their communities.

Their positive reports to their alma maters and to public print media tended to minimize racial problems and a poor clientele in order to promote goodwill, a favorable public image, increased black attendance at medical schools, and cordial relations between whites and blacks. Even the fictional Kenneth Harper tried to ignore racial tensions in Central City, Georgia, in hopes of gaining acceptance and easing whites and blacks through a transitional period of increasing status for Southern blacks. But race did get in the way of success, for Harper and for real-life physicians such as J. Edward Perry, who described it in his autobiography, and for many who did not mention it in letters or reports. Those white physicians who made the effort to welcome and assist their African American colleagues as they might have taken a newly graduated physician of their own race under their wing contributed to the cause of harmony between black and white professionals. But they did not change the mores of Southern society. Whites still dominated; prejudice and segregation still existed. So the success of physicians of color depended not only on their passively receiving welcomes from a few sympathetic white physicians and some local black patients. These physicians had actively to overcome negative white *and* black racial attitudes toward black medical professionals. They did this by practicing good medicine, by proving themselves competent, by becoming leaders in their communities, and by, as will now be shown, addressing directly some of the obstacles others put in their path.

Black physicians fought against professional isolation in several ways. Personal contact with white physicians sometimes helped.[100] More fruitful were activities that sought to circumvent the formal racial isolation imposed by whites. Though these methods simply established parallel segregated institutions for African American physicians, they did provide professional opportunities that were otherwise unavailable. These practitioners acted to improve their situations not only at the local level but also regionally and nationally. A key to all these endeavors was good communication among local black doctors. This, of course, was easier to do in urban areas than out in the country. A glance at city or medical directories of the period reveals the presence of more than one black practitioner in most towns of any size in the South.[101] Numbers allowed them to discuss ways of protecting their interests and to band together in formal and informal ways. Occasionally African American physicians in a city established a local medical society and met regularly for professional or social purposes (see Appendix, Table 8). In May 1911, for example, the physician members of the Falls City (Louisville) Medical Association met and established a fee schedule "in order to secure uniform prices and insure reasonable rates of service to the public."[102] Other physicians simply recognized common needs and acted to assist one another. A black physician in Columbus, Georgia, for instance, helped a recently arrived Leonard Medical School graduate establish his practice in town.[103] In turn-of-the-century Kansas City, Missouri, J. Edward Perry reported in his autobiography that the need for a united front was great:

> Those were tough days and lean pickings for the Negro doctor of Kansas City. We soon learned that the interest of one was the welfare of the other. The objective was to gain a reputation for the efficiency of the brother of color.
>
> Our greatest difficulty was continuing in the service of a patient after having been called. If a patient was stricken in his "tummy" and was not entirely relieved by noon the following day, a white physician was frequently called if per chance the individual had the cash in hand. Ethics were of no significance at all to the white brother. It appeared to be the "survival of the fittest."
>
> Often when an individual became seriously ill with pneumonia or typhoid fever, and one of the group [of black physicians] perchanced to be in the neighborhood, a call would invariably be made upon the patient of a brother physician to see what was "going on" and to evidence interest. If a patient became abruptly, seriously ill and his regular physician was around town on calls, the visit was made by a brother physician, and in case of a collection the amount was readily "turned over," with a note as to findings or impressions of the malady, also information of the remedies administered. We were all for one and one for all.
>
> With sincere service, honesty of opinion and a manifestation of interest in the general welfare of the people, gradually there was observed a broadening of our reputations, a multiplicity of friends and an increase in our practice and income.[104]

Cooperation among black physicians even extended to poor rural areas of the South, if for no other reason than to exchange information about fees and patients. Though perhaps not as well organized or successful as urban groups, these networks appear to have been useful. James Martin's brief statement about the physicians of middle and western Tennessee indicates that such arrangements existed elsewhere as well: "Agreements among negro physicians as to case charges seem to be not very precise; but, in most places where there are two or more practicing, there are such agreements, indefinite and poorly kept as they are."[105]

Forming local societies, arranging fee structures, and providing mutual patient coverage were only some of the actions black doctors took to bolster their professional positions and combat isolation. Another major problem they faced was gaining access to hospitals. So black practitioners established their own, either individually or in groups, where they could care for their patients and perform surgery.[106] When, for example, Cornelius and Alice Woodby McKane arrived in Savannah and found no hospital, they made it a priority to open one. In 1893 the McKane Hospital began accepting patients and continued to care for African Americans using African American physicians long after its founders had left for Africa in 1895 as medical missionaries.[107] The pioneering South Carolina physician

Matilda Evans opened hospitals in Columbia three times between her arrival in 1898, fresh from Women's Medical College in Philadelphia, and 1916.[108] Alonzo McClennan, a Howard graduate, gathered enough black community support to open a hospital and nurse-training school in Charleston in 1897. All but one of the local black physicians joined with McClennan in the project, which gave them their only chance to obtain hospital-operating privileges.[109] An enterprising 1891 Meharry graduate, George S. Burruss, moved to Augusta, Georgia, and in 1901 established a hospital there. Five years later a reporter for a national black magazine described the Burruss Sanitarium for his readers:

> It consists of a large three-story frame building, which contains twenty-seven rooms and one ward. The rooms are well ventilated, handsomely furnished and are provided with electric bells and electric lighting apparatus. The operating room is equipped with all the requisites of modern and asceptic [*sic*] surgery, including the operating table, instrument table, two wheel stretcher, a microscope for examining blood, sputum, etc., and an amphitheater for the convenience of doctors, nurses, and others who are privileged to be present during an operation. Not far from the operating room is the X-ray Department, in which there is an X-ray machine which was installed at a cost of more than $500. The first floor is taken up largely with a drug store, of which Dr. Burruss is sole proprietor, with his private offices and a large public reception room. The Sanitarium, building and equipment, is valued at $10,000 and is free from debt.[110]

The other eleven black physicians in Augusta, according to the writer, offered their "services and active hearty cooperation" to the enterprise.[111]

Of course not all or even most black physician–run hospitals succeeded like Burruss's. Little towns and rural areas required such facilities on a smaller scale. Nor were there always patients to occupy the beds or make use of the equipment. In the seven Tennessee counties he studied, James Martin found three hospitals, only one of which still functioned. In stark contrast to the Burruss Sanitarium, this facility comprised "a large, almost bare house in which there were a number of beds. There were, at the time of this visit, no patients and hence no nurse or caretaker other than the physician whose office was next door."[112] The other two hospitals Martin investigated were cooperative ventures among two or more black physicians.[113] Whether owned individually or by groups, these private hospitals sprang up across the South as physicians of color encountered racial restrictions on their practices.

Like fictional Kenneth Harper of Central City, Georgia, some black physicians had aspirations of becoming experts in surgery in their regions and founded hospitals as the only available means to achieve that goal. Robert C. Burt (Meharry class of 1897) of Clarksville, Tennessee, was such a man. According to biographical sketches in his personal papers, he nourished a "long cherished dream of operating a small hospital and to do surgery on a large scale." So in 1904 he bought some land and by 1906 had converted a house on it into a hospital equipped for surgery. With the support and assistance of black physicians and dentists in the area, Home Infirmary grew over the next few years into a regional hospital caring for hundreds of patients.[114] To help spur on people like Burt, successful African American surgeons such as Daniel Hale Williams and George Cleveland Hall, both of Chicago, traveled through the South in the early twentieth century, holding surgical clinics for fellow practitioners. These men would perform procedures on local patients in order to demonstrate surgical techniques and innovations to African American physicians barred from or unable to attend postgraduate courses and white hospital clinics.[115] Attesting to the influence of surgical clinics and to the felt need for and determination of Southern black practitioners to establish hospitals is Monroe Work's inventory of such institutions in his *Negro Year Book*. In the 1914–15 edition, for example, he listed seventy-seven hospitals in the region, almost all operated by blacks.[116]

Though expensive for practitioners both in direct costs and in lost patient revenues, taking postgraduate courses in the growing specialty areas offered isolated black physicians a chance to improve knowledge and skills, meet new colleagues, and visit large Northern cities such as Chicago, Boston, New York, Washington, D.C., and Philadelphia. These courses were initially held at traditionally white medical schools and were closed to physicians of color, but most institutions had begun to accept blacks, and some African American educational facilities had established postgraduate programs by the decade following 1910.[117] (No Southern black institutions developed postgraduate facilities before 1920.)

These sorts of individual initiatives and cooperative ventures, aimed at overcoming professional isolation, encouraged some African American physicians to link colleagues on an even broader basis. In 1895, enough physicians expressed interest in founding a nationwide medical society that a group met in Atlanta at the Cotton States and International Exposition, the same exposition at which Booker T. Washington gained notice for his famous accommodationist speech, to establish the NMA, with goals similar to those of local groups.[118] And by 1920, virtually every Southern state had a black medical society that sometimes included dentists and pharmacists along with physicians.[119] Such groups met regularly to present medical papers, exchange information and ideas about racial matters, and simply to socialize and become (re)acquainted with colleagues. The fifth annual meeting of the Mississippi Medical and Surgical Association in April 1905 was typical. The Jackson gathering offered those attending case presentations, medical papers and discussions, and a presidential address that stressed, according to a local newspaper report, "promoting friendly co-operation with the white physicians of the state, and spoke in the highest terms of the white physicians generally." In an obvious reference to these remarks, the white newspaper approvingly included in its headlines for the story, "President May Makes a Good Talk in Which He Gives Association Sensible Advice."[120] All these organizations experienced difficult times when membership or attendance at meetings dwindled, but most survived until integration (see Appendix, Table 8).

Black-oriented medical journals also provided a means not only of keeping physicians' knowledge current but also of learning about colleagues' and institutions' activities and of contributing information of one's own. Miles Vandahurst Lynk of Jackson, Tennessee, published the first of these journals, the *Medical and Surgical Observer*, in 1892, just one year after his graduation from Meharry. A forceful and outspoken man on many subjects,[121] Lynk promoted his periodical with advertisements such as this (see figure 22):

> Say, Doctor, have you read the MEDICAL AND SURGICAL OBSERVER, The Organ of the Colored Medical Profession of North America? It recognizes the necessity of a higher standard of medical education in this country, and will put forth its best efforts to raise and maintain the same. It contains all the progressive ideas of the profession—minus the chaff.
>
> Read and endorsed by the profession from the Atlantic to the Pacific and from the Arctic Ocean to Mexico.[122]

In the days before black physicians had organized a national professional association, Lynk's advertisement smacked of hyperbole, but if the letters he published from readers around the country indicate the journal's general reception, then the *Observer* certainly filled a gap. One such letter, from Waco, Texas, read: "I have before my gaze the pride and boast of every Negro doctor—a journal of our own—a counterpart of ourselves—a real living proof of capacity in science and art. In a brief way, allow me to congratulate you for pluck, energy and forethought. The accomplishment of a century in twenty-seven years [since Emancipation]! Who can say (but to be laughed at) that we are not coming one hundred thousand strong? God bless your efforts, provide for the permanence of such a literature and endow the editor with wisdom. My name, accompanied with subscription price of your valuable journal will be forthcoming in a few days."[123] Though lively and interesting, the *Observer* could not (nor could its editor) induce enough black physicians to part with one dollar for a subscription to sustain the publication beyond January 1894. Lynk, however, remained active in the profession, calling for the establishment of a nationwide professional society in 1892 and operating the University of West Tennessee College of Medicine and Surgery almost single-handedly, first in Jackson, then in Memphis, from 1900 to 1923.[124]

Not until 1909 did a second national medical journal by and for black physicians appear. (Alonzo McClennan had published the *Hospital Herald* in Charleston for a few years in the late 1890s, but its audience remained local and oriented toward nursing.)[125] At that time the officers of the NMA began issuing an official *Journal*. It, too, struggled for survival, but endured, strongly promoting the interests of African American physicians. It published papers presented at annual meetings, minutes of the NMA and state society meetings, and advertisements of upcoming black-sponsored medical meetings and events. Individual physicians reading the *Journal of the National Medical Association* (*JNMA*) could feel part of a larger group and learn how and where to participate, if desired.

The *JMNA* published editorials as well, offering opinions on important aspects of black medicine. In 1920 the death of a prominent practitioner, Dr. George W. Cabaniss, provided the editors with an opportunity to look back at the growth of the black medical profession and at the measures of success that African American physicians had been using. They found their colleagues wanting:

> Too many men in the practice of medicine feel that when they have made money and established their economic independence, they have discharged their whole responsibility to their day and generation. . . . Let such a physician stop for a moment and consider how he has made his money,—from whence he has made it. . . . We venture to say that about ninety-nine per cent of [his] practice is among Negroes; and we venture to say further that ninety-five per cent of that ninety-nine percent is among the hard-working class of Negroes, the poor, the lowly, the ignorant—that mass of helpless dependents, many of them absolutely poverty stricken, living from hand to mouth. Doctor, when you drive through the slums in your high-powered, fast-going automobile and look upon this seething mass of disease-ridden, poverty stricken [people], ignorance personified, out of whom you have gained influence and opulence, do you stop for a minute to think that you owe them anything in return?[126]

The editors raised difficult questions for successful practitioners, questions these physicians may have avoided or pushed aside in their pursuit of other goals, but which they would eventually have to confront.[127]

By 1920, Southern black physicians had come a long way in establishing themselves. Though they could never escape the race issue in their dealings with both patients and colleagues, many had earned a good reputation and a good living. As a group they had developed an increasingly strong, active, and accepted body of medical professionals. Their commitment to the general improvement of black health may have suffered in their zeal to establish themselves and provide an enduring presence in a previously white profession. But they had made a good start in accomplishing their other goals.

CHAPTER 20

"A Journal of Our Own"

The Medical and Surgical Observer *in Late-Nineteenth-Century America*

On December 29, 1892, the "Initial Number" of a new medical journal, the *Medical and Surgical Observer* (*MSO*), arrived at the library of the Surgeon General's Office in Washington, D.C. Issues of many medical journals arrived regularly at this large government medical library where John Shaw Billings's staff was compiling the *Index Catalogue*, a comprehensive directory to the world's medical literature. What distinguished the *MSO* from other journals to which the Surgeon General's Library (predecessor of the National Library of Medicine) subscribed was its ownership, audience, and much of its subject matter. At the top of the *MSO* page in the library's "Serials Received" record book, the clerk or librarian wrote: "Only *Negro* M. J. in America."[1]

Miles Vandahurst Lynk, M.D. (1871–1956), editor of the *MSO*, knew that fact quite well. He had established the *MSO* because he believed that black physicians dispersed across the country needed a journal of their own. Although the *MSO* survived for only a little over a year, it served as a vehicle to connect widely scattered and isolated black health professionals with one another, especially in the South, and suggested ways these physicians, dentists, and pharmacists could organize themselves. The *MSO* informed African American physicians of news and practical ideas in the world of medicine. As more and more persons of color entered the white-dominated medical world in an era of growing racism and racial segregation, the new journal did its part, under Lynk's distinctive style of editorship, to promote the development of an African American medical profession.[2] It only partially succeeded. Despite words and letters of encouragement and support from fellow black physicians, Lynk had a difficult time obtaining paid subscriptions for the journal. His editorial call for the organization of a national black physicians' association did succeed, though not until more than two years had elapsed after the *MSO*'s final issue.

Emancipation in the 1860s ostensibly opened many new opportunities for blacks, including the chance to enter professions such as law, the ministry, teaching, and medicine that previously had been the exclusive domain of whites. To educate African Americans, members of both races established schools—primary through college and sometimes beyond—in the former Confederate states. Among the many educational institutions for blacks founded between 1868 and 1900, fourteen offered training for future physicians (see Appendix, Table 4).[3] From those early schools emerged several hundred African American medical practitioners who opened offices in rural areas, towns, and cities, primarily in the South.[4]

The end of Reconstruction brought many changes to the region as black and white Southerners adjusted to race relations after the abrupt termination of slavery. Shifting, unstable political alliances among whites, the enfranchisement of African Americans and the subsequent struggle for their vote and then for their disenfranchisement by whites, the growth of white and black farm tenancy, the burgeoning of towns with increasing numbers of wage earners of both races drawn from the countryside, and the regular contact of whites and blacks in a less structured nonslave society made for rising tensions between the races. As this anxiety expanded in the final decades of the century, resulting in Jim Crow laws, poll taxes, lynchings, and race riots, and as the medical profession became increasingly overcrowded owing to the uncontrolled proliferation of medical schools, the response black physicians received from their white colleagues was not always cordial. Some white doctors viewed physicians of color as economic competitors and as intruders threatening to upset well-established social and professional networks. They devised ways to close ranks against the newly trained black physicians joining their number.[5]

As the profession functioned before the entry of more than a handful of African Americans (a few physicians of color had practiced in the United States during the antebellum period), physicians competed with one another for patients but also worked together by consulting on difficult or puzzling cases, assisting when surgery required an anesthetist or extra hands, and organizing medical societies for professional advancement. At society meetings, physicians established fee structures, exchanged ideas and practical knowledge about treatments, presented problem patients for discussion and possible solutions, and socialized with others having common interests and educational backgrounds. Doctors, individually and in groups, also built hospitals where they could apply the modern surgical techniques newly developed in European and American medical centers. National, state, and local medical societies published their organizations' proceedings, papers presented at monthly meetings, and news of members, often in their own societies' medical journals.

Excluded from the usual activities that bound together most American physicians, late-nineteenth-century black physicians often felt isolated, behind the times, and less technically skilled than their white counterparts. They were barred from joining medical societies and thus from the medical, professional, and social exchanges that occurred at meetings, forced to turn surgical patients over to white physicians at the doors of hospitals that barred them on the basis of skin color, and unable to depend on white physicians for consultation in difficult cases or on their assistance with surgery and anesthesia. Although African American physicians presumably kept up with the latest medical thinking by reading the same journals as white physicians, they could not learn about black professional affairs or comfortably express their ideas and experiences relating to issues of race in white-owned and white-oriented journals. Some black practitioners combated these problems with varying degrees of success by attempting to establish collegial relations with white physicians in their communities, opening their own hospitals and drugstores, forming medical associations with other local black doctors, dentists, and pharmacists, and enrolling in postgraduate courses in the North.[6]

In 1891, Miles Lynk, newly graduated from Meharry Medical College in Nashville, Tennessee, entered this separate and unequal medical world. A scrapper from his youth, Lynk did not let the repressive, segregated race system of the South keep him down. He was, in many ways, a self-made man. Born of former slave parents on June 3, 1871, Lynk grew up on a farm in western Tennessee near Brownsville, Haywood County.[7] He obtained his basic education at rural black schools and then studied more advanced subjects such as algebra, biology, geometry, Latin, and physics with a private tutor. To earn money for medical school tuition, he taught at a rural black summer school in 1888. Sometime during the subsequent year, Jacob C. Hairston, a recently graduated Meharry physician who had opened a practice in Brownsville,[8] became Lynk's preceptor, a common arrangement between medical students and physicians at that time. Lynk's association with Hairston continued on and off for many years. (Hairston moved to Jackson in the early 1890s and joined forces with Lynk in practice for a time, then moved to other Tennessee towns, and eventually to Memphis, where he taught at one of Lynk's later enterprises, the University of West Tennessee College of Medicine and Surgery.)

In the fall of 1889, Lynk enrolled at Meharry Medical College in Nashville. Meharry offered, like most other medical schools of the time, a three-year curriculum. Lynk's prior education with Hairston served him well, allowing him to pass entrance examinations at a high enough level to begin Meharry with the second-year medical class and to impress both Dr. Robert Fulton Boyd, a faculty member at the school, and Dr. George Whipple Hubbard, the school's founder and president. After a successful two-year career at Meharry, Lynk graduated in the spring of 1891 at the age of nineteen, second in a class of thirteen.[9]

Many students at Meharry during Lynk's time there later became leaders in the nascent late-nineteenth-century African American medical community. For example, one of his classmates, Commodore I. Cain of Rome, Georgia, joined the faculty of Chattanooga National Medical College in 1899. William W. Derrick, a soon-to-be instructor at Knoxville College Medical Department and its successor, Knoxville Medical College, was a member of the class just behind Lynk, and Charles Victor Roman, future Meharry faculty member and historian of Meharry and future editor of the *Journal of the National Medical Association*, graduated the year before Lynk. Lynk's acquaintance with these men helped him in his future activities.

Lynk decided to open his practice in home territory, western Tennessee, but in Jackson rather than in the more familiar village of Brownsville. Jackson was larger, numbering 10,039 citizens according to the 1890 census.[10] Its black community, which accounted for just over 40 percent of the town's population (4,160 in 1890), could boast of supporting the founding church (Liberty Church) and some of the administration of a major African American religious denomination, the Colored (later changed to Christian) Methodist Episcopal (CME) Church, and a prominent CME-sponsored black institution of higher learning, Lane College.[11]

Lynk reported in his autobiography that friends tried to dissuade him from moving to Jackson because of recent racial unrest there, including the mobbing of a black woman. Undaunted by this potential danger, however, and invoking his "confidence in the ultimate goodness of human character,"[12] Lynk settled in Jackson in 1891. Perhaps the knowledge that he was born just a few months after and just a few miles from where the CME church was founded, that his parents had been devout CME supporters from the beginning, and that he bore names similar to those of the CME's first two bishops, William Henry Miles and Richard H. Vanderhorst, also pulled Lynk toward Jackson. He thus became the first African American physician in Madison County's seat of government. Between Lynk's open way of dealing with local white physicians and the example one white physician set by extending an immediate warm helping hand to the newly arrived black physician, the young Meharry graduate, as he himself predicted, encountered few problems (then or later, according to Lynk's account) with his white professional brethren.[13]

Winning the trust of African American patients who were skeptical that a person of color could practice good medicine took more effort and time, he recounted, than receiving the endorsement of Jackson's white physicians. Following his motto, "Do all the good you can to all the people you can in all the ways you can," Lynk reported in 1900 that he "soon overcame their scruples and built up a large and lucrative practice."[14]

Success encourages self-confidence. As he progressed in his career, Lynk combined self-confidence with boldness and a willingness to take risks, traits he had possessed and used well before entering medicine. Not content simply to break the race barrier in medicine in Jackson, this physician from rural western Tennessee decided to promote the professionalization and increase the number of African American physicians across the nation and to do what he could to instill self-esteem in his African American brothers and sisters.

Over the next fifteen years, from his home base in the small town of Jackson, Lynk worked on several significant projects. He cofounded a national medical association and founded and ran a medical school that trained students from around the country and abroad. He wrote books and edited a magazine for African Americans on black history, literature, and culture and established a publishing house to print and sell those books and magazines. (That publishing business had an impact on African Americans in his own community because it provided employment to a dozen or more black citizens.) Lynk obtained a law degree, and then opened a law school so other African Americans could become lawyers.[15] It is on the first of his accomplishments after graduating from medical school and opening a practice in Jackson, Tennessee, that we will concentrate here—establishing the *MSO*, the first black medical journal in the United States.

American medical journals of the late nineteenth century virtually ignored the growing but still tiny presence of black physicians in the United States (909 out of 104,391 physicians according to the 1890 census). Few pages contained case reports or articles by physicians of color about their patient experiences, personal notices about African American practitioners, minutes of local black medical societies, or information about medical schools for blacks. Lynk intended to change that situation and begin to bring unity and self-awareness to African American medical professionals.

On December 1, 1892, Lynk, aged twenty-one and just a year and a half out of medical school, formally established a national medical journal. (He undoubtedly had been working on the project before that date.) The *MSO* appeared monthly from December 1892 through January 1894, catering to the interests of African American physicians and other black health professionals around the country. Lynk appears to have overseen the journal's entire operation, from writing and editing its contents to selling advertisements for financial support to printing and mailing each issue. He wrote much of each issue himself, collecting items from correspondence, submitted material, and his growing network of personal contacts. In addition to publishing the articles, news items, and practice tips that African American physicians wrote for the *Observer*, Lynk reprinted articles of medical interest from other journals. (The journals from which Lynk reproduced articles included *Medical News*, *Nashville Journal of Medicine and Surgery*, *Annals of Surgery*, *Memphis Medical Monthly*, *The Post-Graduate*, *Dietetic and Hygienic Gazette*, *St. Louis Medical and Surgical Journal*, *Boston Journal of Health*, *New*

York Therapeutic Review, *New York Medical Journal*, *American Therapist*, *Indian Medical Record*, *Medical Age*, *Archives of Gynecology*, *Buffalo Medical and Surgical Journal*, *Journal of the American Medical Association*, *Harper's Weekly*, *Pacific Medical Journal*, and *Medical World*.)

He adopted a lively, informal style when promoting the journal ("Don't start into [medical] practice before you subscribe for the MEDICAL AND SURGICAL OBSERVER; it's your main agency upon which you are to depend for success"),[16] almost never taking a negative tack, especially when discussing personal and professional matters relating to the African American medical profession. He tried to introduce black physicians, scattered and isolated around the South and the country, to each other through the articles they wrote and through personal notices and to publish other medical gleanings he thought would engage this growing number of American physicians of color.

From the beginning, Lynk made it clear that he was publishing the *MSO* for the black medical profession of the United States. One ad proudly proclaimed: "MEDICAL AND SURGICAL OBSERVER. The only distinctively Negro Medical Journal published in America."[17] Not shy of self-praise, he invited readers of the *MSO*'s first issue "to peruse its pages carefully," as he was "supplying the colored medical profession of the US, with a very necessary weapon in combating disease, ignorance and quackery."[18] "The OBSERVER," Lynk wrote, "like the goddess Minerva [goddess of wisdom], who sprung full-armed from the very head of Jove [Jupiter], fills a long felt want."[19]

The pages of the *MSO* were open to black physicians. Lynk asked in his first editorial that readers "send us information on matters of general interest to the profession,"[20] presumably meaning the African American medical profession. In a later issue, he explained that the material and suggestions readers sent would help make the *MSO* "clean, newsy and fearless." (Lynk's meaning here is unclear. Perhaps it is a misprint and the word he meant to use was "lean.") "This is your journal," he continued. "It will be what you make of it."[21] In another issue he again solicited articles, news, letters, case reports, and practice tips from readers, saying, "Remember, every man knows something that somebody else doesn't know."[22] Lynk remained true to his word: lead articles in every issue were written by practitioners of color, the people mentioned in the news items were, with few exceptions, black, and the medical schools that advertised within the *MSO*'s pages and about whom news was reported were African American. Lynk did what he could to make the *MSO* reflective of and interesting to his black colleagues around the country.

Race was an ever-present, though not usually overt, theme in the *MSO*. Editorials and news items never mentioned race except to compliment successes at one of the black medical schools, advertise the *MSO* as a medical journal for physicians of color, or report on or suggest the need for black medical societies in the United States. Although several of the articles in the journal referred to matters of race, Lynk himself never, in print, solicited articles or comments specifically on race relations among American physicians; never mentioned the race of authors, contributors, or the physicians named in his news reports; and never commented about the problems black physicians faced in the white medical world. He did not need to advertise such issues openly; all *MSO* readers knew the reason for the existence of the journal.

Each issue of the *MSO* contained two main sections, one with longer "Original Communications" and one with briefer news items, editorials, and excerpts from other publications. Although Lynk wished that through the *MSO* "there may be inculcated and fostered among them [physicians of color] a more decided ardor for original research and investigation," the articles he published (both original and selected from other journals) focused on the practical rather than on the scientific research aspects of medicine. They usually emphasized ways to deal with medical and business problems, not medical theories or experimental techniques.

Seventeen of the twenty-four "Original Communications" published in the *MSO*, all written by African American physicians, contained case reports. Topics included malarial fever, chronic metritis, amputation at the wrist joint, endometritis, hysteria, nephritis, placenta previa, sarcoma, dyspepsia, difficult obstetric and gynecological problems, scrofula, and rectal ulceration. These articles read like case reports appearing in other medical journals of the time. A few *MSO* "Original Communications" were general overviews of a subject offering suggestions about diagnosis and treatment, as, for example, "The Importance of Physical Examination in the Disorders of the Pelvic Viscera, in Females,"[23] "Treatment of Summer Complaint,"[24] and "Prevention of Some Diseases from a Practical Hygienic Standpoint."[25] One *MSO* contribution offered "Practical Hints in the Practice of Medicine."[26]

Each of the fifteen authors of major articles in the *MSO* was a graduate of one of the three leading black medical schools of the time: six writers from Meharry Medical College in Nashville, five from Howard University Medical Department in Washington, D.C., and four from Leonard Medical School in Raleigh, North Carolina. They practiced medicine in cities such as Newark, New Jersey; Meridian, Mississippi; San Antonio, Texas; Savannah, Georgia; Washington, D.C.; Petersburg, Virginia; Winston, North Carolina; Hot Springs, Arkansas; Selma, Alabama; and Columbia, South Carolina. These authors tended to be new physicians: eleven of the fifteen had received their medical degrees within the previous five years. Some later became leaders of the profession; two were already well-known; Furman J. Shadd, professor of materia medica at Howard University Medical Department, and Monroe A. Majors, a leader in Texas' Lone Star Medical Association.

The news section of the *MSO* primarily related activities of African American health professionals. Noted black physicians whose endeavors Lynk mentioned numbered only four in the journal's fourteen issues. These people included Ferdinand A. Stewart[27] and Robert F. Boyd,[28] both professors on the Meharry faculty; Lawson A. Scruggs, first graduate of Leonard Medical School;[29] and Cornelius N. Dorsette,[30] an early Alabama practitioner and medical consultant to Booker T. Washington. Most news items were about younger physicians on their way up rather than the more established black practitioners. They were people of Lynk's generation, often Meharry alumni, most of whom the young editor probably knew personally. Typical notices of a personal nature included: "Dr. F. D. G. Harvey, of Brownsville, Tenn. recently took unto himself a lovely bride. Queer indeed are the ways of hymen [the Greek god of marriage]!"[31] And, "The death of Mrs. Dr. F. F. Mckinley has recently been chronicled. Dr. Mckinley is a member of the class of '79, Meharry Medical College. Mrs. Mckinley was cultured, affable and amiable. The doctor has the sympathy of the *Observer* in his sad bereavement."[32] Lynk was clearly not averse to adding his own comments to these stories, especially when he was acquainted with the people involved. In retracting a mistakenly reported story about the marriage of James T. Walton of San Antonio, Lynk, for example, quipped, "The doctor has not been quite so fortunate."[33] He also published brief personal items about, for example, a new "Colored Drug Store" opening in Savannah;[34] successful black medical practitioners in Palestine, Texas, and Helena, Arkansas;[35] the trip of a Brownsville, Tennessee, physician to the bedside of his ailing father in Lawrence, Kansas;[36] the visit of a Chattanooga physician of color to the Chicago World's Fair;[37] and the recovery of a Meridian, Mississippi, physician from "malarial fever."[38]

In addition to these personal stories, Lynk reported on new books and articles by African American physicians, such as Monroe A. Majors's proposed "The Afro-American in Medicine."[39] (The book was never published.) Lawson A. Scruggs's new book, *Women of Distinction*, received a favorable notice and free publicity in the *MSO*.[40] When Charles C. Johnson of Columbia, South Carolina, wished to solicit information from black physicians for a paper he planned to present at the next North Carolina Medical Association meeting on the topic of black physicians' relations with white physicians, Lynk obliged by both printing that request in the *MSO* and relating his own experiences on the subject.[41]

The *MSO*'s longer articles and short pieces informed readers about who among physicians of color was willing to take the time and initiative to write on medical topics, about the kinds of medical and practical business problems fellow physicians (no women physicians were named in any of the fourteen issues) were encountering and the ways others were dealing with them, and about the names and activities of other African American physicians. Lynk's information-gathering network was limited by his short time in the profession, the newness of the journal, and the nature of the journal's readership, but a regular reader could learn about a segment of the African American medical world from the *MSO*'s pages. The journal widened readers' familiarity with some fellow practitioners' names, activities, and to some extent, thoughts.

The journal also acquainted readers with affairs and progress at five of the six medical schools then functioning. Four of them (Howard, Meharry, Leonard, and New Orleans) advertised regularly in the *MSO*, listing their faculty so readers could recognize their names. Lynk's Meharry bias showed in reporting black medical education news. Although he mentioned Leonard, Howard, and New Orleans University (later called Flint) medical schools, he wrote more detailed and affectionate pieces about his alma mater. For example, after stating the number of students at Meharry in one short news item, Lynk added, "The class this year will be a dandy."[42] When it was reported in a white medical journal, the *Medical Review*, that a Dr. Snead of Nashville had died in an accident, Lynk wondered in print if this was the Dr. Snead who, with George W. Hubbard, had founded Meharry in 1876.[43] He included a long description of the 1893 graduating exercises at the school and boasted that the class graduating in 1894 would be "the largest class in the history of the school."[44] When four women enrolled at Meharry, Lynk reported it.[45] Noting in another issue of the *MSO* that Meharry medical students had organized a "Medico-Literary Association," Lynk, himself just recently a student, could not resist commenting on the need "to thoroughly prepare the students for the battle with the great medical problems with which they will have to contend."[46]

The only time Lynk waxed eloquent about another medical school was when the independent, black-owned, and black-operated (rather than church- or federal-government-supported) Louisville National Medical College received recognition as an acceptable medical school by a number of state boards of medical examiners:

> The Louisville National Medical Catalogue has made its appearance on our desk. It will be remembered that this school of medicine was projected solely by colored physicians some six years ago. It will also be remembered that it begun [*sic*] under very discouraging circumstances—everybody hooted at the movement. But we are truly proud to say, not like the Hannibal Medical Institute, of Memphis, it has passed the probationary stage and now its diplomas are recognized by the leading state boards of medical examiners. It has turned out twenty-two graduates, among whom are two ladies. All praise to the manly efforts of [the school's founders] Profs. [William Henry] Fitzbutler, [William A.] Burney and [Rufus] Conrad.[47]

The improvement of standards at five of the six schools earned each a mention in the *MSO* because Lynk saw that better standards meant better educated black physicians and a better black medical profession. Hannibal, an independent school operated, like Louisville National Medical College, by physicians of color, did not meet those standards. It had a poor reputation among both black and white doctors and laypeople, including, apparently, Lynk. He never acknowledged the school's existence in the *MSO* other than in this one backhanded reference as a foil for the Louisville school.[48]

Lynk was very interested in providing opportunities for physicians of color to meet and talk and establish a sense of unity and organization. To that end, he (1) reported on the activities of two existing black statewide medical societies, the Lone Star State Medical Association (founded 1886)[49] and the North Carolina Medical Society (founded 1887),[50] and on the founding of a new association in Arkansas;[51] (2) tried to make the *MSO* the official publishing organ for minutes and papers of the North Carolina group; and (3) called for the establishment of a national association of black physicians.

The idea of establishing a national association of black physicians was clearly on Lynk's mind when he wrote the inaugural issue of the *MSO*. Not only did he mention the need "for thorough organization among the increasing numbers of educated Negro physicians of the U.S." in his first editorial,[52] but also later in that same issue he suggested a way to fulfill that need. Lynk reported that at the third annual meeting of the North Carolina Medical Association in Wilmington the previous May (1892), society members had proposed that African American physicians in neighboring South Carolina and Virginia be invited to the group's fourth annual meeting in hopes of establishing "an interstate organization." The *MSO* editor now, in print, took that idea one step further: "An association of medical men of color, national in its character, we think would have a very inspiring effect upon the profession." The two statewide African American medical societies in Texas and North Carolina could serve as "a nucleus for the foundation of a national association." (Lynk failed to mention, in the pages of the *MSO*, the existence of another medical association for African Americans, the Medico-Chirurgical Society of the District of Columbia, founded in 1884, perhaps revealing his Tennessee and Meharry bias.)[53] Like the need he saw for a black medical journal to help draw the African American medical profession together, Lynk felt it was essential for black physicians to have their own association. He concluded his editorial with a passionate, forceful statement: "This is a dire necessity and we shall, must and will have it."[54]

Surprisingly, Lynk never again broached this subject, one on which he seemed to possess such strong convictions, in the pages of the *MSO*; he apparently held on to the concept for the appropriate moment. That moment did not arise for three more years, until well after the demise of the *MSO*, but Lynk, apparently still intent on bringing a sense of identity and unity to black physicians, was there and ready. He had already spoken several times with his former Meharry teacher Robert Fulton Boyd about forming a national organization. Most black physicians at the time, wrote Lynk in his autobiography, "considered Dr. Boyd the acknowledged [leader] of the profession."[55] The chance to organize arose because an international exposition brought large numbers of African American groups and individuals, including many physicians, together at one location. During the fall of 1895, Atlanta sponsored the Cotton States and International Exposition and invited black organizations and institutions to display their products in a special Negro Building. In an era of worsening race relations and of increasing white supremacist attitudes, the exposition provided a venue to show off the best of the South, black and white. At the opening of the great exposition in September 1895, Booker T. Washington rose to prominence as a leader of African Americans when he delivered a now famous speech, generally interpreted as accommodationist. In it he promoted industrial education for African Americans and accepted the social inequities of a racist South. One of the most eloquent and notorious statements in the speech seemed to foreshadow the goal Miles Lynk had been working toward for more than two years, the formation of a national black physicians' group. Speaking of race relations in the South, Washington said, "In all things that are purely social we can be as separate as the five fingers, yet one as the hand in all things essential to mutual progress."

On the afternoon of November 18, 1895, "Doctors' Day" at the Atlanta Cotton States and International Exposition, a group of black physicians met at the First Congregational Church in Atlanta and formed what later became known as the National Medical Association. Excluded from the more social, but professionally essential, aspects of the white-controlled American medical world, yet working toward the same goal as their white colleagues—better health for all Americans—black physicians had to found their own medical association, "as separate as the five fingers," just as Lynk had had to found a separate black medical journal. Lynk, not surprisingly, was one of the organizers of this nationwide black medical group, and became vice president of this group for Tennessee. Dr. Boyd was chosen as the association's first president.[56]

Although Lynk did not solicit them, he did publish a few articles and letters in the *MSO* that departed from strictly medical topics, in whole or in part, to discuss matters of race as they related to African American physicians' medical practices. At least five articles described, quite directly, race problems in medical practice.

One of these articles, "Consumption among the Colored Race," by L. L. Burwell (Leonard Medical School class of 1889) of Selma, Alabama, dealt with what appeared to be a strictly scientific issue, the prevalence of tuberculosis among African Americans.[57] Burwell, however, discussed the disease in more social terms, explaining why consumption had increased dramatically among blacks since Emancipation. "I have often had the question asked me, what causes the increase of the disease among my race?" He provided answers of both a social and a scientific nature: lack of money to obtain proper medical care or to move to healthier locales with better climates, poor hygiene, poor housing, poor clothing, crowded cities, blacks' poor tolerance of cold compared to whites, little exercise and poor diet, weakening of the body because of the prevalence of syphilis, and weakening of resistance to consumption because of the mixture of white and black blood (mulattoes). Although modern medicine would reject some of these explanations, Burwell was simply passing on to *MSO* readers the commonly held scientific thinking of the time.[58] He stated quite baldly and openly the problems African Americans faced, encouraging readers to discuss and attempt to remedy the very real concern of increased prevalence of tuberculosis among the black population.

The other four *MSO* articles frankly deal with race issues directly concerned with relations between black and white physicians—racial medical politics. One previously mentioned article described Dr. Charles C. Johnson's solicitation from African American physicians of answers to questions about relations between white and black doctors.[59] Johnson, an 1888 graduate of Howard University Medical Department and a practitioner in Columbia, South Carolina, was preparing a paper for delivery at the May 1893 meeting of the North Carolina Medical Association (of which he was the corresponding secretary) titled, "The Professional Relation between Physicians of the Opposite Races in the South." Johnson's questions were quite pointed and provocative:

1) Do you belong to any local medical association?
2) Do you hold consultations with white physicians?
3) Do they recognize you as a reputable practitioner of scientific medicine?
4) Do they carry out the spirit of the code with reference to you?
5) What is the general character of your professional relation to the white physicians of your city?
6) Does the color prejudice enter into their apparent estimate of your professional rights?
7) Is there an appreciable improvement since you have been practicing in regard to their professional courtesy towards you?

To encourage responses on this important topic, Lynk offered, just below Johnson's article, brief and positive reflections on his own experiences with white physicians: "For our part, we have received the highest degree of professional courtesy from our white colleagues. We believe this to be the experience of the average Negro M.D., in the South. His conduct demands it. He has received it." (As far as can be determined, Johnson's paper was never published.)

Furman J. Shadd (1852–1908) held a different view of relations between white and black physicians. A surgeon at Freedmen's Hospital in Washington, D.C., and a highly regarded professor at Howard University's medical department, Shadd published an article in the February issue of the *MSO* titled "Sarcoma."[60] He first

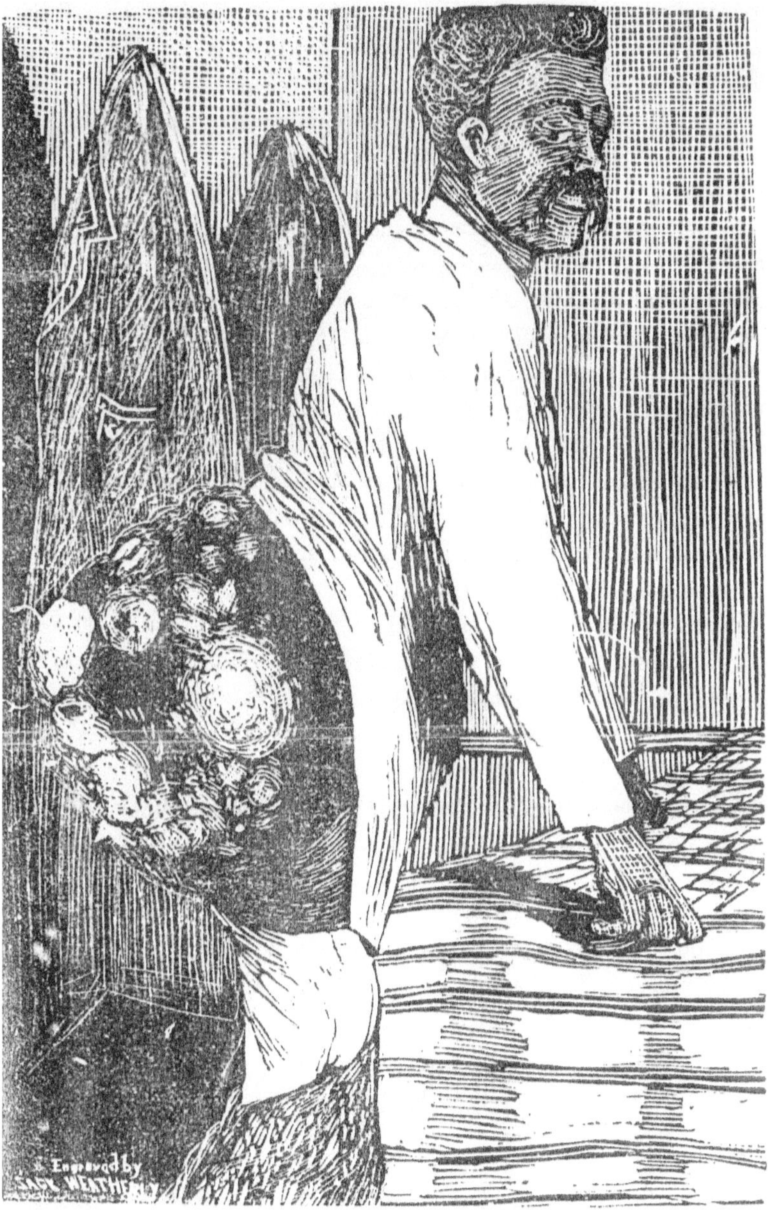

Fig. 21. An illustration that appeared in the *Medical and Surgical Observer* of a patient at Freedmen's Hospital in Washington, D.C., with a sarcoma. The picture appeared without attribution and without the author's permission or knowledge in a well-known textbook of surgery. From *Medical and Surgical Observer* 1 (Feb. 1893): 60.

offered a general medical discussion of sarcomas, then described the case of a patient with sarcoma on the buttocks. He made an engraving of this man's striking "very uncommon and rare" sarcoma, only to find it reproduced, without Shadd's knowledge or permission, in the recently published prestigious and well-known *American Text-book of Surgery*.[61] Shadd complained that Freedmen's Hospital, where the man had obtained medical care for several months and "where the true type of the disease was diagnosed" received no credit in the book.[62]

Using this incident of plagiarism as a springboard for social commentary on antiblack racism in late-nineteenth-century America, Shadd remarked that "courtesy at least should have caused the author [of the textbook] to give credit where it is due, even though the history [of the patient] could only have been gotten through members of a race which has been and is proscribed whenever it suits the whim and inclination of the Anglo-saxon."[63] The black surgeon warmed to his subject, lashing out against whites who threw up barriers against physicians of color simply because of race: "This is only another illustration of class proscription which confronts us at every step up the ladder of professional success. As gold is tried by fire we may be purified and strengthened by rebuffs and opposition. But I, for one, am getting tired of being classed as inferior when every avenue of advancement is locked and barred against me."[64]

Among the avenues of advancement that black physicians found barred against them were the use of hospitals and membership in medical societies. Both of these topics were addressed in *MSO* articles. Dr. S. C. Snelson of Savannah, Georgia, an 1890 graduate of Howard University's medical school and a frequent contributor to the *MSO*, reported in his article "Surgery in General,"[65] appearing in the August 1893 issue, that black patients generally preferred white physicians to black physicians, especially when it came to surgery. White physicians had access to city hospitals, whereas African American physicians could not use those facilities. Black doctors had to turn patients requiring hospitalization (usually for surgery) over to white colleagues, leaving the black doctors with little opportunity to build surgical confidence and skills.

Snelson reported an incident in his city to illustrate the point about black patients' distrust of black physicians, especially when it came to surgery. The family of a patient who had been shot with a pistol called Drs. Snelson and Smalls, both African American, for assistance. These men treated the patient (nonsurgically) and left. "As is quite common," Snelson wrote in his August 1893 *MSO* article, "the [patient's] people called in two white physicians during our absence."[66] Discussions between the white and black physicians centered on whether the patient should undergo surgery at the local hospital or if less invasive treatments would be more advantageous. Snelson and Smalls prevailed, but the competition between the white and black physicians was keen and evident, and mention of black physicians' inability to use hospital facilities unmentioned but implied. Throughout the article, Snelson identified physicians as either white or black, making it quite evident that race was important to him and the physicians with whom he dealt in Savannah. But he made it clear in the article that he wished to maintain cordial relations with the white physicians of Savannah.

Medical societies provided opportunities for physicians to meet with colleagues to discuss difficult cases, get advice, give suggestions, hear scientific papers, and build professional contacts for the future. As stated earlier, African American physicians could not join medical societies in the South during the late nineteenth century, closing another of Dr. Shadd's avenues to professional advancement. In a brief paragraph of the *MSO*'s section called "Spirit of the Medical Profession," the editor Lynk confirmed that restriction on black physicians in one state and praised the solution the state's black physicians had found to combat it: "The State Medical Association of Texas (white) has passed a resolution to the effect that all physicians in the state, that are in good standing, are eligible to membership in said Association, *the negro excepted.* It may be said to the negro's credit that they have formed an association known as the 'Lone Star Medical Association of Texas,' equal to that of the whites, and are consequently independent of the white association."[67] It is interesting to note that Lynk, at the same time that he praised and encouraged the formation of black medical societies in the United States and clearly recognized the existence of segregated medical societies in the Southern states, announced meetings of these same segregated societies in his journal. For example: "The West Tennessee Medical and Surgical Association will convene in this city on the 25th and 26th inst. [May 1893]. A large attendance is expected and an elaborate programme has been arranged."[68] It is not clear if Lynk was accepting these segregated medical societies, black and white, in the same way that Booker T. Washington would later accept segregation in his metaphorical idea of "separate as the five fingers, yet one as the hand."

Articles like these fit with the goals of the *MSO*'s editor—they allowed black physicians entering a profession previously closed to them on account of race to discuss race issues openly and with impunity if they so chose. In fostering community, communication, and cooperation among black physicians, Lynk was encouraging the development of a national black medical profession.

African American physicians who read the *MSO* understood its editor's message. They told him so in letters of support. "I was just thinking of the advisability of such an undertaking," wrote Dr. S. C. Snelson of Savannah, "as there are so many skillful and successful negro physicians and surgeons in our country. . . . It [the *MSO*] is just what we needed."[69] Members of both the North Carolina and Texas black physicians associations wrote Lynk of the need to publicize the activities of their organizations in print so as to, in the words of Marcus W. Alston of Asheville, North Carolina, "afford us development and interest as medical men."[70] John H. Wilkins, a former president of the Lone Star Medical Association, wrote that he had "tried to get the colored physicians [of Texas] to publish a 'journal' three years ago," to no avail.[71] Some of those physicians who recognized the importance of having a medical journal for blacks thanked Lynk for finally taking action: "I highly appreciate your noble effort to enroll the negro's name on the list of medical literature," wrote Dr. D. E. Caldwell of Osceola, Arkansas.[72] The most eloquent letter of thanks came from Dr. Monroe A. Majors of Waco, Texas: "I have before my gaze the pride and boast of every Negro doctor—a journal of our own—a counterpart of ourselves—a real living proof of capacity in science and art. In a brief way, allow me to congratulate you for pluck, energy and forethought."[73]

If the moral support Lynk received in such letters as these is an indication of support for the *MSO*, his new journal filled a need felt among at least some black physicians for a medical publication directed at them. How broadly felt that need was is difficult to determine, however. No records of the *MSO* remain for historians to analyze. Lynk needed more than words of praise and encouragement from a handful of readers to keep the *MSO* in print. He needed money. Letters such as the one from Dr. L. L. Burwell of Selma, Alabama, probably helped lift the editor's spirits: "Dear Sir and Brother—Your spicy little medical journal came before me in today's mail. I was indeed proud to see the effort put forth. I only trust that every colored doctor will subscribe to it." Although Burwell told Lynk to "put me down as a subscriber,"[74] it appears that not many other African American physicians followed his lead.

Lynk needed paid subscribers to sustain the *MSO*. Copies of the inaugural issue went out, gratis, to many black practitioners and to editors of white medical journals as well. In return, Lynk asked readers who found the journal useful and important to "give us a large subscription list" to assure the *MSO*'s success.[75] Subscriptions for the monthly *MSO* cost two dollars per year (later reduced to one dollar) at a time when the weekly *Journal of the American Medical Association* cost five dollars.[76] Mindful of the future, Lynk also sent gratis copies of issue number one to all the black medical schools and charged half the price for student subscriptions.[77]

At first, by reading between the lines of the *MSO*, it appears that subscriptions came in at a reasonable rate. Lynk seemed surprised that prepublication publicity brought in "several actual subscriptions—even before the first number has been issued" and "encouraging letters . . . from scores of colored physicians."[78] Within about two weeks of the first publication, the supply of *MSO*s disappeared, because of both subscriptions and free distribution.[79] In the second issue, published in January 1893, Lynk announced, "So great has been the demand for copies of the initial number of the MEDICAL AND SURGICAL OBSERVER that we are forced to offer 20 cents per copy, in money or credit on subscriptions, for at least 150 copies" of that first issue.[80] People were reading the journal.

But not enough people were subscribing. A request for new subscribers became a regular feature of the *MSO*. In June, Lynk reduced the subscription price to a dollar

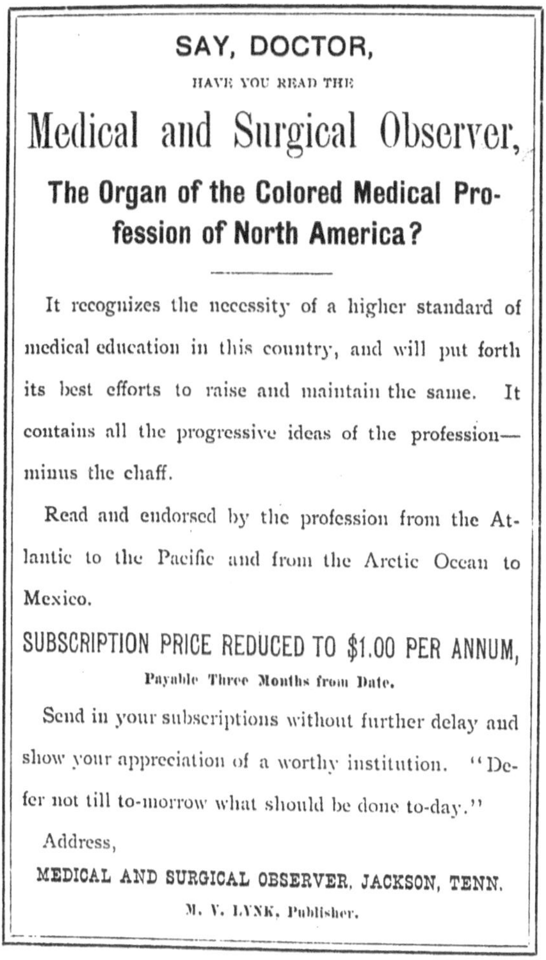

Fig. 22. An advertisement that appeared on the back cover of several issues of the *MSO*, intended to increase subscriptions. From *Medical and Surgical Observer* 1 (July 1893).

and made a special offer: "Subscribe for the OBSERVER. Wanted: Your name now. Dollar, 15th of next October."[81] Between July and November he pushed subscriptions and his special offer with a full-page notice that appeared on the *MSO*'s back cover. The advertisement reflects quite nicely Lynk's writing style, vision of the journal, and need for a stronger financial commitment from fellow and sister physicians. It first accosted physicians with, "Say, Doctor, have you read the MEDICAL AND SURGICAL OBSERVER, The Organ of the Colored Medical Profession of North America?" Referring to letters of praise received after the first issue of the journal, the ad continued: "Read and endorsed by the profession from the Atlantic to the Pacific and from the Arctic Ocean to Mexico." It concluded with an appeal and an offer: "SUBSCRIPTION PRICE REDUCED TO $1.00 PER ANNUM, Payable Three Months from Date. Send in your subscriptions without further delay and show your appreciation of a worthy institution." This advertisement appeared on the back cover of the *MSO* from July 1893 through January 1894.

Lynk claimed in the July issue, under the headline "Our Splendid Success," that the reduced price had caused a "grand rush" on subscriptions. "Today we find ourselves dum-founded [*sic*] because of the numerous applications for back numbers. Those who can furnish us with Nos. 1, 2 and 3, will confer a great honor."[82] A couple of pages later he proclaimed that "Hundreds of physicians have availed themselves of the opportunity to get the newest medical journal published and pay for it three months from date."[83] This boastful statement was followed by an even stronger and more confident one: "Subscribers. Don't fail to keep a file of the OBSERVER and have them bound. It being the first journal of its kind, published in America, will constitute a volume equally rare as it is interesting and instructive. Copies of the first issues are now at a very great premium."[84] By August, he was inserting brief reminders in the journal such as, "He who doesn't subscribe for the MEDICAL AND SURGICAL OBSERVER is a son of a gun,"[85] and, "Everybody reads the OBSERVER. Don't you?"[86] In addition to these methods of increasing subscriptions, Lynk also published letters of support for the journal. No records exist to discover whether people who signed up for the *MSO* in the summer of 1893 actually paid for it in October.

Reducing the *MSO*'s price from two dollars to one dollar may have increased readership and perhaps actual paid subscriptions, but revenues from advertising were also crucial to the financial stability of the journal. At first, a number of companies selling medical products and services, black medical schools, and journals placed advertisements in the *MSO*. Companies included Clemiana Chemical Co. of Atlanta, Georgia, selling medicinal plants; Bowden Lithia Springs Co., selling special water for drinking and bathing; Dr. H. A. Mumaw of Elkhart, Indiana, promoting his monthly listings of physicians', dentists', and druggists' property, books, and equipment available for purchase, rental, or exchange; Lambert Pharmacal Company of St. Louis, Missouri, featuring Listerine; Rumford Chemical Works of Providence, Rhode Island, selling Horsford's Acid Phosphate for Cholera; Parke, Davis & Co. of Detroit, Kansas City, and New York, advertising various medicinal preparations; and "Julius Fehr, M.D., Ancient Pharmacist," of Hoboken, New Jersey, selling his various talcum powders for infants and adults. A few white medical journals as well as two black newspapers (*The Appeal* of Chicago and *Indianapolis Freeman*) placed advertisements in the *MSO*, as did Howard University, Meharry, New Orleans University, and Leonard medical schools. Annual advertising rates listed in the December 1893 and January 1894 issues of the journal ranged from $100 for a full page and $60 for a half page to $35 for a quarter page, payable every three months.

Like paid subscriptions, advertising in the *MSO* appears to have been problematic. Some advertisers may have defaulted on payments. Some advertised for a limited amount of time and then dropped out, while others promoted their products or services from first issue to last. Of the twenty-eight different advertisers who purchased space in the *MSO*, three (Meharry, Leonard, and New Orleans University medical schools) appeared in all fourteen issues, two in thirteen issues, two in twelve issues, and three in ten issues. The remaining eighteen enterprises advertised six or fewer times. (It is not possible chronologically to trace the advertising that appeared in the *MSO* because the ads in the National Library of Medicine's issues were bound out of order at the end of the volume.)

Lynk lost one of his key advertisers after only four issues. Full-page ads on the back cover of the journal by Battle & Co. of St. Louis, a chemical firm that promoted three preparations (a hypnotic, an anodyne, and a combination alterative and uterine tonic), disappeared after April 1893. In May, the back cover of the *MSO* was blank except for the words "THIS SPACE FOR SALE." Lynk never again sold that space and eventually used it to promote the reduced subscription price of the journal and then to try to sell the space to potential advertisers. Using his usual upbeat tone and employing the typical exaggerated promotional language of the time, Lynk wrote, "ADVERTISERS, LOOK HERE! Do you want to advertise with a journal that will pay? Don't you believe for advertising to pay and do the greatest good you must use a medium that reaches the largest number of intelligent, enterprising and thoughtful physicians?" He went on to extol the wide circulation of the *MSO* and the breadth of the territory it covered, "the diameter of which is nearly 450 miles."[87] Starting in March 1893, Lynk, apparently concerned about losing advertisers and anxious to please them, wrote and inserted in the body of the *MSO* short pieces of two or three sentences about some of the regular advertisers:

> We call the special attention of our readers to the advertisement of the specialties kept by G. W. Powell, M.D., Moriah, NY. This is a reliable firm and physicians would do well to investigate his preparations.[88]

> The use of Ch. Marchand's Peroxide of Hydrogen and Glycozone should be tried by all physicians. Write to him at 28 Prince Street, N.Y., for circulars and information.[89]

> Dr. Julius Fehr's Compound Talcum Baby Powder is one of the best preparations that can be used for all affections of the skin. See his "ad" elsewhere.[90]

Unfortunately, these efforts at increasing subscription and advertising revenues did not save Lynk's enterprise from a relatively short life. Fourteen issues of the *MSO* went out to the African American medical profession, to interested white practitioners, to institutional subscribers such as the Surgeon General's library in Washington, D.C.,[91] and to other medical editors on exchange for issues of their journals. Then, following the appearance of the January 1894 issue and without fanfare, the first black medical periodical in the United States simply ceased publication. Hints of problems had emerged over time as the *MSO*'s average monthly length dwindled from a little more than twenty-six pages in the first four issues to half that amount in the next nine issues. The December 1893 edition contained just eight pages. Original articles, which numbered two or three per issue in the beginning months, diminished to one or none as the year progressed. The *MSO*'s final issue contained no explanation for the suspension of operations; it did not even announce the suspension.

What had happened to this promising journal, established with such high expectations and an ambitious agenda, in the space of a year? Why did this journal, which its founder and editor thought fulfilled a real need, disappear so quickly? Had Lynk misunderstood his fellow black physicians? Did he miscalculate the difficulty and time required to produce a medical journal? Had he simply tired of the enterprise?

One dollar seems a small amount to pay for a journal purportedly wanted by African American physicians. Yet even after "the grand rush" in June when the *MSO*'s price was halved, Lynk had to continue soliciting subscriptions. Why? Did the journal really fill the need Lynk felt was there? Lynk reproduced several letters of support for the journal, but these may not have represented the true feelings of the majority of the African American medical community of the time.

Did most black physicians want a journal of their own? In the distrustful and sometimes volatile racial climate of the early 1890s South, physicians of color may not have wished to single themselves out as unique or having special interests apart from the rest of the medical profession. They may have hoped for integration or at least little notice at a time when Lynk was promoting just the opposite. Perhaps the standard medical journals were sufficient for their need to keep up with the latest innovations and ideas, and they therefore felt little need for a separate, race-oriented periodical. Where Lynk saw two professions, one white and one black, other black doctors may have seen just one. African American physicians were trying to succeed in a previously and still overwhelmingly white medical professional world and may not have wished to draw attention to themselves.

Was Lynk's timing off? The *MSO* preceded the establishment of a national association of black physicians and failed perhaps because it arrived on the scene before a separate African American medical profession could manifest and organize itself. Black physician support for an African American medical journal did eventually develop after the National Medical Association had had a chance to form and gain strength. The *Journal of the National Medical Association* succeeded from its inception in 1909.

One outside force that may have affected the fortunes of the *MSO* was the financial panic of 1893. That economic catastrophe took its toll on most Americans, including, presumably, Lynk, *MSO* advertisers and subscribers, and black patients who could not pay their black physicians, who, in turn, lost spendable income. Furthermore, Lynk may have tired of the enterprise and wished to move on to another of the many projects that seemed to engage his interest during that first decade or so after becoming a physician. Certainly, overseeing the publication of a monthly journal required much time and effort. Lynk hinted at this problem in his autobiography, published in 1951: "[I]t was a pioneering venture. Pioneers clear the trees, throw up the highways and make straight the paths. Their tasks are hard because the average person hasn't caught the vision."[92]

Did others catch the vision? Lynk thought so. Looking back on his enterprise almost sixty years later, Lynk saw that what he had started in 1892 had made a difference in the history of African American physicians: "While the *Observer* has not been in the fight throughout, yet it is a scientific fact that a chain reaction is set in motion by the initial cause, sometimes apparently small."[93] If, by the term "chain reaction," Lynk meant the founding of other medical journals for African Americans, the evidence is not conclusive. It took only a few years—until 1898—for another pioneering African American physician, Alonzo McClennan of Charleston, South Carolina, to begin publishing the second black medical journal, the *Hospital Herald* (December 1898 through May 1900). McClennan, however, did not mention in the pages of the *Herald* that the *MSO* had served as a model or inspiration for his new enterprise. He also limited the scope of his journal to Charleston and the state of South Carolina rather than attempting to market it nationwide.[94] Several years later, in 1909, some members of the organization the *MSO* had called for in December 1892 and that Lynk had helped to found in 1895, the National Medical Association, produced the first issue of the *Journal of the National Medical Association*. The editors did not mention the *MSO* either.

The reasons that moved Lynk to cease publication of the *MSO* at the start of its second year may never be discovered. Nor is it possible to determine what effect the *MSO* had on the establishment of subsequent African American medical publications. Lynk may have laid the groundwork that, by example, quietly encouraged McClennan and the National Medical Association to attempt medical periodicals of their own. Whether openly acknowledged at the time or not, however, the *MSO* did influence a number of African American physicians to think about the needs and position of blacks in the medical profession during the late nineteenth century.

CHAPTER 21

Walking the Color Line

Alonzo McClennan, the Hospital Herald, *and Segregated Medicine*

The February 1899 issue of *The Hospital Herald* (*HH*), a black-owned monthly published in Charleston, South Carolina, carried a potentially inflammatory cover photograph. Replacing the previous cover picture of a refurbished nearly century-old Charleston-style building that housed a hospital and nurse-training school for African Americans was a photo of two physicians, one light-skinned, the other dark-skinned, at the bedside of a hospitalized African American patient, with African American nurses standing on the other side of the bed. This picture captured the *HH*'s multiple missions in racially tense late-1890s South Carolina: support of African American health professionals and medical institutions; education of African American laypeople about health, disease, and the need to patronize black health professionals and medical institutions; and biracial cooperation in matters of health. For a year and half, from December 1898 to May 1900, as segregation tightened around the state, the *HH* published articles promoting these causes.

Just how aptly this cover scene represented the journal's mission was revealed in the *HH*'s fifth issue (April 1899), in which the editor included an explanation of the picture. A year before the photograph was first published, on the evening of Monday, February 21, 1898, a mob of whites set fire to the black postmaster's home in Lake City, near Florence, South Carolina, then shot family members as they tried to escape from the burning building, killing the postmaster and his infant son and injuring the man's wife and three other children. This violence occurred because Lake City's white citizens strongly opposed the federal appointment of a black postmaster in their town. By Friday evening of that week the surviving members of the Baker family were residing and receiving medical care

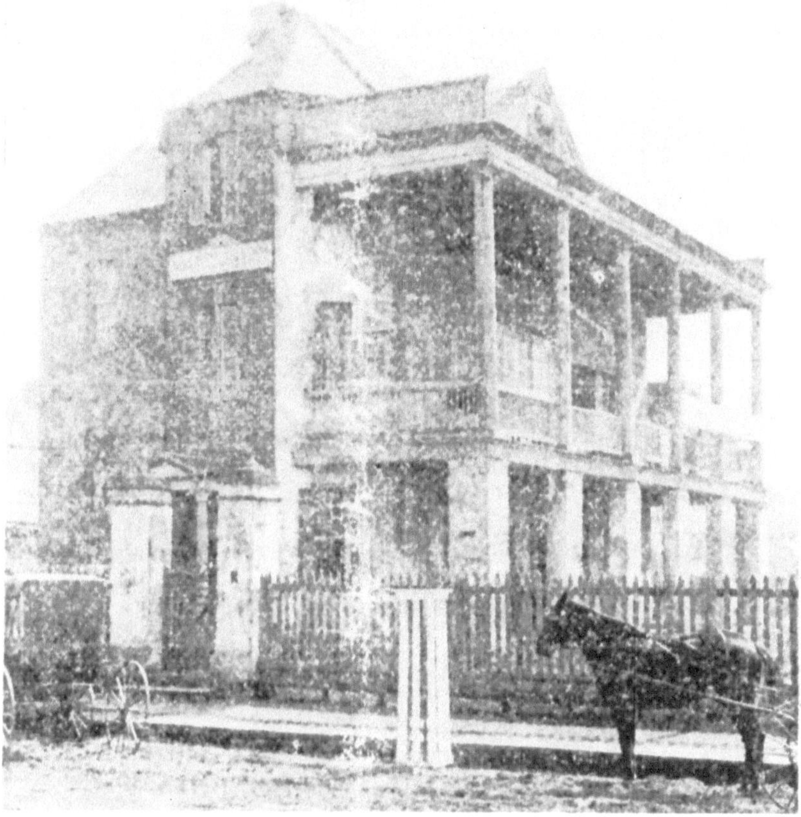

Fig. 23. Photograph of the Hospital and Training School for Nurses in Charleston that appeared on the cover of the first two issues (December 1898 and January 1899) of the *Hospital Herald*. From the *Hospital Herald* 1:6 (May 1899).

at the recently established black hospital in Charleston pictured on the first two *HH* covers. Mrs. Lavinia Baker, the murdered postmaster's wife, was the patient shown on the revised cover,[1] and the light-skinned physician was the African American founder of both the hospital and the *HH*, Alonzo C. McClennan (1855–1912). The nurses in the picture were students at the black nurse-training school McClennan had established two years earlier, in January 1897. McClennan used those two cover photographs to announce the presence of a black hospital, black nurse-training school, black journal, and black medical practitioners to his fellow citizens, African American and white, in segregated, sometimes violent, race-conscious South Carolina. In publishing the Baker picture, McClennan walked a fine line between speaking out against injustice and retaining biracial support for the black medical enterprises he was developing.

McClennan was not the first black physician to publish a health-related journal dedicated to serving African Americans. A few years earlier, between

The Hospital Herald.

A MONTHLY JOURNAL DEVOTED TO HOSPITAL WORK, NURSE TRAINING, DOMESTIC AND PUBLIC HYGIENE.

TERMS, 50 CENTS PER YEAR IN ADVANCE. SINGLE COPIES 5 CENTS.

VOL. I. JUNE, 1899. No. 7

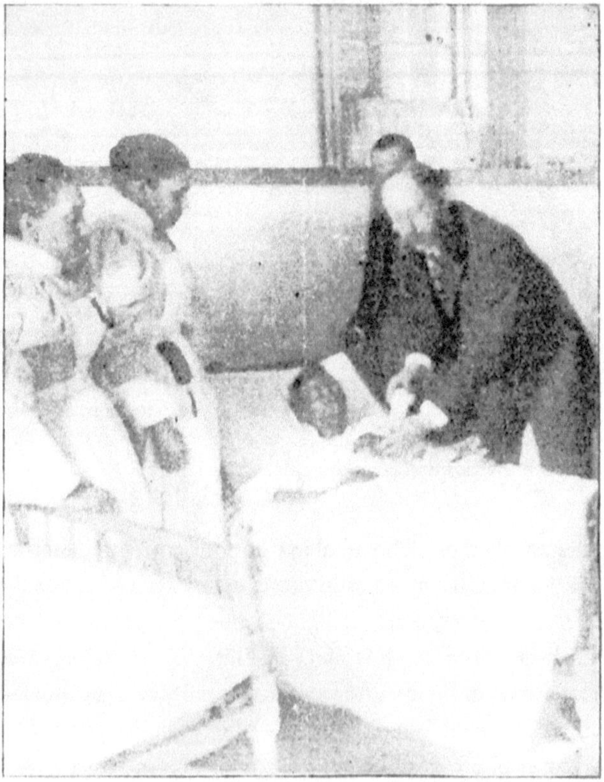

Fig. 24. Photograph that appeared on the cover of the third and several subsequent *Hospital Herald* issues of Dr. Alonzo McClennan (foreground), another African American physician, and two African American nursing students caring for Lavinia Baker at the Hospital and Training School for Nurses, Charleston. From the *Hospital Herald* 1:7 (June 1899).

December 1892 and January 1894, Miles Vandahurst Lynk (1871–1956), a recent graduate (1891) of Nashville's Meharry Medical College, had produced fourteen issues of the *Medical and Surgical Observer* [*MSO*] in Jackson, Tennessee.[2] Lynk's goal had been different from McClennan's: he intended from the start to publish a national journal aimed at black physicians, hoping to fill a gap he saw in contemporary medical journals. No local, state, or national medical journal focused on the needs of African American doctors. Until the appearance of the *MSO*, this group had no "journal of our own," as one subscriber wrote to Lynk after receiving his first issue. Articles in the *MSO* contained medical information for physician care of patients and news about other black physicians around the country and region. Only a few articles overtly broached issues of poverty, antiblack bias, and the everyday concerns African American physicians and patients faced in a white-dominated society. Lynk used the pages of the *MSO* to call for the establishment of a national medical organization for black doctors (the National Medical Association [NMA] was founded just a few years later, with Lynk as one of its leaders) and to serve as the official organ for an association of North Carolina African American physicians. He aimed the messages and articles at a professional audience.

McClennan, in contrast, had more local goals in mind. In the increasingly tense and exclusionary racial climate of 1890s South Carolina, he acted firmly and determinedly to provide the means, in the sphere he knew best—medicine—for African American laypeople, health professionals, and medical institutions in his city and state to survive and perhaps even to move forward. Between 1896 and 1900, McClennan established or helped establish a statewide physicians' association, a nurse-training school, a hospital, and a monthly journal to support and promote those organizations. Two statements on the *HH*'s masthead summarized McClennan's intentions: "A journal devoted to hospital work, nurse training, domestic and public hygiene," and, beginning with issue 8, July 1899, "Official Organ of the Association of Colored Physicians of South Carolina." The *HH* was not, strictly speaking, a medical journal. It published no scientific articles on the latest advances in medicine, surgery, drug therapy, or dentistry. The *HH* informed its eclectic readership of laypeople and various health professionals about matters such as good health practices in the home, fund-raising efforts for McClennan's hospital and nurse-training school, hospital and nursing school activities, hospital board and area black physician association meetings, and the effect of local and regional race issues on African American citizens' health.

The problem McClennan and Lynk and all other African Americans faced in the late-nineteenth-century South was exclusion from the white-dominated medical establishment. Hospitals either excluded or segregated black patients and barred black physicians from admitting and thus caring for their patients who required surgery or other advanced supervised medical care. Nurse-training and medical schools refused admission to African American students. Hospitals also prevented black nursing and medical students from gaining clinical experience on their wards, even when those facilities were publicly supported by white and black citizens' tax dollars. Local, state, and national medical societies refused to accept African Americans as members. Medical journals failed to address concerns of African American physicians and rarely reported on black physicians' activities. There would have been no need for the establishment of separate black medical journals, nurse-training schools, hospitals, medical schools, or medical societies had the racial climate in the South been different. But, owing to racial exclusion, African Americans in the various health fields had to establish their own networks and institutions in parallel with and duplicative of those already in existence in the white medical world.[3]

South Carolina in the 1890s was one of the most racially repressive and unwelcoming states for black health professionals and institutions in the nation. In 1890 it ranked second from the bottom among Southern states (only Alabama was lower) in the ratio of African American citizens per African American physician. Thirty years later it held that same ranking (see Appendix, Table 7).[4] Black medical students and physicians knew the state's reputation, and most chose to practice elsewhere. As Charles F. Meserve, the white president of Leonard Medical School in Raleigh, North Carolina, explained in an 1897 letter to a citizens' group in one South Carolina town hoping to recruit a graduating medical student to settle there: "I appreciate what you say about the need of a Colored physician in your locality. The fact is, Colored physicians do not desire to settle in South Carolina. You, of course, understand why without my saying anything further. I wish it were not so."[5]

Alonzo McClennan, however, disregarded the state's reputation and, after completing his education, chose to return to his South Carolina roots to practice medicine. He had encountered racial problems during his educational career. Born in Columbia, South Carolina, in 1855, McClennan was orphaned young and raised by his uncle, a well-known local barber. He received sporadic schooling, including brief attendance at Columbia's Benedict Institute, before becoming a page for a black state legislator in 1872. When that legislator won election to Congress he appointed McClennan, who had taken the competitive qualifying examination, to the Naval Academy in Annapolis in 1873. The young cadet, the third African American to win a place at the Naval Academy, had a difficult time dealing with the open racism he experienced at the hands of cadets and faculty. He withdrew under trying circumstances in January 1874, enrolled for a short time at Wesleyan Academy in Massachusetts, and finally matriculated at South Carolina College (the future University of South Carolina) in his hometown of Columbia. McClennan entered South Carolina College when it was integrated in 1875, but had to leave a year later when the collapse of Reconstruction allowed

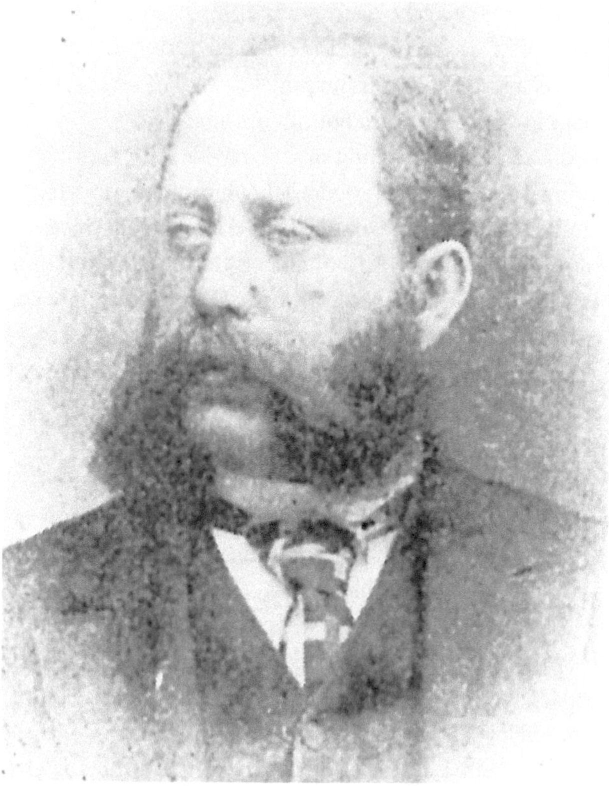

Fig. 25. Dr. Alonzo C. McClennan, founder and editor-in-chief of the *Hospital Herald*, founder and surgeon-in-charge of the Hospital and Training School for Nurses, Charleston. From the *Hospital Herald* 2:2 (February 1900).

the school to become a segregated institution once again. Concluding that, as he wrote in an 1897 autobiographical statement for the Charleston *Sunday News*, "there were some other places in this country where it was a little more comfortable" to obtain an education than Columbia, McClennan made a new career choice and decided "to take the train and go to Washington [D.C.] to commence the study of my chosen life-work—medicine."[6]

McClennan spent three years at Howard University, studying medicine from 1877 to 1880 and pharmacy from 1879 to 1880.[7] Equipped with both M.D. and Phar.D. degrees, he entered private practice in Augusta, Georgia, where he met and in 1883 married Ida V. Ridley, a schoolteacher from a socially prominent local black family. The following year the couple moved to Charleston where the light-skinned, blue-eyed, fair-haired physician and his light-skinned wife became part of the city's black aristocracy. McClennan's practice flourished, as did his People's Pharmacy, opened in 1892.[8] Despite these successes, McClennan, like his African American medical contemporaries throughout the South, could not escape the issue of race as the color line stiffened during the 1890s. In response, McClennan took a leadership role, helping to establish several medical institutions for blacks in Charleston and South Carolina.

He first assisted in the founding of a statewide African American medical association. As a physician of color, McClennan could not join the local or state medical societies.[9] Exclusion meant that he and his African American colleagues were barred from meetings in which members developed professional relationships and learned from exchanges of information, both formal and informal. (White physicians also, of course, lost out, missing the collegiality and experiences of black physicians.)[10] In an attempt to remedy this isolation of the approximately thirty African American physicians distributed across South Carolina in the 1890s, McClennan and three colleagues organized in 1896 the Association of Colored Physicians of South Carolina (also referred to as the South Carolina Association of Colored Physicians, in 1900 renamed the Palmetto Association of Physicians, Pharmaceutists and Dentists of South Carolina).[11]

The idea of forming statewide black medical societies as a means of supporting African American physicians did not originate in South Carolina. In 1886, black Texas physicians founded the Lone Star State Medical Association in Galveston;[12] in 1887, a similar group established the North Carolina Medical Association (later renamed the Old North State Medical Society);[13] and in 1893, the Colored Medical Association of Arkansas was organized.[14] All three groups received coverage in Miles Lynk's *MSO*. Charles Catlett Johnson (1860–1928) of Columbia, the prime force behind the South Carolina Association of Colored Physicians, was a member and corresponding secretary of the North Carolina Medical Association as early as 1893 and a subscriber to the *MSO* when the North Carolina Medical Association invited Virginia and South Carolina health professionals to the 1893 annual meeting "for the purpose of considering the advisability of an inter-state organization,"[15] and when Lynk called for the founding of a national black physicians' organization. Johnson was concerned about the problems black physicians faced as they entered a profession previously dominated by white physicians and felt the need to found a medical association in South Carolina.[16]

Johnson may have been encouraged by the existence of these three other state organizations and the founding of the NMA in 1895 in Atlanta to propose establishing such a group in South Carolina the following year. The four founders of the Association of Colored Physicians of South Carolina were Johnson, James R. Levy of Florence, Lawrence A. Earle of Anderson, and Alonzo C. McClennan of Charleston.[17] McClennan inserted reports and encouraging editorials about the association in the *HH*, providing most of what is known about the group between late 1898 and mid-1900.

The second and third black medical institutions that McClennan founded, and that the *HH* supported, a nurse-training school and a hospital in Charleston, had their inception in the same year as the establishment of the Association of Colored Physicians of South Carolina. They were an early part of a wave of black nurse-training-school and hospital foundings around the country. Just as the growth of black physician numbers in the 1880s and 1890s spurred the recognition of a need for African American medical societies, so too the rapid development of nursing as a profession to assist physicians and patients both in homes and hospitals spurred appreciation among many African Americans of the need for black nurses. Black women also saw nursing as an economic opportunity. The Charleston nurse-training school was the ninth black institution of its kind in the country.[18]

The Charleston school had its beginnings in the fall of 1896 when McClennan, seeing "an imperative need for an institution in Charleston to train colored young women as nurses,"[19] brought together the five other African American physicians then practicing in Charleston to discuss the possibility of establishing a nurse-training school. They, with one exception, pledged to support the work, as did the one black dentist in town. On January 15, 1897, the Charleston Training School for Colored Nurses opened, offering lectures in a room at the Wallingford Academy on Meeting Street.[20] The white-owned *Charleston News and Courier* predicted success for the school based in part on McClennan's good reputation: "Dr. McClennan has many friends among the white race in this city and they will watch with the closest interest his work for the Training School."

Problems arose, however, regarding race and the clinical training of black nursing students. "We soon saw," McClennan recalled a few years later, "that it would be impossible to properly instruct those who came to us for training without giving practical demonstration at the bedside."[21] The initial plan to provide clinical training using patients of the physicians involved in the school failed. McClennan then proposed to the local commissioners of public lands that the school provide medical and nursing care for inmates at the Ashley River Asylum (also known as the Old Folks' Home) where, according to a newspaper report, "the physicians connected with the Training School will be willing to attend the negroes in the Home free of charge, the same as the [white] Medical College physicians attend the sick at the City Hospital."[22] The commissioners turned McClennan down, as did the city authorities when he asked that a ward in the city hospital be made available to the nurse-training school.[23] (A year later, in 1898, the city council appropriated $4,500 for a white nurse-training school at the city hospital and allowed nurse-training students from this school, called the Charleston Training School for Nurses, to assist in the care of patients at the city-owned Riverside Infirmary.)[24] In response, McClennan felt "compelled" to establish another parallel medical institution for African Americans—the hospital pictured on the cover of the *HH*'s first two issues that came to be known as the Cannon Street Hospital.[25]

Opening and operating a hospital proved to be a much greater undertaking than starting a nurse-training school. A permanent building equipped for patient care as well as for education and student residence was now needed. McClennan mobilized his allies and reached out to the black and white communities of Charleston for help. He formed a corporation that obtained a charter for the school and hospital and organized a Hospital Association to support the institution. The group located a suitable building and refurbished it. Churches, individuals, and business and professional people, primarily black but also some white, donated money and needed items, including beds, linens, furniture, supplies, and food to the cause. The building, at 135 Cannon Street, cost $4,500, $1,500 of which was required at purchase, and $500 annually thereafter, plus interest. The owner relented somewhat on the contract and allowed immediate transfer of the property to the Hospital Association with payment of $500 of the $1,500 on the promise of paying the other $1,000 within a year. By early November 1897 the building was ready to receive patients and nurse-trainees.[26]

A reporter for the *Charleston News and Courier* visited the hospital just after it opened. "With the opening of the Hospital a new field of labor is afforded the better class of colored people, and it promises to be fruitful of good results," he wrote. "The purpose of the school is to train colored men and women, so that they can be placed in charge of hospital wards, and give the same careful attention to patients as white nurses." He described the inside of the building, mentioning a "comfortable office," nurses' dining room, kitchen, operating and lecture rooms, male and female wards, "ward for the nurses [living in the hospital]," and a moderately well-stocked dispensary for outpatient care. The reporter also mentioned the many donations already made and the continuing need for more: "The school wants one more upward pull. It was a hard struggle to raise the money to buy a building and equip it for a hospital. This, however, has been done and with a little more assistance it will be made complete in every respect."[27] Money would always be an issue for the hospital and school. Alonzo McClennan emphasized this theme as well as issues of race and the health of African Americans when, just over a year after dedicating the hospital and nurse-training school building, he launched his next undertaking, the *HH*, a medical journal to support all the black institutions he had so far helped create in South Carolina.

The initial issue of the *HH* greeted readers shortly after Christmas 1898. After a quick perusal of its contents, readers could readily identify the journal as a production of people deeply involved with Charleston's black Hospital and Training School for Nurses: the cover displayed a photograph of the refurbished hospital and nurse-training school building, the masthead announced the *HH* as "A Monthly Journal Devoted to Hospital Work, Nurse Training and Domestic

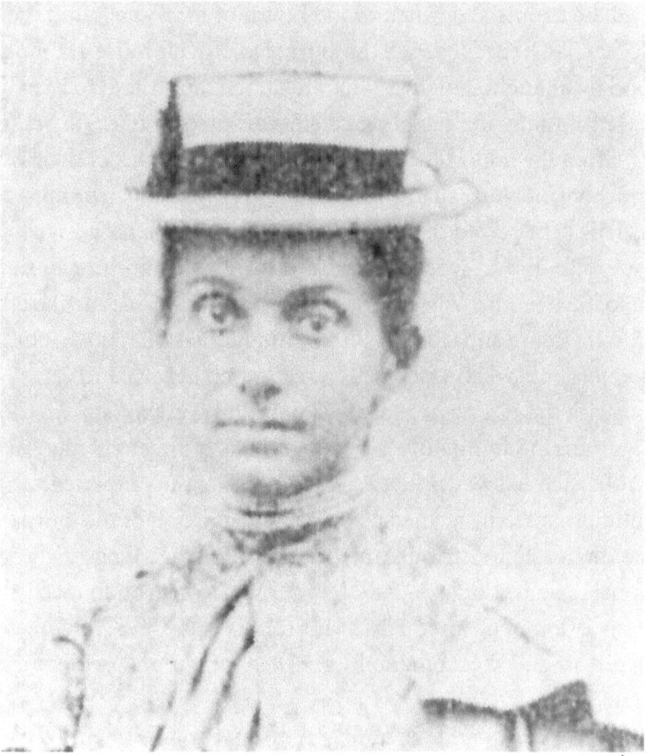

Fig. 26. Dr. Lucy H. Brown, assistant editor of the *Hospital Herald* and faculty member at the Hospital and Training School for Nurses, Charleston. From the *Hospital Herald* 1:10 (September 1899).

and Public Hygiene," and one full page listed Hospital Association officers, executive committee and advisory board members, Training School faculty, and hospital staff. Further confirming this connection, the names of the editor-in-chief (Alonzo C. McClennan, M.D., Phar.D.) and two associate editors (Lucy Hughes Brown, M.D., and Robert J. Macbeth, D.D.S.) also appeared on the list of Hospital Association officers/executive committee members and of the Training School faculty (McClennan taught surgical nursing and hygiene, Brown taught obstetrical nursing and care of infants, and Macbeth taught anatomy and physiology). Every subsequent *HH* issue contained this same information (though the cover picture changed, as mentioned earlier, pushing the hospital building picture to an inside page and eventually entirely out of the journal) along with a one-page "Announcement to the Public" about the hospital/training school's founding, purpose and patient charges, and a list of the enterprise's financial needs.[28]

McClennan set the tone for the journal in his "Greeting" on page one. "It is not the object of the *Hospital Herald*," he wrote, to seek "comparison with . . . the great journals of medical science" already in existence. Rather, "the *Hospital*

Herald will be a journal devoted to the health of individuals and the community." McClennan hoped through the journal to provide nurse-training students with "food for thought and digestion" and at the same time "to keep before the [medical] profession and the public the necessity for *trained* nurses to care for the sick." Given the importance of trained nurses, the work of the Hospital and Training School for Nurses had great significance. McClennan promised that "the public will be kept posted through these columns of the progress of the work." In that way also, those "who are giving [donations] from time to time will be gratified to learn . . . that what they give is bearing fruit." He thanked those who donated to the cause and closed with a reminder that "the subscription price of the *Hospital Herald* will be fifty cents a year payable in advance."[29]

Fitting with the *HH*'s practical and community orientation, McClennan invited physicians to submit not research or scholarly pieces but manuscripts that shared with "their fellow workers . . . the benefits of their experience."[30] Though the promotion of scientific medicine was not a mission of the journal, promotion of South Carolina's African American physicians and their newly established professional organization was. The *HH* was, McClennan announced, the "organ of the Association of Colored Physicians of this State" and would include each month a picture and short biographical sketch "of one of the colored physicians in the State."[31]

For their five-cents-an-issue or fifty-cents-a-year investment *HH* readers received a bound and printed pamphlet of approximately sixteen pages containing three or four pages of advertisements from local and regional white and black business sponsors, eight to ten pages of text, an information sheet about the Hospital and Training School for Nurses, and occasional fillers such as train schedules and Charleston monthly mortality returns by race. They could count on reading a lengthy and provocative editorial about some current health issue often relating to race. Shorter articles or sections contained practical information for healthy living and discussions of community and public health needs, as well as hospital and nursing school news. Always there were mentions of fund-raising wants and successes. Physicians and nurses could find professional notes and activities of the state association of colored physicians. With so broad a mission and so mixed a readership the *HH* faced an editorial challenge much different from the *MSO*'s, with its clearly defined audience of African American physicians.

HH articles about African American health addressed a variety of subjects directed at these different audiences. Some took the form of editorials aimed at revealing health and health care disparities between the races and at motivating black laypeople to use black health care personnel and institutions. Others explained medical conditions or provided medical advice. Some were a sentence or two in length, others continued for several pages. The editors tried to educate African American laypeople about basic good health practices, nursing students about the provision of good patient care, and physicians about patient needs and expectations. Pithy pieces of health advice were mixed with articles about, for example, the importance of the trained nurse, the care and preservation of teeth, the value of massages, the need to cleanse one's spirit as well as one's body each spring, the physician's dilemma of when to inform family members of a patient's impending death, the significance of water to the body, the nature of influenza, and rules for physicians governing consultations.

In addition to health matters affecting African Americans, two other sometimes overlapping and conflicting subjects found their way into every issue of the journal: money and race. Confronting race issues in the *HH* too bluntly could undermine McClennan's carefully crafted biracial fund-raising efforts to support black medical institutions.

Money

Because the city contributed nothing toward the maintenance of the hospital and nurse-training school, the expense for this project, which duplicated already existing facilities and institutions in Charleston, fell almost entirely to the black community. Keeping the nurse-training program running and the hospital from defaulting on its mortgage payment each year were McClennan's and thus the *HH*'s chief concerns. Secondary but by no means minor concerns addressed in the *HH* included furnishing the hospital with food, medical supplies, linens, operating room equipment, gas, electricity, and telephone lines. Every issue of the *HH* discussed some aspect of these matters.

By unrelentingly yet inventively mentioning financial matters whenever it could be slipped into an article or notice, the *HH* made the survival of the Hospital and Training School for Nurses a community project and a matter of pride for African Americans around the region. The Hospital Association served as fund-raising arm and governing board. It was composed of leading black citizens, while its advisory board included both blacks and whites, all of whom contributed their own financial and human resources but also reached out to gain support from others in the general public. The *HH*'s arrival added a new dimension to these efforts, supplementing word-of-mouth, community fair, and buttonholing approaches already in use. McClennan's journal publicized the work to a larger, more literate, geographically wider, and probably wealthier audience than before, thus enlarging the "community" from which funds could be raised.[32] The Hospital Association's president recognized the *HH*'s contribution in his annual report for 1899: "The advent of *The Hospital Herald* has been very timely. It has not only been the medium of information of our work, but has brought in much funds to the Association. Long may it live to continue its good work."[33]

McClennan's editorial skills created a sense of community ownership of the Hospital and Training School for Nurses. He included in each issue of the *HH* a statement called "The Needs of the Hospital" that asked readers to search their consciences: "In asking for means to carry on this work we feel that we only have to appeal to the common sense and love of fair play that characterizes the best people of this country." A list of the specific amounts required for various aspects of the hospital's operations then followed. He concluded with an appeal to people's hearts and to race consciousness ("Every penny you give will do something toward the relief of suffering and toward training some deserving colored woman in an honorable and useful profession"), but also with an unspoken invitation to become part of a community striving together toward an admirable and attainable goal ("Who will send us ten dollars, five dollars or one dollar to assist in liquidating this indebtedness. This great work is dependent upon the gifts of friends for its support and the expenses can be met in no other way").[34]

McClennan promoted the cause wherever and however he could. The *HH* reported on trips he made to Washington, D.C.,[35] Tuskegee, Alabama,[36] and cities around South Carolina,[37] where, even if conducting other business, he always managed to make a fund-raising pitch for the hospital and school. McClennan was skillful in creating a sense of belonging among those who donated and those who read his journal or heard him speak. He also made people feel they were donating to a worthy cause that would improve the lives of all. On the first anniversary of the *HH*, he emphasized that "in this work, where we expect the pennies and the dimes to count up [to] the hundreds and the thousands, we must have every one feel that they are giving a helping hand."[38]

That all-embracing style may have made contributors of both races and at all economic levels feel comfortable regardless of the amount or kind of donation they gave. Gifts of money, goods, or services were equally recognized in the *HH*'s columns. Everyone who gave, it seemed, was mentioned and thanked by name.[39]

The *HH* brought in one form of revenue that would otherwise not have been available to the Hospital Association—advertising dollars. Every issue of the journal contained an array of thirty to forty advertisements from both black and white business owners and from the two leading African American medical schools in the country, Howard and Meharry. Even if the ads did not bring in large sums of money to the *HH* (no mention of advertising rates appeared in the journal), the message of community was again broadcast to readers: these advertisers were supporters of the black-owned and black-run hospital and nurse-training school in Charleston, South Carolina.

McClennan used advertising to obtain materials for a free children's clinic sponsored by the hospital he planned to open in mid-1899. He solicited and received drugs and medical supplies from Northern pharmaceutical companies whose names he readily acknowledged in the *HH*: "The donation of surgical supplies sent by Messrs. Johnson & Johnson, of New Jersey, is the largest received. This firm is certainly generous and is deserving of the patronage they receive from all parts of the country."[40] Other companies that sent medicines received endorsement of their products.[41]

The Hospital Association sponsored an annual fund-raising fair each fall, publicized even more widely when the *HH* began publication. The *HH*'s pages contained public thanks to those who participated or gave large contributions and used stories from the fair to encourage others to donate. Editor McClennan particularly singled out two white members of the Hospital Association's advisory board for recognition, apparently in hopes of motivating other white Charleston citizens of means to become involved. Of one he wrote: "Mr. A. C. Kaufman . . . is large hearted and is interested in all institutions that are being established for the uplifting of our people. It is a great pity that we did not have a thousand in Charleston that think and act as he does."[42] McClennan also thanked a local white businessman, J. F. Lochrey, manager of the Atlantic and Pacific Tea Store, who "left a wad before he left distributed with the table holders, raffle books and voting lists. Our people should patronize this business, and show that we appreciate his liberality."[43]

The community enterprise nurtured in the pages of the *HH* included one other group whose contributions the journal regularly recognized—students. According to Surgeon-in-Charge McClennan's annual report for 1898–99, published in the *HH*, the hospital had two sources of revenue: fees collected from patients admitted for treatment and funds collected from "nurse service in private families and in the St. Francis [Xavier] Infirmary" (a Catholic hospital run by the Sisters of Our Lady of Mercy). The "nurse service" was staffed by nurse-trainees from the school when they were not in class or fulfilling their regular responsibilities at the hospital. The income earned from that employment went not to the students but to the Hospital and Training School to pay for board, lodging, uniforms, shoes, and laundry.[44] Any of those funds not applied to student expenses were directed toward supporting the hospital's other needs. The *HH* recognized students for their efforts in both bringing income to the institution and conveying a positive image of the Training School to their (usually white) employers, who were, of course, potential donors. Typical of McClennan's comments in the *HH* was, "Mrs. Catherine Bowen who was nursed by Miss Whaley [a student] when so critically ill has returned to Boston, Mass. She promises to stir up Boston in behalf of the hospital and the *Herald*."[45] Another notice read: "Drs. J. S[omers] Buist and John L. Dawson expressed themselves as highly pleased with our student nurses who have been recently with patients of theirs."[46] The nursing students gave an additional gift to the institution, as announced in the *HH* just before the first class graduated in the spring of 1899: "The 'Gatling Gun' Club of nurses are making great preparation for their entertainment. The proceeds of the entertainment will

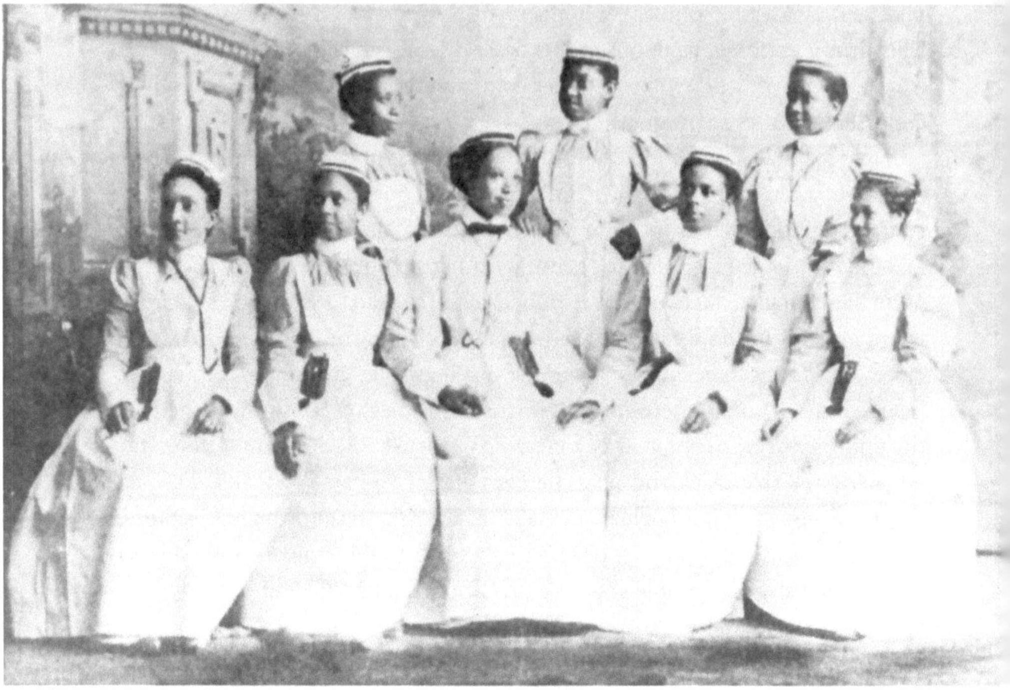

Fig. 27. The first graduating class of the Hospital and Training School for Nurses, Charleston, 1899. From the *Hospital Herald* 1:7 (June 1899).

be devoted to the purchase of an operating table. This will be the donation of the present graduating class as a parting gift to the Hospital."[47] The succeeding class planned to raise money to purchase a sterilizer for the operating room.[48]

The other regular source of revenue for the hospital, in addition to collections from the nurse service, was patient fees.[49] The "Announcement to the Public" inserted into every issue of the *HH* stated that "the object of this institution is not for the purpose of making money, and charges for medicines, nourishments, nursing, etc., are made merely to meet the ordinary running expenses of an institution of this kind." However small the fees charged, patients in the hospital meant income to run the hospital as well as clinical experience for the nurse-trainees. Notices in the *HH* named new patients and encouraged black and white physicians and trained nurses in the region to send patients to the hospital. Those who did received a public thank you in the journal and thus became part of the support community.[50]

One white Charleston physician stood out to McClennan and the Hospital Association as a sustaining ally. Charles W. Kollock specialized in ophthalmology and performed cataract and other surgeries on patients at the hospital, always without charge.[51] In the last issue of the *HH*, McClennan recognized Kollock, this time, however, "for the remarks he made in the white Medical Association commending our work and advising physicians to patronize the Hospital. Dr. Kollock has given valuable aid to our work."[52]

Financial support for the Hospital and Training School for Nurses extended beyond the borders of South Carolina, often north of the Mason-Dixon line. Though the financial panic and depression of the 1890s, the temporal distance from Reconstruction, and urban problems caused by a rapid increase in immigration from central and eastern Europe had diverted Northern attention and money from the former slaves' needs, some groups and individuals continued to help.[53]

McClennan, however, hoped to raise most of the money for the hospital from within South Carolina. In July 1899 he wrote an editorial strongly opposing the plan recently revealed by members of the black community in Columbia to organize a nurse-training program there. Fearing that such an effort would drain funds from the Charleston project and leave the state with no black hospital or nursing school at all, McClennan called for cooperation rather than rivalry. He believed that "there is a desire on the part of the people of this State to contribute towards the fund to purchase the [Charleston hospital] building and to assist in establishing and supporting the work." Rather than using money obtained from the North, McClennan argued for local fund-raising so South Carolina's citizens could say that "one [black] institution at least was paid for through money collected from them. We are not opposed to Northern philanthropy or the blessed charity that has been bestowed upon the South since the end of the civil war up to the present time. But let us exhaust our efforts at home before we go beyond the borders of the State."[54] A few months later the *HH* reported that "Rev. Richard Carrol, who sometime ago published that he intended opening a hospital and training school in connection with his work at Columbia, . . . had abandoned the project and would do what he could for our work."[55]

By the following February, McClennan had changed his view about funding. In another editorial he announced, "We have found it impossible to raise all the money needed to meet our obligations from local contributions, and we now appeal to those outside our city and State who are able and willing to help a deserving cause."[56] Once again McClennan used the pages of his journal to create a biracial sense of community, this time an even more far-flung one, to save the parallel medical institutions he had been forced to create in the harsh racial climate of South Carolina.

Race

Whereas readers of Miles Lynk's *MSO* could go for many pages before being reminded about the matter of race, *HH* readers could not avoid it. The *HH* could not be mistaken for anything but an African American journal. For the most part, McClennan wrote about race matters neutrally (e.g., matter-of-factly mentioning the skin color of individuals in articles about nonracial topics) or positively, showing the best side of African American health practitioners and institutions and promoting interracial cooperation for the good of both groups. But McClennan and other *HH* authors also spoke out in the journal about perceived racial injustices in health and medicine, though they had to keep in mind the interracial financial and moral support the journal, hospital, and nurse-training school received.

The *HH* published several pieces on Charleston's striking black/white mortality rate differential, beginning in the journal's first issue (December 28, 1898), with a commentary titled "Negro Mortality," by Robert J. Macbeth, a prominent black dentist in Charleston and strong supporter of McClennan's projects. Macbeth set a tone of frankness in *HH* editorials by challenging city health authorities on two counts. First, noting that the mortality rate for blacks at city health facilities was twice that of whites at the hospital and more than three times the white rate at the dispensary (a free or low cost outpatient clinic), he concluded that "hospital and dispensary treatment are much more fatal to colored than to white patients." Macbeth argued that the higher death rate among African Americans had to do with inadequate living conditions: "The poor people and especially the colored live in the low lying sections of the city, where the drainage is poor, and often in alleys where the well, the [privy] vault and the drain are within a few feet of each other." Their poverty forced them to eat "tainted meat, stale vegetables, and fish that is smelt long before it is seen." He concluded, "It is not strange" that the [African American] death rate is large under such conditions."[57]

Four months later, the *HH* pushed these issues one step further when the city health department's 1898 annual report showed a worsening from the previous year of the comparative mortality between Charleston's black and white populations, both overall and in the city's hospitals and dispensaries. The *HH* challenged health authorities to act rather than just report or lament this problem: "We trust that those who profess to be interested in the welfare of our people, may study the facts and figures we have given, and see if something can be done to lower this alarmingly high death rate."[58]

McClennan drove home his point the following month in a third editorial, three pages in length. He conceded that though poverty and "ignorance and a disregard of the laws of hygiene" were certainly causes of the high death rate among the poor in cities like Charleston, it was, however, "in the power of the city governments ...

to see that these places [where people live] are kept in a strictly sanitary condition, that they have an abundant supply of good wholesome water, and that they are not overcrowded." In addition to looking more carefully at the sanitary condition of their city so that the poor are healthier, McClennan suggested, Charleston city authorities should, based on the differential in mortality statistics for whites and blacks at city health institutions, scrutinize the medical care provided the poor at these facilities. Though he was careful to say that he was "not making the charge that it *does*" cause more harm than good among Charleston's black citizens, McClennan did put the idea before his readers that the failings of the city dispensary system was an issue to be pursued. "We could pile up instances upon instances where it has come to our knowledge of [dispensary physicians] giving inhuman and indifferent treatment to cases that should have special care and attention."[59] McClennan was walking a fine line here between advocating for his constituents and antagonizing powerful members of the white community who supported and even donated to his hospital and nurse-training school.

Another issue of racial justice raised in the *HH* involved perceived bias against African American candidates standing for state medical licensure exams around the country. Dr. J. A. Lightner, a recent graduate of Leonard Medical School in Raleigh who had opened a practice in Camden, South Carolina, wrote an article in the January 1900 *HH* calling for a national licensing exam in order to eliminate what he believed were unfair practices in many state licensing boards against black and poor white candidates. "Had all physicians had my personal experience [not described in the article] they would do all in their power to have a Federal Medical Law." Besides being unfair to African American graduates of medical schools, he wrote, the bias he asserted occurred in some states deprived black patients of medical care: "There are many Northern cities crying for negro doctors and because of these . . . State boards the [black] doctors cannot go to the call." Lightner called for an open discussion of the issue in the pages of the *HH*,[60] but a brief editorial note in the next issue of the *HH* seemed to indicate that other African American physicians in the state were either unwilling to address the issue openly or not as concerned about this matter as Lightner. "Colored men have made a good record before the State board," McClennan wrote, "and the percentage of failure and success compare favorably with white candidates." McClennan indicated that black physicians in South Carolina "are perfectly satisfied to go into the examinations . . . as long as there is no discrimination on account of color."[61] No other responses appeared in the journal. Was McClennan covering up an issue, choosing his battles carefully, walking a tightrope, or dismissing a matter that, from his perspective, simply was not a concern?

The *HH* editors were in an awkward position with regard to race issues. They were rightfully concerned about the city of Charleston's and the rest of white South Carolina's commitment to maintaining or improving the health of its

African American citizens, especially as the color line openly hardened during the late 1890s in all aspects of life, including health. Yet the *HH*'s fund-raising efforts on behalf of the hospital and nurse-training school depended on the generosity and goodwill of whites. Perversely, the very necessity for fund-raising, that is, the establishment and maintenance of a parallel medical system for South Carolina's black citizens, was directly related to the racist attitudes of whites. McClennan and his colleagues courted whites on the one hand and cautiously spoke out against white racism on the other. They provided readers with examples of interracial cooperation on area health concerns, listing names of white contributors to the nurse-training school, hospital, and journal and identifying white physicians who sent patients to the hospital, but also wrote editorials exposing racist attitudes and practices.

Some *HH* articles reflected the editors' awareness of the need to raise funds from South Carolina's segregated society. When, for example, McClennan called on the then current president and fellow founder of the South Carolina Association of Colored Physicians, Dr. Lawrence Earle, in Earle's hometown of Anderson, in 1899, the *HH* story about the visit emphasized interracial ties: "We were welcomed cordially, especially by the white people, who seemed to have a special interest in the hospital and training school. Dr. Earle has the good will of *all* the white people, and the good will and *all* the practice of the colored people."[62] The need to raise funds among Anderson's whites appeared to be lurking just beneath the surface of this article. When that same year McClennan visited Dr. James Babcock, superintendent of the state's hospital for the insane in Columbia, an institution that had a poor reputation for its care of African American citizens, the *HH* article had nothing but praise for Babcock, calling the state "fortunate in having at the head of this institution a physician who has all the elements that make the good physician and humanitarian." It made note of "the excellent care and treatment our people receive in this model institution" and announced that the superintendent "has promised his cooperation in our work and we hope to have one of his nurses take the course at our hospital." The need to ignore race differences in care provided at the asylum in order to promote a possible relationship between the Charleston and Columbia institutions apparently outweighed McClennan's desire to speak out against the asylum's inferior conditions for blacks.[63] The editors walked cautiously along the color line in their need to maintain parallel medical institutions for African Americans in Charleston and South Carolina.

Another financial issue with racial overtones was the concern of black physicians, nurses, pharmacists, and dentists in South Carolina for gaining the patronage of reluctant black citizens. African American health professionals, most only recently graduated, along with the hospitals, schools, and organizations needed to support them in the increasingly segregated South had to win the confidence of a clientele unused to them. Black physicians faced a two-front battle against disease and death, Dr. Charles C. Johnson of Columbia told the first graduating class at the black Hospital and Training School for Nurses in Charleston in 1899. They had to "fight against the unjust prejudice in the opposite race and the silly lack of confidence still to some extent found among some members of our own race."[64] *HH* articles took two tacks in dealing with this issue, touting the success and competence of black practitioners and medical institutions while also urging black citizens to utilize practitioners and medical institutions of their own race.

The first pages of the February 1899 *HH* contained a strongly worded editorial urging support of fellow African Americans. It began by referring readers to an article several pages later: "We reprint in another column resolutions adopted at the Preachers Union in Columbia calling upon the citizens to patronize the colored drug store in that city." McClennan praised the union's act as a sign that "in one part of the State at least the effort is being made by united action to assist a business that has so much to contend with in opposition and depends almost entirely upon race patronage." Too often, he explained, leaders say one thing and do another, as, for example, urging people to "patronize your own," but then not doing so themselves. "We cannot hope to amount to much as a people, especially in business and the professions," McClennan warned, "unless we have a sufficient interest in our own young men who depend upon us to give them encouragement and support." Generally, he continued, "If it were not for the poorer classes who have always shown more loyalty to our enterprises, much more so than those who are fortunate to be in better circumstances, the professional and business man would be failures."[65]

Dr. C. C. Johnson of Columbia pursued this theme a few pages later in an article titled "The Need of Colored Physicians." In the early years of their practices, white doctors "get their entire support from our people. We feed and clothe them and furnish them cases for experimental purposes while they are getting themselves advertised among whites." Once they achieve status and gain white clientele, he continued, "they begin to drop the colored. They have climbed by a ladder and they kick it away after they do not need it any more." Black physicians, he argued, did not have that option. Their clientele was fixed. "The colored physician must begin and, whether he wants to or not, must end with colored patrons." Since the state had passed a law in 1898 requiring segregated seating on railway coaches[66] "there is at least one white physician in Columbia who has set up a jim crow waiting room at his office." That action "should cause sober thought" to African Americans and encourage them to choose physicians of color over white doctors.[67]

Continuing this black self-help theme, McClennan included in the same *HH* issue an editorial criticizing people who opposed or who failed to assist institutions that educated trained nurses. Writing, no doubt, with his own struggling nursing school in mind, McClennan asserted it was "the duty of every one to do all in his power to lend a hand in making" such institutions a success because "these institutions are doing inestimable good to communities" and because "in cases that require skillful nursing and handling their services cannot be estimated."[68]

McClennan reprinted sympathetic articles from other publications to reinforce his cause of supporting black medical undertakings. A story he quoted from the *Aiken Herald* about the opening of the 1899–1900 term at and the recent graduation of nine new nurses from McClennan's nurse-training school, for example, publicized the school's significance for African Americans and hoped that the institution would "become fully known and appreciated by every intelligent colored family in this State. It is an opening into new fields of activity for young women who aspire to independence and self-support."[69] An article reproduced from the *Charleston Messenger*, a local African American newspaper, offered additional reasons why "every self-respecting negro in the city" should support "the Colored Hospital on Cannon street" and demonstrated how intertwined the success of black health professionals and black health institutions were. Because black physicians could not practice at the city hospital, the Cannon Street facility allowed black physicians "an opportunity of diagnosing critical cases," broadening their clinical experience, and thus of honing their clinical skills to be better physicians to their patients. "Therefore," the article concluded, "the destiny of the colored physicians rests within the walls of the Colored Hospital and should be encouraged."[70]

Many issues of the *HH* described instances of African American medical patronage or opportunities for such patronage. Some items simply mentioned the patients who were admitted to the Cannon Street hospital or the names of the African American or white physicians or nurses who had referred them.[71] Others were full descriptions or articles. When, for example, John McFall graduated from the Philadelphia College of Pharmacy and opened his own business in Charleston, McClennan announced it in the *HH* in the form of a challenge: "This store will offer an excellent opportunity to some of our race men to give this young man a mite of the share of prescriptions and assist our own when it is needed and appreciated."[72] Lawson Scruggs, one of the first graduates of Leonard Medical School in Raleigh (1886), wrote an article about the value of sanitariums in arresting or curing tuberculosis and ended it with an invitation to those readers affected by the disease to visit his establishment at Southern Pines, North Carolina. Scruggs was the general manager and founder of the Pickford Sanitarium for Consumptive Negroes. McClennan endorsed Scruggs's work a few pages later, saying the Raleigh physician "has succeeded in establishing an institution where colored persons can go and receive scientific treatment when suffering with consumption. Dr. Scruggs is the only colored physician in this country who has made a special study of the germ theory, as it relates to tuberculosis."[73] Six months later McClennan again added a word of his own, urging black physicians to send their patients to Pickford: "We hope that colored physicians will take pride in recommending this institution as the only one in this country where negroes are received and given special treatment."[74]

This matter of establishing and supporting black medical enterprises was obviously a keen concern of McClennan's. He led a discussion on the question "Should we encourage the establishing of hospitals for our people?" at the second annual meeting of the Association of Colored Physicians of South Carolina in April 1898[75] and, in the anniversary issue of the *HH* in November 1899 answered that question with an emphatic yes: "The time has come when it is a necessity for colored physicians to establish hospitals and infirmaries in towns where there are three or four physicians."[76] A long article a few months earlier provided *HH* readers with an example of such an undertaking in Washington, D.C., and of the person behind its success, Dr. John R. Francis.[77]

The sixteenth and last issue of the *HH* appeared in May 1900. The editors nowhere in that issue hinted that this would be its last. Whereas Miles Lynk's *MSO* showed signs of failure toward the end of its run in the early 1890s by its shorter length, constant editorial appeals for more subscribers, reduction of subscription price, fewer advertisers, and increased number of reprinted articles from other journals, the *HH* exhibited none of those indicators, save occasionally appealing for new subscribers and skipping publication in December 1899 and April 1900. McClennan wrote no farewell editorial. Did the work of editing and producing a lively, readable publication month after month become more than he could sustain? Did age or illness cause him to cease publishing? That some people understood and appreciated the *HH*'s goals is revealed in a letter to the editor from a Manning, South Carolina, resident, Robert A. Stewart, dated January 2, 1900, and printed in the January issue. Stewart wrote to explain why he was sending money for a subscription to the journal. His first reason was for general principles, "as a contribution towards carrying on the humane work it represents." His second reason was more practical: "Because it enables me to gain such information, as will enable me at times to keep the doctor away," by "taking advantage of its hints and advices." Stewart's final reason related to race: "For the general information it sends forth of new progress and its ascendant aims to better the race and develop race enterprises and its much needed patronage on all sides, it should have and deserves the aid of every one of us."[78]

McClennan tried, in the sixteen issues of his journal, to balance interracial cooperation on needed local black health enterprises forced to exist because of racial bias and segregation with reporting of perceived racial injustices in matters of health. Though the *HH* lasted only a short time, the Cannon Street Hospital and nurse-training school continued operating into the 1950s, and the Palmetto Medical Society is still in existence.

Appendix

Table 1

Leading Known Causes of Death In Virginia, 1850[a], by Race[b]

White (N = 8,014)[c]	Percentage	Slave (N = 6,284)[c]	Percentage	Free Black (N = 558)[c]	Percentage
1. Tuberculosis[d]	13.8	1. Respiratory diseases[e]	16.1	1. Cholera[j]	17.2
2. Respiratory diseases[e]	9.2	2. Tuberculosis[d]	10.7	2. Tuberculosis[d]	13.8
3. Nervous system diseases[f]	8.6	3. Nervous system diseases[f]	7.9	3. Respiratory diseases[e]	10.0
4. Diarrhea[g]	8.5	4. Old age	7.3	4. Old age	7.9
5. Scarlet fever[h]	6.9	5. Dropsy[i]	6.0	5. Dropsy[i]	7.5
6. Dropsy[i]	5.5	6. Typhoid[k]	5.7	6. Nervous system diseases[f]	6.5
7. Cholera[j]	4.9	7. Diarrhea[g]	5.5	7. Diarrhea[g]	5.9
8. Typhoid[k]	4.7	8. Cholera[j]	5.5	8. Accidents[n]	5.8
9. Old age	4.5	9. Accidents[n]	4.5	9. Typhoid[k]	2.9
10. Digestive system diseases[l]	4.5	10. Digestive system diseases[l]	3.2	10. Digestive system diseases[l]	2.5
11. Diphtheria[m]	3.5	11. Diphtheria[m]	2.3	11. Whooping cough	2.5
12. Accidents[n]	3.4	12. Suffocation[q]	2.2	12. Maternity[o]	2.0
13. Maternity[o]	2.1	13. Scarlet fever[h]	2.0	13. Worms	2.0
14. Measles	1.5	14. Worms	1.8	14. Teething	1.3
15. Whooping Cough	1.4	15. Maternity[o]	1.8	15. Diphtheria[m]	1.1
16. Neoplasms[p]	1.2	16. Measles	1.6	16. Intemperance	1.1
17. Heart disease	0.8	17. Teething	1.5	17. Malaria[r]	0.7
18. Teething	0.8	18. Whooping cough	1.5	18. Scarlet fever[h]	0.7
19. Worms	0.8	19. Homicide	0.9	19. Measles	0.5
20. Erysipelas	0.7	20. Heart disease	0.6	20. Homicide	0.5
Fevers (unclassifiable)[s]	6.5	Fevers (unclassifiable)[s]	5.5	Fevers (unclassifiable)[s]	4.6

a. Includes figures from the entire state. Compiled from *Mortality Statistics of the Seventh Census of the United States, 1850* (Washington, D.C., 1855), 291–95.

b. All figures are percentages of the total number of deaths for that race during the designated time period. Causes listed as "unknown" were excluded from the computations.

c. The numbers in parentheses reflect the total number of deaths from all known causes for that race. Only leading causes are listed for each race.

d. Consumption, scrofula

e. Asthma, bronchitis, catarrh, catarrhal fever, influenza, disease of lungs, pleurisy, pneumonia

f. Apoplexy, disease of brain, chorea, congestion of brain, convulsion, epilepsy, brain fever, inflammation of brain, insanity, neuralgia, paralysis, disease of spine

g. Cholera infantum, diarrhea, dysentery, summer complaint

h. Scarlet fever, disease of throat, quinsy

i. Dropsy, hydrothorax, ascites

j. Cholera epidemics struck Virginia during the period covered by this census.

k. Typhoid was referred to as typhus fever in the list of causes of death in the 1850 census.

l. Disease of bowels, colic, cramp, dyspepsia, hernia, inflammation of bowels, inflammation of stomach, jaundice, disease of liver, piles, disease of stomach

m. Croup

n. Burns, drownings, scaldings, explosions, shootings, railroad, unspecified

o. Childbirth, puerperal fever

p. Cancer, tumor

q. Many of these deaths are probably attributable to what is know now as crib death or Sudden Infant Death Syndrome (SIDS).

r. Intermittent fever, remittent fever

s. Bilious fever, congestive fever, inflammatory fever, fever not specified

Table 2. North Carolina Mutual Life Insurance Company of Raleigh : Data Sheet on Slave and White Policies, 1850–64

For year ending	6/20/ 1850	6/20/ 1851	6/20/ 1852	6/20/ 1853	1854	5/31/ 1855	5/31/ 1856	5/31/ 1857	5/31/ 1858	5/31/ 1859	5/31/ 1860	5/31/ 1861	5/31/ 1862	5/31/ 1863	5/31/ 1864
Total policies in force	610	1,161	1,464		2,083	2,288	2,308	2,193	2,167	2,239	2,200		1,528	1,394	1,206
White policies in force								500	492		501			425	387
Slave policies in force								1,693	1,675		1,699			969	819
# White losses[1]	1	1	5	6	6	10	10	8	6	5	8	7	7	9	8
# Slave losses[1]	1	10	10	17	25	21	31	17	23	19	25	20	16	13	17
White losses/ 100 white policies								1.60	1.20		1.60			2.12	2.07
Slave losses/ 100 slave policies								1.00	1.37		1.47			1.34	2.08
Money on hand	23,565	46,117	60,911	75,419	91,346	89,754	100,250	114,113	142,180	175,198	191,516		202,027	214,603	209,505
Paid on white losses[1]	1,000	5,000	17,000	22,000	19,000	34,200	25,968	28,283	15,716	14,350	26,000	25,500	19,000	39,000	24,000
Paid on slave losses[1]	400	5,288	5,660	9,132	14,170	13,712	19,116	11,300	14,433	13,200	17,816	14,666	12,533	10,567	14,366
Average paid / white loss	1,000	5,000	3,400	3,667	3,167	3,420	2,597	3,535	2,619	2,870	3,250	3,643	2,714	4,333	3,000
Average paid / slave loss	400	529	566	537	567	653	617	665	628	695	713	733	783	813	845

Information was drawn from annual reports and manuscipt minutes of the company. Blank spaces indicate that information was not available.

1. The company paid losses ninety days following claim. Deaths filed later than March 31 of each year (beginning in 1852) were included with figures for the following fiscal year (which began on June 1)

Table 3. Slave Life Insurance Premiums of Franklin Slaughter, Insurance Broker (1849)* and North Carolina Mutual Life Insurance Company (1849, 1851, 1852)**

Annual Premium per $100 of Insurance

	For One Year				For Five Years			
	Franklin Slaughter	N.C. Mutual			Franklin Slaughter	N.C. Mutual		
Age at Next Birthday	1849	1849	1851	1852	1849	1849	1851	1852
10	$1.28	$1.18	$1.37	$1.60	$1.64	$1.30	$1.51	$1.77
20	1.36	1.24	1.44	1.67	1.73	1.38	1.61	1.88
30	1.57	1.41	1.65	1.93	1.98	1.59	1.85	2.18
40	1.95	1.77	2.07	2.41	2.35	1.97	2.30	2.68
50	2.98	2.70	3.14	3.66	3.49	3.00	3.50	4.18
60	5.65	5.10	5.95	6.94	6.26	5.66	6.60	7.70

*Grinnan Family Papers, Box 8, Folder 20, Manuscript Department, University of Virginia Library, Charlottesville

**North Carolina Mutual Life Insurance Company, *Life Insurance: Its Principles, Operations and Benefits* (Raleigh, N.C.: 1849), 23; North Carolina Mutual Life Insurance Company, *Second Annual Report* (Raleigh, N.C.: 1851), 22; *Third Annual Report* (Raleigh, N.C.: 1852), 21.

Table 4. Black Medical Colleges, 1868–1923

Name	City	Year Opened	Year Discontinued	Affiliation
Howard University Medical Dept.	Washington, D.C.	1868	—	None
Lincoln University Medical Dept.	Oxford, Pa.	1870	1874	Presbyterian (local)
Straight University Medical Dept.	New Orleans, La.	1873	1874	American Missionary Assn.
Meharry Medical College	Nashville, Tenn.	1876	—	Methodist Episcopal
Leonard Medical School of Shaw Univ.	Raleigh, N.C.	1882	1918	Baptist
Louisville National Medical College	Louisville, Ky.	1888	1912	Independent
Flint Medical College of New Orleans University	New Orleans, La.	1889	1911	Methodist Episcopal
Hannibal Medical College	Memphis, Tenn.	1889	1896	Independent
Knoxville College Medical Dept.	Knoxville, Tenn.	1895	1900	Presbyterian
Chattanooga National Medical College	Chattanooga, Tenn.	1899	1904	Independent
State University Medical Dept.	Louisville, Ky.	1899	1903 (merged with LNMC)	Colored Baptist (Ky.)
Knoxville Medical College	Knoxville, Tenn.	1900	1910	Independent
University of West Tennessee College of Medicine and Surgery	Jackson	1900	1907	Independent
University of West Tennessee College of Medicine and Surgery	Memphis	1900	1923	Independent
Medico-Chirurgical and Theological College of Christ's Institution	Baltimore, Md.	1900	1908?	Independent

Table 5. UWT Graduates[1] by Year of Graduation

1904 (3)	
Cason, Willis	Weldon, Ark.
Christopher, F. E.	Gregory, Ark.
West, Edward W.	Ferguson, Ark.
1905 (6)	
Burnley, F.[2]	Wynnwood, Okla.
Hargrove, S. H.	Helena, Ark.
Henry, L. H.	Tatums, Okla.
Lowe, J. J.	Tatums, Okla.
Mitchell, C. G.	Tenn.
Shelton, G. A.	Whiteville, Tenn.
1906 (4)	
Bryant, D. W.	Dorceyville, La.
Chandler, J. J.	Wewaka, Okla.
Lee, William A.	Mantee, Okla.
Wall, T. L.	Taft, Okla.
1907 (3)	
Banks, G. W.	Newelton, La.
Paxton, William A.	Weldon, Ark.
Thomas, A. W.	Trenton, Tenn.
1908 (9)	
Cook, F. L.	Hartshorn, Okla.
Dorman, P. J.	Mantee, Okla.
Hawkins, E. T.	Atlantic City, N.J.
Haynes, G. W.	Braggs, Okla.
Henderson, N. H. C.	Memphis, Tenn.
Hose, J. W.	Memphis, Tenn.
Newman, F. R.	Memphis, Tenn.
Waytes, W. J.	Jackson, Tenn.
Winchester, John W.	Memphis, Tenn.
1909 (8)	
Davis, D. W.	Somerville, Tenn.
Howard, Z. M.	Halls, Tenn.
Jones, Elisha H.	Talladega, Ala.
Lavender, T. H.	Florence, Ala.
Leftwich, L. W.	White Springs, Fla.
Richards, S. W.	Ark.
Thompson, E. N.	Memphis, Tenn.
West, T. H.	Holdenville, Okla.
1910 (6)	
Carr, J. D.	
Dunbar, Mason W.	
Prince, S. H.	Memphis, Tenn.
Smith, Oncey H.	Ardmore, Okla.
Tinsley, Conn.	
Young, Wm. E.	

1911 (8)

Freeland, J. B.	Dyersburg, Tenn.
Jones, D. W.	
Mitchell, B. A.	
Scurry, B. C.	
Smith, C. E.	
Thomas, H. A.	Memphis, Tenn.
Vaughn, L. E.	
Williams, E. J.	

1912 (9)

Dillard, C. E.	
Heman, T. W.	Columbia, S.C.
McNeil, L. W.	
Moore, C. M.	
Moore, W. R.	Cartersville, Ga.
Ransom, T. M.	
Thomas, D. J.	Memphis, Tenn.
Wakefield, M. H.	
Walker, M. G.	Somerville, Tenn.

1913 (13)

Arrington, B. L.	
Beckett, J. W.	Memphis, Tenn.
Borum, S. A.	
Cannady, N. O.	
Douglass, F. L.	
McComb, W. S.	
Myers, L. H.	Jacksonville, Fla.
Priece, Joseph Antonia	Bocas del Toro, Panama
Richardson, C. W.	
Roberts, J. A.	
Ross, F. K.	
Strother, W. A.	
Williams, J. R.	

1914 (25)

Brakeen, Thomas C.	Beaumont, Tex.
Branch, Dennis[3, 4]	Newport, Tenn.
Edwards, James T.[3]	St. Louis, Mo.
Felder, W. W.	
Fortune, Fred W.[3]	Philadelphia, Pa.
Green, Henry H., Jr.[3]	
Greenlee, B. N.	
Gregg, E. J.[3]	St. Louis, Mo.
Hatcher, Bernard M.[3]	Baltimore, Md.
Howell, Raymond G.[3]	
Johnson, George W.[3]	
Lane, Willard M.[3]	Washington, D.C.[3]
Martin, Prince E.[3]	
McCleave, Benjamin F.[3]	Memphis, Tenn.
McMillan, Henry T.	Memphis, Tenn.
Moore, Samuel E.[3]	St. Louis, Mo.
Patterson, R. H.	

Pope, J. E.	
Reese, Thomas H.[3]	
Seabrook, Herbert U.[3]	
Smith, R. Stillmon[3] [5]	Macon, Ga.
Walker, Theodore L.[3]	St. Louis, Mo.
Walthall, Solomon L.[3]	
Watson, Norman M.	Memphis, Tenn.
Wooden, Henry W.[3]	
1915 (26)	
Bell, James E.[3]	
Blize, Parham	British Honduras
Bridges, William Cullen[3]	St. Louis, Mo.
Buckley, D. W.	
Cheeseborough, W. B.	
Crosby, E. W.	
Dancy, W. C.	Sedalia, Mo.
DeVane, William P.[3]	Oxford, N.C.[6]
Dorsey, Jackson S.[3]	
Harris, James T.[3]	
Jaques, Jefferson S.[3]	St. Louis, Mo.
King, D. W.	Wichita Falls, Tex.
Levy, James W., Jr.[3]	
Madison, Waite H.	Marshall, Mo.
Moore, I. E.	
Pack, Seba E.[3]	Louisville, Ky.
Patterson, ?	Bastrop, La.
Perry, John Sinclair[3] [7]	Washington, D.C.
Richardson, Reginald G.	Jefferson City, Mo.
Robertson, Samuel P.	New Orleans, La.
Speight, William O., Jr.[3] [8]	Memphis, Tenn.
Thurman, F. D.	St. Louis, Mo.
White, James E.[3]	
Wilder, J. L.	St. Louis, Mo.
Wilkerson, James W.[3]	St. Louis, Mo.
Wilkinson, G. D.	
1916 (10)	
Blii, Maa	Cape Palmas, Liberia
Cox, T. E.	Washington, D.C.
Grandberry, Dorsey B.	
Horrington, M. H.[3]	
Johnson, Leandrew A.	Memphis, Tenn.
Lewis, Motea M.	Richmond, Va.
Moore, F. A.	
Mynns, F. A.	Brocton, Mass.
Prioleaux, S. W.[3]	
Rickman, W. T.	
1917 (4)	
Ellis, N. D.	
Etter, E. A.	Galveston, Tex.
Harrel, B. D.	Memphis, Tenn.
Kennedy, E. A.	Washington, D.C.

1918 (6)	
Alston, L. C.	Mesa, Ariz.
Capehart, LeRoy R.	Chattanooga, Tenn.
Elmore, J. W.	
Lacey, W. P.	Brownsville, Tenn.
Lemore, J. H.	Murfreesboro, Tenn.
Red, R. K.	Pueblo, Colo.
1919 (4)	
Magsino, Margarette	Lippa, Phillipines
Mallari, Ysabella	Mexico, Lonce, Phillipines
Sanders, Hobart M.	Haskell, Okla.
Wood, J. L.	Newbern, Tenn.
1920 (1)	
Ford, Cosby	Taft, Okla.
1921 (6)	
Briggs, D. W.	
Cobb, Jackson Silas	Pueblo, Colo.
Henry, Edna P.	Taft, Okla.
Lee, T. H.	
Outten, E. C.	Memphis, Tenn.
Tirado, P. A.	
1922 (4)	
Hawkins, Clayton L.	Denver, Co.
Lewis, C. E.	
Lewis, W. M.	
Wyksell, J. C.	Brazil

1. Source: Memphis *Tri-State Defender,* Jan. 1, 1955, 9.

2. Not on alumni list in Memphis *Tri-State Defender,* Jan. 1, 1955, 9. Name found on alumni list in UWT Catalog, 1906–07, 14.

3. Transferred from Leonard Medical School in 1914

4. *Journal of the National Medical Association* 50 (1958): 387.

5. *Journal of the National Medical Association* 58 (1966): 145–47.

6. Lynk, *Sixty Years,* 78–87.

7. *Journal of the National Medical Association* 55 (1963): 83–84.

8. *Journal of the National Medical Association* 50 (1958): 387; 57 (1965): 71.

Table 6. Black and White Physicians in Southern States and Selected Southern and Northern Cities, 1890 and 1920

Location	1890			1920		
	Black Physicians* (no.)	White Physicians (no.)	Black Physicians (% of all physicians)	Black Physicians (no.)	White Physicians (no.)	Black Physicians (% of all physicians)
United States	909†‡	103,482†	0.9†‡	3,495†	125,666†	2.7†
Southern States						
Alabama	28	1,798	1.5	106	2,137	4.7
Arkansas	70	2,224	1.8	150	2,183	6.4
Delaware	2	231	0.9	7	253	2.7
Florida	12	620	1.9	118	1,261	8.6
Georgia	40	2,343	1.7	228	3,027	7.0
Kentucky	42	3,214	1.3	155	2,844	5.2
Louisiana	38	1,212	3.0	94	1,816	4.9
Maryland	37	1,663	2.2	66	2,186	2.9
Mississippi	34	1,624	2.1	66	1,576	4.0
Missouri	28	5,225	0.5	200	5,614	3.4
North Carolina	46	1,488	3.0	125	1.983	5.9
Oklahoma	0	217	0	122	2,424	4.8
South Carolina	30	1,099	2.7	85	1,257	6.3
Tennessee	102	3,283	3.0	327	2,851	10.3
Texas	54	4,286	1.2	217	5,783	3.6
Virginia	39	1,892	2.0	178	2,179	7.6
West Virginia	4	1,022	0.4	56	1,653	3.3
Southern Cities						
Atlanta, Ga.	6†	205†	2.8†	41	456	8.2
Baltimore, Md.	28	764	3.5	53	1,381	3.7
Kansas City, Mo.	10	473	2.1	52	891	5.5
Louisville, Ky.	12	400	2.9	47	484	8.9
Memphis, Tenn.	14†	140†	9.1†	83	329	20.1
Nashville, Tenn.	24	187	11.4	68	218	23.8
New Orleans, La.	18	281	6.0	30	598	4.8
Richmond, Va.	6	144	4.0	28	317	8.1
St. Louis, Mo.	2	787	0.3	106	1,607	6.2
Washington, D.C.	87	642	11.9	130	998	11.5
Northern Cities						
Boston, Mass.	8†	1,156†	0.7†	31	1,681†	1.8†
Chicago, Ill.	11	1,783	0.6	209†	5,143†	3.9†
Cleveland, Ohio	6	482	1.2	27	854	3.1
Detroit, Mich.	3	372	0.8	28	1,291	2.1
Indianapolis, Ind.	8†	307†	2.5†	29	612	4.7

Location	1890 Black Physicians* (no.)	1890 White Physicians (no.)	1890 Black Physicians (% of all physicians)	1920 Black Physicians (no.)	1920 White Physicians (no.)	1920 Black Physicians (% of all physicians)
New York (Manhattan)	14	3,192	0.4	78†	5,517†	1.4†
Philadelphia, Pa.	15	2,095	0.7	95†	3,309†	2.8†
Pittsburgh, Pa.	4	340	1.2	27	976	2.7

Source: U.S. Census, 1890 and 1920.

Note: Unless otherwise indicated, figures are for males only. In only a few states and cities did the published census data provide statistics for female physicians by race. In 1890, 4.3 percent of white and 12.7 percent of "colored" physicians were female. In 1920, 2.7 percent of white and 1.9 percent of black physicians were female.

* The occupation listings of the 1890 Census grouped blacks, Indians, and persons of Chinese and Japanese descent into one racial category labeled "colored." (California alone listed 260 "colored" physicians, most of whom must have been of Asian descent. Most "colored" physicians in the South were of Negro descent.)

† Includes both males and females

‡ The 1890 Census distinguished "Negroes" and "Colored" in this instance.

Table 7. Black and White Citizens per Black and White Physicians in Southern States and Selected Southern and Northern Cities, 1890 and 1920

Location	Black Citizens per Black Physician 1890*	Black Citizens per Black Physician 1920	Change in Ratio (%)	White Citizens per White Physician 1890	White Citizens per White Physician 1920	Change in Ratio (%)
United States	8,403†‡	2,994†	-64.4	531†	755†	+42.2
Southern States						
Alabama	24,232	8,497	-64.9	464	677	+45.9
Arkansas	7,728	3,148	-59.3	368	586	+59.2
Delaware	14,193	4,334	-69.5	606	761	+25.6
Florida	13,848	2,792	-79.8	363	506	+39.4
Georgia	21,470	5,291	-75.4	418	558	+33.5
Kentucky	6,383	1,522	-76.2	495	767	+54.9
Louisiana	14,716	7,450	-49.4	461	604	+31.0
Maryland	5,829	3,704	-36.5	497	551	+10.9
Mississippi	21,840	14,169	-35.1	335	542	+61.8
Missouri	5,364	891	-83.4	484	574	+18.6
North Carolina	12,196	6,107	-49.9	709	900	+26.9
Oklahoma	0	1,225	0	271	751	+177.1
South Carolina	22,964	10,173	-55.7	420	651	+55.0
Tennessee	4,222	1,382	-67.3	407	662	+62.7
Texas	9,040	3,418	-62.2	407	683	+67.8
Virginia	16,293	3,877	-76.2	539	743	+37.8
West Virginia	8,173	1,542	-81.1	714	842	+17.9
Southern Cities						
Atlanta, Ga.	4,683	1,532	-67.3	183†	302	+65.0
Baltimore, Md.	2,397	2,044	-14.7	481	453	-5.8
Kansas City, Mo.	1,370	591	-56.9	251	329	+31.1
Louisville, Ky.	2,388	853	-64.3	331	402	+21.5
Memphis, Tenn.	2,050†	737	-64.0	255†	307	+20.4
Nashville, Tenn.	1,224	524	-57.2	250	379	+51.6
New Orleans, La.	3,583	3,364	-6.1	631	478	-24.2
Richmond, Va.	5,388	1,930	-64.2	341	371	+8.8
St. Louis, Mo.	13,433	659	-95.1	540	437	-19.1
Washington, D.C.	869†	846	-2.6	241†	328	+36.1
Northern Cities						
Boston, Mass.	1,016†	527†	-48.1	381†	435†	+14.2
Chicago, Ill.	1,297	524†	-59.6	609	503†	-17.4
Cleveland, Ohio	498	1,276	+156.2	536	892	+66.4
Detroit, Mich.	1,144	1,459	+27.5	544	737	+35.5
Indianapolis, Ind.	1,142†	1,196	+4.7	314†	457	+45.5
New York (Manhattan)	1,686	1,399	-17.0	467	393	-15.8
Philadelphia, Pa.	2,652	1,413	-46.2	480	510	+6.3
Pittsburgh, Pa.	1,963	1,397	-28.8	678	564	-16.8

Source: U.S. Census, 1890 and 1920.

Note: Unless otherwise indicated, figures are for males only. (See note, Figure 23.)

* The occupation listings of the 1890 Census grouped blacks, Indians, and persons of Chinese and Japanese descent into one racial category labeled "colored."

† Includes both males and females

‡ The 1890 Census distinguished "Negroes" and "Colored" in this instance.

Table 8. Black Medical Societies in the United States, 1914–15

National
- National Medical Association

State and Regional
- Alabama Medical, Dental, and Pharmaceutical Association
- Arkansas Medical Association
- Central Pennsylvania Medical Society
- Flat Top Medical Association of West Virginia
- Florida Medical, Dental, and Pharmaceutical Association
- Georgia State Medical Society
- Indiana Association of Physicians, Dentists, and Pharmacists
- Kentucky Medical, Dental, and Pharmaceutical Association
- The Lone Star Medical, Dental, and Pharmaceutical Association (Texas)
- Louisiana Medical, Dental, and Pharmaceutical Association
- Maryland Medical, Dental, and Pharmaceutical Association
- Massachusetts Medical, Dental, and Pharmaceutical Association
- Mississippi Medical, Dental, Pharmaceutical, and Surgical Association
- North Carolina Medical, Pharmaceutical, and Dental Association
- North Jersey Medical Society of New Jersey
- Ohio Medical Association
- Palmetto Medical Association (South Carolina)
- Pan-Missouri Medical Association
- Tennessee Medical Association
- Tidewater Medical Society of Virginia
- Tri-State Medical, Dental, and Pharmaceutical Association of Florida, Georgia, and Alabama
- Tri-State Medical Association of Indiana, Kentucky, and Ohio
- West Virginia State Medical Society

City
- The Aesculapian Society of Indianapolis, Indiana
- Aesculapian Society of New York
- The Atlanta Association of Negro Physicians, Dentists, and Pharmacists
- Bluff City Medical, Dental, and Pharmaceutical Society, Memphis, Tennessee
- Charleston County Medical Association, Charleston, South Carolina
- Dallas Negro Medical, Dental, and Pharmaceutical Association
- The Falls City Medical Association, Louisville, Kentucky
- Freedman's Hospital Medical Society, Washington, D.C.
- Medico-Chirurgical Society of Greater New York
- Medico-Chirurgical Society of the District of Columbia
- Mound City Medical Association, St. Louis, Missouri
- Philadelphia Academy of Medicine and the Allied Sciences
- The Physicians, Dentists, and Pharmacists Club of Chicago
- Raleigh Medical Association, Raleigh, North Carolina
- The Richmond Medical Society of Richmond, Virginia
- Rock City Academy of Medicine and Surgery, Nashville, Tennessee
- South Atlantic Medical Society, Savannah, Georgia

Source: Monroe N. Work, ed., *The Negro Year Book, An Annual Encyclopedia of the Negro, 1914–15* (Tuskegee, Ala.: Negro Year Book Publishing, 1914), 335–38.

Notes

1. Smothering and Overlaying of Virginia Slave Children

This chapter originally appeared as "Smothering and Overlaying of Virginia Slave Children: A Suggested Explanation," *Bulletin of the History of Medicine* 49 (1975): 400–404.

The author is indebted to Carole L. Savitt for calling to his attention the article that led him to connect Sudden Infant Death Syndrome with overlaying and to Willie Lee Rose, now of Johns Hopkins University, for originally posing the problem of slave smothering. This publication was supported in part by NIH Grant 1 RO1 LM 02071 from the National Library of Medicine, 1973–76.

1. Virginia, Register of Deaths (manuscript on microfilm), 1853–1860, Southampton County, Augusta County, Petersburg Town, Staunton Town, at Virginia State Library, Richmond, Virginia; United States, Bureau of the Census, *Mortality Statistics of the Seventh Census of the United States, 1850* (Washington, D.C.: GPO, 1855), 290–295. The infant mortality rate for the entire country, according to the 1850 Census, was 16.4 percent, and 18.3 percent for the slaveholding states.

2. U.S. Department of Health, Education and Welfare, *Vital Statistics of the United States* (Washington, D.C.: GPO, 1967), IIA, 2–31.

3. In 1999, pneumonia and influenza were responsible for only 3.1 percent of infant deaths between one and eleven months, a substantial reduction from when this article was first published in the mid-1970s. Robert N. Anderson, "Deaths: Leading Causes for 1999," in U.S. Department of Health and Human Services, Centers for Disease Control and Prevention, National Center for Health Statistics, *National Vital Statistics Reports* 49 (Oct. 12, 2001): 12.

4. Abraham B. Bergman, J. Bruce Beckwith, and C. George Ray, eds., *Sudden Infant Death Syndrome: Proceedings of the Second International Conference on Causes of Sudden Death in Infants* (Seattle, 1970), 18.

5. J. Bruce Beckwith, "Defining the Sudden Infant Death Syndrome," *Archives of Pediatric and Adolescent Medicine* 157 (2003): 286–94.

6. Anderson, "Deaths," 76.

7. J. Bruce Beckwith and Abraham B. Bergman, "The Sudden Death Syndrome of Infancy," *Hospital Practice* 2 (Nov. 1967): 44.

8. Nathaniel Ryan, Saratoga, Buckingham County, Virginia, to Edmund W. Hubard, Washington, D.C., Dec. 15, 1841, Hubard Papers, Southern Historical Collection, University of North Carolina, Chapel Hill, N.C. (hereafter cited as Hubard Papers).

9. Robert T. Hubard, Rosny, Buckingham County, Virginia, to Edmund W. Hubard, Washington, D.C., Dec. 21, 1841, Hubard Papers.

10. Beckwith and Bergman, "Sudden Death Syndrome," 50–51. See also, on the history of SIDS, Todd L. Savitt, "The Social and Medical History of Crib Death," *Journal of the Florida Medical Association* 66 (1979): 853–59; Warren G. Guntheroth, "The Thymus, Suffocation, and Sudden Infant Death Syndrome—Social Agenda or Hubris?" *Perspectives in Biology and Medicine* 37 (Autumn 1993): 2–13; Warren G. Guntheroth, *Crib Death: The Sudden Infant Death Syndrome*, 3d ed. (Armonk, N.Y.: Futura Publishing, 1995); Abraham B. Bergman, *The "Discovery" of Sudden Infant Death Syndrome: Lessons in the Practice of Political Medicine* (New York: Praeger Publishers, 1986); Susan M. Beal, "The Rise and Fall of Several Theories," in *Sudden Infant Death Syndrome: Problems, Progress and Possibilities*, ed. Roger W. Byard and Henry F. Krous (New York: Oxford Univ. Press, 2001), 238.

11. Beckwith, "Defining the Sudden Infant Death Syndrome," 287.

12. Abraham B. Bergman, C. G. Ray, M. A. Pomeroy, P. W. Wahl, and J. B. Beckwith, "Studies of the Sudden Infant Death Syndrome in King County, Washington. III. Epidemiology," *Pediatrics* 49 (1972): 863; John W. Melton, Abdullah Fatteh, and Geoffrey Mann, "Sudden and Unexpected Deaths in Infancy," *Virginia Medical Monthly* 95 (1968): 64–65.

13. Virginia, Register of Deaths (manuscript on microfilm), 1853–1860, Accomac, Albemarle, Amelia, Arlington, Augusta, Bedford, Botetourt, Brunswick, Cumberland, Essex, Fairfax, Fauquier, Floyd, Frederick, Greene, Greensville, Halifax, Hanover, Henrico, Henry, Isle of Wight, Lancaster, Pittsylvania, and Southampton Counties; Petersburg and Staunton Towns, at Virginia State Library, Richmond, Va. The oldest child in the survey to die of suffocation was six years old.

14. For current thinking on the causes of SIDS, see Byard and Krous, *Sudden Infant Death Syndrome*, and Guntheroth, *Crib Death*.

15. Anderson, "Deaths," 76, 77.

16. M. Valdes-Dapena, L. J. Birle, J. A. McGovern, J. F. McGillen, and F. H. Colwell, "Sudden Unexpected Death in Infancy: A Statistical Analysis of Certain Socioeconomic Factors," *Journal of Pediatrics* 73 (1968): 390–92. A researcher discussing the epidemiology of SIDS in 2001 wrote, "One explanation for the higher rate of SIDS among African Americans is the higher concentration of socioeconomic risk factors commonly associated with SIDS, such as young maternal age, single marital status, lower education and poverty. The effect of race was eliminated in one study after controlling for family income and maternal education. In another study, where only infants of college educated couples were included, there were no differences in the rates of SIDS, despite the twice higher incidence of low birth weight in African-American infants. The higher rate of SIDS can also be explained, in part, by higher usage of the prone sleeping position by black mothers (43 percent) compared with white mothers (22 percent). Other practices such as bed-sharing, which is more common among African Americans, may also contribute to the higher rate." Fern R. Hauck, "Changing Epidemiology," in Byard and Krous, eds., *Sudden Infant Death Syndrome*, 33–35.

17. N. S. Weiss, D. Green, and D. E. Krueger, "Problems in the Use of Death Certificates to Identify Sudden Unexpected Infant Deaths," *Health Services Reports* 88 (1973): 555–58.

18. Thomas Affleck, "On the Hygiene of Cotton Plantations and the Management of Negro Slaves," *Southern Medical Reports* 2 (1851): 435.

19. Bureau of the Census, *Mortality Statistics, 1850*, 28.

20. See, for instance, the case of Opha Jane in the Powhatan County, Virginia, Order Book no. 29, 1851–1856, 501 (Apr. 7, 1856), at Virginia State Library, Richmond, Va.

21. Michael P. Johnson demonstrated in 1981 that differing rates of smothering, overlaying, and suffocation of enslaved children around the South correlated with differing labor demands on pregnant women. Though he took his argument in a different direction (because at that time SIDS researchers still believed that it was extremely unlikely that children could be accidentally smothered by their mothers), the evidence he provided could now be used to show that exhausted enslaved mothers could have accidentally overlaid and smothered their infant children. Thus not all antebellum infant deaths among the enslaved attributed to smothering, overlaying, and suffocation were instances of SIDS. See Johnson, "Smothered Slave Infants: Were Slave Mothers at Fault?" *Journal of Southern History* 47 (1981): 493–520.

2. Filariasis (Elephantiasis) in the United States

This chapter originally appeared as "Filariasis [Elephantiasis] in the United States," *Journal of the History of Medicine and Allied Sciences* 32 (1977): 140–50.

Research and publication of this article were supported in part by National Institutes of Health Grant LM 02477 from the National Library of Medicine, 1973–76.

1. Alfred W. Crosby Jr., *The Columbian Exchange: Biological and Cultural Consequences of 1492* (Westport, Conn.: Greenwood, 1972), 35–63, 122–64. See also P. M. Ashburn, *The Ranks of Death: A Medical History of the Conquest of America*, ed. Frank D. Ashburn (New York: Coward-McCann, 1947). The origin of syphilis is still a matter of controversy among medical historians. Some argue for a European and others for an American origin and some for neither. See, for example, Crosby, *Columbian Exchange*, 122–64; Jon Arrizabalaga, "Syphilis," in *The Cambridge Historical Dictionary of Disease*, ed. Kenneth F. Kiple (New York: Cambridge Univ. Press, 2003), 312–17; C. Meyer, C. Jung, T. Kohl, A. Poenicke, A. Poppe, and K. W. Alt, "Syphilis 2001—A Palaeopathological Reappraisal," *Homo* 53 (2002): 39–58; B. M. Rothschild, F. L. Calderon, A. Coppa, and C. Rothschild, "First European Exposure to Syphilis: The Dominican Republic at the Time of Columbian Contact," *Clinical Infectious Diseases* 31 (2000): 936–41; Guy A. Settipane, ed., *Columbus and the New World: Medical Implications* (Providence, R.I.: OceanSide Publications, 1995).

2. R. Hoeppli, *Parasitic Diseases in Africa and the Western Hemisphere: Early Documentation and Transmission by the Slave Trade* (Basel, Switz.: Verlag für Recht und Gesellschaft, 1969). See also entries for these diseases in Kiple, *Cambridge Historical Dictionary of Disease;* Kenneth F. Kiple, *The Caribbean Slave: A Biological History* (New York: Cambridge Univ. Press, 1984); Kiple, ed., *The African Exchange: Toward a Biological History of Black People* (Durham, N.C.: Duke Univ. Press, 1988).

3. Charles Wilcocks and P. E. C. Manson-Bahr, *Manson's Tropical Diseases*, 17th ed. (Baltimore, Md.: Williams and Wilkins, 1972), 192–217; Larry S. Roberts and John Janovy Jr., *Foundations of Parasitology*, 6th ed. (Boston: McGraw-Hill: 2000), 447–51. On the history of filariasis, see Todd L. Savitt, "Filariasis," in *Cambridge World History of Human Disease*, ed. Kiple, 724–30; W. D. Foster, *A History of Parasitology* (Edinburgh: E. and S. Livingston, 1965).

4. Hoeppli, *Parasitic Diseases*, 31–41.

5. Wilcocks and Manson-Bahr, *Manson's Tropical Diseases*, 192–217; Roberts and Janovy, *Foundations of Parasitology*, 447–51.

6. Wilcocks and Manson-Bahr, *Manson's Tropical Diseases*, 193; James M. Gordon,

"Elephantiasis—Its History, Symptomatology, Aetiology and Pathology, With a Report of a Case and Successful Treatment," *Southern Medical and Surgical Journal,* n.s., 6 (1850): 67.

7. Gordon, "Elephantiasis," 66–67; J. Scott, "Elephantiasis Arabum," *The Cyclopaedia of Practical Medicine* (Philadelphia: Lea and Blanchard, 1845), 2:770–71; Aldo Castellani and Albert J. Chalmers, *Manual of Tropical Medicine* (London: Baillière, Tindall and Cox, 1919), 1597–98; B. R. Laurence, "'Barbadoes Leg': Filariasis in Barbados, 1625–1900," *Medical History* 33 (1989): 480–88.

8. Peter H. Wood, *Black Majority: Negroes in Colonial South Carolina, from 1670 through the Stono Rebellion* (New York: Knopf, 1974), xiii–xiv, 152.

9. Marcus W. Lyon Jr., "Filariasis: Report of Two Cases in the District of Columbia, and Analysis of the Cases Reported for Eastern North America," *Journal of the American Medical Association* (hereafter cited as *JAMA*) 68 (1917): 119.

10. Edward Francis, *Filariasis in Southern United States* (Washington, D.C.: United States Public Health Service, Hygienic Laboratory Bulletin No. 117, June 1919), 17–19; Roberts and Janovy, *Foundations of Parasitology,* 447–51.

11. Wood, *Black Majority,* 24, 45–46, describes the settlement and development of South Carolina by Barbadians. For mention of the continuing intercourse between these two areas, see John Guitéras, "The Filaria Sanguinis Hominis in the United States—Chyluria," *Medical News (Phila.)* 48 (1886): 400. The interesting speculation of Dr. I. Snapper (Hoeppli, *Parasitic Diseases,* 122–24) that a boatload of Brazilian Jews seeking refuge from the Inquisition carried *W. bancrofti* to Charleston in the 1650s cannot be correct because few, if any, Jews actually settled in Charleston at that time. Most emigrated to Holland, and a small number moved to the West Indies, to England, and to New Amsterdam. The one or two families that might have gone to Charleston could not have caused the development of endemic filariasis. See Jacob R. Marcus, *The Colonial American Jew, 1492–1776* (Detroit: Wayne State Univ. Press, 1970), 1:81, 343–45.

12. Bernard Romans, *A Concise Natural History of East and West Florida* (1775; repr., New Orleans: Pelican Publishing Company, 1961), 170–71.

13. On other causes of elephantiasis, see Rudolph Matas, "The Surgical Treatment of Elephantiasis and Elephantoid States Dependent upon Chronic Obstruction of the Lymphatic and Venous Channels," *American Journal of Tropical Diseases and Preventive Medicine* 1 (1913): 60–67; Robert Berkow, ed., *The Merck Manual of Diagnosis and Therapy,* 16th ed. (Rahway, N.J.: Merck Research Laboratories, 1992), 1746; F. Dudley Hart, ed., *French's Index of Differential Diagnosis,* 12th ed. (Bristol, U.K.: John Wright and Sons, 1985), 752.

14. Francis, *Filariasis in Southern United States,* 13, 15–16; Ernest Carroll Faust, "Parasitism in Southeastern United States: History of Human Parasitic Infections," *Public Health Reports* 70 (1955): 963. There is no mention of elephantiasis in John Duffy, ed., *The Rudolph Matas History of Medicine in Louisiana,* 2 vols. (Baton Rouge: Louisiana State Univ. Press, 1958–62), and only one death attributed to elephantiasis in Savannah between 1854 and 1869 (William Duncan, *Tabulated Mortuary Record of the City of Savannah, From January 1, 1854, to December 31, 1869* [Savannah: Morning News Steam-Power Press, 1870]).

15. There were cases of elephantiasis reported in the North throughout the nineteenth and early twentieth centuries, though most were either imported or of nonfilarial origin. A few may have been true filariasis contracted from some unknown source. See, for example, David Hosack, *Essays on Various Subjects of Medical Science* (New York: J. Seymour, 1830), 3:442–45; Isaac Parrish, "Tumour of the Left Labium, Resembling Elephantiasis, Removed from a Negress," *Medical Examiner (Phila.)* 3 (1840): 229; J. W. Webster, "Elephantiasis," *New England Journal of Medicine and Surgery* 9 (1820): 213–20; Lyon, "Filariasis," 118.

16. J. M. W. Picton, "A Case of Elephantiasis Scroti, With Successful Operation," *New Orleans Medical and Surgical Journal* 2 (1845–46): 316–21.

17. Joseph Jones, "Observations on the African Yaws . . . and on Leprosy . . . in Insular and Continental America," *New Orleans Medical and Surgical Journal*, n.s., 5 (1878): 690; Jones, *Medical and Surgical Memoirs: Containing Investigations on the Geographical Distribution, Causes, Nature, Relations and Treatment of Various Diseases* (New Orleans: n.p., 1876–90), 2:1188–89, 1287–1332.

18. V. H. Taliaferro, "Remarks upon Elephantiasis," *Atlanta Medical and Surgical Journal* 2 (1856–57): 647–51; Anonymous, "Service of Dr. Jones—Elephantiasis," *Atlanta Medical and Surgical Journal* 4 (1859): 341–42; Juriah Harriss, "Report of a Case of Elephantiasis," *Savannah Journal of Medicine*, n.s., 5 (1866): 12–15; S. W. Francis, "Report of Case of Elephantiasis Arabum," *Medical and Surgical Reporter* 14 (1866): 284–86; D. W. Hammond, "Elephantiasis," *Transactions of the Medical Association of Georgia* 28 (1877): 109–12.

19. J. L. Dawson, "Return of Deaths in the City of Charleston," *Charleston Medical Journal and Review* 10 (1855): 747; 11 (1856): 574; 13 (1858): 282; 14 (1859): 138.

20. Charles Witsell, "Pathology and Treatment of a Discharge of Chyloserous Urine," *Charleston Medical Journal and Review* 10 (1855): 621–25.

21. William Fletcher Holmes, "Two Cases of Pneumonia, Illustrating the Comparative Efficacy of Mercury and Tartar Emetic, in the Treatment of That Disease," *Charleston Medical Journal and Review* 4 (1849): 176–79.

22. Clarence A. Fripp, "An Essay on Elephantiasis" (M.D. thesis, Medical College of the State of South Carolina, 1855), 3, Waring Historical Library, Medical University of South Carolina, Charleston. Fripp's paper included discussions of both elephantiasis (Elephantiasis Arabum) and leprosy (Elephantiasis Graecorum). The mention of a paucity of cases in previous years and an increase in recent times probably referred to leprosy.

23. Ibid., 7–8. Leprosy, Fripp observed, occurred more often among whites than blacks in South Carolina.

24. Ibid., 13.

25. F. Galvez, "Case of Elephantiasis of Scrotum," *Charleston Medical Journal and Review* 14 (1859): 124.

26. T. L. Ogier, "Ligature of the Femoral Artery for the Cure of Elephantiasis of the Leg and Foot," *Charleston Medical Journal and Review* 15 (1860): 191–95.

27. Charleston, S.C., *Annual Reports of the Officers of the City Government, to the City Council of Charleston, For the Year Ending . . . 1870*, 36, 39, 40; *1873*, 45, 48, 54, 58; *1874*, 44; *1876*, 46; Charleston, S.C., *Year Book*, 1882, 83; 1883, 83.

28. Guitéras, "Filaria Sanguinis Hominis," 399.

29. Ibid.

30. P. G. De Saussure, "A Clinical History of Twenty-two Cases of Filaria Sanguinis Hominis, Seen in Charleston, S.C., From 1886 to May, 1890," *Medical News (Phila.)* 56 (1890): 704.

31. Ibid., 704–7.

32. Charleston, S.C., *Year Book*, 1891, 51; 1893, 83; 1894, 91–92; 1896, 86, 89; 1899, 72; 1903, 83, 86; 1906, 170; 1912, 189.

33. Patrick Manson, *Tropical Diseases: A Manual of the Diseases of Warm Climates* (London: Cassell and Company, 1898), 448; W. M. Mastin, "The History of the Filaria Sanguinis Hominis, Its Discovery in the United States, and Especially the Relationship of the Parasite to Chylocele of the Tunica Vaginalis Testis," *Annals of Surgery* 8 (1888): 339–41, 346–47; Lyon, "Filariasis," 118–19.

34. Francis B. Johnson, "Filarial Infection: An Investigation of Its Prevalence in Charleston, S.C.," *Southern Medical Journal* 8 (1915): 630–34.

35. Francis, *Filariasis in Southern United States*, 11.

36. Some of these cases were undoubtedly duplicates, i.e., the same cases reported by more than one physician. Johnson, "Filarial Infection," 634.

37. See, for instance, Mastin, "History of the Filaria Sanguinis Hominis," 339–41; Lyon, "Filariasis," 118–19; R. M. Slaughter, "Filaria Sanguinis Hominis: The Discovery and Prevalence of the Disease in the United States," *Transactions of the Medical Society of Virginia* (1891): 239–45.

38. The cities were Columbia, Beaufort, and Georgetown, South Carolina; Milledgeville and Savannah, Georgia; Jacksonville and Tampa, Florida; Mobile, Alabama; and New Orleans, Louisiana.

39. Francis, *Filariasis in Southern United States*, 16.

40. Leon Banov, *As I Recall: The Story of the Charleston County Health Department* ([Columbia, S.C.]: R. L. Bryan, 1970), 56–57; Charleston, S.C., *Year Book*, 1924, 204; 1925, 198.

41. George Cheever Shattuck, *Diseases of the Tropics* (New York: Appleton-Century-Crofts, 1951), 508.

42. Ernest Carroll Faust, *Human Helminthology: A Manual for Physicians, Sanitarians, and Medical Zoologists*, 3d ed. (Philadelphia: Lea and Febiger, 1949), 499.

3. Race, Medicine, and the Discovery of Sickle Cell Anemia

1. James B. Herrick, "Peculiar Elongated and Sickle-Shaped Red Blood Corpuscles in a Case of Severe Anemia," *Archives of Internal Medicine* 6 (1910): 517–21.

2. R. E. Washburn, "Peculiar Elongated and Sickle-Shaped Red Blood Corpuscles in a Case of Severe Anemia," *Virginia Medical Semi-Monthly* 15 (1911): 490–93.

3. For more on the history of sickle cell anemia, see C. Lockard Conley, "Sickle-Cell Anemia—The First Molecular Disease," in *Blood, Pure and Eloquent: A Story of Discovery, of People, and of Ideas*, ed. Maxwell M. Wintrobe (New York: McGraw-Hill, 1980), 319–72; Todd L. Savitt and Morton Goldberg, "Herrick's 1910 Case Report of Sickle Cell Anemia—The Rest of the Story," *JAMA* 83 (1989): 266–71; Keith Wailoo, "'A Disease *Sui Generis*: The Origins of Sickle Cell Anemia and the Emergence of Modern Clinical Research, 1904–1924," *Bulletin of the History of Medicine* 65 (1991): 185–208. On social and political aspects of sickle cell anemia, see Keith Wailoo, *Dying in the City of the Blues: Sickle Cell Anemia and the Politics of Race and Health* (Chapel Hill: Univ. of North Carolina Press, 2001), and Melbourne Tapper, *In the Blood: Sickle Cell Anemia and the Politics of Race* (Philadelphia: Univ. of Pennsylvania Press, 1999). For a comprehensive overview of clinical, epidemiological, historical, and other aspects of sickle cell anemia, see Graham R. Serjeant and Beryl E. Serjeant, *Sickle Cell Disease*, 3d ed. (Oxford, U.K.: Oxford Univ. Press, 2001).

4. Jerome E. Cook and Jerome Myer, "Severe Anemia with Remarkable Elongated and Sickle-Shaped Red Blood Cells and Chronic Leg Ulcers," *Archives of Internal Medicine* 16 (1915): 644–51; V. R. Mason, "Sickle Cell Anemia," *JAMA* 79 (1922): 1318–22.

5. V. P. Sydenstricker, W. A. Mulherin, R. W. Houseal, "Sickle Cell Anemia: Report of Two Cases in Children, with Necropsy in One Case," *American Journal of Diseases of Children* 26 (1923): 132–54; J. G. Huck, "Sickle Cell Anaemia," *Johns Hopkins Hospital Bulletin* 34 (1923): 335–44; V. P. Sydenstricker, "Sickle Cell Anemia," *Southern Medical Journal* 17 (1924): 177–83; W. H. Taliaferro and J. G. Huck, "The Inheritance of Sickle-Cell Anaemia in Man," *Genetics* 8 (1923): 594–98; T. B. Cooley and P. Lee, "The Sickle Cell Phenomenon," *American Journal of Diseases of Children* 32 (1926): 334–40; C. S. Johnson, "Sickle Cell Anemia," *JAMA* 254 (1985): 1958–63.

4. Herrick's 1910 Case Report of Sickle Cell Anemia, Chicago, Illinois

This chapter originally appeared as "Herrick's 1910 Case Report of Sickle Cell Anemia," *JAMA* 261 (1989): 266–71, and it appears here with the permission of Morton F. Goldberg, M.D., original coauthor.

This investigation was supported in part by the Sickle Cell Eye Clinic and the Comprehensive Sickle Cell Center at the University of Illinois at Chicago; by grant HL 15168 from the National Heart, Lung, and Blood Institute and Ophthalmic Research Center Core Grant EY 01792 from the National Eye Institute, National Institutes of Health, Bethesda, Md.; and by unrestricted grants from Research to Prevent Blindness, Inc., New York, and a Senior University Scholar Award from the University of Illinois at Chicago.

The authors wish to thank the following persons for their suggestions and assistance: Norman Gevitz, Ph.D., and Patrician Spain Ward, M.A., University of Illinois at Chicago; Michael Grace, M.A., Loyola University Archives, Chicago; Mary Hudall and Judy Stewart, Loyola University School of Dentistry, Maywood, Illinois; William Kona, M.A., and Mary Jane Kirchner, Rush-Presbyterian-St. Luke's Medical Center Archives, Chicago; Janet Kinney, M.D., Rush Presbyterian-St. Luke's Medical Center, Chicago; Micaela Sullivan-Fowler, M.S., American Medical Association Library, Chicago; Terence Norwood, M.A., Cook County Hospital Archives, Chicago; Robert J. Adelsperger, M.S., University of Illinois at Chicago Special Collections Library; Margaret Kaiser and staff, History of Medicine Division, National Library of Medicine, Bethesda, Maryland; Denise Campbell and staff, Supreme Court Registry, St. George's, Grenada; the staff at the Registrar-General's Office, St. George's, Grenada; Agatha Clarke, Pathology Laboratory, General Hospital, St. George's, Grenada; Virginia Withers, special assistant to Morton Goldberg; and Loretta Kopelman, Ph.D., Reider Lie, M.D., Ph.D., and John Moskop, Ph.D., Department of Medical Humanities, East Carolina University School of Medicine, Greenville, North Carolina.

The name of Walter Clement Noel is used with permission of Noel's step-grandnephew, Cosmore St. Bernard, St. George's, Grenada.

1. James B. Herrick, "Peculiar Elongated and Sickle-Shaped Red Blood Corpuscles," *Archives of Internal Medicine* 6 (1910): 517–21.

2. Ibid.; James B. Herrick Papers, University of Chicago Library, Manuscript Division (hereafter cited as Herrick Papers). This collection contains a complete typewritten list of all Herrick's publications, files of correspondence Herrick received, and folders on many of his published articles. The sickle cell folder holds a working draft of the 1910 sickle cell paper; original hospital records on Walter Clement Noel, including blood smear slides; Herrick's and Irons's notes on the case and on Irons's visits to the patient after his discharge from the hospital; and bibliographic references to other articles as Herrick searched the medical literature.

3. Presbyterian Hospital Register of Admissions, Dec. 26, 1904, Rush-Presbyterian-St. Luke's Medical Center Archives, Chicago, Ill.

4. *Presbyterian Hospital, 22nd Annual Report* (1905), Rush-Presbyterian-St. Luke's Medical Center Archives, Chicago.

5. Herrick Papers.

6. James B. Herrick, "Peculiar Elongated and Sickle-Shaped Red Blood Corpuscles in a Case of Severe Anemia," *Transactions of the Association of American Physicians* 25 (1910): 553–61. Several physicians, including Herrick, participated in a discussion after the next paper, by Alexander McPhedran on pernicious anemia, but no one mentioned Herrick's presentation. See ibid., 567–69.

7. Herrick, "Peculiar Elongated and Sickle-Shaped Red Blood Corpuscles."

8. Chicago Medical Society, *History of Medicine and Surgery and Physicians and Surgeons of Chicago* (Chicago: Biographical Publishing, 1922); *The Lakeside City Directory* (Chicago: Polk, 1904–8); T. N. Bonner, *Medicine in Chicago, 1850–1950: A Chapter in the Social and Scientific Development of a City* (Madison, Wisc.: American History Research Center, 1957); E. E. Irons, "James Bryan Herrick, 1861–1954," *Transactions of the Association of American Physicians* 57 (1954): 15–19; James B. Herrick, *Memories of Eighty Years* (Chicago: Univ. of Chicago Press, 1949); James B. Herrick, M.D., Editorial, *Chicago Clinical Review* 5 (1896): 495–96; W. H. Holmes, *James Bryan Herrick: An Appreciation* (Chicago: Central Interurban Clinical Club, 1935); R. R. Ross, "A Parlous State of Storm and Stress: The Life and Times of James B. Herrick," *Circulation* 67 (1983): 955–59.

9. Herrick Papers; A. M. Harvey, "Classics in Clinical Science: From Horse and Buggy Doctor to Clinical Investigator: The Story of James Bryan Herrick," *American Journal of Medicine* 68 (1980): 639–41; P. S. Rhoads, "James B. Herrick, M.D, Born August 11, 1861—Died March 7, 1954," *Proceedings of the Institute of Medicine of Chicago* 35 (1982): 3–6; Irons, "James Bryan Herrick," 15–19; Herrick, *Memories of Eighty Years;* Herrick, Editorial, *Chicago Clinical Review,* 495–96; Holmes, *Herrick;* Ross, "Parlous State," 955–59; "James Bryan Herrick," *National Cyclopaedia of American Biography* (New York: James T. White and Co., 1958), 42:595–96; J. C. Bay, "James B. Herrick: Youth in Man Makes History," *Proceedings of the Institute of Medicine of Chicago* 14 (1942): 288–98; J. Bowman, *Good Medicine: The First 150 Years of Rush-Presbyterian-St. Luke's Medical Center* (Chicago: Chicago Review Press, 1987).

10. Bowman, *Good Medicine;* "The President-elect: Dr. Ernest Edward Irons," *JAMA* 137 (1948): 870; "Ernest E. Irons," *Current Biography* (New York: H. W. Wilson Co., 1950), 293–94; "Ernest Edward Irons, Obituaries," *JAMA* 169 (1959): 520–21; F. B. Kelly, "Ernest Edward Irons, 1877–1959," [Rush Medical College] *Medical Alumni Bulletin* (Winter 1959): 7; B. G. Rosenkrantz, "On the Spot: A History of Focal Infection: The Fielding H. Garrison Lecture" (read before the American Association for the History of Medicine, Philadelphia, May 1, 1987).

11. Irons, "James Bryan Herrick," 15–19; Kelly, "Ernest Edward Irons," 7; Evan Barton, M.D. (an intern under and later a colleague of Irons), telephone interview with author, Chicago, June 30, 1987; Stanton A. Friedberg, M.D., interview with author, Chicago, July 2, 1987.

12. *The Lakeside City Directory* (Chicago: Polk, 1904–08).

13. Herrick Papers.

14. G. H. Coleman, "Internal Medicine," in *History of Medical Practice in Illinois,* ed. D. J. Davis (Chicago: Illinois State Medical Society, 1955), 108–52; C. E. Black, ed., *General Index to the Transactions of the Illinois State Medical Society, 1850–1898* (Springfield: Illinois Medical Journal, 1913), 38.

15. D. D. Bishop, "General Microscopic Examination of the Blood—Its Importance as a Diagnostic Measure," *Transactions of the Illinois State Medical Society* 45 (1895): 496–512.

16. J. B. Herrick, "The Practical Value of Blood Examinations," *Illinois Medical Journal* 6 (1904–5): 619–21.

17. H. Rolleston, "The History of Hematology," *Proceedings of the Royal Society of Medicine* 27 (1933–34): 31–48; J. C. Sabine, "A History of the Classification of Human Blood Corpuscles," *Bulletin of the History of Medicine* 8 (1940): 696–720, 785–805; C. Dreyfus, *Some Milestones in the History of Hematology* (New York: Grune and Stratton, 1957), 3–45; M. L. Verso, "The Evolution of Blood-Counting Techniques, *Medical History* 8 (1964): 149–58; P. M. Ness and J. M. Stengle, "Historical Introduction," in *The Red Blood Cell,* 2d ed., ed. D. N. Surgenor (Orlando, Fla.: Academic Press, 1974), 1:2–50; A. D. Farr, "Some Problems in the History of Haemoglobinometry (1878–1931)," *Medical History* 22 (1978): 151–60; M. M. Wintrobe, *Hematology, the Blossoming of a Science: A Story of Inspiration*

and Effort (Philadelphia: Lea and Febiger, 1985); M. M. Wintrobe, "Milestones on the Path of Progress," in *Blood, Pure and Eloquent,* ed. Wintrobe, 1–32; J. V. Dacie, "The Life Span of the Red Blood Cell and Circumstances of Its Premature Death," in *Blood, Pure and Eloquent,* ed. Wintrobe, 211–56; W. B. Castle, "The Conquest of Pernicious Anemia," in *Blood, Pure and Eloquent,* ed. Wintrobe, 283–318.

18. Bishop, "General Microscopic Examination of the Blood," 496–512; F. C. Shattuck and R. C. Cabot, "Examination of the Blood; Plethora; Anemia," in *A System of Practical Medicine by American Authors,* ed. A. L. Loomis and W. G. Thompson (Philadelphia: Lea Brothers and Co., 1897), 2:633–78; J. B. Herrick, "Relation of the Clinical Laboratory to the Practitioner of Medicine," *JAMA* 48 (1907): 1915–19; R. C. Cabot, "The General Pathology of the Blood-Forming Organs: Pernicious and Secondary Anaemia, Chlorosis, and Leukaemia," in *Modern Medicine: Its Theory and Practice,* ed. W. Osler (Philadelphia: Lea and Febiger, 1908), 4:595–680.

19. On the history of medical schools that trained African Americans, see the chapters in Part 3 of this volume as well as the references in those chapters. On African American nursing history, see M. E. Carnegie, *The Path We Tread: Blacks in Nursing, 1854–1984* (Philadelphia: J. B. Lippincott, 1986), and D. C. Hine, *Black Women in White: Racial Conflict and Cooperation in the Nursing Profession, 1890–1950* (Bloomington: Indiana Univ. Press, 1989).

20. H. M. Morais, *The History of the Negro in Medicine* (New York: Publishers Co., 1967); T. L. Savitt, "Entering a White Profession: Black Physicians in the New South, 1880–1920," *Bulletin of the History of Medicine* 61 (1987): 507–40; T. J. Ward Jr., *Black Physicians in the Jim Crow South* (Fayetteville: Univ. of Arkansas Press, 2003).

21. Morais, *History of the Negro in Medicine;* Helen Buckler, *Doctor Dan: Pioneer in American Surgery* (Boston: Little, Brown and Company, 1954).

22. American Medical Association, *American Medical Directory* (Chicago: American Medical Association, 1906–20).

23. G. Brizan, *Grenada, Island of Conflict: From Amerindians to People's Revolution, 1498–1979* (London: Zed Books, 1984); Colonial Secretary, comp., *The Grenada Handbook, Directory, and Almanac* (London: various publishers, 1895–1921), available in Library of Congress, Washington, D.C.; F. M. Coard, "Grenada, An Island State: Its History and Its People," *Caribbean Quarterly* 20 (1974): 5–43. *The Grenada Handbook,* published annually in London from 1895 to 1921, contains a chronicle of the past year's events; Grenada's history; a descriptive sketch of the colony; lists of civil servants, business people, and professionals; information about schools, hospitals, roads, clubs, mail, telephones, duties, laws, crops, and vegetation; and a directory of important people on the island.

24. "Register of Births, 1884," Registers of Births and Deaths, Registrar-General's Office, St. George's, Grenada.

25. Philip Alexis (Walter Clement Noel's step-nephew), interview with author, on Duquesne Estate, Grenada, July 29, 1987.

26. Will of Mary Justina King, Supreme Court Registry, St. George's, Grenada; Philip Alexis, interview.

27. Registers of Births and Deaths, Registrar-General's Office, St. George's, Grenada. Births and deaths are listed by year in separate books. Available records indicate that Clement, as Walter Clement Noel was known, was the youngest of Mary Justina's and John Cornelius's four children. Henry Cornelius, born in 1874, and Jane Cecilia, born in 1882, were the Noel siblings with whom Clement grew up on Duquesne. A daughter, name not known, was born to the couple in 1875, but presumably died in childhood, as she is not mentioned in John Cornelius's 1886 will. Cosmore St. Bernard, a step-grandnephew of Walter Clement Noel, recalled in an interview on July 27, 1987, in St. George's, another child, Julia ("Jules"), younger than Clement, who drowned in her youth in the lagoon of

St. George's Bay. The author could locate no record of her birth or death, however. Within a few years of Walter Clement Noel's father's death in 1886, Mary Justina married Samuel O'Connell King, son of the teacher at the Sauteurs, Grenada, Anglican Church School, and began a second family. Clement's half-siblings included Mary Ethelina ("Lena," born in 1891), Edith Unice (born in 1893), and Philip Norbert (born in 1895).

28. Will of John Cornelius Noel, Supreme Court Registry, St. George's, Grenada.

29. Transcript of W. C. Noel from Harrison College, Barbados, and letters to Chicago College of Dental Surgery, in W. C. Noel file, Dean's Office, Loyola University School of Dentistry, Maywood, Ill. In his 1910 article and in the Presbyterian Hospital admission notes found in the Herrick Papers at the University of Chicago, Herrick states that Noel ended his education at age seventeen. However, Noel's file in the Loyola University Dental School contains an official transcript from Harrison College, Bridgetown, Barbados, for January 1901 through March 1903, when Noel would have been eighteen years old.

30. L. Braithwaite, "The Development of Higher Education in the British West Indies," *Social and Economic Studies* 7 (1958): 1–64; I. Oxaal, *Black Intellectuals and the Dilemma of Race and Class in Trinidad* (Cambridge, Mass.: Schenkman, 1972), 62; D. S. Lamb, ed., *Howard University Medical Department, Washington, D.C.: A Historical, Biographical and Statistical Souvenir* (Washington, D.C.: Beresford, 1900); Catalogs (1870–1920) of Meharry Medical School (Nashville, Tenn.), Howard University Medical Department (Washington, D.C.), Leonard Medical School ([Shaw University Library] Raleigh, N.C.), Flint Medical College of New Orleans University, Louisville National Medical College, and the University of West Tennessee College of Medicine and Surgery (Memphis). Catalogs for the last three named are available in the National Library of Medicine, History of Medicine Division (Bethesda, Md.).

31. Lamb, *Howard University Medical Department,* 233.

32. Arthur is listed in the professional registry of *The Grenada Handbook.*

33. Transcript of W. C. Noel from Harrison College, Barbados, and letters, Oliver Arthur to Truman Brophy, June 16 and July 28, 1904, and Brophy to Arthur, Aug. 10, 1904, in W. C. Noel file, Dean's Office, Loyola University School of Dentistry, Maywood, Ill.

34. Chicago Medical Society, *History of Medicine of Chicago;* T. W. Brophy, "History of Chicago College of Dental Surgery," in *Medical and Dental Colleges of the West, Historical and Biographical, Chicago,* ed. H. G. Cutler (Chicago: Oxford, 1896), 411–24; J. Jackson and E. Jackson, *Dentists to the World: Illinois's Influence on the Growth of the Profession* (Chicago: Quadrangle Books, 1964), 91–106.

35. Mary Justina King, Duquesne Estate, to Dr. Truman Brophy, Chicago College of Dental Surgery, Aug. 26, 1904, in Noel File, Loyola University School of Dentistry.

36. Passenger and Crew Lists of Vessels Arriving at New York, 1897–1942, Record Group 85, Records of the Immigration and Naturalization Service, National Archives, Washington, D.C.

37. Presbyterian Hospital Register of Admissions, Dec. 26, 1904, Rush-Presbyterian-St. Luke's Medical Center Archives, Chicago.

38. Catalogs of the Chicago College of Dental Surgery, Loyola University Archives, Chicago; *The Bur* 10 (1905): 1–9, Loyola University Health Sciences Library, Maywood, Ill. *The Bur* was the Dental School's magazine for students, faculty, and alumni.

39. Presbyterian Hospital was just diagonally across Congress Street from Noel's lodgings, along the route he probably took many mornings on his way to classes at CCDS. Possibly one or two friends, both senior dental students, Yott Edward Whitmore of Arkansas and Henry Clifton Wands of Chippewa Falls, Wisconsin, accompanied Noel to the hospital. Their names appear in the Presbyterian Hospital register of admissions for December 26, 1904, as personal references for Noel. Whitmore lived just down the street from Noel at 255 Hermitage Avenue.

40. Herrick, "Peculiar Elongated and Sickle-Shaped Red Blood Corpuscles," 517–21; Herrick Papers.

41. Herrick Papers.

42. Chicago College of Dental Surgery, *24th Annual Announcement, Session of 1905–6*, 31, Loyola University Archives, Chicago.

43. Herrick, "Peculiar Elongated and Sickle-Shaped Red Blood Corpuscles," 517–21; Herrick Papers.

44. Herrick, "Peculiar Elongated and Sickle-Shaped Red Blood Corpuscles," 517–21.

45. Herrick Papers. The four articles were T. M. R. Leonard, "Ankylostomiasis or Uncinariasis [in Grenada]," *JAMA* 45 (1905): 588–94; A. Castellani, "Further Observations on Parangi (Yaws)," *British Medical Journal* 2 (1905): 1330–31; A. Lingard, "The Significance of the Pyriform Circular and Irregular Shaped Bodies Present in the Circulation, Organs, or Tissues, in Various Forms of Disease in Man and Animals, With Suggestions Regarding Their Identification and Classification," *Indian Medical Gazette* 40 (1905): 333–38, 381–84; M. Löwit, "Der Nachweis sichelförmiger Gebilde im myelämischen Blute bei Giemsa-Färbung," *Zentralblatt für Bakteriologie, Parasitenkunde, Infektionskrankheiten und Hygiene* 39 (1905): 274–76.

46. Irons, "James Bryan Herrick," 15–19.

47. Herrick, "Peculiar Elongated and Sickle-Shaped Red Blood Corpuscles," 517–21.

48. For more on the subsequent history of sickle cell anemia after 1910, see citations in chapter 3 and in chapters 5 and 6.

49. Chicago College of Dental Surgery, *Catalog, 1907–1908*, 40, Loyola University Archives; *The Bur* 12 (1907): 160–67, 178, available at Loyola University Health Sciences Library, Maywood, Ill. The author could locate no record of Noel's grades or comments from faculty on his medical problems, absences from school, or academic performance at the Loyola University School of Dentistry, Loyola University Archives, or Valparaiso University Archives. (CCDS was part of Valparaiso University before joining with Loyola.)

50. Noel is listed in the professional registry of post-1907 editions of *The Grenada Handbook*. Information about his office and living accommodations was obtained from Mary Justina King's will and from interviews with Enid MacLeish (July 28, 1987, St. George's, Grenada), Philip Alexis (July 29, 1987, Duquesne Estate, Grenada), and Cosmore St. Bernard (July 27–31, 1987, St. George's, Grenada).

51. Enid MacLeish, interview.

52. Will of Walter Clement Noel.

53. Registers of Births and Deaths, Registrar-General's Office, St. George's, Grenada.

54. Cosmore St. Bernard, interview.

55. Will of Walter Clement Noel. Noel left most of his assets to his family, but his dental instruments to his assistant, Eldon Marksman. Marksman (b. 1892) attended Howard University Dental School, but soon switched to the medical school. After graduation in 1926, he practiced general medicine in Princess Anne, Maryland, for many years. Cosmore St. Bernard, interview, and various editions of the *American Medical Directory*.

56. Herrick, "Peculiar Elongated and Sickle-Shaped Red Blood Corpuscles," 517–21; Registers of Births and Deaths, Registrar-General's Office, St. George's, Grenada.

5. Washburn's 1911 Case Report of Sickle Cell Anemia, Charlottesville, Virginia

This chapter originally appeared as "The Second Reported Case of Sickle Cell Anemia: Charlottesville, Virginia, 1911," *Virginia Medical Quarterly* 124 (1997): 2–10.

I wish to acknowledge the help of a number of people who helped me track down leads in the search for information about Ellen Anthony and Benjamin E. Washburn. In particular, Samuel D. Ogden of Altavista, Virginia, who was working on a history of Lynch Station, opened his home and his vast knowledge of places, events, and local residents to me during several visits to central Virginia. Through him I met and interviewed more people than space will allow me to name. My thanks to them all, including Lillian Andrew, Lou Ethel Edwards Anthony, Calvin P. Carter, Hester Faulkner, Samuel Faulkner, Arnita Gertrude Anthony Franklin, Anna Keller, Clarissa Mormon, Mary Parsons, J. B. Payne, and T. J. Wilkinson. Others who provided assistance in the course of this project include, in Rutherfordton, North Carolina, Edith Atchley, Delores Cordell, Nancy Ellen Ferguson, and Joyce Tate; and in Charlottesville, Virginia, Joan Echtenkamp Klein (Special Collections Librarian at the University of Virginia Health Sciences Library), Dr. Daniel Mohler, Jeanne Pardee of the University of Virginia Archives, and Charles Williams (director of medical records at the University of Virginia Hospital). Kenneth Rose at the Rockefeller Archive Center was most helpful in opening to me the papers of Benjamin Earl Washburn.

1. Washburn, "Peculiar Elongated and Sickle-Shaped Red Blood Corpuscles," 490–93. The first reported case was Herrick, "Peculiar Elongated and Sickle-Shaped Red Blood Corpuscles," 517–21.

2. Savitt and Goldberg, "Herrick's 1910 Case Report," 266–71, reproduced with some revisions in chapter 3 of this book.

3. Benjamin Earle Washburn, *To Every Thing a Season: Rutherfordton—Long, Long Ago* (Spindale, N.C.: Spindale Press, [1960?]), 135.

4. On Washburn's early years in Rutherfordton and the family's financial situation, see Washburn, *To Every Thing a Season,* esp. 42–45. On John Rutherford Washburn, see a brief obituary in the *News,* Oct. 6, 1932, 4, cols. 2–3, located in the Benjamin Washburn Papers, Rockefeller Archive Center, Pocantico Hills, North Tarrytown, N.Y. (hereafter cited as Washburn Papers), Box 8, Folder 54.

5. Washburn, *To Every Thing a Season,* 76–78.

6. University of North Carolina (hereafter cited as UNC), *Yakety Yak, 1906* [student yearbook], 45.

7. Washburn, *To Every Thing a Season,* 79.

8. Ibid., 110–11.

9. Ibid., 111–14; UNC, *Catalog,* 1908–9, 177, 198; *Catalog,* 1909–10, 207, 208; UNC, *Yakety Yak, 1908,* 125, 126; *Yakety Yak, 1909,* 128, 129.

10. Benjamin E. Washburn, "The Uncle Remus Stories" (M.A. thesis, University of North Carolina, 1909). A copy of this thesis is shelved in the North Carolina Room of the Louis Round Wilson Library at UNC.

11. Washburn, *To Every Thing a Season,* 116. On the state of medical education and medical facilities at the University of North Carolina Medical Department in Raleigh, see Isaac Hall Manning Sr. and Walter Reece Berryhill, "Medical Education at the University of North Carolina," in *Medicine in North Carolina: Essays in the History of Medical Science and Medical Service, 1524–1960,* ed. Dorothy Long (Raleigh: North Carolina Medical Society, 1972), 382–87; John H. Felts, "Abraham Flexner and Medical Education in North Carolina," *North Carolina Medical Journal* 56 (1995): 534–39.

12. Washburn, *To Every Thing a Season,* 116.

13. Ibid., 118–20.

14. There are virtually no records or documents other than the official register of the University of Virginia Hospital that name Ellen Anthony. The manuscript censuses for 1880, 1900, 1910, and 1920 (1890 is not available) do not mention her. The Commonwealth of Virginia's birth and death registers do not mention her. (Thanks to Sandra G. Treadway of the Virginia State Library for verifying this information.) Campbell County registers in the courthouse at Rustburg do not mention Ellen Anthony or her father, Richard Anthony.

Her exact age cannot be determined from the hospital records, as no birth date is given, and each admission lists a different age.

15. Information about the life of Ellen Anthony was gleaned primarily from statements in Washburn's article reporting Anthony's case of sickle cell anemia, data provided in the University of Virginia Hospital admissions books for 1907–18, and interviews with various citizens of Campbell County as indicated. No family papers, church or local hospital records, or physicians' files could be located. Washburn states in his article (490n2) that "the patient . . . , a native of Southwestern Virginia, . . . has lived there all of her life."

16. R. H. Early, *Campbell Chronicles and Family Sketches: Embracing the History of Campbell County, Va., 1782–1926* (Lynchburg, Va.: J. P. Bell Company, 1927), 107–17.

17. University of Virginia (hereafter cited as UVa) Hospital Admissions Books, patient #1567 (4/7/09), #3802 (10/25/10), and #5077 (8/22/11), located on microfilm in the Medical Records Department, University of Virginia Hospital, Charlottesville.

18. The 1880 manuscript census for the Otter River District of Campbell County, 113b, household number 204, includes a Richard Anthony, listed as a black male laborer age forty; his wife, Polly, age forty-one, a housewife; and five daughters ages three to nineteen, none named Ellen or anything close to that name. In 1900 (the 1890 manuscript census is not available), Richard Anthony is listed (133b, household number 121) as a black male farmer, born September 1833, sixty-six years old, married for thirty years. His family then consisted of his wife Polly, a black female, born October 1836, sixty-three years old, married for thirty years, having borne eight children, three of whom were still living; and an unmarried son, John, a black male farm laborer, born May 1875, twenty-five years old. The 1910 census (6th Supervisor's District, 25th Enumeration district, sheet 19a, household number 351) lists Richard Anthony as a sixty-eight-year-old black male farmer, married twenty years; his wife, Polly, aged sixty-five, having borne seven children, three of whom were still living; and a twenty-year-old single son, John, who was a laborer.

19. Washburn, "Peculiar Elongated and Sickle-Shaped Red Blood Corpuscles," 490.

20. Ibid., 490–91.

21. The author conducted numerous interviews with people throughout the area who might have known the Anthonys. Mr. T. J. Wilkinson Jr. of Lynch Station remembered, during an interview on September 10, 1993, that two African American residents of Lynch Station, Haynes and Josephine Arnold, took in Richard and Ellen Anthony to live with them. There are other African American Anthonys in southern Campbell County, but in tracing their family trees, none could be found who were related to Ellen or Richard Anthony.

22. Washburn, "Peculiar Elongated and Sickle-Shaped Red Blood Corpuscles," 490; UVa Hospital Admissions Book, patient #433 (3/30/08), #1567 (4/7/09), #2153 (9/18/09), #3802 (10/25/10), #5077 (8/22/11), #9078 (10/27/13).

23. Washburn, "Peculiar Elongated and Sickle-Shaped Red Blood Corpuscles," 490.

24. Ibid., 491.

25. UVa Hospital Admissions Book, patient #433 (3/30/08).

26. American Medical Association, *American Medical Directory* (Chicago: American Medical Association, 1909), 1179, and (1912), 1242; Anna Keller, Lynchburg, Virginia, telephone interview with author, May 25, 1993.

27. Wilhelm Moll and Todd L. Savitt, "The Early Years of the University of Virginia Hospital: An Analysis of Patients' Records," *Virginia Medical Monthly* 102 (1975): 544–45, 716–18; Stephen H. Watts, "The University of Virginia Hospital," *Alumni Bulletin of the University of Virginia*, 3d ser., 1 (1908): 313–16.

28. Keller, interview.

29. Washburn, "Peculiar Elongated and Sickle-Shaped Red Blood Corpuscles," 491. Though some patient charts for this early period of the hospital are available on microfilm,

Ellen Anthony's chart could not be located. Anthony's other admissions to UVa Hospital occurred as follows: patient #433 (3/30/08—6/18/08); patient #1567 (4/7/09—6/9/09); patient #2153 (9/18/09—7/9/10); patient #3802 (10/25/10—4/1/11); patient #5077 (8/22/11—11/18/11); patient #6817 (8/10/12—1/15/13); patient #9078 (10/27/13—5/14/14); patient #11271 (10/28/14—4/30/15); patient #12896 (7/3/15—12/15/15); patient #17397 (1/2/17—5/19/17); patient #20784 (1/26/18—5/5/18); patient #21760 (5/14/18—6/27/18).

30. UVa Hospital Admissions Books, patient #433 (3/30/08); Washburn, "Peculiar Elongated and Sickle-Shaped Red Blood Corpuscles," 491.

31. Washburn, "Peculiar Elongated and Sickle-Shaped Red Blood Corpuscles," 491; UVa Hospital Admissions Books, patient #2153 (9/18/09).

32. M. Price Margolies, "Sickle Cell Anemia: A Composite Study and Survey," *Medicine* 30 (1951): 360–61; Conley, "Sickle-Cell Anemia," 322. Thanks to Daniel Mohler, M.D., of Charlottesville, for first relating this story to me. No records of this incident are extant at either the University of Virginia or the Johns Hopkins University archives.

33. Washburn, "Peculiar Elongated and Sickle-Shaped Red Blood Corpuscles," 491n2; UVa Hospital Admissions Book, patient #1567 (4/7/09).

34. Washburn, "Peculiar Elongated and Sickle-Shaped Red Blood Corpuscles," 491.

35. UVa Hospital Admissions Book, patient #2153 (9/18/09). Lynches, Lynches Station, and Lynch Station are three names for the same town.

36. Washburn, *To Every Thing a Season*, 118–24.

37. Washburn, "Peculiar Elongated and Sickle-Shaped Red Blood Corpuscles," 491.

38. Ibid., 492.

39. Herrick, "Peculiar Elongated and Sickle-Shaped Red Blood Corpuscles."

40. Washburn, *To Every Thing a Season*, 135.

41. Wyndham B. Blanton, *Medicine in Virginia in the Nineteenth Century* (Richmond, Va.: Garrett and Massie, 1933), 27, 30.

42. Washburn, *To Every Thing a Season*, 125.

43. See masthead of the journal for Davis's name as a member of the editorial board.

44. In Washburn, "Peculiar Elongated and Sickle-Shaped Red Blood Corpuscles," 492, he provides the results of a blood examination dated January 8, 1911.

45. Herrick, "Peculiar Elongated and Sickle-Shaped Red Blood Corpuscles," 517.

46. Washburn, "Peculiar Elongated and Sickle-Shaped Red Blood Corpuscles," 490.

47. Washburn, *To Every Thing a Seaon*, 132.

48. Washburn, "Peculiar Elongated and Sickle-Shaped Red Blood Corpuscles," 492.

49. Ibid., 493.

50. Washburn wrote about his experiences during this time period (1912–13) in his book *A Country Doctor in the South Mountains* (Spindale, N.C.: Spindale Press, 1955).

51. For more on Washburn's life, see Washburn, *To Every Thing a Season; The Heritage of Rutherford County, North Carolina* (Winston-Salem, N.C.: Genealogical Society of Old Tryon County, 1984), 1:421–22; B. E. Washburn, *As I Recall: The Hookworm Campaigns Initiated by the Rockefeller Sanitary Commission and the Rockefeller Foundation in the Southern United States and Tropical America* (New York: Rockefeller Foundation, 1960); Washburn Papers; files on Washburn in the North Carolina Collection and in the Alumni Office at the University of North Carolina at Chapel Hill; William S. Powell, *North Carolina Lives: The Tar Heel Who's Who* (Hopkinsville, Ky.: Historical Record Association, 1962), 1275.

52. On the history of this era, see, for example, Richard Harrison Shryock, *The Development of Modern Medicine: An Interpretation of the Social and Scientific Factors Involved* (1936; repr., Madison: Univ. of Wisconsin Press, 1979), and Roy Porter, *The Greatest Benefit to Mankind: History of Humanity from Antiquity to the Present* (London: Hammersmith, 1997), 245–461.

53. Savitt and Goldberg, "Herrick's 1910 Case Report," 270.

54. Washburn, *To Every Thing a Season,* 134.

55. C. Vann Woodward, *The Strange Career of Jim Crow* (New York: Oxford Univ. Press, 1955); Edward L. Ayers, *The Promise of the New South: Life after Reconstruction* (New York: Oxford Univ. Press, 1992), 132–59. On African Americans in the medical profession, see Savitt, "Entering a White Profession," 507–40, reproduced in chapter 19 of this book; Edward H. Beardsley, *A History of Neglect: Health Care for Blacks and Mill Workers in the Twentieth-Century South* (Knoxville: Univ. of Tennessee Press, 1987); and Ward, *Black Physicians.*

56. For more information on Walter Clement Noel, see Savitt and Goldberg, "Herrick's 1910 Case Report."

6. Sickle Cell Anemia: The Invisible Malady

This chapter originally appeared as "The Invisible Malady: Sickle Cell Anemia in America: 1910–1970," *Journal of the National Medical Association* 73 (1981): 739–46.

1. James B. Herrick, "Peculiar Elongated and Sickle-Shaped Red Blood Corpuscles in a Case of Severe Anemia," *Archives of Internal Medicine* 6 (1910): 517–21.

2. Charles W. Triche and Diane S. Triche, *The Sickle Cell Hemoglobinopathies: A Comprehensive Bibliography,* 2 vols. (Troy, N.Y.: Whitston, 1973–76); Conley, "Sickle-Cell Anemia," 319–72.

3. John C. Lane and Robert B. Scott, "Awareness of Sickle Cell Anemia among Negroes of Richmond, Virginia," *Public Health Reports* 84 (1969): 949–53; F. N. Cooper and Robert B. Scott, "The Virginia Sickle Cell Anemia Awareness Program (VASCAP): Education, Screening, and Counseling," *MCV Quarterly* 13 (1977): 151–53.

4. R. A. Binder and S. R. Jones, "Prevalence and Awareness of Sickle Cell Hemoglobin in a Military Population," *JAMA* 214 (1970): 909–11; M. S. Greenberg, "Need to Identify Sickle-Cell Trait," *New England Journal of Medicine* 282 (1970): 629–30; M. L. Hampton, J. Anderson, B. S. Lavizzo, and A. B. Bergman, "Sickle Cell 'Nondisease': A Potentially Serious Public Health Problem," *American Journal of Diseases of Children* 128 (1974): 58–61; P. Desai and G. R. Serjeant, "Awareness of Sickle Cell Disease among High School Students in Kingston, Jamaica," *Public Health Reports* 91 (1976): 265–67.

5. Robert B. Scott, "Health Care Priority and Sickle Cell Anemia," *JAMA* 214 (1970): 731–34.

6. F. I. D. Konotey-Ahulu, "Hereditary Qualitative and Quantitative Erythrocyte Defects in Ghana: An Historical and Geographical Survey," *Ghana Medical Journal* 7 (1968): 118–19, 167.

7. J. R. Young, "Malaria in the South, 1900–1930" (Ph.D. diss., University of North Carolina, 1972).

8. Todd L. Savitt, *Medicine and Slavery: The Diseases and Health Care of Blacks in Antebellum Virginia* (Urbana: Univ. of Illinois Press, 1978), 7–25.

9. Ibid.

10. A. C. Allison, "Aspects of Polymorphism in Man," *Cold Spring Harbor Symposia on Quantitative Biology* 20 (1955): 239–55; A. C. Allison, "Notes on Sickle-Cell Polymorphism," *Annals of Human Genetics* 19 (1954–55): 39–57; P. L. Workman, "Gene Flow and the Search for Natural Selection in Man," *Human Biology* 40 (1968): 260–79; C. Stern, *Principles of Human Genetics* (San Francisco: Freeman, 1960) 234–35; Georges C. Benjamin, "Sickle-Cell Anemia," in *The Cambridge World History of Human Disease,* ed. Kenneth F. Kiple (Cambridge, U.K.: Cambridge Univ. Press, 1993), 1006; Serjeant and Serjeant, *Sickle Cell Disease,* 16–30.

11. See, for example, John H. Morgan, "An Essay on the Causes of Production of Abortion among Our Negro Population," *Nashville Journal of Medicine and Surgery* 19 (1860): 117–23; E. M. Pendleton, "On the Comparative Fecundity of the Caucasian and African Races," *Charleston Medical Journal and Review* 6 (1851): 351–56.

12. W. J. Williams, E. Beutler, A. J. Erslev, and R. W. Rundles, eds., *Hematology* (New York: McGraw-Hill, 1972), 418; Serjeant and Serjeant, *Sickle Cell Disease*, 413–15.

13. Arno G. Motulsky, "Frequency of Sickling Disorders in U.S. Blacks," *New England Journal of Medicine* 288 (1973): 31–33; Serjeant and Serjeant, *Sickle Cell Disease*, 23–28.

14. See, for example, Robert W. Gibbes, "Southern Slave Life," *De Bow's Review* 24 (1858): 323; John Duffy, "Eighteenth-Century Carolina Health Conditions," *Journal of Southern History* 18 (1952): 300.

15. Sherwin A. Kabins and Charles Lerner, "Fulminant Pneumococcemia and Sickle Cell Anemia," *JAMA* 211 (1970): 467–71; Serjeant and Serjeant, *Sickle Cell Disease*, 170–84.

16. J. Thomson, *A Treatise on the Diseases of Negroes, as They Occur in the Island of Jamaica* (Jamaica: A. Aikman, 1820), 107.

17. R. Lebby, "Case of Absence of the Spleen," *Southern Journal of Medicine and Pharmacy* (Charleston) 1 (1846): 481–83; Graham Serjeant and Beryl Serjeant, "Sickle-Cell Anaemia before Herrick," *Lancet* 1 (1972): 746–47.

18. Conley, "Sickle-Cell Anemia," 318–71; Serjeant and Serjeant, "Sickle-Cell Anaemia before Herrick," 746–47; A. Adeloye, "Sickle-Cell Anaemia," *British Medical Journal* 2 (1973): 304. See also Wailoo, "'Disease *Sui Generis*,'" 185–208, esp. 195–98.

19. Washburn, "Peculiar Elongated and Sickle-Shaped Red Blood Corpuscles," 490–93; P. G. Firth, "Anaesthesia for Peculiar Cells—A Century of Sickle Cell Disease," *British Journal of Anaesthesia* 95 (2005): 287–99.

20. Cook and Myer, "Severe Anemia," 644–51; Mason, "Sickle Cell Anemia," 1318–22.

21. V. E. Emmel, "A Study of the Erythrocytes in a Case of Severe Anemia with Elongated and Sickle-Shaped Red Blood Corpuscles," *Archives of Internal Medicine* 20 (1917): 586–98; Sydenstricker, Mulherin, and Houseal, "Sickle Cell Anemia," 132–54; Sydenstricker, "Sickle Cell Anemia," 177–83; Huck, "Sickle Cell Anaemia," 335–44. See also Wailoo, "Disease *Sui Generis*," and Keith Wailoo, "Detecting 'Negro Blood': Black and White Identities and the Reconstruction of Sickle Cell Anemia," in *Drawing Blood: Technology and Disease Identity in Twentieth-Century America* (Baltimore, Md.: Johns Hopkins Univ. Press, 1997), 134–44.

22. G. S. Graham and S. H. McCarty, "Notes on Sickle Cell Anemia," *Journal of Laboratory and Clinical Medicine* 12 (1927): 536–47; Cooley and Lee, "Sickle Cell Phenomenon," 334–40; K. Miyamoto and J. H. Korb, "Meniscocytosis (Latent Sickle Cell Anemia): Its Incidence in St. Louis," *Southern Medical Journal* 20 (1927): 912–16; L. W. Diggs, C. F. Ahmann, and J. Bibb, "The Incidence and Significance of the Sickle Cell Trait," *Annals of Internal Medicine* 7 (1933–34): 769–78.

23. W. B. Stewart, "Sickle Cell Anemia: Report of a Case with Splenectomy," *American Journal of Diseases of Children* 34 (1927): 72–80.

24. Sydenstricker, "Sickle Cell Anemia."

25. Cooley and Lee, "Sickle Cell Phenomenon," 340.

26. E. Vernon Hahn and Elizabeth B. Gillespie, "Sickle Cell Anemia: Report of a Case Greatly Improved by Splenectomy," *Archives of Internal Medicine* 39 (1927): 233–54; B. Steinberg, "Sickle Cell Anemia," *Archives of Pathology and Laboratory Medicine* 9 (1930): 876–97; Margolies, "Sickle Cell Anemia," 357–443, esp. 358–59.

27. Stewart, "Sickle Cell Anemia"; Margolies, "Sickle Cell Anemia," 361–63; Taliaferro and Huck, "Inheritance of Sickle Cell Anaemia in Man," 493–98.

28. Margolies, "Sickle Cell Anemia," 362. See also Diggs, Ahmann, and Bibb, "Incidence and Significance."

29. Julian H. Lewis, *Biology of the Negro* (Chicago: Univ. of Chicago Press, 1942), 236. See also W. W. Anderson and R. L. Ware, "Sickle Cell Anemia," *JAMA* 99 (1932): 902–5.

30. Diggs, Ahmann, and Bibb, "Incidence and Significance"; J. V. Neel, "The Inheritance of Sickle Cell Anemia," *Science* 110 (1949): 64–66; Margolies, "Sickle Cell Anemia."

31. Conley, "Sickle-Cell Anemia." See also Wailoo, "Disease *Sui Generis*"; Wailoo, "Detecting 'Negro Blood'"; and Wailoo, *Dying in the City of the Blues.*

32. Cyrus C. Sturgis, *Hematology,* 2d ed. (Springfield, Ill.: Charles C. Thomas, 1955), 468.

33. Sydenstricker, "Sickle Cell Anemia"; Miyamoto and Korb, "Meniscocytosis."

34. Margolies, "Sickle Cell Anemia," 401–4; Sturgis, *Hematology,* 483–84; P. K. Switzer and H. H. Fouche, "The Sickle Cell Trait: Incidence and Influence in Pregnant Colored Women," *American Journal of the Medical Sciences* 216 (1948): 330–32.

35. L. Pauling, H. A. Itano, S. J. Singer, and I. C. Wells, "Sickle Cell Anemia: A Molecular Disease," *Science* 110 (1949): 543–48.

36. Conley, "Sickle-Cell Anemia." See also Wailoo, *Dying in the City of the Blues,* and Tapper, *In the Blood.*

37. Conley, "Sickle-Cell Anemia."

38. Sydenstricker, "Sickle Cell Anemia," 182.

39. See, for example, J. P. Baker, "Sickle Cell Anemia," *Virginia Medical Monthly* 69 (1942): 208–12.

40. Sydenstricker, "Sickle Cell Anemia," 182.

41. Cooley and Lee, "Sickle Cell Phenomenon"; U.S. Department of Labor, Division of Negro Economics, *Negro Migration in 1916–1917* (Washington, D.C., 1919; repr., Westport, Conn.: Greenwood Press, 1969); R. A. Moser and W. J. Shaw, "Sickle-Cell Anemia in the Northern Negro," *JAMA* 84 (1925): 507–8.

42. Stewart, "Sickle Cell Anemia"; Baker, "Sickle Cell Anemia"; T. Winsor and G. E. Burch, "Sickle Cell Anemia: 'A Great Masquerader,'" *JAMA* 129 (1945): 793–96; B. C. Halpern and H. K. Faber, "The Cardiopathology of Sickle Cell Anemia and Its Differentiation from Rheumatic Carditis," *Journal of Pediatrics* 30 (1974): 289–94.

43. J. F. Hamilton, "A Case of Sickle Cell Anemia," *U.S. Veteran's Bureau Medical Bulletin* 2 (1926): 497–500.

44. "Clinicopathologic Conference. A Patient with Sickle Cell Anemia Surviving Forty-Eight Years," *American Journal of Medicine* 48 (1970): 226–34.

45. Anderson and Ware, "Sickle Cell Anemia," 905.

46. J. T. Givens, "Sickle-Cell Anemia," *Journal of the National Medical Association* 37 (1945): 133.

47. Marian M. Torchia, "The Tuberculosis Movement and the Race Question, 1890–1950," *Bulletin of the History of Medicine* 49 (1975): 152–68.

48. Lewis, *Biology of the Negro,* 228–250; S. J. Holmes, *The Negro's Struggle for Survival: A Study in Human Ecology* (Berkeley: Univ. of California Press, 1937); Gunnar Myrdal, *An American Dilemma: The Negro Problem and Modern Democracy* (New York: Harper and Brothers, 1944); "The Health Status and Health Education of Negroes in the United States," *Journal of Negro Education* (Yearbook Issue) 6 (1937): 259–587; "The Health Status and Health Education of Negroes in the United States," *Journal of Negro Education* (Yearbook Issue) 18 (1949): 197–443.

49. Editorial, "Race and Disease," *Journal of the National Medical Association* 40 (1948): 259.

50. George W. Gray, "Sickle-Cell Anemia," *Scientific American* 185 (Aug. 1951): 56–69; Anthony C. Allison, "Sickle Cells and Evolution," *Scientific American* 195 (Aug. 1956): 87–94.

51. Myron C. Golton, "Sickle Cell Anemia: The Race Malady," *Negro Digest* 13 (Dec. 1963): 73–77; Lydia Allen DeVilbiss, "Sickle Cell Anaemia," *American Mercury* 89 (Aug.

1959): 129–32; M. A. Walker, "I'm Living on Borrowed Time," *Ebony* 14 (Jan. 1959): 40–46; "The Sickle Threat," *Time* 73 (Jan. 19, 1959): 42.

52. "Mechanism of a Fatal Anemia," *Life* 64 (June 21, 1968): 51–52; "Incurable 'Negro Disease' Strikes Five in Family," *Ebony* 21 (May 1966): 154–62; Dick Campbell, "Sickle Cell Anemia and Its Affect on Black People," *The Crisis* 73 (Jan.–Feb. 1971): 7–9; "Discriminating Disease," *Time* 96 (Dec. 21, 1970): 41; A. H. Pettigrew and T. F. Pettigrew, "Race, Disease and Desegregation: A New Look," *Phylon* 24 (1963): 315–33. See also Wailoo, *Dying in the City of the Blues*, 147–48.

53. Pettigrew and Pettigrew, "Race, Disease and Desegregation"; C. Putnam, *Race and Reason: A Yankee View* (Washington, D.C.: Public Affairs Press, 1961), 46, 50; T. F. Pettigrew, *A Profile of the Negro American* (Princeton, N.J.: D. Van Nostrand, 1964), 90–92. See also Tapper, *In the Blood.*

54. But Wailoo, *Dying in the City of the Blues*, describes some community activities in Memphis.

55. Robert B. Scott, "Sickle-Cell Anemia—High Prevalence and Low Priority," *New England Journal of Medicine* 282 (1970): 164–65; Scott, "Health Care Priority."

56. Scott, "Health Care Priority," 731.

57. Roland B. Scott, "A Commentary on Sickle Cell Disease," *Journal of the National Medical Association* 63 (1971): 1–2, 60. See also Editorial, "Sickle Cell Anemia," *JAMA* 214 (1970): 749.

58. Barbara J. Culliton, "Sickle Cell Anemia: The Route from Obscurity to Prominence," *Science* 178 (1972): 138–42. See also, in addition to the articles cited earlier, Greenberg, "Need to Identify Sickle-Cell Trait," 629–30; Doris L. Wethers, Letter to the Editor, *New England Journal of Medicine* 282 (1970): 630; William J. Stone, "Sickle-Cell Trait," [Letter to the Editor], *New England Journal of Medicine* 282 (1970): 1157–58; William C. Mentzer Jr., Bertram H. Lubin, and David G. Nathan, "Screening for Sickle-Cell Trait and G-6-PD Deficiency," *New England Journal of Medicine* 282 (1970): 1155–56; "Counterattack on a Killer: Blacks Fight to End Tragic Toll of Sickle Cell Anemia," *Ebony* 26 (Oct. 1971): 84–93; R. M. Nalbandian, N. L. Henry, J. M. Lusher, F. R. Camp Jr., and N. F. Conte, "Sickledex Test for Hemoglobin S: A Critique," *JAMA* 218 (1971): 1679–80; R. M. Nalbandian, B. M. Nichols, A. E. Heustis, W. B. Prothro, and F. E. Ludwig, "An Automated Mass Screening Program for Sickle Cell Disease," *JAMA* 218 (1971): 1680–82; L. W. Diggs, "New Strategy for Sickle Cell Disease," *JAMA* 218 (1971): 1693–94.

59. For more on social and political issues surrounding sickle cell anemia in the twentieth century, see Wailoo, *Dying in the City of the Blues*, and Tapper, *In the Blood.*

7. Black Health on the Plantation

This chapter originally appeared as "Black Health on the Plantation: Masters, Slaves and Physicians," in *Science and Medicine in the Old South*, ed. Ronald L. Numbers and Todd L. Savitt (Baton Rouge: Louisiana State Univ. Press, 1989), 327–55.

1. This chapter is extracted in large part from Savitt, *Medicine and Slavery*, 1–184. Citations in this chapter are only for direct quotes or references or are to pertinent sources appearing since the publication of *Medicine and Slavery.*

Except in the first section of this chapter, which is a general overview of black-related diseases, the focus is on Virginia from the Revolutionary War to the Civil War. Health conditions in the Old Dominion at that time were, in many respects, typical of those prevailing throughout the antebellum South. Residents suffered from malaria, parasitic worm diseases, and dysentery just as Mississippians and Georgians did. Yellow fever struck the state's major ports, though usually not so severely or so frequently as at Charleston, Mobile, or New Orleans. Virginia's position on the northern fringe of the slaveholding South perhaps lessened the intensity and duration of warm-weather diseases, but not enough to render its diseases significantly different from those in the lower South.

During the time span under consideration, the black population and the health picture in Virginia were relatively stable. The slave trade had ended, there was little black "immigration" into the state, and tropical diseases brought from Africa and unable to survive in the new environment had all but disappeared.

2. Editorial, *Monthly Stethoscope and Medical Reporter* 1 (1856): 162–63.

3. These medical differences and other diseases and conditions are discussed in Kenneth F. Kiple and Virginia Himmelsteib King, *Another Dimension to the Black Diaspora: Diet, Disease, and Racism* (Cambridge, U.K.: Cambridge Univ. Press, 1981). See also Kiple, *Caribbean Slave;* Kiple, *African Exchange;* Darrett B. Rutman, Charles Wetherell, and Anita H. Rutman, "Rhythms of Life: Black and White Seasonality in the Early Chesapeake," *Journal of Interdisciplinary History* 11 (1980): 29–53; Richard H. Steckel, "A Peculiar Population: The Nutrition, Health, and Mortality of American Slaves from Childhood to Maturity," *Journal of Economic History* 46 (1986): 721–41; Susan E. Klepp, "Seasoning and Society: Racial Differences in Mortality in Eighteenth-Century Philadelphia," *The William and Mary Quarterly,* 3d ser., 51 (1994): 473–506. On the life and thought of one Southern medical thinker, see Reginald Horsman, *Josiah Nott of Mobile: Southerner, Physician, and Racial Theorist* (Baton Rouge: Louisiana State Univ. Press, 1987).

4. For a discussion of the Southern disease environment from colonial times to the present, see Albert Cowdrey, *This Land, This South: An Environmental History* (Lexington: Univ. Press of Kentucky, 1983). See also K. David Patterson, "Disease Environments of the Antebellum South," in *Science and Medicine in the Old South,* ed. Ronald L. Numbers and Todd L. Savitt (Baton Rouge: Louisiana State Univ. Press, 1989), 152–65. On malaria and immunity, see Kevin Marsh, "Immunology of Malaria," in *Essential Malariology,* ed. David A. Warrell and Herbert M. Gilles, 4th ed. (London: Arnold, 2002), 252–67.

5. Kiple and King, *Another Dimension,* emphasize dietary considerations in their explanations of many slave health problems.

6. John H. Van Evrie, *Negroes and Negro "Slavery"* (New York: Van Evrie, Horton, and Co., 1861), 25. A recent discussion of racial differences in susceptibility to frostbite is W. H. Candler and H. Ivey, "Cold Weather Injuries among U.S. Soldiers in Alaska: A Five-Year Review," *Military Medicine* 162 (1997): 788–91.

7. Van Evrie, *Negroes and Negro "Slavery,"* 251, 256.

8. Peripherally related to the matter of differences in electrolyte retention between whites and blacks is the issue of white and black differences in the incidence of hypertension. For a discussion and references to the debate over this issue, see Jay S. Kaufman and Susan A. Hall, "The Slavery Hypertension Hypothesis: Dissemination and Appeal of a Modern Race Theory," *Epidemiology* 14 (2003): 111–18. Commentaries and a rejoinder by the authors may be found in ibid., 118–26.

9. For examples of the political use some white Southerners made of the relative immunity of blacks to yellow fever and of blacks' ability to labor in humid heat, see Jo Ann Carrigan, "Yellow Fever: Scourge of the South," in *Disease and Distinctiveness in the American South,* ed. Todd L. Savitt and James Harvey Young (Knoxville: Univ. of Tennessee Press, 1988), 55–78. On yellow fever immunity, see Donald B. Cooper and Kenneth F. Kiple, "Yellow Fever," in *Cambridge Historical Dictionary of Disease,* ed. Kiple, 3.

10. "Medico-Chirurgical Society of Richmond, [Mar. 1, 1853]," *Virginia Medical and Surgical Journal* 1 (1853): 35.

11. Recent historical discussions of SIDS and slavery include Kiple and King, *Another*

Dimension, 107–10, and Johnson, "Smothered Slave Infants," 493–520. See chapter 1 of this book for a more detailed discussion and more references to recent scholarship on the history of SIDS.

12. E. M. Pendleton, "On the Susceptibility of the Caucasian and African Races to the Different Classes of Disease," *Southern Medical Reports* 1 (1849): 336–37.

13. Editorial, "The Medical Society of Virginia," *Virginia Medical and Surgical Journal* 4 (1855): 256–58.

14. On the matter of Southern medical nationalism, see James O. Breeden, "States-Rights Medicine in the Old South," *Bulletin of the New York Academy of Medicine* 52 (1976): 348–72; John Duffy, "Medical Practice in the Antebellum South," *Journal of Southern History* 25 (1959): 53–72; and John Harley Warner, "A Southern Medical Reform: The Meaning of the Antebellum Argument for Southern Medical Education," *Bulletin of the History of Medicine* 57 (1983): 364–81; Warner, "The Idea of Southern Medical Distinctiveness: Medical Knowledge and Practice in the Old South," in *Science and Medicine in the Old South*, ed. Numbers and Savitt, 179–205.

15. Richard Allen Williams, ed., *Textbook of Black-Related Diseases* (New York: McGraw-Hill, 1975).

16. For an example of typical planters' writings on the management of the enslaved, see James O. Breeden, ed., *Advice among Masters: The Ideal of Slave Management in the Old South* (Westport, Conn.: Greenwood Press, 1980).

17. Kiple and King, *Another Dimension.* See also Robert A. Margo and Richard H. Steckel, "The Heights of American Slaves: New Evidence on Slave Nutrition and Health," *Social Science History* 6 (1982): 516–38; Steckel, "Peculiar Population"; Steckel, "A Dreadful Childhood: The Excess Mortality of American Slaves," *Social Science History* 10 (1986): 427–66.

18. Shirley in the James Farm Journals, June 23, 1825, Library of Congress, Washington, D.C.

19. Quoted in Wyndham B. Blanton, *Medicine in Virginia in the Eighteenth Century* (Brooklyn, N.Y.: AMS Press, 1931), 161 (Blanton cites no source).

20. Charles R. Kemper, "Case of Injury from the Penetration of a Hay Fork into the Abdomen—with Recovery," *Stethoscope and Virginia Monthly Gazette* 4 (1854): 9–11.

21. Interview of William Lee, n.d., in WPA Folklore File, Manuscript Room, Alderman Library, University of Virginia, Charlottesville.

22. White Hill Plantation Books, July 6–20, 1849, Southern Historical Collection, University of North Carolina at Chapel Hill Library.

23. On enslaved women's and children's health conditions, see also Kiple and King, *Another Dimension;* Steckel, "Dreadful Childhood"; J. Campbell, "Work, Pregnancy, and Infant Mortality among Southern Slaves," *Journal of Interdisciplinary History* 14 (1984): 793–812; Deborah Gray White, *Ar'n't I a Woman? Female Slaves in the Plantation South* (New York: Norton, 1985), 79–87, 124–26; Wilma King, *Stolen Childhood: Slave Youth in Nineteenth-Century America* (Bloomington: Indiana Univ. Press, 1995), 9–16; Marie Jenkins Schwartz, *Born in Bondage: Growing Up Enslaved in the Antebellum South* (Cambridge, Mass.: Harvard Univ. Press, 2000); Schwartz, *Birthing a Slave: Motherhood and Medicine in the Antebellum South* (Cambridge, Mass.: Harvard Univ. Press, forthcoming 2006). More general studies on antebellum Southern medicine that include discussions of enslaved women's and children's situations include Steven M. Stowe, "Obstetrics and the Work of Doctoring in the Mid-Nineteenth-Century American South," *Bulletin of the History of Medicine* 64 (1990): 540–66; Sally G. McMillen, *Motherhood in the Old South: Pregnancy, Childbirth and Infant Rearing* (Baton Rouge: Louisiana State Univ. Press, 1990); McMillen, "Antebellum Southern Fathers and the Health Care of Children," *Journal of Southern History* 60 (1994): 513–32; McMillen, "'No Uncommon Disease': Neonatal Tetanus, Slave Infants, and the Southern Medical Profession," *Journal of the History of Medicine and Allied Sciences* 46 (1991): 291–314.

24. Alban S. Payne, "Report of Obstetrical Cases," *Stethoscope and Virginia Monthly Gazette* 3 (1853): 204.

25. Fredrick Law Olmsted, *A Journey in the Seaboard Slave States, with Remarks on Their Economy* (New York: Dix and Edwards, 1856), 190.

26. Thomas Jefferson to Joel Yancey, Jan. 17, 1819, in *Thomas Jefferson's Farm Book, with Commentaries and Relevant Extracts from Other Writings*, ed. Edwin M. Betts (Princeton, N.J.: Princeton Univ. Press, 1953), 43. On women feigning illness, see Sharla M. Fett, *Working Cures: Healing, Health, and Power on Southern Slave Plantations* (Chapel Hill: Univ. of North Carolina Press, 2002), 179–86.

27. There were, of course, exceptions to these statements. See, for example, Johnson, "Smothered Slave Infants," 511–20.

28. Adelaide M. Hunter, "The Punishment of Crimes in Virginia" (master's thesis, Duke University, 1947), 15; *Commonwealth v. Sall and Creasy*, Apr. 14, 1806, described in James Hugo Johnson, *Race Relations in Virginia and Miscegenation in the South, 1776–1860* (Amherst: Univ. of Massachusetts Press, 1970), 22; Governor Henry Wise, "Message IV Relative to Reprieves and Pardons, to the General Assembly of Virginia," Dec. 7, 1857, in Virginia, *Governor's Message and Reports of the Public Officers of the State, of the Boards of Directors, and of the Visitors, Superintendents, and Other Agents of Public Institutions or Interests of Virginia*, 1857–58, part 1, doc. 1, clxxvi; Legislative Petitions, Richmond [City], Dec. 23, 1857, Virginia State Library, Richmond.

29. Steckel, "Dreadful Childhood," 427–29.

30. John Walker Diary, Apr. 23, 1853, Southern Historical Collection, University of North Carolina at Chapel Hill Library; *The Diary of Colonel Landon Carter of Sabine Hall, 1752–1778*, ed. Jack P. Greene (Charlottesville: Univ. Press of Virginia, 1965), 1:377 (entry for Mar. 31, 1770); *Journal and Letters of Phillip Vickers Fithian, 1773–1774: A Plantation Tutor of the Old Dominion*, ed. Hunter Dickinson Farish (Williamsburg, Va.: Colonial Williamsburg, 1957), 182.

31. For an excellent look at these issues and at slave self-care, see Fett, *Working Cures.*

32. Catherine C. Hopley, *Life in the South: From the Commencement of the War* (London: Chapman and Hall, 1863), 1:103.

33. On the healing roles of white women on the plantation, see Catherine Clinton, *The Plantation Mistress: Women's World in the Old South* (New York: Pantheon, 1982), 28, 43, 187. See also Fett, *Working Cures*, 65–67, 111–41, esp. 115–17, 134–35; Schwartz, *Born in Bondage;* McMillen, *Motherhood in the Old South.*

34. For more examples of such notes, see Todd L. Savitt, ed., "Patient Letters to an Early Nineteenth Century Virginia Physician," *Journal of the Florida Medical Association* 69 (1982): 688–94.

35. The best treatment of Thomsonianism in a Southern state is James O. Breeden, "Thomsonianism in Virginia," *Virginia Magazine of History and Biography* 82 (1974): 150–80. On the national Thomsonian movement, see John S. Haller Jr., *The People's Doctors: Samuel Thomson and the American Botanical Movement, 1790–1860* (Carbondale: Southern Illinois Univ. Press, 2000); Alex Berman and Michael A. Flannery, *America's Botanico-Medical Movements: Vox Populi* (New York: Pharmaceutical Products Press, 2001), esp. 69–93.

36. James L. Hubard to Robert T. Hubard, Aug. 4, 1857, in Hubard Papers; Greene, *Diary of Landon Carter*, 2:812 (entry for May 20, 1774).

37. G. Lane Corbin, "Collodion on Stumps of Amputated Limbs," *Stethoscope and Virginia Monthly Gazette* 1 (1851): 489.

38. L. G. Cabell to Bowker Preston, Oct. 8, 1834, in John Hook Collection, Manuscript Room, Alderman Library, University of Virginia, Charlottesville.

39. W. S. Morton, "Causes of Mortality amongst Negroes," *Monthly Stethoscope and Medical Reporter* 1 (1856): 290.

40. John W. H. Trugien, "A Case of Wound of the Left Ventricle of the Heart—Patient Survived Five Days—with Remarks," *American Journal of the Medical Sciences*, n.s., 20 (1850): 99–102.

41. See, for more information and references, Lawrence W. Levine, *Black Culture and Black Consciousness: Afro-American Folk Thought from Slavery to Freedom* (New York: Oxford Univ. Press, 1977), 55–80; Fett, *Working Cures.*

42. Richard S. Cauthorn, "A New Anti-Periodic and a Substitute for Quinia," *Monthly Stethoscope and Medical Reporter* 2 (1857): 7–14.

43. For more on conjuring and herbal and folk remedies among antebellum African Americans, see Fett, *Working Cures*, 60–108; and Elliott J. Gorn, "Black Magic: Folk Beliefs of the Slave Community," in *Science and Medicine in the Old South*, ed. Numbers and Savitt, 295–326.

44. John M. Galt, *Practical Medicine: Illustrated by Cases of the Most Important Diseases* (Philadelphia: Barrington and Haswell, 1843), 295–96.

45. [William McKean to James Dunlap], July 17, 1810, in Roslin Plantation Records, Virginia State Library, Richmond.

46. Interview of Virginia Hayes Shepherd, 1939, in WPA Folklore File, Alderman Library, University of Virginia, Charlottesville.

47. Interview of Uncle Bacchus White, 1939, in WPA Folklore File, Alderman Library, University of Virginia, Charlottesville. Much of Fett's book *Working Cures* deals with enslaved women as healers.

48. White Hill Plantation Books, 1:8, Southern Historical Collection, University of North Carolina at Chapel Hill Library. See also White, *Ar'n't I a Woman?* 125.

49. Louise Clarke Pyrnelle, *Diddie, Dumps, and Tot; or, Plantation Child-Life* (New York: Harper, 1882), quoted in Blanton, *Medicine in Virginia*, 49.

50. See also White, *Ar'n't I a Woman?* 111–24. Free black women also practiced midwifery in parts of the Old South. See, for example, Suzanne Lebsock, *The Free Women of Petersburg: Status and Culture in a Southern Town, 1784–1860* (New York: Norton, 1984).

8. Medical Experimentation and Demonstration on Blacks in the Old South

This chapter originally appeared as "The Use of Blacks for Medical Experimentation and Demonstration in the Old South," *Journal of Southern History* 48 (1982): 331–48.

1. J. Walter Fisher, "Physicians and Slavery in the Antebellum Southern Medical Journal," *Journal of the History of Medicine and Allied Sciences* 23 (1968): 45. W. Montague Cobb discussed a similar theme in "Surgery and the Negro Physician: Some Parallels in Background," *Journal of the National Medical Association* 43 (May 1951): 145–52, esp. 147–48.

2. David C. Humphrey, "Dissection and Discrimination: The Social Origins of Cadavers in America, 1760–1915," *Bulletin of the New York Academy of Medicine* 49 (1973): 819–27; John B. Blake, "Anatomy," in *The Education of American Physicians: Historical Essays*, ed. Ronald L. Numbers (Berkeley: Univ. of California Press, 1980), 34–35, 37. See also Suzanne M. Shultz, *Body Snatching: The Robbing of Graves for the Education of Physicians in Early Nineteenth Century America* (Jefferson, N.C.: McFarland, 1992); Michael Sappol, *A Traffic of Dead Bodies: Anatomy and Embodied Social Identity in Nineteenth-Century America* (Princeton, N.J.: Princeton Univ. Press, 2002); Richardson, *Death, Dissection and the Destitute* (London: Routledge and Kegan Paul, 1987).

3. John Duffy, "A Note on Ante-Bellum Southern Nationalism and Medical Practice," *Journal of Southern History* 34 (1968): 274–76; John S. Haller Jr., "The Negro and the Southern Physician: A Study of Medical and Racial Attitudes, 1800–1860," *Medical History*

16 (1972): 247–51; Savitt, *Medicine and Slavery*, 7–17. See also Warner, "Idea of Southern Medical Distinctiveness," 186; and Warner, "Southern Medical Reform," 223.

4. Commenting on this irony, the anatomist W. Montague Cobb, himself African American, wrote in 1951, "[O]ur [white] colleagues recognized in the Negro [on the dissecting table] a perfection in human structure which they were unwilling to concede when structure was animated by the vital spark." Cobb, "Surgery and the Negro Physician," 148.

5. On the ideas and importance of the Paris school of hospital medicine, see Erwin H. Ackerknecht, *Medicine at the Paris Hospital, 1794–1848* (Baltimore, Md.: Johns Hopkins Press, 1967); Michel Foucault, *The Birth of the Clinic: An Archaeology of Medical Perception* (New York: Pantheon Books, 1973). On the influence of the Paris school on American medicine, see Shryock, *Development of Modern Medicine*, 170–91; Gerald N. Grob, *Edward Jarvis and the Medical World of Nineteenth-Century America* (Knoxville: Univ. of Tennessee Press, 1978), 37–38; John Harley Warner, *Against the Spirit of System: The French Impulse in Nineteenth-Century American Medicine* (Baltimore, Md.: Johns Hopkins Univ. Press, 1998).

6. Robert Peter, *The History of the Medical Department of Transylvania University* (Louisville, Ky.: J. P. Morton and Company, 1905), 61; catalogues of the Medical Department of Transylvania University, 1829–1855, in the library at Transylvania University, Lexington, Kentucky; "Preamble and Resolutions of the Dissecting Class [of Transylvania Medical College, 1837/38]," Appendix to Thomas D. Mitchell, "Transylvania Catalogue of Medical Graduates, with an Appendix, Containing a Concise History of the School from Its Commencement to the Present Time," *Transylvania Journal of Medicine and the Associate Sciences* 11 (Jan.–Mar. 1838): 229–30. For a discussion of the history of anatomy in antebellum Kentucky, see Wayne C. Williams, "The Teachers and Teaching of Anatomy in the Medical Department of Transylvania University, 1799–1857" (paper in Savitt's possession), 7–16. Mr. Williams was director of the Audiovisual Department, East Carolina University School of Medicine. See also John H. Ellis, *Medicine in Kentucky* (Lexington: Univ. Press of Kentucky, 1977), 13.

7. Quoted in Franklin M. Garrett, *Atlanta and Environs: A Chronicle of Its People and Events* (New York: Lewis Historical, 1954), 1:395–96 (quotation on 395, from *Atlanta Weekly Intelligencer*, Oct. 12, 1855). See also Gerald L. Cates, "Medical Schools in Ante-Bellum Georgia" (M.A. thesis, University of Georgia, 1968), 92–93.

8. J. G. Westmoreland, "Report of Medical Clinic, Continued," *Atlanta Medical and Surgical Journal* 1 (Feb. 1856): 329 (first two quotations), 331 (third quotation). On the use of blacks and indigent whites in Alabama, see W. Taylor, "Annual Oration," *Transactions of the Medical Association of the State of Alabama* 8 (Feb. 1855): 121.

9. *Charleston Courier*, Nov. 14, 1837.

10. Ibid., Nov. 16, 1837.

11. *Annual Circular of the Trustees and Faculty of the Medical College of the State of South Carolina . . . Session of 1840–41* (Charleston, S.C.: n.p., 1841), 5–6.

12. "A Plan of Organization for the Roper Hospital. Adopted by the Medical Society, Jan. 3, 1846," *Rules and Regulations for the Government of the Trustees and Officers of the Roper Hospital* (Charleston, S.C.: Evans and Cogswell, 1861), 11–12; *Annual Circular of the Trustees and Faculty of the Medical College of the State of South Carolina . . . Session of 1857–58*, 17. See also Joseph Ioor Waring, *A History of Medicine in South Carolina, 1825–1900* ([Charleston?]: South Carolina Medical Association, 1967), 75–76, 79n.

13. "An Address to the Public in Regard to the Affairs of the Medical Department of Hampden-Sydney College, by Several Physicians of the City of Richmond, 1853," quoted in Blanton, *Medicine in Virginia*, 38–39; *Richmond Enquirer*, May 8, 1860; "Notes of the Hampden-Sydney Medical Department Minutes," in William T. Sanger, *Medical College of Virginia before 1925, and University College of Medicine 1893–1913* (Richmond, Va.: Medical College of Virginia Foundation, 1973), 8; Editorial, "A State General Hospital," *Virginia*

Medical and Surgical Journal 1 (1853): 173–74; Editorial, "The Virginia Free Hospital," *Virginia Medical and Surgical Journal* 3 (1854): 273–75. For more descriptive details see Savitt, *Medicine and Slavery*, 282–86.

14. Of 109 patients mentioned in Richmond medical journals between 1851 and 1860, 63.3 percent (69) were black. For a listing of the pertinent journal articles, see Savitt, *Medicine and Slavery*, 286.

15. See, for example, *Richmond Daily Dispatch*, July 21, 1854; William W. Brown, *Clotel, or, The President's Daughter: A Narrative of Slave Life in the United States* (London: Partridge and Oakey, 1853), 123–24, cited in Gladys-Marie Fry, *Night Riders in Black Folk History* (Knoxville: Univ. of Tennessee Press, 1975), 175–76; Keith A. Winsell, "Black Identity: The Southern Negro, 1830–1895" (Ph.D. diss., University of California at Los Angeles, 1971), 188.

16. *Circular of the Transylvania University Medical Department, Session of 1846–47*, 4. For a vivid description of the popular image of distasteful hospital life, see Thomas Jefferson to Joseph C. Cabell, May 16, 1824, in *Early History of the University of Virginia as Contained in the Letters of Thomas Jefferson and Joseph C. Cabell*, ed. Nathaniel F. Cabell (Richmond, Va.: J. W. Randolph, 1856), 310.

17. Henry A. Ramsay, "Gastro-Enteritis of Twelve Months Duration, Exhibiting in Autopsy an Entire Absence of the Spleen, and Calcareous Depositions in Both Lungs," *Charleston Medical Journal and Review* 5 (1850): 728–32 (quotation on 732).

18. Roper Hospital Case Book #2, 1858–62, 432, in possession of Dr. Robert Jordan, Sanford, North Carolina (microfilm copy at Waring Historical Library, Medical University of South Carolina, Charleston). See also Walter Brice, "Typhoid Fever, as It Prevailed in Fairfield District, South-Carolina," *Charleston Medical Journal and Review* 6 (1851): 671.

19. George B. Jenkins, "The Legal Status of Dissecting," *Anatomical Record* 7 (1913): 378–88; John B. Blake, "The Development of American Anatomy Acts," *Journal of Medical Education* 30 (1955): 434.

20. Harriet Martineau, *Retrospect of Western Travel* (London: Saunders and Otley, 1838), 1:140, quoted in Humphrey, "Dissection and Discrimination," 819.

21. Henry M. Dowling, "Case of Verminose Disease," *Transylvania Journal of Medicine and the Associate Sciences* 2 (1829): 250.

22. L. H. Anderson, "Report on the Diseases of Sumterville and Vicinity," *Transactions of the Medical Association of the State of Alabama* 7 (1854): 61–66.

23. Richard Jarrot, "Amputation for Gangrene of the Foot, Successfully Performed on a Negro, at the Advanced Age of One Hundred and Two Years," *Charleston Medical Journal and Review* 4 (1849): 301–3.

24. P. N. Cilley, "Diseases of Lowndesboro and Vicinity," *Proceedings of the Medical Association of the State of Alabama* 5 (Dec. 1851): 91–95.

25. A Young Practitioner, "Report of a Case of Disease Supposed to be Peritonitis," *Monthly Stethoscope and Medical Reporter* 1 (1856): 364.

26. *Milledgeville Statesman and Patriot*, Aug. 16, 1828. The author wishes to thank Professor Larry Morrison, History Department, Virginia Polytechnic Institute and State University, for bringing this newspaper article to his attention.

27. Kentucky House of Representatives, *Journal of the House of Representatives of the Commonwealth of Kentucky* (Frankfort, Ky., 1833), 107, 122–23, 177–78. See also John D. Wright Jr., "Robert Peter and Early Science in Kentucky" (Ph.D. diss., Columbia University, 1955), 61, 70; F. Garvin Davenport, *Ante-Bellum Kentucky: A Social History, 1800–1860* (Oxford, Ohio: Mississippi Valley Press, 1943), 23.

28. Savitt, *Medicine and Slavery*, 290–93; James O. Breeden, "Body Snatchers and Anatomy Professors: Medical Education in Nineteenth-Century Virginia," *Virginia Magazine of History and Biography* 83 (1975): 321–45.

29. Lane Allen, "Grandison Harris, Sr.: Slave, Resurrectionist and Judge," *Bulletin of the Georgia Academy of Science* 34 (1976): 192–99. A more recent piece on Harris attempts (with mixed success) a broader view of the man and his work: Tanya Telfair Sharpe, "Grandison Harris: The Medical College of Georgia's Resurrection Man," in *Bones in the Basement: Postmortem Racism in Nineteenth-Century Medical Training*, ed. Robert L. Blakely and Judith M. Harrington (Washington, D.C.: Smithsonian Institution Press, 1997), 206–24.

30. Fry, *Night Riders*, 173–74.

31. Faculty Minutes, Medical College of the State of South Carolina, May 8, 1876, at the Waring Historical Library, Medical University of South Carolina, Charleston. For reference to similar attitudes at the Medical College of Georgia in Augusta, see Cates, "Medical Schools in Ante-Bellum Georgia," 32, and various essays in Blakely and Harrington, eds., *Bones in the Basement*. On the use of blacks for dissection in an Alabama medical school, see Howard L. Holley, "Dr. Phillip Madison Shepard and His Medical School," *De Historia Medicinae* 2 (Feb. 1958): 1–5. For an instance in Kentucky, see "Autobiography of Dr. Charles A. Hentz" (typescript), 10:108, Hentz Family Papers (Southern Historical Collection, University of North Carolina, Chapel Hill, N.C.). This autobiography has been published recently. See Steven M. Stowe, ed., *A Southern Practice: The Diary and Autobiography of Charles A. Hentz, M.D.* (Charlottesville: Univ. Press of Virginia, 2000), 468.

32. Robert Wilson, "Their Shadowy Influence Still Hovers about Medical College," *Charleston Sunday News Courier*, Apr. 13, 1913. The author wishes to thank Mrs. Anne Donato of the Waring Historical Library, Medical University of South Carolina, Charleston, for bringing this article to his attention.

33. George P. Rawick, ed., *The American Slave: A Composite Autobiography*, vol. 2, *South Carolina Narratives* (Westport, Conn.: Greenwood, 1972), pt. 2, 175–76 (quotation on 176).

34. Fry, *Night Riders*, 170–211.

35. There is evidence to indicate that bodies of persons of color from the South were regularly shipped to Northern medical schools during the post–Civil War era. See Frederick C. Waite, "Grave Robbing in New England," *Bulletin of the Medical Library Association* 33 (1945): 283–84; Cobb, "Surgery and the Negro Physician," 148.

36. *The Scribe of the Medical Society of South Carolina* 1 (Dec. 1951): 17. The author is again indebted to Mrs. Anne Donato, Waring Historical Library, Medical University of South Carolina, Charleston, for this reference.

37. Theodore Dwight Weld, *American Slavery as It Is: Testimony of a Thousand Witnesses* (New York: American Anti-Slavery Society, 1839), 170.

38. For a broad overview of this subject, see Richard H. Shryock, "Empiricism versus Rationalism in American Medicine, 1650–1960," *Proceedings of the American Antiquarian Society*, n.s., 79, pt. 1 (Apr. 15, 1969): 99–150.

39. T. S. Hopkins, "On Nitric Acid in the Treatment of Asthma," *Charleston Medical Journal and Review* 5 (1850): 749–52 (quotation on 750).

40. Joseph Evelyn May, "On the Remedial Use of Sulphate of Quinine in Large Doses," *Transylvania Journal of Medicine and the Associate Sciences* 10 (1837): 218–19. See also Albert Russell, "Remarks on the Use of Cold Water in the Congestive and Collapsed Forms of Fever," *Transylvania Journal of Medicine and the Associate Sciences* 6 (1833): 96–97; Richard D. Arnold, "On the Epidemics of Savannah, Geo., in 1847 and 1848," *Charleston Medical Journal and Review* 4 (1849): 149; Alexander Somervail, "On the Efficacy of a Mixture of Camphor and Muriate of Ammonia in the Treatment of Suppression of Urine," *American Journal of the Medical Sciences* 14 (1834): 113–15; Savitt, *Medicine and Slavery*, 298–301.

41. Ronald L. Numbers, "William Beaumont and the Ethics of Human Experimentation," *Journal of the History of Biology* 12 (Spring 1979): 113–35. See also Chester R. Burns, "Medical Ethics in the United States before the Civil War" (Ph.D. diss., Johns Hopkins

Univ. Press, 1969), 83. For an early expression of this attitude toward blacks as experimental subjects in South Carolina, see Edmund Berkeley and Dorothy S. Berkeley, *Dr. Alexander Garden of Charles Town* (Chapel Hill: Univ. of North Carolina Press, 1969), 95–96. For a full description of Beaumont's work, see James T. Flexner, *Doctors on Horseback: Pioneers of American Medicine* (New York: Viking Press, 1937), 237–89. For an overview of the history of human experimentation in the United States, see Susan E. Lederer, *Subjected to Science: Human Experimentation in America before the Second World War* (Baltimore, Md.: Johns Hopkins Univ. Press, 1995).

42. Weymouth T. Jordan, *Ante-Bellum Alabama: Town and Country* (Tallahassee: Florida State Univ. Press, 1957), 34–35.

43. *Charleston Mercury*, Oct. 12, 1838, reprinted in Weld, *Slavery as It Is*, 171.

44. Louis A. Chamerovzow, ed., *Slave Life in Georgia: A Narrative of the Life, Sufferings, and Escape of John Brown, a Fugitive Slave Now in England* (London: W. M. Watts, 1855), 45–48, cited in F. Nash Boney, "Doctor Thomas Hamilton: Two Views of a Gentleman of the Old South," *Phylon* 28 (1967): 288–92 (quotation on 291).

45. James Marion Sims, *The Story of My Life* (New York: D. Appleton and Company, 1884), 226–46; Seale Harris, *Woman's Surgeon: The Life Story of J. Marion Sims* (New York: Macmillan, 1950), 82–93, 99–103, 108–10; J. Marion Sims, *Silver Sutures in Surgery* (New York: Wood, 1858), 55; Sims to Dr. H. V. Wooten, Jan. 23, 1850, Hardy Vickers Wooten Papers, Manuscripts Division, Alabama Department of Archives and History, Montgomery, Ala. Sims is a controversial figure in the history of human experimentation. Some people argue that no enslaved person could have given truly voluntary consent to any experimental medical procedure and that there thus had to have been an element of coercion in the conduct of Sims's experiments. Others argue that there is no evidence to indicate coercion and that vesico-vaginal fistula was sufficiently repulsive and foul that the three slave women would have willingly undergone these multiple surgeries for relief of so intolerable a condition. See, for example, Deborah Kuhn McGregor, *From Midwives to Medicine: The Birth of American Gynecology* (New Brunswick, N.J.: Rutgers Univ. Press, 1998), esp. 33–68. Lewis L. Wall, an obstetrician/gynecologist at Washington University in St. Louis, has presented papers on Sims's development of vesico-vaginal fistula surgery and the use of slave women, but as of this writing has not published his research.

46. Nathan Bozeman, "Remarks on Vesico-Vaginal Fistule, with an Account of a New Mode of Suture, and Seven Successful Operations," *Louisville Review* 1 (1856): 75–101. Bozeman and Sims became bitter rivals. See McGregor, *From Midwives to Medicine*, 62–66. For information on a Virginia physician's earlier attempts to cure vesico-vaginal fistula using white and black patients, see Savitt, *Medicine and Slavery*, 297–98.

47. Samuel D. Gross, "Report of the Committee on Surgery," Kentucky State Medical Association, *Transactions* 2 (1852): 104–6; Cobb, "Surgery and the Negro Physician," 148.

48. [Minutes of Annual Meeting, Apr. 14, 1853], Medical Society of the State of Georgia, *Transactions* 4 (1853), 7; C[rawford] W. Long, "An Account of the First Use of Sulphuric Ether by Inhalation as an Anesthetic in Surgical Operations," *Southern Medical and Surgical Journal*, n.s., 5 (1849): 710–11.

49. John M. B. Harden, "Some Experiments to Determine the Relative Areas of the Trunks and Branches of Arteries," *Southern Medical and Surgical Journal*, n.s., 2 (1846): 330–33. The author wishes to thank Professor Lester Stephens of the History Department, University of Georgia, for bringing this article to his attention.

50. R[obert] P. Harris, "The Operation of Gastro-Hysterotomy, Viewed in the Light of American Experience and Success; with the History and Results of Sewing up the Uterine Wound; and a Full Tabular Record of the Cæsarean Operations Performed in the United States," *American Journal of the Medical Sciences*, n.s., 75 (1878): 336–39. For more detail on Caesarean section cases in Virginia, see Savitt, *Medicine and Slavery*, 118–19.

51. R[obert] P. Harris, "Special Statistics of the Caesarian Operation in the United States, Showing the Successes and Failures in Each State," *American Journal of Obstetrics* 14 (1881): 347.

9. Slave Life Insurance in Virginia and North Carolina

This chapter originally appeared as "Slave Life Insurance in Virginia and North Carolina," *Journal of Southern History* 43 (1977): 583–600.

The author's research was supported in part by a grant from the National Institutes of Health Grant LM 02477 from the National Library of Medicine, 1973–76.

1. Drewry to Buford, Jan. 20, Apr. 14, 1854, John Buford Papers, Duke University Library, Durham, N.C. (hereafter cited as Buford Papers).

2. See, for example, C. F. Wills to John McCue, Dec. 7, 1852, McCue Family Papers, University of Virginia Library, Charlottesville (hereafter cited as McCue Family Papers); Insurance Policies of slaves Austin and Mary Jane, June 1, 7, 1860, Haxall Family Papers (items 235 and 236), Virginia Historical Society, Richmond (hereafter cited as Haxall Family Papers).

3. Virginia Legislative Petitions, City of Richmond, Feb. 9, 1854, Virginia State Library, Richmond; Josiah C. Nott, "Statistics of Southern Slave Population, with Especial Reference to Life Insurance," *De Bow's Review* 4 (Nov. 1847): 275, 286–87; Robert S. Starobin, *Industrial Slavery in the Old South* (New York: Oxford Univ. Press, 1970), 71–74.

4. For general histories of the life insurance industry, see J. Owen Stalson, *Marketing Life Insurance: Its History in America* (Cambridge, Mass.: Harvard Univ. Press, 1942); Mildred F. Stone, *A Short History of Life Insurance* (Indianapolis: Insurance Research and Review Service, 1947); Terence O'Donnell, comp., *History of Life Insurance in Its Formative Years* (Chicago: American Conservation Company, 1936). Figures are from Stalson, *Marketing Life Insurance*, 784–86.

5. Stalson, *Marketing Life Insurance*, 784–86.

6. Virginia Legislative Petitions, City of Richmond, Feb. 9, 1854.

7. Starobin, *Industrial Slavery*, 71, states that "slave underwriting dated back to at least the turn of the nineteenth century." The proofs he cites, however (254n88), are a series of South Carolina court cases relating to insurance in the international and domestic slave trade. And his example of Jacob, an enslaved boatman (71), is misleading inasmuch as the insurer was an individual rather than a company.

8. Ibid., 71.

9. Ibid., 72. For more on white resistance to slave life insurance, see W. P. Burrell, "The Negro in Insurance," *Proceedings of the Hampton Negro Conference* 8 (1904): 14–15.

10. Eugene D. Genovese, "The Medical and Insurance Costs of Slaveholding in the Cotton Belt," *Journal of Negro History* 45 (July 1960): 146–47, 155.

11. It appears that a much higher ratio of bondsmen engaged in certain particularly hazardous pursuits was protected. All five enslaved workers, for example, killed in an 1859 explosion at the Bright Hope Coal Pits in Chesterfield County, Virginia, were insured, as were some forty bondsmen purchased by the Cape Fear and Deep River Navigation Company (North Carolina) in 1855, and many of the bondsmen hired to the Great Dismal Swamp Land Company and to John Buford, the contractor building the Virginia and Tennessee Railroad. *Petersburg (Va.) Daily Express*, Apr. 15, 1859; Cape Fear and Deep River Navigation Company, Account Books, vol. 21, 72; vol. 25, 10, 14, 34, in Henry Adolphus London Papers, Southern Historical Collection, University of North Carolina Library, Chapel Hill (hereafter cited as London Papers); Samuel Drewry to John Buford, Jan. 20, Apr. 14, May 18, Dec. 30, 1854, Buford Papers.

12. Nott, "Statistics," 286–87.

13. Virginia Executive Papers, Governor Floyd, June 1851, Virginia State Library (Richmond Fire Association policy); Folder 9, London Papers (North Carolina Mutual Life Insurance Company policies); *Woodfin v. Asheville Mutual Insurance Company,* 6 Jones (N.C.) 558 (1859); C. F. Wills to John McCue, Dec. 7, 1852, McCue Family Papers (Lynchburg Hose and Fire Insurance Company); Joseph Adolph Linn Papers (hereafter cited as Linn Papers), 1855, Southern Historical Collection (Greensborough Mutual Life Insurance and Trust Company policy). For examples of other Southern companies insuring lives of bondspeople, see *Savannah Morning News,* Dec. 16, 1851 (Southern Mutual Insurance Company); O'Donnell, *History of Life Insurance,* 744–46 (Phenix Insurance Company of St. Louis); *Affleck's Southern Rural Almanac, 1851,* 47 (general statement about slave life insurance).

14. C. F. Wills to Buford, Feb. 25, 1854, Buford Papers.

15. *Petersburg Daily Express,* Aug. 13, 1859; North Carolina Mutual Life Insurance Company Minute Book, Feb. 5, 1849, Archives, State Division of Archives and History, Raleigh, N.C. (hereafter cited as NC Mutual Minutes); Jordan to J. M. Hirah, Jan. 2, 1855, Orin Datus Davis Papers, Southern Historical Collection, University of North Carolina Library, Chapel Hill. For a similar case, see NC Mutual Minutes, Aug. 20, 1851.

16. C. F. Wills to John McCue, Dec. 7, 1852, McCue Family Papers.

17. See, for example, M. W. Davenport to John McCue, July 1, 1852, McCue Family Papers; *Petersburg Daily Express,* Aug. 13, 1859.

18. Slaughter to Grinnan, Dec. 15, 1852, Grinnan Family Papers, University of Virginia Library (hereafter cited as Grinnan Family Papers).

19. A. Alexander Little to Andrew G. Grinnan, Feb. 8, 1851, Grinnan Family Papers; M. W. Davenport to John McCue, July 1, 1852, McCue Family Papers; NC Mutual Minutes, July 5, 1856.

20. *Petersburg Daily Express,* Feb. 2, 1859.

21. James F. Jordan Jr. to W. T. B. Haynesworth, Mar. 21, 1851, James F. Jordan Papers, Archives, North Carolina Division of Archives and History (hereafter cited as Jordan Papers); M. W. Davenport to John McCue, July 1, 1852, McCue Family Papers.

22. NC Mutual Minutes, Feb. 9, 1858 (hernia); May 12, Aug. 4, 1857 (unsound); Oct. 31, 1849, and Nov. 6, 1857 (pregnancy).

23. A. C. Mitchell to Buford, Apr. 7, 1854, Buford Papers. For instances from other states of physical examinations for slave life insurance, see *Bloodgood v. Wilson,* 10 La. Ann. 302 (1855); *Murphy v. Mutual Benefit Life and Fire Insurance Company,* 6 La. Ann. 518 (1851); *Durham v. Broddus,* 26 Ga. 524 (1855).

24. Drewry to Buford, Apr. 14, May 18, 1854, Buford Papers.

25. Drewry to Buford, Apr. 14, 1854; Jno. H. Baker to Buford, Feb. 17 1855, Buford Papers.

26. *Richmond Enquirer,* Jan. 27, 1860; printed circular of Franklin Slaughter, General Broker [1849], Grinnan Family Papers, Box 8, Folder 20; North Carolina Mutual Life Insurance Company, *Life Insurance: Its Principles, Operations and Benefits* (Raleigh, N.C.: S. Gales, 1849), 23, Pamphlet Collection, Duke University Library (hereafter cited as NC Mutual, *Life Insurance*).

27. Franklin Slaughter circular, Grinnan Family Papers.

28. See, for example, slave insurance policies in Linn Papers, 1855; Virginia Executive Papers, Governor Floyd, June 1851; Haxall Family Papers, items 235 and 236.

29. For more on the diseases and acclimation of bondspeople of African descent in the antebellum South, see Todd L. Savitt, "Sound Minds and Sound Bodies: The Diseases and Health Care of Blacks in Antebellum Virginia" (Ph.D. diss., University of Virginia, 1975), 16–48, 518–28; Savitt, *Medicine and Slavery,* 8–47; and Kiple and King, *Another Dimension.*

On insurance premiums in the lower South, see Genovese, "Medical and Insurance Costs of Slaveholding," 146–47. The insurance premium quoted for New Orleans was taken from a slave policy reproduced in Richard Hooker, *Aetna Life Insurance Company: Its First Hundred Years, A History* (Hartford, Conn.: Aetna Life Insurance Company, 1956), 14–15. On Northern companies' experiences with slave insurance, see Hooker, *Aetna Life Insurance Company,* 12–13; James M. Hudnut, *Semi-Centennial History of the New York Life Insurance Company, 1845–1895* (New York: The Company, 1895), 22–23; Shepard B. Clough, *A Century of American Life Insurance: A History of the Mutual Life Insurance Company of New York, 1843–1943* (New York: Columbia Univ. Press, 1946), 96; Mildred F. Stone, *Since 1845: A History of the Mutual Benefit Life Insurance Company* ([New Brunswick, N.J.]: Rutgers Univ. Press, 1957), 19–20, 41–42.

30. Insurance policy of slave George, owned by Joseph Myers, Apr. 3, 1858, Confederate Museum, Richmond, Va.

31. NC Mutual Minutes, July 4, Nov. 24, 1851; Sept. 2, 1857; Jan. 12, 1858.

32. Franklin Slaughter circular, Grinnan Family Papers; NC Mutual, *Life Insurance,* 17.

33. C. F. Wills to John Buford, Feb. 25, 1854, Buford Papers.

34. M. W. Davenport to John McCue, July 1, 1852, McCue Family Papers.

35. See, for example, slave policies in Linn Papers, 1855.

36. See, for example, the forms enclosed in a letter from Jno. H. Baker to John Buford, Feb. 17, 1855, Buford Papers; insurance policy of slave George, Apr. 3, 1858; NC Mutual Minutes, Sept. 6, 1851.

37. Draft of a certificate on death of slave Bill, n.d., Folder 5, Linn Papers.

38. James F. Jordan Jr. to W. T. B. Haynesworth, Mar. 21, 1851, Jordan Papers.

39. James F. Jordan Jr. to W. T. B. Haynesworth, Mar. 21, 1851, Jordan Papers; NC Mutual Minutes, passim.

40. NC Mutual Minutes, July 7, 1849; July 1, 1850.

41. North Carolina Mutual Life Insurance Company, *Eighth Annual Report* (Raleigh, N.C., 1857), 8 (hereafter annual reports of the company will be cited as NC Mutual, *AR,* preceded by the number and followed by the year in parentheses, then the page number. All are located in the North Carolina Room, University of North Carolina Library, Chapel Hill).

42. NC Mutual, *Life Insurance,* 12.

43. NC Mutual Minutes, Aug. 29, Sept. 7, 1849.

44. Ibid., July 1, 1850; Dec. 27, 1849; NC Mutual, *2d AR* (1851), 5.

45. NC Mutual, *2d AR* (1851), 5–6; NC Mutual Minutes, June 7, July 5, 1851.

46. NC Mutual, *2d AR* (1851), 20.

47. NC Mutual Minutes, Sept. 6, 1851.

48. Ibid., Jan. 3, 1852. For more on the health of free blacks in the antebellum South, see Savitt, *Medicine and Slavery,* 139–46, 207–17.

49. NC Mutual Minutes, July 3, 1852; NC Mutual, *3d AR* (1852), 4. The figures in Table 2 add up to $11,348, but the directors of the company recorded these losses as $14,713 in the minutes of their meeting on July 3, 1852. Available records do not clarify this discrepancy.

50. NC Mutual, *7th AR* (1856), 5–6.

51. NC Mutual Minutes, Feb. 4, 1854.

52. NC Mutual, *6th AR* (1855), 5, 7.

53. NC Mutual, *7th AR* (1856), 5–6; NC Mutual Minutes, July 5, 1856; NC Mutual, *9th AR* (1858), 11; James F. Jordan Jr. to W. T. B. Haynesworth, Mar. 21, 1851, Jordan Papers.

54. NC Mutual, *8th AR* (1857), 6–7.

55. NC Mutual Minutes, July 1, 1854. It is unclear, owing to incomplete records, why the company found it necessary to charge higher premiums for enslaved black people than for whites, since both groups demonstrated approximately equal mortality rates.

56. NC Mutual, *6th AR* (1855), 31; NC Mutual Minutes, Jan. 7, 1860.

57. NC Mutual Minutes, Jan. 6, 1855.

58. NC Mutual *2d AR* (1851), 7; *3d AR* (1852), 9; *4th AR* (1853), 5; *6th AR* (1855), 10; *7th AR* (1856), 8–9; *8th AR* (1857), 9–10; *9th AR* (1858), 8–9; *11th AR* (1860), 8–9.

59. See, for example, slave policies in Linn Papers, 1855, and London Papers, 1855–56.

60. NC Mutual, *11th AR* (1860), 3–4.

61. NC Mutual Minutes, Aug. 6, 1866.

62. The highest policy number listed in the *15th AR* (1864), 6, was 7,227.

10. The Georgia Freedmen's Bureau and the Organization of Health Care, 1865–66

This chapter originally appeared as "Politics in Medicine: The Georgia Freedmen's Bureau and the Organization of Health Care, 1865–1866," *Civil War History* 28 (1982): 45–64.

1. Quoted in Alan Conway, *The Reconstruction of Georgia* (Minneapolis: University of Minnesota Press, 1966), 64.

2. Georgia, Surgeon-in-Chief, Letters Received Unentered, 1865–67, Box 1, Records of the Bureau of Refugees, Freedmen, and Abandoned Lands, National Archives, Washington, D.C. (hereafter cited as Ga LRU).

3. For discussions of the Medical Department's activities in other states, see Martin L. Abbott, *The Freedmen's Bureau in South Carolina, 1865–1872* (Chapel Hill: Univ. of North Carolina Press, 1967), 48–50; Jude Thomas May, "The Medical Care of Blacks in Louisiana during Occupation and Reconstruction, 1862–1868: Its Social and Political Background" (Ph.D. diss., Tulane University, 1971), 81–177; May, "A Nineteenth-Century Medical Care Program for Blacks: The Case of the Freedmen's Bureau," *Anthropological Quarterly* 56 (July 1973): 160–71; Alan Raphael, "Health and Social Welfare of Kentucky Black People, 1865–1870," *Societas* 2 (1972): 143–47; Marshall Scott Legan, "Disease and the Freedmen in Mississippi during Reconstruction," *Journal of the History of Medicine and Allied Sciences* 28 (1973): 257–67; Howard N. Rabinowitz, *Race Relations in the Urban South, 1865–1890* (New York: Oxford Univ. Press, 1978), 128–31; Gail S. Hasson, "Health and Welfare of Freedmen in Reconstruction Alabama," *Alabama Review* 35 (1982): 94–110; Gaines M. Foster, "The Limitations of Federal Health Care for Freedmen, 1862–1868," *Journal of Southern History* 48 (1982): 349–72; Randy Finley, "In War's Wake: Health Care and Arkansas Freedmen, 1863–1868," *Arkansas Historical Quarterly* 51 (1992): 135–63; Paul A. Cimbala, *Under the Guardianship of the Nation: The Freedmen's Bureau and the Reconstruction of Georgia, 1865–1870* (Athens: Univ. of Georgia Press, 1997), 98–104; Reggie L. Pearson, "'There Are Many Sick, Feeble, and Suffering Freedmen': The Freedmen's Bureau's Health-Care Activities during Reconstruction in North Carolina, 1865–1868," *North Carolina Historical Review* 79 (2002): 141–81.

4. Conway, *Reconstruction of Georgia,* 18; C. Mildred Thompson, "The Freedmen's Bureau in Georgia in 1865–66: An Instrument of Reconstruction," *Georgia Historical Quarterly* 5 (1921): 42; Jerry Thornberry, "Northerners and the Atlanta Freedmen, 1865–69," *Prologue* 6 (1974): 236–44; Cimbala, *Under the Guardianship of the Nation,* 22–42.

5. Conway, *Reconstruction of Georgia,* 10–13.

6. "Report of the Commissioner of the Bureau of Refugees, Freedmen and Abandoned Lands" [BRFAL], in U.S. Congress, *House Executive Documents,* 39th Cong., 1st sess., no. 11, 18 (serial 1255); George R. Bentley, *A History of the Freedmen's Bureau* (Philadelphia: Univ. of Pennsylvania, 1955), 76.

7. Bentley, *Freedmen's Bureau,* 68. For an explanation of Saxton's seeming neglect of Georgia, see Cimbala, *Under the Guardianship of the Nation,* 247n20.

8. This was General Howard's population estimate, in Howard to E. M. Stanton, Secretary of War, in U.S. Congress, *Senate Executive Documents,* 39th Cong., 2d sess., no. 6, 1 (serial 1276). Thompson, "Freedmen's Bureau in Georgia," 42; Bentley, *Freedmen's Bureau,* 68–70; Cimbala, *Under the Guardianship of the Nation,* 27.

9. Caleb W. Horner, chief medical officer, BRFAL, to J. W. Lawton, Sept. 12, 1865, Ga LRU; *The War of the Rebellion: A Compilation of the Official Records of the Union and Confederate Armies,* 128 vols. (Washington, D.C.: GPO, 1880–1901), ser. 1, vol. 38, 2:522, 536, 576, 578–80 (hereafter cited as *OR*); "Report of the Chief Medical Officer BRFAL," in *House Executive Documents,* 39th Cong., 1st sess., no. 11, 18–19 (serial 1255).

10. "Circular No. 14, Instructions to Medical and Other Officers," in *House Executive Documents,* 39th Cong., 1st sess., no. 11, 50 (serial 1255).

11. Lawton to Surgeon B. Mc[clun?], Dist. Columbus, Georgia, Sept. 15, 1865, Georgia, Surgeon-in-Chief, Letters Sent, Sept. 15, 1865–July 26, 1867, vol. 52, 1 (hereafter cited as Ga 52 LS).

12. Lawton to Horner, Sept. 17, 1865, Ga 52 LS, 3.

13. Georgia, Surgeon-in-Chief, Station Book of Officers, vol. 56 (hereafter cited as Ga 56 SB); Georgia, Surgeon-in-Chief, Roster of Medical Officers, June 1863–Feb. 1867, vol. 57 (hereafter cited as Ga 57 R); Georgia, Surgeon-in-Chief, Contracts Made and Annulled [with Physicians], vol. 58 (hereafter cited as Ga 58 C). Little information could be located about Dr. C. H. Taylor.

14. Ga 57 R; "Report of the Chief Medical Officer BRFAL," in *House Executive Documents,* 39th Cong., 1st sess., no. 11, 18–19 (serial 1255).

15. Dr. A. T. Augusta to Lawton, Sept. 26, 1865, Ga LRU; Lawton to [Augusta], Ga 52 LS, 10.

16. Lawton to [?], Oct. 1, 1865, Ga 52 LS, 11; Ga 56 SB.

17. Lawton to Drs. L. Carter and J. Bettison, Oct. 4, 1865, Ga 52 LS, 13; Lawton to Capt. W. W. Drane, Oct. 4, 1865, Ga 52 LS 14; Ga 57 R; Ga 58 C.

18. Lawton to Dr. G. W. Southwick, Sept. 29, 1865, Ga 52 LS, 17.

19. See, for instance, Dr. J. L. Mulford to Horner, referred to Lawton, Oct. 21, 1865, Ga LRU; and Lawton to Horace N. Howland, Sept. 15, 1865, Ga 52 LS, 2.

20. Lawton to Dr. Louis Masson, Oct. 4, 1865, Ga 52 LS, 12.

21. Masson to Lawton, Sept. 23, 1865, Ga LRU. Augusta later taught anatomy at the newly opened Howard University Medical Department in Washington, D.C. For a biographical sketch, see William Montague Cobb, "Alexander Thomas Augusta," *Journal of the National Medical Association* 44 (1952): 327–29.

22. Lawton to Masson, Oct. 4, 1865, Ga 52 LS, 12. Masson appears to have taken a position as a physician for the Freedmen's Bureau in North Carolina in 1865, but had his contract annulled after five months on the job owing to misconduct. See Pearson, "Freedmen's Bureau's Health-Care Activities in North Carolina," 160.

23. Dr. H. H. Buck to Lawton, Oct. 13, 1865, Ga LRU; Frank K. Boland, "Early History of Medicine in Atlanta," *Atlanta Historical Bulletin* 5 (1940): 256–57; Dr. Noel D'Alvigny to [Lawton], Jan. 1, 1866, Ga LRU; Ga 56 SB; Ga 57 R; Ga 58 C.

24. Capt. P. Slaughter to Lawton, Oct. 2, 1865, Ga LRU; Ga 57 R; Ga 58 C.

25. *OR,* ser. 2, vol. 5:753.

26. Tuggle to Lawton, Jan. 1, 1866, Ga LRU; Carter to Lawton, Nov. 3, 1865, Ga LRU; D'Alvigny to [Lawton], Jan. 1, 1866, Ga LRU; L. A. Edwards to J. V. DeHanne, Oct. 26, Nov. 28, 1866, Ga LRU; J. B. L. Baker to DeHanne, Nov. 20, Dec. 29, 1866, Ga LRU; circular letter regarding oath sent by DeHanne, July 5, 1867, Ga 52 LS.

27. Lawton to Brig. Gen. E. A. Wild, Sept. 14, 1865, Ga LRU.

28. Lawton to Maj. D. D. [Kinsman?], asst. adj. gen., Sept. 19, 1865, Ga 52 LS, 4; Lawton to Horner, Sept. 29, 1865, Ga 52 LS, 8–9.

29. Lawton to Horner, Sept. 29, 1865, Ga 52 LS, 8–9; Ga 57 R; Augusta to Lawton, Sept. 26, 1865, Ga LRU; Lawton to [Augusta], Sept. 29, 1865, Ga 52 LS, 10; Dr. Richard Arnold to Mrs. W. C. Cosens [his daughter], Aug. 18, 1865, in Richard H. Shryock, ed., *Letters of Richard D. Arnold, M.D., 1808–1876, Mayor of Savannah, Georgia, First Secretary of the American Medical Association* (Durham, N.C.: Duke Univ. Press, 1929), 125–26; Lawton to Horner, Oct. 17, 1865, Ga 52 LS, 19.

30. Conway, *Reconstruction of Georgia,* 28; Lawton to Surgeon B. Mc[clun?], Sept. 15, 1865, Ga 52 LS, 1; Carter to Lawton, Oct. 31, 1865, Ga LRU; Bettison to Lawton, Sept. 29, 1865, Ga LRU; Dr. Frank Matlack to Lawton, July 21, 1866, Ga LRU.

31. Tuggle to Lawton, Nov. 3, 1865, Ga LRU; Slaughter to Lawton, Oct. 2, 1865, Ga LRU.

32. D'Alvigny to Lawton, Oct. 28, Nov. 26, 1865, Ga LRU.

33. D'Alvigny to Lawton, Dec. 24, 1865, Ga LRU.

34. Arthur Reed Taylor, "From the Ashes: Atlanta during Reconstruction, 1865–1876" (Ph.D. diss., Emory University, 1973), 122–23.

35. D'Alvigny to [Lawton], Mar. 9, 1866, Ga LRU.

36. Lawton to [Tuggle], Oct. 14, 1865, Ga 52 LS, 15; Philip C. Davis, medical purveyor at Hilton Head, to Lawton, Dec. 27, 1865, Ga LRU; Tuggle to Lawton, [Oct. 12, 1865], Ga LRU.

37. "Circular No. 14, Instructions to Medical and Other Officers," in *House Executive Documents,* 39th Cong., 1st sess., no. 11, 50 (serial 1255); Horner to Lawton, Mar. 31, 1866, Ga LRU.

38. Carter to Lawton, Oct. 21, Nov. 24, 1865, Ga LRU.

39. Dr. Augustus Mitchell to Lawton, May 22, 1866, Ga LRU; E. B. Carling, Quartermaster's Office, Savannah, to Lawton, July 27, 1866, Ga LRU.

40. Tuggle to Lawton, Jan. 18, 1866, Ga LRU.

41. D'Alvigny to Lawton, Jan. 8, 1866, Ga LRU.

42. Tuggle to Lawton, Jan. 1, 1866, Ga LRU. See also Lawton to [Tuggle], Oct. 14, 1865, Ga LRU; Tuggle to Lawton, Nov. 3, 1865, Ga LRU.

43. Carter to Lawton, Oct. 31, 1865, Ga LRU.

44. Henry W. Bellows to Lawton, Oct. 7, 1865, Ga LRU; Mitchell to Lawton, June 28, 1866, Ga LRU.

45. D'Alvigny to [Lawton], Feb. 8, Mar. 9, 1866, Ga LRU.

46. W. C. Spencer, Surgeon General's Officer, to Col. John Campbell, medical director [of military forces in Georgia], Feb. 3, 1866, Ga LRU; D'Alvigny to [Lawton], Oct. 28, Nov. 26, 1865, Ga LRU.

47. Campbell to [Lawton], Feb. 9, 1866, Ga LRU; Carter to Lawton, Feb. 26, Mar. 7, 1866, Ga LRU; Campbell to Lawton, May 3, 1866, Ga LRU.

48. Horner to Lawton, Mar. 15, 1866, Ga LRU.

49. Augusta to Lawton, Mar. 21, [1866], Georgia, Subordinate Offices, Savannah, Letters Sent, Dec. 1865–Sept. 1868, vol. 354 (hereafter cited as Ga 354 LS); Tuggle to Lawton, Mar. 26, 1866, Ga LRU; D'Alvigny to Lawton, Mar. 23, 1866, Ga LRU; Carter to Lawton, Mar. 26, 1866, Ga LRU.

50. Carter to Lawton, Apr. 9, 1866, Ga LRU.

51. Arnold to Miss M. W. Houston, Madison, Georgia, Oct. 8, 1866, in *Letters of Arnold,* ed. Shryock, 131.

52. R. S. Taylor, judge of the Inferior Court, Clark Co., to Gen. Davis Tillson, assistant commissioner of the BRFAL, Jan. 25, 1866, Ga LRU.

53. "Report of the Chief Medical Officer BRFAL," in *House Executive Documents,* 39th Cong., 1st sess., no. 11, 21 (serial 1255).

54. Lawton to Horner, Sept. 28, 1865, Ga 52 LS, 8–9.

55. Augusta to Lawton, Dec. 3, 1865, Ga LRU.

56. D'Alvigny to Lawton, Oct. 28, Nov. 26, 1865; Jan. 8, Apr. 14, 1866, Ga LRU; The Committee of the Colored Benevolent Society to D'Alvigny, Apr. [Feb.?] 14, 1866, Ga LRU. See also Taylor, "From the Ashes," 122.

57. Carter to Lawton, Apr. 10, 1866, Ga LRU; Tuggle to Lawton, Mar. 10, 1866, Ga. LRU.

58. Lawton to Horner, Sept. 29, 1865, Ga 52 LS, 9; "Report of the Assistant Commissioner of the State of Georgia," in *Senate Executive Documents,* 39th Cong., 2d sess., no. 6, 60 (serial 1276).

59. Conway, *Reconstruction of Georgia,* 68.

60. Augusta to Lawton, Nov. 7, 1865, Ga LRU; Ga 58 C.

61. Col. H. F. Sickles to Lawton, Nov. 19, 1865, Ga LRU.

62. Lawton to Augusta, Nov. 21, 1865, Ga LRU.

63. Augusta to Lawton, Nov. 24, 1865, Ga LRU; Augusta to Sickles, Nov. 28, 1865, Ga LRU; Augusta to Lawton, Dec.[?] 28, 1865, Ga LRU; Horner to Lawton, Nov. 29, 1865, Ga LRU; Assistant Surgeon G. W. Southwick to Lawton, Jan. 31, 1866, Ga LRU.

64. Carter to Lawton, Apr. 23, 28, May 2, 1866, Ga LRU; Dr. Travis's attorney to DeHanne, June 11, 1867, Georgia, Surgeon-in-Chief, Registers of Letters Received and Endorsements Sent and Received, July 1867–Jan. 1869, vol. 49, 16 (hereafter cited as Ga 49 REG); Bowes to DeHanne, Feb. 3, 1867, Ga LRU; M. J. Jones to Col. Sibley, Jan. 28, 1867, Ga LRU.

65. "Report of Surgeon J. W. Lawton . . . from September 1st 1865 to October 1st 1866," 3, Georgia, Office of the Assistant Commissioner, Operations Reports Sent to Commissioner Howard, 1866–1868 (hereafter cited as Ga 640); Dr. J. Dillsworth to Lawton, July 31, 1866, Ga LRU; Dr. C. H. Andrus to Lawton, Jan. 5, 1866, Ga LRU. For a more complete discussion of the problems freed people encountered in writing medical care provisions into labor contracts, see Pearson, "Freedmen's Bureau's Health-Care Activities in North Carolina," 167–70.

66. "Report of Surgeon J. W. Lawton . . . from September 1st 1865 to October 1st 1866," 8, Ga 640; "Annual Report of the Operations of the Medical Department . . . from October 1st 1866 to September 30th 1867," 1–22, Ga 640.

67. See, for example, DeHanne to Lawton, Dec. 26, 1865, Ga LRU; Dr. R. D. Moore to Lawton, Jan. 14, 1866, Ga LRU; R. S. Taylor to Tillson, Jan. 25, 1866, Ga LRU; John Calvin Johnson, clerk, Inferior Court, to Lawton, Jan. 6, 1866, Ga LRU. For other, later examples, see W. F. White to DeHanne, Mar. 7, 1867, Ga LRU; Dr. F. J. Gould to James M. Laing, Feb. 10, 1868; and Laing to Gould, Feb. 13, 1868, Ga 49 REG.

68. Andrew Clark to Laing, Nov. 11, 1867, 55, Ga 49 REG.

69. George Wagner to Capt. W. W. Dean, Oct. 20, 1866, Ga LRU.

70. Dalton to DeHanne, Mar. 18, 1867, Ga LRU.

71. See, for example, Horner to Lawton, May 1, 1866, Ga LRU; Augusta to Lawton, May 8, 1866, Ga LRU; Carter to Lawton, Dec. 30, 1865, Ga LRU.

72. D'Alvigny to Lawton, Nov. 26, 1865, Ga LRU.

73. The activities of the Medical Department of the Freedmen's Bureau in other states paralleled those in Georgia. (See references in note 3.) A similar emphasis on providing temporary health care, primarily in urban areas, with little attempt at establishing a permanent system or medical professional education that included black citizens, prevailed. For a different interpretation of this philosophy of the Medical Department of the Freedmen's Bureau in Georgia, see Cimbala, *Under the Guardianship of the Nation,* 104.

11. The Rise and Decline of African American Medical Schools

1. On the education of freed people see, for example, Henry Allen Bullock, *A History of Negro Education in the South, from 1619 to the Present* (Cambridge, Mass.: Harvard Univ. Press, 1967); James M. McPherson, *The Abolitionist Legacy, from Reconstruction to the NAACP* (Princeton, N.J.: Princeton Univ. Press, 1975); James D. Anderson, *The Education of Blacks in the South, 1860–1935* (Chapel Hill: Univ. of North Carolina Press, 1998); Jacqueline Jones, *Soldiers of Light and Love: Northern Teachers and Georgia Blacks, 1865–1873* (Athens: Univ. of Georgia Press, 1992); Robert C. Morris, *Reading, 'Riting, and Reconstruction: The Education of Freedmen in the South, 1861–1870* (Chicago: Univ. of Chicago Press, 1982); William Preston Vaughan, *Schools for All: The Blacks and Public Education in the South, 1865–1877* (Lexington: Univ. Press of Kentucky, 1974); Adam Fairclough, *Teaching Equality: Black Schools in the Age of Jim Crow* (Athens: Univ. of Georgia Press, 2001).

2. Some Northern schools that graduated black physicians in the late nineteenth century include the University of Pennsylvania, Long Island Hospital Medical College, Woman's Medical College of Pennsylvania, Temple University, the University of Vermont, the University of Illinois, and the University of Michigan. Consult medical directories of the early twentieth century for more information about graduates.

3. On the history of Howard University Medical Department, see Lamb, *Howard University Medical Department;* D. B. Nichols, "The Genesis of Howard University," in *Twenty-Fifth Anniversary of the Organization of Howard University, March 2, 1892, Historical Papers* (Washington, D.C.: Howard Univ. Press, 1895); Walter Dyson, "Founding of the School of Medicine of Howard University, 1868–1873," *Howard University Studies in History* 10 (1929); Walter Dyson, *Howard University, The Capstone of Negro Education: A History, 1867–1940* (Washington, D.C.: The Graduate School, Howard University, 1941); Lafayette C. Loomis, *Address . . . Delivered at the Opening of the First Course of Lectures, November 5th, 1868* (Washington, D.C.: GPO, 1868); Rayford Logan, *Howard University: The First Hundred Years, 1867–1967* (New York: New York Univ. Press, 1969); Gloria Moldow, *Women Doctors in Gilded-Age Washington: Race, Gender, and Professionalization* (Urbana: Univ. of Illinois Press, 1987); Howard R. Epps, "The Howard University Medical Department in the Flexner Era: 1910–1929," *Journal of the National Medical Association* 81 (1989): 885–911. On the history of Meharry Medical College, see James Summerville, *Educating Black Doctors: A History of Meharry Medical College* (University: Univ. of Alabama Press, 1983); Charles Victor Roman, *Meharry Medical College: A History* (Nashville, Tenn.: Sunday School Pub. Board of the National Baptist Convention, 1934); Darlene Clark Hine, "The Pursuit of Professional Equality: Meharry Medical College, 1921–1938, A Case Study," in *New Perspectives on Black Educational History,* ed. Vincent P. Franklin and James D. Anderson (Boston: G. K. Hall, 1978), 173–92; Leslie A. Falk, "Meharry Medical College: A Century of Service," *Southern Exposure* 6 (Summer 1978): 14–17; Leslie A. Falk and N. A. Quaynor-Malm, "Early Afro-American Medical Education in the United States: The Origins of Meharry Medical College in the Nineteenth Century," *Proceedings of the XXIII International Congress of the History of Medicine, London, 2–9 September 1972* (London: Wellcome Institute of the History of Medicine, 1974), 346–56. On the history of Lincoln University Medical Department, see Todd L. Savitt, "Lincoln University Medical Department: A Forgotten Black Medical School," *Journal of the History of Medicine and Allied Sciences* 40 (1985): 42–65 (revised version is chapter 12 of the present book). On the history of Leonard Medical School, see Todd L. Savitt, "The Education of Black Physicians at Shaw University, 1882–1918," in *Black Americans in North Carolina and the South,* ed. Jeffrey J. Crow and Flora J. Hatley (Chapel Hill: Univ. of North Carolina Press, 1984), 160–88 (revised version is chapter 14 of the present book); Darlene Clark Hine,

"The Anatomy of Failure: Medical Education Reform and the Leonard Medical School of Shaw University, 1882–1920," *Journal of Negro Education* 54 (1985): 512–25; Todd L. Savitt, "Training the 'Consecrated, Skillful, Christian Physician': Documents Illustrating Student Life at Leonard Medical School, 1882–1918," *North Carolina Historical Review* 75 (1998): 250–76 (revised version is chapter 15 of the present book). On Flint Medical College of New Orleans University, see Desha P. Rhodes, "A History of Flint Medical College, 1889–1911" (master's thesis, University of New Orleans, 1999). On Knoxville College Medical Department, see Todd L. Savitt, "Money versus Mission at an African-American Medical School: Knoxville College Medical Department, 1895–1900," *Bulletin of the History of Medicine* 75 (2001): 680–716 (revised version is chapter 17 of the present book).

4. On the histories of Louisville National Medical College, Hannibal Medical College, Chattanooga National Medical College, and the University of West Tennessee College of Medicine and Surgery, see Todd L. Savitt, "Four African-American Proprietary Medical Colleges: 1888–1923," *Journal of the History of Medicine and Allied Sciences* 55 (2000): 203–55 (revised version is chapter 16 of the present book). On the history of Knoxville Medical College, see Savitt, "Money versus Mission," 711–16.

5. Freedmen's Aid Society of the Methodist Episcopal Church, *Tenth Annual Report, 1876–77*, 7.

6. Abraham Flexner, *Medical Education in the United States and Canada: A Report to the Carnegie Foundation for the Advancement of Teaching* (New York: Carnegie Foundation for the Advancement of Teaching, 1910), 180–81.

7. Little will be discussed about State University Medical Department or the Medico-Chirurgical and Theological College of Christ's Institution owing to lack of information.

12. Lincoln University Medical Department

This chapter originally appeared as "Lincoln University Medical Department: A Forgotten Black Medical School," *Journal of the History of Medicine and Allied Sciences* 40 (1985): 42–65.

The author acknowledges with gratitude the assistance of Mrs. Sophy Cornwell, Special Collections Librarian, Lincoln University, Pennsylvania. Research for this publication was supported in part by National Institutes of Health Grant LM 03413 from the National Library of Medicine, 1980–82.

1. Horace Mann Bond, *Education for Freedom: A History of Lincoln University, Pennsylvania* (Lincoln University, Pa.: Lincoln University, 1976), 203–56, 469.

2. The fact that LU had a medical school is not widely known. Horace Mann Bond mentions it only peripherally and fleetingly in his fine, thoughtful history of the university, *Education for Freedom*, 432, 434. None of the published historical discussions of black medical education, including Herbert M. Morais's *The History of the Afro-American in Medicine* (Cornwells Heights, Pa.: Publishers Agency, 1976), touch on Lincoln. Dr. W. Montague Cobb, the "dean" of black medical history, remarked in conversation on Lincoln's existence but did not look at the school's records as he had on so many other topics relating to African American medical history. Harold J. Abrahams, a historian interested in the defunct medical schools of Philadelphia and its vicinity (Harold J. Abrahams, *Extinct Medical Schools of Nineteenth Century Philadelphia* [Philadelphia: Univ. of Pennsylvania Press, 1966]), did some research in the early 1960s on Lincoln but never published his findings. The only evidence we have of his interest is a series of three letters written in March and April 1963 to Abrahams from Dr. Donald C. Yelton, librarian and former (1960–62) acting president of Lincoln University, providing detailed information about the medical department. Donald C. Yelton to Harold

J. Abrahams, Mar. 14, Apr. 5, 9, 1963, Lincoln University Archives (hereafter cited as Yelton, date, page). Yelton spent much effort poring through presidential annual reports, faculty and trustees minute books, college catalogs, and other archival materials, many of which are no longer available at LU and are presumed lost or destroyed. Yelton's comments on and quotations from the original documents are the only source of information on some crucial aspects of the medical department's operations and are thus cited in the footnotes of this chapter as historical sources.

3. Bond, *Education for Freedom,* 257–66, 447–55; American Council of Learned Societies, *Dictionary of American Biography* (New York: Scribners, 1928).

4. For a discussion of African Americans' health conditions in the Reconstruction South, see chapters 10 and 11 of this book.

5. Bond, *Education for Freedom,* 274–75, 432. It is interesting to note how closely in time development of programs at the newly created Howard University in Washington paralleled those at Lincoln. The former was founded in 1867 and opened medical and law departments in 1868. Horace Mann Bond asserted in his history of LU (*Education for Freedom,* 264) that Gen. O. O. Howard "most certainly took the idea of establishing Howard University, chartered in 1867, from the Lincoln University whose board he joined in 1866."

6. Memorial of the Faculty of Lincoln University to the Board of Trustees, in Trustees Minutes, Sept. 25, 1874, quoted in Yelton, Apr. 5, 1963, 3–4.

7. *Annual Catalog of Lincoln University,* no. 11, June 1868, 6; no. 12, June 1869, 6, 23 (hereafter cited as LU, *Catalog,* issue number, date, page).

8. LU, *Catalog,* no. 12, June 1869, 19. Hutchison's name also appears in the records as Hutchinson.

9. Yelton, Apr. 9, 1963, 2–3.

10. Yelton, Apr. 9, 1963, 2.

11. LU, *Catalog,* no. 13, Apr. 1870, 20; also quoted in Yelton, Apr. 9, 1963, 2.

12. LU, *Catalog,* no. 13, Apr. 1870, 20.

13. LU, *Catalog,* no. 14, June 1871, 32.

14. LU, *Catalog,* no. 15, Aug. 1872, 40–45; no 16, Aug. 1873, 36–40.

15. Martin Kaufman, "American Medical Education," in *The Education of American Physicians: Historical Essays,* ed. Numbers, 15–16. See also Kenneth M. Ludmerer, *Learning to Heal: The Development of American Medical Education* (New York: Basic Books, 1985), 50, 53, 56, 74.

16. LU, *Catalog,* no. 14, June 1871, 32.

17. LU, *Catalog,* no. 15, Aug. 1872, 43.

18. Ibid.

19. Ibid., 42–43.

20. On the condition of medical education in the last third of the nineteenth century, see Martin Kaufman, *American Medical Education: The Formative Years, 1765–1920* (Westport, Conn.: Greenwood Press, 1976); Robert P. Hudson, "Abraham Flexner in Perspective: American Medical Education, 1865–1910," *Bulletin of the History of Medicine* 56 (1972): 545–61; Numbers, *Education of American Physicians;* Ludmerer, *Learning to Heal.*

21. Bond, *Education for Freedom,* 225.

22. Ibid., 259.

23. Ibid., 429–30, 449–57, 469–76.

24. Yelton, Mar. 14, 1963, 1–3; Apr. 9, 1963, 1; LU annual catalogs.

25. William B. Atkinson, *The Physicians and Surgeons of the United States* (Philadelphia: C. Robson, 1878), 66–67; LU annual catalogs.

26. LU, *Catalog,* no. 11, June 1868, 6; no. 12, June 1869, 23; no. 13, 1870, 30; no. 14, June 1871, 38; no. 15, Aug. 1872, 16.

27. LU, *Catalog,* no. 12, June 1869, 19; no. 13, 1870, 21; no. 14, June 1871, 7, 21.

28. Lisabeth M. Holloway, comp., *Medical Obituaries: American Physicians' Biographical Notices in Selected Medical Journals before 1907* (New York: Garland, 1981), 251a.

29. LU, Trustees Minutes, Sept. 7, 1871, Lincoln University Archives; LU, *Catalog,* no. 15, Aug. 1872, 6.

30. For more biographical information, see, on Allen, Howard A. Kelly and Walter L. Burrage, eds., *American Medical Biographies* (Baltimore, Md.: Norman, Remington Company, 1920), 15–17; and Atkinson, *Physicians and Surgeons of the United States,* 675; on Hartshorne, see Kelly and Burrage, American Council of Learned Societies, *American Medical Biographies,* 499–500; Atkinson, *Physicians and Surgeons of the United States,* 458–59; and American Council of Learned Societies, *Dictionary of American Biography;* on Wood, see Martin Kaufman, Stuart Galishoff, and Todd L. Savitt, eds., *Dictionary of American Medical Biography* (Westport, Conn.: Greenwood Press, 1984), 820–21; G. E. de Schweinitz, "Reminiscences of an American Pioneer in Experimental Medicine: Dr. Wood as a Medical Teacher," *Transactions of the College of Physicians of Philadelphia* 42 (1920): 155–257; and G. B. Roth, "An Early American Pharmacologist, Horatio C. Wood," *Isis* 30 (1930): 38–45.

31. Yelton, Mar. 14, 1963, 1–3; Apr. 9, 1963, 1; LU annual catalogs.

32. LU, Trustees Minutes, Jan. 13, 1872.

33. Ibid.; Yelton, Mar. 14, 1963, 2a.

34. LU, Trustees Minutes, Sept. 21, 1874; Yelton, Apr. 9, 1963, 2.

35. Yelton, Mar. 14, 1963, 2a–6.

36. Yelton, Mar. 14, 1963, 3.

37. Kelly and Burrage, *American Medical Biographies,* 500.

38. Yelton, Mar. 14, 1963, 3.

39. Yelton, Mar. 14, 1963, 2a, 2b, 3; LU, Trustees Minutes, Mar. 20, 1873.

40. LU, *Catalog,* no. 14, June 1871, 32.

41. Bond, *Education for Freedom,* 434, 449–57, 469–76.

42. Yelton, Mar. 14, 1963, 3–4; LU, Faculty Minutes, Sept. 17, 24, 1874, Lincoln University Archives.

43. "Excerpts from Memorial of the Faculty . . . September 25, 1874," quoted in Yelton, Apr. 5, 1963, 1–2.

44. Yelton, Mar. 14, 1963, 4.

45. LU, *Catalog,* no. 14, June 1871, 22; no. 15, Aug. 1872, 40; no. 16, Aug. 1873, 35; [no. 21], 1878, 29–34.

46. Yelton, Mar. 14, 1963, 7.

47. LU, *Catalog,* no. 15, Aug. 1872, 41–42.

48. Ibid., 44–45.

49. Yelton, Mar. 14, 1963, 5–6.

50. LU, Board of Trustees, Summary of Operations Book, 1853–92, 22, Lincoln University Archives.

51. Yelton, Mar. 14, 1963, 4.

52. Yelton, Mar. 14, 1963, 5.

53. On the early years of Howard University Medical Department, see Lamb, *Howard University Medical Department;* Nichols, "Genesis of Howard University"; Dyson, "Founding of the School of Medicine of Howard University"; Dyson, *Howard University;* Loomis, *Address . . . Delivered at the Opening of the First Course of Lectures.*

54. LU, *Catalog*, [no. 21], 1878, 29–34; Lamb, *Howard University Medical Department*, 170–71, 183–84. See also medical directories of the period.

55. LU, *Catalog*, [no. 21], 1878, 29–34; Yelton, Mar. 14, 1963, 62. Some information on Brooks is in Fanny Jackson-Coppin, *Reminiscences of School Life, and Hints on Teaching* (Philadelphia: A. M. E. Book Concern, 1913), 157–58. Information on Smith and Henderson is contained in letters from Judith A. Schiff, Yale University Library, to Todd L. Savitt, Nov. 5, 1981, and Wesley H. Poling, Yale Alumni Records Office, to Todd L. Savitt, Nov. 18, 1981; obituary notice, *JAMA* 27 (1896): 503.

56. "Excerpts from Memorial of the Faculty," 4.

13. Straight University Medical Department

This chapter originally appeared as "Straight University Medical Department: The Short Life of a Black Medical School in Reconstruction New Orleans," *Louisiana Historical Quarterly* 41 (2000): 175–201.

1. On the history of New Orleans University Medical Department, later known as Flint Medical College, see Rhodes, "History of Flint Medical College."

2. John W. Blassingame, *Black New Orleans, 1860–1880* (Chicago: Univ. of Chicago Press, 1973), 126.

3. Joe M. Richardson, *Christian Reconstruction: The American Missionary Association and Southern Blacks, 1861–1890* (Athens: Univ. of Georgia Press, 1986), 133. Joe Gray Taylor, *Louisiana Reconstructed, 1863–1877* (Baton Rouge: Louisiana State Univ. Press, 1974), 477, somewhat more accurately states that the medical school, though included in Straight University's charter, did not function at all.

4. His plan began by establishing a church school, which grew to a normal school and evolved into a full-blown university in the course of six months.

5. The AMA founded seven colleges around the South between 1866 and 1869.

6. On Healy, the AMA, and the founding of Straight University, see Jacquelyn Slaughter Haywood, "The American Missionary Association in Louisiana during Reconstruction" (Ph.D. diss., University of California, Los Angeles, 1974), 127–73; *American Missionary* 14 (1870): 170–71; American Missionary Association, *Annual Report of the American Missionary Association, 1869*, (New York: Missionary Association, 1869), 57; Straight University, *Charter, Board of Trustees and Faculty* (New Orleans: n.p., 1870), item 45869 in American Missionary Association Archives, Amistad Research Center, New Orleans, Louisiana (hereafter cited as AMA Archives); Blassingame, *Black New Orleans*, 124–31 (caution: contains several inaccurate statements about the medical department); Richardson, *Christian Reconstruction*, 131–33, 295n31; Howard A. White, *The Freedmen's Bureau in Louisiana* (Baton Rouge: Louisiana State Univ. Press, 1970), 190; James M. McPherson, *The Struggle for Equality: Abolitionists and the Negro in the Civil War and Reconstruction* (Princeton, N.J.: Princeton Univ. Press, 1964), 406.

7. Haywood, "American Missionary Association in Louisiana," 35–36, 127–37. Straight's letterhead stationery reads: "Commission House of McFarland, Straight & Co., Nos. 44, 46 and 48 New Levee Street, New Orleans" with a second smaller imprint in the left corner containing the words: "Straight, Deming & Co. Wholesale Grocers and Commission Merchants, Cincinnati, Ohio." See, for example, Seymour Straight to Rev. George Whipple, Apr. 5, 1870, AMA Archives, item 45826.

8. J. W. Healy to (?), n.d. [probably 1869], AMA Archives, item 45801.

9. J. W. Healy to (?), n.d. [probably 1869], AMA Archives, item 45801; Straight University, *Charter, Board of Trustees and Faculty*, AMA Archives, item 45869; Haywood, "American Missionary Association in Louisiana," 137, 162.

10. Haywood, "American Missionary Association in Louisiana," 136–37. On the history of Howard University Medical Department, see references in chapter 11 of the present book, note 3.

11. J. W. Healy to Brethren, Oct. 6, 1869, AMA Archives, item 45800.

12. Haywood, "American Missionary Association in Louisiana," 138–42.

13. Walter L. Fleming, *Louisiana State University, 1860–1896* (Baton Rouge: Louisiana State Univ. Press, 1936), 150–59; Roger A. Fischer, *The Segregation Struggle in Louisiana, 1862–77* (Urbana: Univ. of Illinois Press, 1974), 105–6.

14. *Acts Passed by the General Assembly of the State of Louisiana at the Third Session of the First Legislature, Begun and Held in New Oleans, January 3, 1870, and at the Extra Session, Begun and Held in the City of New Orleans, March 7, 1870* (New Orleans, La.: A. L. Lee, 1870), Act 81, 111–12.

15. Fleming, *Louisiana State University,* 158.

16. Ibid., 157.

17. Seymour Straight to George Whipple, Apr. 5, 1870, AMA Archives, item 45826.

18. *Official Journal of the Proceedings of the House of Representatives of the State of Louisiana, 1870,* 266, 271, 313; J. W. Healy to My Dear Brother, Feb. 23, 1870, AMA Archives, item 45821.

19. Act 81, *Acts of Louisiana, 1870,* 111–12; Straight University, *Catalog of the Officers and Students of Straight University with the Courses of Study for the Academic Year 1870–1871* (New Orleans, La.: Pelican Print, 1871), 43.

20. Seymour Straight to George Whipple, Apr. 5, 1870, AMA Archives, item 45826.

21. *Official Journal of the Proceedings of the Senate of the State of Louisiana, 1870,* 303, 306, 324; *Louisiana House Journal, 1870,* 377. The contents of Senate Bill 226 is not available because the governor vetoed it. Thus it never became an act and was never published. Unpublished records relating to that bill could not be located in the Archives of the State of Louisiana.

22. J.W. Healy to My Dear Brother, May 25, 1870, AMA Archives, item 45835.

23. Seymour Straight to George Whipple, June 2, 1870, AMA Archives, item 45836.

24. *American Missionary* 14 (1870): 182.

25. Other named faculty members were Frederick Bernard Albers, R. C. Richardson, Julius Homberger, and V. O. King. Straight University, *Charter, Board of Trustees and Faculty,* AMA Archives, item 45869; Straight University, *Catalog, 1870–71,* 5. Some of these physicians are listed in Samuel W. Butler, *The Medical Register and Directory of the United States* (Philadelphia: Office of the Medical and Surgical Reporter, 1874), and in *Medical and Surgical Directory of the United States* (Detroit: R. L. Polk and Co., 1886) (hereafter cited as *Polk's Medical Directory*). See also Gordon E. Gillson, *Louisiana State Board of Health: The Formative Years* ([New Orleans?]: n.p., [1967?]), 132–56; Duffy, *Rudolph Matas History of Medicine,* 2:211, 328–29, 361–64, 390, 440, 462; Louisiana, *Annual Report of the Board of Health of the State of Louisiana to the General Assembly,* for 1868 through 1876.

26. J. W. Healy to Brethren, Sept. 9, 1870, AMA Archives, item 45851; Sept. 10, 1870, plus enclosure, AMA Archives, items 45850 and 45853.

27. "Report of Straight University . . . for the Month of February 1871," AMA Archives, item 45880, lists students in all departments, but does not mention a medical department. J. F. Fuller to Mr. Cravath, Apr. 8, 1871, AMA Archives, item 45887, also lists students in other departments and indicates "0" next to "Medical." The Straight University catalog for 1870–71, published in 1871, lists no medical students and speaks of the future opening of a medical department on page 43. See also the *New Orleans Semi-Weekly Louisianian,* June 22, 1871.

28. *Louisiana Senate Journal, 1871,* 7; Charles Vincent, *Black Legislators in Louisiana during Reconstruction* (Baton Rouge: Louisiana State Univ. Press, 1976), 92.

29. "*State of Louisiana ex rel. Board of Trustees of Straight University v. James Graham, Auditor,*" in Louisiana Supreme Court, *Reports of Cases Argued and Determined in the Supreme Court of Louisiana* 25 (1873): 441.

30. A dispensary was a medical facility similar to today's outpatient clinic, providing medical attention to patients who could not afford to pay a physician but who also did not require hospital care. For more on nineteenth-century dispensaries, see Charles Rosenberg, "Social Class and Medical Care in Nineteenth-Century America: The Rise and Fall of the Dispensary," *Journal of the History of Medicine and Allied Sciences* 29 (1974): 32–54.

31. Richardson, *Christian Reconstruction,* 66; Blassingame, *Black New Orleans,* 166.

32. *Acts of Louisiana, 1871,* 186.

33. J. W. Healy to My Dear Brethren, Mar. 9, 1871, AMA Archives, item 45881. See also Richardson, *Christian Reconstruction,* 66.

34. *New Orleans Semi-Weekly Louisianian,* Apr. 23, 1871. For more on Gunn and Allen, see Bowman, *Good Medicine,* 27, 30; Chicago Medical Society, *History of Medicine and Surgery and Physicians and Surgeons of Chicago* (Chicago: Biographical Pub. Corp., 1922), 61–62, 68–69. Bonner, *Medicine in Chicago,* 34, calls Gunn "the most famous surgeon in Chicago in the 1870s."

35. J. T. Newman, M.D., to Rev. E. M. Cravath, July 2, 1874, AMA Archives, item 46258.

36. The New Orleans city directories cease listing him in 1926. (Thanks to the staff at the Dillard University [descendent of New Orleans University] Archives for assistance in tracking down this information.) When, in 1882, the Louisiana Board of Health required the registration of all physicians practicing in the state, Newman told authorities he had no diploma. Under provisions of the new law that year, he received permission to continue practicing medicine because he had "more than five years practice without a diploma." Louisiana Board of Health, *Physicians and Surgeons of Louisiana, Registered by the Secretary of the Board of Health of the State of Louisiana, in Accordance With Provisions of Act 31 of 1882* (Baton Rouge: n.p., 1885). Newman altered his statements about medical credentials in 1890 and 1893, submitting information to *Polk's Medical Directory.* At this time he indicated that he had, in fact, received a medical diploma, graduating from the University of Toronto in Ontario, Canada, in 1865. For the 1896, 1898, and 1900 editions of *Polk's Medical Directory,* Newman, now a faculty member of the New Orleans University Medical Department, again submitted different information, claiming this time to be an 1893 graduate of the school where he now taught. He once more changed his medical pedigree for the 1902, 1904, and 1906 editions of *Polk's Medical Directory,* stating that he had graduated from both the University of Toronto (giving the year now as 1868 rather than 1865) and New Orleans University. Even more confusing, annual catalogs for these two schools fail to list Newman either as a student or as a graduate at any time in their histories. Archival records at the University of Toronto contain no mention of his presence at the Canadian school. Newman continued to list himself as an 1868 graduate of the University of Toronto in *Polk's Medical Directory* for 1908, 1910, and 1912–13, and as an 1893 medical graduate of New Orleans University in American Medical Association directories (American Medical Association, *American Medical Directory* [Chicago: American Medical Association, 1906]) at least through 1925. See, for example, *Polk's Medical Directory* (1886), 417; (1890), 491; (1893), 535; (1896), 623; (1898), 698; (1900), 768; (1902), 867; (1904), 853; (1906), 897; (1908), 825; (1910), 813; (1912–13), 728, and *American Medical Directory* (1914), 620; (1923), 687; (1925), 686. Newman's name does not appear in "List of Former Pupils," Toronto School of Medicine, in affiliation with the University of Toronto, *Annual Announcement, 29th Session (1871–72),* 15–18, or on lists of current students for 1863–64 and 1864–65. These are the only extant lists of students for the Toronto School of Medicine, and they, according to Harold Averill of the University of Toronto Archives, are complete only for graduates of the school, not for those who attended but did not finish

the course and receive degrees. Mr. Averill checked the very complete lists of students and graduates of the Victoria College Medical Department in Toronto and was unable to find Newman's name. Newman is not on the list of graduates up to 1885 that appeared in the *Annual Announcement of Trinity Medical School, Toronto, Session 1885–6,* 38–43. The University of Toronto Archives has no record of Henry T. Newman attending the school. Annual catalogs of the New Orleans University Medical Department from 1889 through 1911 mention Newman only as a faculty member, not as a student or graduate.

37. *American Medical Directory* (1914), 620, gives his birth year as 1847.

38. "Venomous Bites," *Chicago Medical Journal* 24 (1867): 368; "Opium and Stramonium," *Chicago Medical Journal* 25 (1868): 758; "Prolonged Retention of Life by Infants Who Have Not Breathed," *Chicago Medical Journal* 25 (1868): 638–39; "Senile Gangrene," *Chicago Medical Journal* 25 (1868): 205; "Opium and Belladonna," *Chicago Medical Journal* 24 (1867): 529–32; Letter to the Editor, *Chicago Medical Journal* 25 (1868): 60–61; "Digitalis: Its Use in Suppression of Urine," *Chicago Medical Journal* 25 (1868): 790–92; "Electricity: Its Use in Hysteria," *Chicago Medical Journal* 26 (1869): 48–50; "Relations between the Sense of Touch, the Sense of Temperature, and the Sense of Pain," *Chicago Medical Journal* 25 (1868): 57–58; "Senile Gangrene," *Chicago Medical Times* 1 (1869): 111; James Newman, "Acute Bronchitis. The Use of Aconite in Bronchitis and Croup. Extract de la Tribune Medicale. Translated for the *Chicago Medical Times*," *Chicago Medical Times* 1 (1869): 214–15. After his arrival in New Orleans, Newman seems to have published no more articles in medical journals. For more on the Eclectic medical sect, see John S. Haller, *Medical Protestants: The Eclectics in American Medicine, 1825–1939* (Carbondale: Southern Illinois Univ. Press, 1994).

39. Newman, "Acute Bronchitis."

40. Charity Hospital of New Orleans, *Annual Report* (1872), 3; (1873), 5; (1874), 5; (1875), 9; (1876), 9; Louisiana Board of Health, *Annual Report* (1874), 3, 5, 178; (1875), 3, 87–102; (1876), 4.

41. *American Missionary* 15 (1871): 230; Hathaway Home Accounts, 1871, AMA Archives, item 45876; "Report of James T. Newman, Physician and Surgeon of Hathaway Home, December 31, 1872," AMA Archives, item 45968. The American Missionary Association Archives contains many bills and receipts with Newman's name on them during this period. See also Blassingame, *Black New Orleans,* 129, 166; and Richardson, *Christian Reconstruction,* 66, 132.

42. *American Missionary* 16 (1872): 178.

43. "*State of Louisiana ex rel. Board of Trustees of Straight University v. James Graham, Auditor,*" 440–41.

44. *American Missionary* 17 (1873): 177–78.

45. Ibid.

46. "*State of Louisiana ex rel. Board of Trustees of Straight University v. James Graham, Auditor,*" 440–43.

47. Blassingame, *Black New Orleans,* 125; Fleming, *Louisiana State University,* 192–200, 264.

48. *New Orleans Republican,* Oct. 21, 1873.

49. An eleventh student was registered for the medical course, but he died during the summer while teaching in a public school. S. S. Ashley to E. M. Cravath, Sept. 24, 1873, AMA Archives, item 46096. On student numbers and gender, see S. S. Ashley, "Report of Straight University School . . . for the Month of Apr. 1874," AMA Archives, item 46222. On the racial identity of the law students, see Richardson, *Christian Reconstruction,* 132.

50. James T. Newman, "Inaugural Address," *New Orleans Republican,* Oct. 26, 1873.

51. Richardson, *Christian Reconstruction,* 136.

52. Samuel S. Ashley to Rev. E. M. Cravath, Sept. 24, 1873, AMA Archives, item 46096.

53. J. T. Newman to Rev. E. M. Cravath, Oct. 27, 1873, AMA Archives, item 46122.

54. Newman, "Inaugural Address"; J. T. Newman to Rev. E. M. Cravath, Oct. 27, 1873, AMA Archives, item 46122.

55. Samuel S. Ashley to Rev. E. M. Cravath, Sept. 24, 1873, AMA Archives, item 46096.

56. J. D. Lichtenberger to Dear Doc, Oct. 3, 1873, item 46108; J. D. Lichtenberger to Dear Doc, Oct. 23, 1873, item 46118; James T. Newman to C. F. Hart, M.D., Nov. 26, 1873, item 46138, all in AMA Archives.

57. M. A. Ashley to Rev. E. M. Cravath, Oct. 31, 1873, AMA Archives, item 46124.

58. S. S. Ashley to Rev. E. M. Cravath, Nov. 13, 1873, AMA Archives, item 46133.

59. J. D. Lichtenberger to Dear Doc, Oct. 3, 1873, AMA Archives, item 46108.

60. J. T. Newman to Rev. E. M. Cravath, Oct. 27, 1873, AMA Archives, item 46122.

61. J. T. Newman to Rev. E. M. Cravath, Oct. 27, 1873, AMA Archives, item 46122.

62. J. T. Newman to Rev. E. M. Cravath, Nov. 26, 1873, AMA Archives, item 46137.

63. J. T. Newman to Rev. E. M. Cravath, Dec. 10, 1873 (item 46149); Dec. 23, 1873 (item 46158); Jan. 10, 1874 (item 46168); Feb. 10, 1874 (items 46189 and 46190); Apr. 2, 1874 (item 46206), all in AMA Archives.

64. J. T. Newman to Rev. E. M. Cravath, Apr. 2, 1874, AMA Archives, item 46206.

65. S. S. Ashley to E. M. Cravath, Apr. 2, 1874, AMA Archives, item 46207.

66. Other African American medical schools founded by Northern missionary groups during the late nineteenth century were also expected to be self-supporting.

67. S. S. Ashley to (?), Apr. 16, 1874, AMA Archives, item 46216.

68. James A. Martling to E. M. Cravath, Apr. 6, 1874, AMA Archives, item 46212.

69. J. T. Newman to E. M. Cravath, July 22, 1874, AMA Archives, item 46264. On the white medical schools and the state of white medical education in New Orleans during Reconstruction, see Duffy, *History of Medicine in Louisiana,* 2:529–35, and John Duffy, *The Tulane University Medical Center: One Hundred and Fifty Years of Medical Education* (Baton Rouge: Louisiana State Univ. Press, 1984), 47–58.

70. The only letter with such remarks against Newman that appears in the AMA Archives is James A. Martling to E. M. Cravath, Apr. 6, 1874, item 46212.

71. J. T. Newman, M.D., to Rev. E. M. Cravath, June 4, 1874, AMA Archives, item 46248.

72. J. T. Newman, M.D., to Rev. E. M. Cravath, July 2, 1874, AMA Archives, item 46258.

73. J. T. Newman to E. M. Cravath, July 22, 1874, AMA Archives, item 46264; Duffy, *History of Medicine in Louisiana,* 2:529–35; Duffy, *Tulane University Medical Center,* 47–58; Charity Hospital Medical College of New Orleans, *Circular, 1877–78,* available at Tulane University Medical School Library History Collection (thanks to Ms. Patsy Copeland for her assistance). Charity Hospital Medical College opened in 1873 and was extinct by 1877.

74. J. T. Newman to E. M. Cravath, July 22, 1874, AMA Archives, item 46264.

75. J. T. Newman to E. M. Cravath, July 22, 1874, AMA Archives, item 46264.See also Duffy, *History of Medicine in Louisiana,* 2:529–35, and Duffy, *Tulane University Medical Center,* 47–58.

76. Professor J. A. Adams to E. M. Cravath, Oct. 31, 1874, AMA Archives, item 46301. Prof. J. A. Adams, "Straight University, New Orleans," *American Missionary* 19 (1875): 209–10, contains a report on activities at the school during the 1874–75 academic year and omits any mention of the medical department or Newman. The failure of Straight University Medical Department did not signal the end of Dr. James T. Newman's efforts to provide New Orleans with a medical school for African Americans. Determined to establish such an institution, the former SU medical school dean turned for help to another Northern missionary group—the Methodist Episcopal Church—and became involved with the founding of New Orleans University's medical department several years later. Rhodes, "History of Flint Medical College."

77. On aspects of Newman's later medical career in New Orleans, see Rhodes, "History of Flint Medical College," 11.

14. The Education of Black Physicians at Shaw University, 1882–1918

This chapter originally appeared as "The Education of Physicians at Shaw University, 1882–1918: Problems of Quality and Quantity," in *Black Americans in North Carolina and the South,* ed. Jeffrey J. Crow and Flora J. Hatley (Chapel Hill: Univ. of North Carolina Press, 1984), 160–88.

This publication was supported in part by National Institutes of Health Grant LM 03413 from the National Library of Medicine, 1980–82, and by University of Florida Seed Money and Biomedical Research grants, 1979–80. Thanks are extended to Mr. Clarence Toomer, Ms. Robena Bradley, and the staff at the Shaw University Library for their assistance in locating and using early records of the school.

1. *Annual Catalog of the Officers and Students of the Leonard Medical School . . . for the Academic Year Ending May Thirty-first Nineteen Hundred and Twelve,* 9, Shaw University Archives, Raleigh, N.C. (hereafter Leonard Medical (or Shaw University) catalogs will be cited as *Leonard [or Shaw] Catalog,* followed by academic year and page number). Broken runs of these catalogs may also be found at the National Library of Medicine, Bethesda, Md., and the American Baptist Historical Society Archives, Rochester, N.Y.

2. Abraham Flexner, *Medical Education in the United States and Canada: A Report to the Carnegie Foundation for the Advancement of Teaching* (New York: Carnegie Foundation for the Advancement of Teaching, 1910), 180.

3. For background on this subject, see chapter 11 of this volume, especially note 1.

4. For a comprehensive history of Shaw University, see Wilmoth A. Carter, *Shaw's Universe: A Monument to Educational Innovation* (Raleigh, N.C.: Shaw University, 1973).

5. Henry L. Morehouse, *H. M. Tupper, D.D.: A Narrative of Twenty-Five Years' Work in the South, 1865–1890* (New York: American Baptist Home Mission Society, 1890), 8.

6. Ibid., 5–10; Carter, *Shaw's Universe,* 1–9.

7. Morehouse, *Narrative,* 13.

8. *Shaw Catalog,* 1876–77, 18; 1877–78, 19; 1878–79, 18; 1879–80, 18. The quotation appears in each catalog.

9. Dyson, *Howard University,* 301–34; Morais, *History of the Afro-American in Medicine,* 42–43.

10. Bullock, *History of Negro Education in the South,* 33; Morais, *History of the Afro-American in Medicine,* 44; Summerville, *Educating Black Doctors,* 1–20.

11. *Shaw Catalog,* 1876–77, 18–19; 1877–78, 19; 1878–79, 18.

12. Henry M. Tupper to Dr. S. S. Cutting [Corresponding Secretary of the ABHMS], ca. Dec. 1878, in Charles F. Meserve, "A History of Shaw University, Raleigh, North Carolina, 1865–1930" (unpublished typescript at American Baptist Historical Society, Rochester, N.Y., unpaginated).

13. *Shaw Catalog,* 1878–79, 18.

14. *Shaw Catalog,* 1879–80, 18; *Baptist Home Mission Monthly* 2 (1880): 35.

15. *Baptist Home Mission Monthly* 2 (1880): 105.

16. Ibid., 155.

17. Ibid., 35, 155.

18. Ibid., 219; *Baptist Home Mission Monthly* 3 (1881): 15; Meserve, "History of Shaw."

19. *Laws and Resolutions of the State of North Carolina, Passed by the General Assembly at Its Session, 1881* (Raleigh: J. Turner Jr., 1881), c. 149; Carter, *Shaw's Universe,* 27–28.

20. Meserve, "History of Shaw"; *Baptist Home Mission Monthly* 3 (1881): 191; 4 (1882): 216.

21. *Baptist Home Mission Monthly* 4 (1882): 216.

22. Ibid.

23. *Baptist Home Mission Monthly* 2 (1880): 105.

24. American Baptist Home Mission Society Executive Board Minutes, June 11, 1883, book 9, 438, at American Baptist Historical Society, Rochester, N.Y.; Shaw University Trustees Minutes, Apr. 30, 1903, and Feb. 4, 1910, in Shaw University Archives.

25. *Shaw Catalog*, 1881–82, 22.

26. *Baptist Home Mission Monthly* 5 (1883): 101.

27. *President's Annual Report to the Board of Trustees of Shaw University and to the Secretary of the American Baptist Home Mission Society* [Dec. 1883], 6, Shaw University Archives (hereafter cited as *Shaw Annual Report*). See also John F. Slater Fund, *Annual Report*, for these years; these are published and available in most university research libraries.

28. *Medical News* 43 (1883): 76.

29. *North Carolina Medical Journal* 12 (1883): 220.

30. Ibid. LMS was actually one of the first (if not *the* first) medical schools to establish a four-year graded curriculum for its students. See *Leonard Catalog*, 1885–86, 9, where Dr. Keen is quoted from the *Medical News* article saying, "They [the Leonard faculty] have wisely decided that, in view of the limited early education of the colored people, the medical course shall be four years, both to give a thorough graded course, and the opportunity to study Latin and other branches in the academic department."

31. *North Carolina Medical Journal* 12 (1883): 221.

32. *Baptist Home Mission Monthly* 14 (1892): 271.

33. Ibid., 5 (1883): 196; *Raleigh Farmer and Mechanic*, Jan. 30, 1884; *Leonard Catalog*, 1885–86, 8.

34. *Leonard Catalog*, 1885–86, 8; *Shaw Annual Report*, 1885, 6.

35. *African Expositor*, Apr. 1886. Copies of this school newspaper may be found in the North Carolina Collection, Wilson Library, University of North Carolina at Chapel Hill.

36. Ibid., 2, 4.

37. Ibid., 3. Scruggs later opened his own hospital in Southern Pines, North Carolina, called the Pickford Sanitarium for Consumptive Negroes. See chapter 19 of the current volume. For biographical information on Scruggs, see Elizabeth Reid Murray, "Scruggs, Lawson Andrew," in *Dictionary of North Carolina Biography*, ed. William S. Powell (Chapel Hill: Univ. of North Carolina Press, 1994), 5: 307–8.

38. *Shaw Annual Report*, 1886, 3. See also *Baptist Home Mission Monthly* 8 (1886): 146. On the history of the North Carolina State Board of Medical Examiners, see Ivan M. Proctor, Joseph J. Combs, and Dorothy Long, "The State Board of Medical Examiners," in *Medicine in North Carolina: Essays in the History of Medical Science and Medical Service, 1524–1960*, ed. Dorothy Long (Raleigh: North Carolina Medical Society, 1972), 1:215–31.

39. *Shaw Annual Report*, 1888, 3; 1889, 2; 1891, 4; 1893, 3; *Baptist Home Mission Monthly* 15 (1893): 254–55.

40. *Shaw Annual Reports*, 1887–93, passim.

41. *Baptist Home Mission Monthly* 9 (1887): 64.

42. *Baptist Home Mission Monthly* 16 (1894): 2.

43. *Shaw Annual Report*, 1894, 3.

44. *Raleigh News and Observer*, Sept. 29, 1895.

45. *Baptist Home Mission Monthly* 8 (1886): 56.

46. *Baptist Home Mission Monthly* 10 (1888): 125.

47. Ibid., 219.

48. Ibid., 333, 350–53.

49. Ibid., 16 (1894): 103. This change in attitude and missionary priorities is well demonstrated in the pages of the *Baptist Home Mission Monthly* for that period.

50. C. F. Meserve to J. L. M. Curry, Jan. 9, 1895, in Meserve Letter Book, 43, Shaw University Archives.

51. C. F. Meserve to J. L. M. Curry, Jan. 9, 1895, in Meserve Letter Book, 46.

52. C. F. Meserve to J. L. M. Curry, Jan. 9, 1895, in Meserve Letter Book, 45.

53. See Slater Fund *Annual Reports* for these years.

54. C. F. Meserve to Gen. T. J. Morgan, Mar. 23, 1895, in Meserve Letter Book, 317; *Shaw Annual Report*, 1895, 3–6.

55. For background information on the history of medical education up to 1910, see Kaufman, *American Medical Education;* Hudson, "Abraham Flexner in Perspective," 545–61; Ludmerer, *Learning to Heal.*

56. See annual education issues of *JAMA* for those years.

57. Flexner, *Medical Education in the United States,* 280–81.

58. See *Leonard Catalogs* for these years.

59. E. Richard Brown, *Rockefeller Medicine Men: Medicine and Capitalism in America* (Berkeley: Univ. of California Press, 1979), 153, 165–66.

60. See, for instance, William A. Mapp, M.D., to C. F. Meserve, Dec. 30, 1896; J. H. G. Williams, M.D., to same, May 12, 1904; B. F. Hutchins, M.D., to same, Apr. 26, 1904, all in Letters Received Files, Shaw University Archives.

61. *Journal of the National Medical Association* 10 (1918): 126.

62. For more on the struggle to keep black medical schools, including LMS, open after the publication of the Flexner Report, see chapter 18 of the current volume.

15. Training the "Consecrated, Skillful, Christian Physician"

This chapter originally appeared as "Training the 'Consecrated, Skillful, Christian Physician': Documents Illustrating Student Life at Leonard Medical School, 1882–1918," *North Carolina Historical Review* 75 (1998): 250–76.

1. *Leonard Catalog,* 1898, 5; 1909, 7. Leonard Medical School did not accept female students, though other medical schools for African Americans, such as Howard and Meharry, did.

2. On the establishment of medical schools for African Americans in the late nineteenth and early twentieth centuries, see chapter 11 of the current volume. On the motivations and attitudes of white missionary groups and philanthropists for founding and supporting African American colleges in the late nineteenth century, see articles by Roy E. Finkenbine, J. M. Stephen Peeps, and Sandy Dwayne Martin, reprinted in *African Americans and Education in the South, 1865–1900,* ed. Donald G. Nieman (New York: Garland Publishing, 1994), 70–86, 293–311, 228–45. On the education of freed people, see, for example, Bullock, *History of Negro Education in the South;* McPherson, *Abolitionist Legacy;* Anderson, *Education of Blacks in the South;* Jones, *Soldiers of Light and Love;* Morris, *Reading, 'Riting, and Reconstruction;* Vaughan, *Schools for All;* Fairclough, *Teaching Equality.*

3. On the importance of religion at Knoxville College Medical Department, see Savitt, "Money versus Mission," 680–716.

4. On student life at predominantly white medical schools of the late nineteenth and early twentieth centuries, see, for example, Thomas Neville Bonner, *Becoming a Physician: Medical Education in Britain, France, Germany, and the United States, 1750–1945* (New York: Oxford Univ. Press, 1995), 316–19; Robert H. Shikes and Henry N. Claman,

The University of Colorado School of Medicine: A Centennial History, 1883–1983 (Denver: Univ. of Colorado School of Medicine, 1983), 81–111; Horace W. Davenport, *Fifty Years of Medicine at the University of Michigan, 1891–1941* (Ann Arbor: Univ. of Michigan Medical School, 1986), 17–33; Duffy, *Tulane University Medical Center,* 89–92, 102.

5. Todd L. Savitt, "Abraham Flexner and the Black Medical Schools," in *Beyond Flexner: Medical Education in the Twentieth Century,* ed. Barbara M. Barzansky and Norman Gevitz (Westport, Conn.: Greenwood Press, 1992), 65–81 (a revised version appears as chapter 18 of the current volume).

6. On the history of Leonard Medical School, see Savitt, "Education of Black Physicians at Shaw University," 160–88; and Hine, "Anatomy of Failure," 512–25. For a comprehensive history of Shaw University, see Carter, *Shaw's Universe.*

7. For more on general educational conditions in the New South, see references in note 2 of this chapter.

8. On rising standards and medical education reform, see Kaufman, *American Medical Education;* Hudson, "Abraham Flexner in Perspective," 545–61; Ludmerer, *Learning to Heal;* Bonner, *Becoming a Physician,* 251–308.

9. [Student], Philadelphia, to Charles F. Meserve, Nov. 27, 1896, Letters Received, 1896–1897, 1904, 1905, Shaw University Records, University Archives, Shaw University Library, Raleigh (hereafter cited as Shaw Archives). For reasons of confidentiality, students' names are excluded from citations.

10. [Student], John A. Dix School, Dinwiddie, Va., to "Prin. of Pshaw University," Sept. 7, 1905, Letters Received, Shaw Archives.

11. [Student], Greenville, S.C., to Meserve, Sept. 8, 1905, Letters Received, Shaw Archives.

12. [Student], Lakewood, N.J., to Meserve, n.d., 1905, Letters Received, Shaw Archives.

13. [Student], Prestonville, N.C., to Meserve, Jan. 20, 1897, Letters Received, Shaw Archives.

14. [Student], Philadelphia, to Meserve, Apr. 19, 1904, Letters Received, Shaw Archives.

15. [Student], Louisville, Ky., to Meserve, Apr. 6, 1904, Letters Received, Shaw Archives.

16. [Student], Orangeburg, S.C., to Meserve, Sept. 29, 1896, Letters Received, Shaw Archives.

17. [Student], Waycross, Ga., to Meserve, Apr. 8, 1904, Letters Received, Shaw Archives.

18. [Student], Alcorn College, Westside, Miss., to Meserve, Dec. 6, 1896, Letters Received, Shaw Archives.

19. Meserve to [Student], Manchester, Va., Nov. 8, 1895, Meserve Letter Books, 1894–95, 1897, 1898, Shaw Archives.

20. Meserve to L. J. Barrett, President, Jackson College, Jackson, Miss., Aug. 21, 1903, Letters Received, Shaw Archives.

21. Meserve to [Student], Greenland, Fla., Feb. 6, 1897, Meserve Letter Books, Shaw Archives.

22. Meserve to [Student], Jackson College, Jackson, Miss., Feb. 4, 1895, Meserve Letter Books, Shaw Archives.

23. [Student], Washington, D.C., to Meserve, Sept. 13, 1905, Letters Received, Shaw Archives.

24. Meserve to [Student], Equality, S.C., Sept. 24, 1895, Meserve Letter Books, Shaw Archives.

25. Meserve to [Student], Bessemer, Ala., Apr. 26, 1895, Meserve Letter Books, Shaw Archives.

26. *Leonard Catalog,* 1897–98, 17.

27. [Student], Newberry, S.C., to Meserve, Sept. 2, 1896, Letters Received, Shaw Archives.

28. [Student], McKenney, Va., to Meserve, Aug. 28, 1905, Letters Received, Shaw Archives.

29. [Student], Asbury Park, N.J., to Meserve, Sept. 9, 1905, Letters Received, Shaw Archives.

30. Meserve to C. Ayer, Clifton Springs, N.Y., Feb. 4, 1895, Meserve Letter Books, Shaw Archives.

31. See, for example, Meserve to [Student], Hampton Institute, Hampton, Va., Jan. 19, 1895, Meserve Letter Books, Shaw Archives.

32. *Leonard Catalog,* 1881–82, 28; 1912–13, 17–19. The cost of attending Tulane Medical School in 1889–90, for example, was $320, including room and board, according to Duffy, *Tulane University Medical Center,* 89n.

33. [Student], New York, N.Y., to Meserve, Sept. 21, 1905, Letters Received, Shaw Archives.

34. [Student], Birmingham, Ala., to Meserve, Sept. 23, 1905, Letters Received, Shaw Archives.

35. [Student], Beaufort, S.C., to Meserve, Sept. 7, 1905, Letters Received, Shaw Archives.

36. [Student], Philadelphia, to Meserve, Sept. 1, 1896, Letters Received, Shaw Archives.

37. Meserve to [Student], Philadelphia, Sept. 9, 1896, Letters Received, Shaw Archives.

38. Meserve to Hope Bros. and Co., Knoxville, Tenn., Apr. 5, 1897, Meserve Letter Books, Shaw Archives.

39. Meserve to Pullman Car Company, n.p., Mar. 25, 1895, Meserve Letter Books, Shaw Archives.

40. Meserve to R. C. Wagner, Wagner-Palace Car Co., Mott Haven, New York City, Mar. 7, 1898, Meserve Letter Books, Shaw Archives.

41. [Student], Warsaw, N.C., to Meserve, Dec. 14, 1896, Letters Received, Shaw Archives.

42. [Student], Louisville, Ky., to Meserve, Jan. 20, 1897, Letters Received, Shaw Archives.

43. [Student], Garysburg, N.C., to Meserve, Sept. 6, 1896, Letters Received, Shaw Archives.

44. Meserve to J. L. M. Curry, Jan. 9, 1895, and to Gen. T. J. Morgan, Mar. 23, 1895, Meserve Letter Books, Shaw Archives; *Shaw Annual Report* 1895, 3–6.

45. Meserve to [Student], Warsaw, N.C., Nov. 27, 1895, Meserve Letter Books, Shaw Archives.

46. Meserve to [Student], Virginia Beach, Va., Sept. 24, 1895, Meserve Letter Books, Shaw Archives.

47. Meserve to [Student], Savannah, Ga., Sept. 24, 1895, Meserve Letter Books, Shaw Archives.

48. Meserve to Mrs. I. McLaurie Cummings, Salt Lake City, Utah, Feb. 28, 1898, Meserve Letter Books, Shaw Archives.

49. Meserve to [Student], Knoxville, Tenn., May 7, 1897, Meserve Letter Books, Shaw Archives.

50. *Shaw Annual Report,* 1885–86, 2.

51. Charles F. Meserve, *The Negro Physician* (Raleigh, N.C.: n.p., 1910), 6, in Shaw University Scrapbook, Shaw Archives.

52. Charles F. Meserve, "Christianity and Character at Shaw University," *Baptist Home Mission Monthly* 23 (1901): 13.

53. See, for example, *Baptist Home Mission Monthly* 24 (1902): 79; *The Workers* [Shaw University student magazine] 3, Feb.–Mar. 1907, 18; Richard H. Lewis, "The Urgent Need of Hospitals for the Colored People of the South," and James McKee, "Leonard Medical School," in Meserve, "History of Shaw."

54. See, for example, *Leonard Catalog,* 1887–88, 16.

55. *Leonard Catalog,* 1911–12, 21.

56. *Leonard Catalog,* 1899–1900, 17.

57. Henry M. Tupper, "The Leonard Medical School, Shaw University—Its Endowment a Necessity," *Baptist Home Mission Monthly* 8 (1886): 56.

58. *Shaw Annual Report*, 1885–86, 2.

59. See, for example, *The Workers* 3 (Dec. 1906–Jan. 1907): 13, and 3 (Feb.–Mar. 1907): 14.

60. Flyers and programs may be found in the Shaw University Scrapbook, Shaw Archives.

61. For flyers and newspaper clippings, see Shaw University Scrapbook, Shaw Archives.

62. Shaw University Scrapbook, Shaw Archives.

63. *The Workers* 1 (Jan. 1905): 15, and 3 (Feb.–Mar. 1907): 11, 13. See also "Dr. C. C. Boone," in Meserve, "History of Shaw."

64. *The Workers* 1 (Jan. 1905): 14.

65. Entry of Dec. 31, 1912, Leonard Medical School Faculty Minutes, in "Medical School, Leonard Building," Miscellaneous Papers, Shaw Archives. Every Leonard Medical School catalog contained a similar statement.

66. *African Expositor* [Shaw University newspaper], Apr. 1886.

67. *Baptist Home Mission Monthly* 10 (1888): 125; *The Workers* 2 (June–July 1906): 1; *Missions* 2 (1911): 538. *Missions* was the successor to the *Baptist Home Mission Monthly*.

68. *The Workers* 3 (Dec. 1906–Jan. 1907): 2.

69. [Student], Raleigh, to Meserve, Sept. 14, 1905, Letters Received, Shaw Archives.

70. "To the President of Shaw University," Jan. 26, 1897, Letters Received, Shaw Archives.

71. "To the President of Shaw University," Jan. 26, 1897, Letters Received, Shaw Archives. This latter request seems to have been a perennial one. See, for example, Leonard Medical School Faculty Minutes, Feb. 26, 1909, and Mar. 7, 1913, Miscellaneous Papers, Shaw Archives.

72. Meserve to 15 Members of Sophomore Class, Leonard Medical School, Feb. 1898, Meserve Letter Books, Shaw Archives.

73. Meserve to 15 Members of Sophomore Class, Leonard Medical School, Feb. 1898, Meserve Letter Books, Shaw Archives. Meserve made a similar statement and refused to see a group of students in January 1914 when an undergraduate was dismissed for marrying. See *Raleigh News and Observer*, Jan. 3, 1914.

74. Meserve to 15 Members of Sophomore Class, Leonard Medical School, Feb. 1898, Meserve Letter Books, Shaw Archives.

75. *Leonard Catalog*, 1896–97, 14.

76. *Leonard Catalog*, 1908–9, 19.

77. *Leonard Catalog*, 1897–98, 5–6, and 1898–99, 19.

78. Meserve, "History of Shaw."

79. In the early years at Leonard, students had to obtain a minimum grade of 60 percent in each subject but an overall average of 75 percent. In 1890 both those numbers were raised to 80 percent. *Leonard Catalog*, 1885–86, 11, and 1890–91, 10–11.

80. James M. Pickel Roll book, 1906–10, 11, Chemistry Class Rollbooks for Leonard Medical School, 1896–1913, J. M. Pickel Papers, Private Collections, North Carolina State Archives, Raleigh (hereafter cited as Pickel Papers).

81. "Plan of Teaching Chemistry to the Leonard Medical Students," Pickel Roll book, 1900–1901, Pickel Papers.

82. Entry of Oct. 28, 1913, Leonard Medical School Faculty Minutes, Miscellaneous Papers, Shaw Archives; Leonard Medical School Composite Grade Sheets, 1908–14, in "Medical School, Leonard Building," Miscellaneous Papers, Shaw Archives.

83. Davenport, *Fifty Years of Medicine*, 26–27; Shikes and Claman, *University of Colorado School of Medicine*, 99; Duffy, *Tulane University Medical Center*, 90.

84. [Student], Saratoga Springs, N.Y., to Meserve, May 16, 1904, Letters Received, Shaw Archives. See also Meserve to George Williams, Philadelphia, May 24, 1895, Meserve Letter Books, Shaw Archives.

85. Pickel Roll books, 1901–2, 2, and 1904–6, 10, Pickel Papers. On deficiencies of students at white medical schools, see, for example, Duffy, *Tulane University Medical Center,* 102, and Shikes and Claman, *University of Colorado School of Medicine,* 82–83, 109.

86. Pickel Roll books, passim, Pickel Papers.

87. Pickel Roll books, passim, Pickel Papers.

88. Leonard Medical School Composite Grade Sheets, 1908–14, Miscellaneous Papers, Shaw Archives. Similar statements can be found in this record, the Pickel Roll books, and the Leonard Medical School Faculty Minutes.

89. Meserve to [Student's brother], Lynchburg, Va., May 10, 1897, Meserve Letter Books, Shaw Archives.

90. Meserve to [Student], Shaw University, Mar. 23, 1895, Meserve Letter Books, Shaw Archives.

91. Meserve to [Student's brother], Lynchburg, Va., May 10, 1897, Meserve Letter Books, Shaw Archives.

92. Meserve to [Student], Shaw University, Mar. 5, 1895, Meserve Letter Books, Shaw Archives.

93. Meserve to [Student], Philadelphia, May 24, 1895, Meserve Letter Books, Shaw Archives.

94. Meserve to [home office], New York, N.Y., Apr. 4, 1895, Meserve Letter Books, Shaw Archives.

95. [Student], Chicago, to Meserve, Mar. 30, 1904, Letters Received, Shaw Archives.

16. Four African American Proprietary Medical Colleges, 1888–1923

This chapter originally appeared as "Four African-American Proprietary Medical Colleges: 1888–1923," *Journal of the History of Medicine and Allied Sciences* 55 (2000): 203–55.

I thank the staff members of the History of Medicine Division at the National Library of Medicine in Bethesda for their collegiality and assistance on this project during the year I served there as Visiting Historical Scholar (1991–92). I thank Dwayne Cox and Sherrill Redmon for their help in locating materials on Louisville National Medical College, and several people for their invaluable assistance in conveying and locating information on Hannibal Medical College: Mary H. Teloh of the Special Collections Division at the Vanderbilt University Medical Center Library in Nashville; Anne Carroll Bunting of the Health Sciences Library at the University of Tennessee in Memphis; Edwina Walls of the Health Sciences Library at the University of Arkansas for Medical Sciences in Little Rock; Wayne Moore of the Public Service Section at the Tennessee State Library and Archives in Nashville; Sandy Stratton of the Territorial Museum in Guthrie, Oklahoma; and Dr. S. R. Bruesch and Arthur Webb of Memphis. I also thank Calvin McBride of Jackson, Tennessee, for his help in gathering material and sharing information about the University of West Tennessee and about his family's connections with that institution; Patricia LaPointe of the Memphis Shelby County Public Library and Information Center for her help and encouragement in locating medical history resources in Memphis; and Ruth Crenshaw, president of the Health Sciences Museum Foundation of Memphis, for sharing the only copy of the 1907–08 *UWT Catalogue* known to exist.

1. These schools included Yale, the University of Pennsylvania, Harvard, Women's Medical College of Pennsylvania, Western Reserve University, Northwestern University, Detroit Medical College, Bennett Medical College, Illinois Medical College, Medical College of Indiana, and Long Island College Hospital. According to W. E. B. Du Bois, ed., *The Health and Physique of the Negro American* (Atlanta, Ga.: Atlanta Univ. Press, 1906), 99, there were

at least 213 graduates of Northern medical schools practicing in 1906. See also Daryl Keith Daniels, "African-Americans at the Yale University School of Medicine: 1810–1960" (M.D. thesis, Yale University, 1991), 51, 109; [W. Montague Cobb], "Nathan Francis Mossell, M.D., 1856–1946," *Journal of the National Medical Association* 46 (1954): 122.

2. Todd L. Savitt, "Training the 'Consecrated, Skillful, Christian Physician': Documents Illustrating Student Life at Leonard Medical School, 1882–1918, *North Carolina Historical Review* 75 (1998): 270.

3. For more on the history of medical education during the late nineteenth and early twentieth centuries, see Flexner, *Medical Education in the United States,* 3–19; Kaufman, *American Medical Education,* esp. 109–82; Ludmerer, *Learning to Heal;* Regina Markell Morantz-Sanchez, *Sympathy and Science: Women Physicians in American Medicine* (New York: Oxford Univ. Press, 1985), 64–89; and Moldow, *Women Doctors in Gilded-Age Washington,* 37–74.

4. No records of any of the black proprietary schools have been located. Unlike the mission schools, which had affiliations with universities or with religious organizations, Louisville National, Chattanooga National, and the others answered to no other record-keeping organization. Official records of these schools appear to no longer exist, or, if they do, have not been put in the public domain. The discussions in this article are based primarily on college catalogs and other published primary source material.

5. H. C. Weeden, *Weeden's History of the Colored People of Louisville* (Louisville, Ky.: H. C. Weeden, 1897), 57. On black life and community in Louisville during this period, see George C. Wright, *Life behind a Veil: Blacks in Louisville, Kentucky, 1865–1930* (Baton Rouge: Louisiana State Univ. Press, 1985). See also Lawrence H. Williams, *Black Higher Education in Kentucky, 1879–1930: The History of Simmons University* (Lewiston, N.Y.: Edwin Mellen Press, 1987).

6. For biographical information on Fitzbutler, see W. Montague Cobb, "Henry Fitzbutler," *Journal of the National Medical Association* 44 (1952): 403–7; Leslie L. Hanawalt, "Henry Fitzbutler: Detroit's First Black Medical Student," *Detroit in Perspective* 1 (1973): 126–40; Obituary, *Louisville National Medical College Catalogue* (hereafter *LNMC Catalogue*), 1901–2, 32, found in the National Library of Medicine, Bethesda, Md.; Weeden, *History of Colored People,* 26, 44, 57.

7. Conrad is listed in *Polk's Medical Directory,* 1886, 399; 1890, 496. Conrad later (1892) took courses at the Hahnemann Medical College in Chicago. His advertised specialty in *Polk's Medical Directory* (1893, 510) was diseases of women and children.

8. A brief historical statement about LNMC's founding appears in *LNMC Catalogue,* 1891–92, 8. One of Fitzbutler's preceptees, William T. Peyton, was principal of the Western Colored Public School for many years (see, for example, *Louisville City Directory,* 1877, 333). Another student, Richard Harper, as the history section of the *LNMC Catalogue* explains, had been a student at Meharry before going to Louisville in about 1885 to study medicine with Dr. Conrad. Little information is available for others who formed what the *LNMC Catalogue* described as "a nucleus for medical education . . . in the cities of the Ohio Falls." Ms. Janet Meyer, Kornhauser Health Sciences Library, Univ. of Louisville, has collected information on the founders and deposited documents at the Kornhauser Library.

9. *LNMC Catalogue,* 1891–92, 8; 1894–95, 7; Kentucky General Assembly, *Session Acts of the General Assembly,* 1888, 443 (chapter 1234); "Medical Laws of Kentucky," Apr. 25, 1888, Sec. 3, printed in *Polk's Medical Directory,* 1890, 457.

10. Weeden, *History of Colored People,* 26, 57; *LNMC Catalogue,* 1894–95, 7.

11. See faculty lists in LNMC catalogs.

12. Ibid.; *Polk's Medical Directory.*

13. *LNMC Catalogue,* 1902–3, 7.

14. *LNMC Catalogue,* 1891–92, 9; 1889–90, 5–7.

15. No LNMC catalog for 1890–91 is extant. See historical descriptions in subsequent catalogs (for example, 1896–97, 4).

16. *LNMC Catalogue,* 1891–92, 5, 6.

17. F. H. Gerrish, "Report of the Committee," *Bulletin of the American Academy of Medicine* 19 (1894): 435–39.

18. *LNMC Catalogue,* 1891–92, quotes on 11, 5.

19. *LNMC Catalogue,* 1891–92, 6; 1902–3, 5; *State University Catalogue,* 1892–93, 32, found at the National Library of Medicine, Bethesda, Md.; *LNMC Catalogue,* 1890–91, 4, 9.

20. *LNMC Catalogue,* 1894–95, 3.

21. Obituary, *Louisville Courier-Journal,* Apr. 13, 1893, 7.

22. *LNMC Catalogue,* 1895–96, 8.

23. *Louisville Courier-Journal,* Apr. 10, 1891, 8; Apr. 7, 1893, 5; Apr. 11, 1894, 6; Apr. 9, 1896, 8; Apr. 6, 1898, 6.

24. *Medical and Surgical Observer* 1 (1893): 161. On the history of the *Medical and Surgical Observer,* see Todd L. Savitt, "'A Journal of Our Own': The *Medical and Surgical Observer* at the Beginnings of an African-American Medical Profession in Late Nineteenth-Century America," *Journal of the National Medical Association* 88 (1996): 52–59, 115–22 (reproduced as chapter 20 in the current volume).

25. See, for example, *LNMC Catalogue,* 1898–99, 11; 1905–6, 8–9.

26. See George M. Kober, "The Past and Present Status of Medical Education in This Country," *Proceedings of the Association of American Medical Colleges* (1907): 35. On LNMC's adherence, see *LNMC Catalogue,* 1894–95, 4; 1903–4, 5–6; 1897–98, 9. Association of American Medical Colleges, Constitution, Art. III, Sec. 4, *Bulletin of the American Academy of Medicine* 22 (1894): 538; *LNMC Catalogue,* 1894–95, 4.

27. *LNMC Catalogue,* 1897–98, 3.

28. *LNMC Catalogue,* 1891–92, 11; 1895–96, 3; 1897–98, 3; 1896–97, 15.

29. *LNMC Catalogue,* 1898–99, 8–10.

30. Ibid., 6.

31. Each catalog through 1897–98 contained summary statements about the graduation exercises up to that year.

32. *LNMC Catalogue,* 1899–1900, 5; 1907–8, 38.

33. See, for example, lists of staff and board members in *LNMC Catalogue,* 1901–2, 11, 15; 1902–3, 27.

34. *LNMC Catalogue,* 1901–2, 12; 1899–1900, 6; 1902–3, 17.

35. Obituary, *LNMC Catalogue,* 1902–3, 32; Obituary, *JAMA* 38 (1902): 120.

36. *LNMC Catalogue,* 1902–3, 6, 7.

37. *LNMC Catalogue,* 1905–6, 13.

38. See, for example, *LNMC Catalogue,* 1907–8, 38–39. No catalogs beyond 1907–8 could be located.

39. *LNMC Catalogue,* 1907–8, 39.

40. The national failure rate for all medical graduates during those same years was 17.2 percent; for black medical school graduates it was 46.5 percent. State board results were published annually in *JAMA.* Alabama placed LNMC on its unacceptable list in 1910. See *Journal of the National Medical Association* 2 (1910): 306; *JAMA* 59 (1912): 642.

41. Flexner, *Medical Education in the United States,* 230, 180–81.

42. Ibid., 307.

43. Tennessee, *Acts of the State of Tennessee Passed by the General Assembly, 1875* (Nashville: n.p., 1875), 232–36, chap. 142, "An Act to Provide for the Organization of Corporations."

44. *Polk's Medical Directory,* 1886, 859.

45. See Philip M. Hamer, ed., *The Centennial History of the Tennessee State Medical Association, 1830–1930* (Nashville: Tennessee State Medical Association, 1930), 90–103; and minutes of the Medical Association of the State of Tennessee for the 1880s, printed annually in the Association's *Transactions.*

46. The 1889 law was printed in full in the *Transactions of the Medical Society of the State of Tennessee,* 1891, 231–36.

47. United States Census Office, Manuscript Census, 1870, Marshall County, Mississippi, range 2, 568; Obituary, *Memphis Commercial Appeal,* Oct. 28, 1899, 7.

48. John McLeod Keating, *History of the City of Memphis and Shelby County, Tennessee* (Syracuse, N.Y.: D. Mason, 1888), 2:96; *Polk's Medical Directory,* 1890, 1056; *Meharry Medical College Catalogue,* 1880–81, 6; 1882–83, 6.

49. *Polk's Medical Directory,* 1890, 1056.

50. No literature from the school, which later became Shorter College, hints at the existence of a medical department, nor do the standard histories of medical education in Arkansas, the Little Rock city directories for those years, or three official surveys of American medical schools in 1889, 1890, and 1891, mention Bethel Medical Department or Southwestern University. See John H. Rauch, *Report on Medical Education, Medical Colleges and the Regulation of the Practice of Medicine in the United States and Canada, 1765–1890* (Springfield, Ill.: Rokker [for Illinois State Board of Health], 1890), 143; Rauch, *Medical Education, Medical Colleges and the Regulation of the Practice of Medicine in the United States and Canada, 1765–1891* (Springfield, Ill.: Rokker [for Illinois State Board of Health], 1891), 3–4; W. David Baird, *Medical Education in Arkansas, 1879–1978* (Memphis, Tenn.: Memphis State Univ. Press, 1979).

51. Keating, *History of Memphis,* 2:96; "Dr. Cottrell's Death," *The Christian Index* (Jackson, Tennessee), Nov. 18, 1899, 4; *Memphis City Directory* (Dow), 1885, 293; *Memphis City Directory* (Shole), 1885, 509 (boldface and capital letters). (Different city directories were published in Memphis during these years and are cited hereafter by the publisher.)

52. "Charter of Incorporation for Hannibal Medical College," filed in Book O, 124, Domestic Charters, Tennessee State Library and Archives, Nashville (hereafter cited as Charter of HMC).

53. *Memphis City Directory* (Dow), 1886, 172.

54. "Elias Cottrell," in *Who's Who of the Colored Race,* ed. Frank Lincoln Mather (Chicago: n.p., 1915), 77; "Bishop E. Cottrell, Holly Springs, Miss.," in G. P. Hamilton, *Beacon Lights of the Race* (Memphis, Tenn.: E. H. Clarke and Brother, 1911), 7–17; Othal Hawthorne Lakey, *The History of the CME Church* (Memphis, Tenn.: CME Publishing, 1985), 128, 258, 265, 289, 382–83, 651, 671; *Encyclopedia of World Methodism* (Nashville, Tenn.: United Methodist Publishing, 1974), 592; Isaac Lane, *Autobiography of Bishop Isaac Lane, L.L.D.* (Nashville, Tenn.: Publishing House of the M.E. Church, South, 1916), 163–64 (with photograph); *Central Tennessee College Catalogue,* 1879–80, 20, found in the Meharry Medical College Archives, Nashville, Tenn.

55. Fields's name appears in Memphis city directories only twice between 1884 and 1894. *Memphis City Directory* (Dow), 1885, 781; *Memphis City Directory* (Shole), 1885, 17.

56. G. P. Hamilton, *The Bright Side of Memphis: A Compendium of Information Concerning the Colored People of Memphis, Tennessee* (Memphis, Tenn.: n.p., 1908), 152; *Memphis City Directory,* 1888, 389.

57. Humes's name appears on the Charter of HMC as "H. H. Hennes." The city directories are confusing concerning Humes, as he is sometimes listed without his middle initial, sometimes as J. Humes, and sometimes twice, as both Henry and Henry H., in the same year. Possibly there were two people with the same name living in Memphis or he had a relative living there.

58. Alonzo L. Hall, *The Ancient, Mediaeval and Modern Greatness of the Negro* (Memphis, Tenn.: Striker Printers, 1907), 44–45. See also David M. Tucker, *Black Pastors and Leaders: The Memphis Clergy, 1819–1972* (Memphis, Tenn.: Memphis State Univ. Press, 1975), 59.

59. For the 1889–90 academic year, both the school and Cottrell were located at 317 2d Street. In 1890–91, the school was at 73 Madison Street, and Cottrell's office was at 315 2d Street. In 1891–92, both HMC and Cottrell's office were located at 130 Beale Street. In 1892–93, the school was at 34 Winchester, and Cottrell had his office listed in the 1893 directory at 518 Orleans. The display ad in the 1893 directory directed those wishing further information to write or call on Cottrell at 446 Main Street, his home address according to the directory. From 1893 until the last listing in the city directory, 1895, HMC was located at 121 Beale Street, the same as Cottrell's office and residence. See Memphis city directories and *Polk's Medical Directory* for these years.

60. *Memphis City Directory* (Polk), 1892, 1097 (street listing), 272, 447, 572, 687, 720 (name listing), 18 (advertisement for Morgan and Young); *Memphis City Directory* (Dow), 1892, 466 (Fernandis listing). Another year, 1893–94, 121 Beale Street housed HMC, the offices of three lawyers, a barbershop, and the medical office and residence of Tarleton C. Cottrell. *Memphis City Directory*, 1894, 968 (street listing), 240 (name listing), 722, 790, 880 (business listings).

61. *Memphis City Directory*, 1894, 5.

62. Ibid., 54–55; Sanborn Fire Insurance maps of Memphis, 1897, no. 143, found in the Memphis Shelby County Public Library and Information Center, Memphis, Tenn.

63. Rauch, *Report on Medical Education, 1890*, 143; Rauch, *Medical Education, 1891*, 150.

64. For faculty rosters, see *Memphis City Directory* (Polk), 1892, 65–66; 1893, 56; 1894, 54–55; 1895, 73; 1896, 67.

65. Rauch, *Report on Medical Education, 1890*, 143; Rauch, *Medical Education, 1891*, 150. If Cottrell and Anderson were two of the three M.D. holders on the faculty, then at least one of the two whites must not have been a physician, or must have practiced in Memphis without an M.D. degree. Perhaps one was a lawyer who taught medical jurisprudence, a course Rauch lists as offered at HMC. Unfortunately, no evidence to help identify these two individuals is extant.

66. Two African American ministers associated with medicine and with Hannibal resided in Memphis in 1889—Hall and Jacob Palmer Jay. Jay had, throughout the 1880s, served as a pastor, first at Salem Church, then at Gilfield Church. He had also, for some of those same years, operated a drugstore (see Memphis city directories for the 1880s). Jay appears on the first available HMC faculty roster, for 1891–92 (*Memphis City Directory* [Polk], 1892, 65–66), and could possibly have taught from 1889 until that date. Two facts argue against this, however. First, he appears to have held an M.D. degree, as he signed an 1879 article on yellow fever published in an Eclectic medical journal as "J. P. Jay, M.D., Memphis" (J. P. Jay, "Yellow Fever," *Eclectic Medical Journal of Pennsylvania* 17 (1879): 196–97. This article is cited in Abrahams, *Extinct Medical Schools of Nineteenth-Century Philadelphia*, 520). The location of Jay's medical training cannot be determined. Second, though Jay's name appears in the 1889 city directory, it disappears from the 1890 and 1891 editions, each compiled during each previous respective autumn. Thus Jay was probably not living in Memphis during the 1889–90 or 1890–91 school terms. If the directories were inaccurate (they were not always reliable), and if none of the white faculty members were M.D. physicians, then Jay could have been the third M.D. physician at HMC. Were Jay the third M.D., however, the as-yet-unidentified non-M.D. minister would have to have been one of the two whites on the faculty, an unlikely circumstance, as that minister, now that Jay has been eliminated because he claimed to have held an M.D., was probably Hannibal cofounder Alonzo L. Hall.

67. See annual reports of the board, reprinted in the *Transactions of the Medical Society of the State of Tennessee* in 1890, 1891, and 1892.

68. *Physicians', Dentists', and Druggists' Directory of Alabama, Georgia, Louisiana, Mississippi, South Carolina and Tennessee* (New Orleans: Galen Gonser and Co., 1891), 215; Hamilton, *Bright Side of Memphis*, 152; *Polk's Medical Directory*, 1893, 1184; American Medical Association, *American Medical Directory* (Chicago, Ill.: American Medical Association, 1906), 1909, 1098; 1912, 1165; *Memphis City Directory*, 1894, 5; 1895, 73, 67 (for faculty lists).

69. *Memphis City Directory* (Dow), 1892, 627; *Memphis City Directory* (Polk), 1892, 530; *Polk's Medical Directory*, 1893, 1037; *Memphis City Directory* (Polk), 1894, 5.

70. *Polk's Medical Directory*, 1893, 1037. Guthrie, Oklahoma, city directories do not list Jeter as a resident between 1890 and 1896, though he may well have lived in a nearby rural area, as was the case in 1898 (*The Business and Residence Directory of Guthrie and Logan County Oklahoma for the Year Commencing January 1, 1898* [Guthrie, Okla.: Rooney and Hamilton, n.d.], 129, located at the Territorial Museum, Guthrie, Oklahoma), and thus not have been listed in the directory. By 1898, Jeter, born in Alabama, was practicing in the small African American town of Evansville, Oklahoma, and then in nearby Luther. In 1900, though practicing far from Memphis, in Luther, Oklahoma, Jeter was proud enough of his previous connection with HMC to advertise in a national medical directory that he was "Ex Professor of Physiology and Hygiene" at the school. "Oklahoma Register of Physicians," 171, offices of the State Board of Medical Licensure and Supervision, Oklahoma City, Okla. The register lists his name as John Troy Jeter.

71. *Polk's Medical Directory*, 1900, 1461; Charles James Bate, *"It's Been a Long Time" (And We've Come a Long Way): A History of the Oklahoma Black Medical Providers (The Black Healers)* (Muskogee, Okla.: Hoffman, 1986), 152, 290.

72. *Memphis City Directory* (Dow), 1891, 723; (Dow), 1892, 790; (Polk), 1892, 66, 719, 720; 1893, 56; 1894, 55; 1895, 73; 1896, 67.

73. On medical sectarianism and the rivalry between allopaths and "irregular" practitioners in the nineteenth century, see William G. Rothstein, *American Physicians in the Nineteenth Century: From Sects to Science* (Baltimore, Md.: Johns Hopkins Univ. Press, 1972); Norman Gevitz, ed., *Other Healers: Unorthodox Medicine in America* (Baltimore, Md.: Johns Hopkins Univ. Press); James C. Whorton, *Nature Cures: The History of Alternative Medicine in America* (New York: Oxford Univ. Press, 2002).

74. It is possible that Chiles arrived in Memphis in 1889 and was one of the two whites on HMC's faculty whom Rauch listed in his 1890 report. He does not, however, appear in either the 1888 or 1890 city directories. (The relevant alphabetical pages are missing from the 1889 directory, but he is not included in the physician listings that year. See Memphis city directories and *Polk's Medical Directory* for the 1880s and 1890s and *Physicians', Dentists', and Druggists' Directory of Alabama . . . and Tennessee*, 214.) Chiles maintained a private practice in Memphis during the early 1890s, departing, according to Memphis city directories, perhaps as early as 1894 (Chiles's name disappears from city directories beginning with the 1895 edition, published in late 1894). He continued his practice in the small town of Pecan Point, Arkansas. See *Polk's Medical Directory*, 1898, 224. On the Physio-Medical movement in general and the Physio-Medical College of Indiana in particular, see John S. Haller Jr., *Kindly Medicine: Physio-Medicalism in America, 1836–1911* (Kent, Ohio: Kent State Univ. Press, 1997).

75. Clifford Hickman's brother, Benjamin Hickman Jr., graduated two years later. Their father was the longtime and highly respected janitor of the Eclectic Medical Institute until his death in 1900. See Harvey Wickes Felter, *History of the Eclectic Medical Institute, Cincinnati, Ohio, 1845–1902* (Cincinnati, Ohio: Alumni Association of the Eclectic Medi-

cal Institute, 1902), 191, 192, 78, 64; *Eclectic Medical Journal* (Cincinnati) 49 (1889): 309; 60 (1900): 232. The Eclectic Medical Institute, according to William Rothstein, *American Physicians,* 227, "compared favorably with the better medical schools of all sects." Even Dr. T. J. Happel, secretary of the Tennessee State Board of Medical Examiners, admitted to a gathering of state medical society members in 1892 "with some degree of shame, that the regular medical profession is apparently being outstripped" in medical education by the two major medical sects of the time, homeopathy and eclecticism. "Address to the Tennessee State Medical Society," *Transactions of the Medical Society of the State of Tennessee, Knoxville, 1892,* 292. On the Eclectic movement and on the Eclectic Medical Institute, see Haller, *Medical Protestants.* Hickman is listed in Memphis city directories from 1891 through 1894 and then disappears. *Polk's Medical Directory,* 1898, 1278, places him in Cincinnati, and the obituary notice on his father in the *Eclectic Medical Journal* 60 (1900): 232, puts him in South Bend, Indiana.

76. See listings in medical directories, 1886–1900, and in Memphis, Tennessee, and Evansville, Indiana, city directories for the 1880s and 1890s. For more on Jay, see note 66.

77. *Memphis Commercial Appeal,* Oct. 18, 1935, and June 22, 1990; *Memphis Daily News,* June 25, 1990; *Interactions* (University of Michigan College of Pharmacy), Spring 1991, 18; Roberta Church and Ronald Walter, *Nineteenth Century Memphis Families of Color, 1850–1900* (Memphis, Tenn.: Church-Walter, 1987), 63; Patricia M. LaPointe, *From Saddlebags to Science: A Century of Health Care in Memphis, 1830–1930* (Memphis, Tenn.: Health Sciences Museum Foundation of the Memphis and Shelby County Medical Society Auxiliary, 1984), 106; Tennessee Historical Commission highway marker at 159 Beale Street, Memphis; University of Michigan School of Pharmacy, *Catalogue,* 1891–92, found in the National Library of Medicine, Bethesda, Md.; John Parascandola, *The Development of American Pharmacology: John J. Abel and the Shaping of a Discipline* (Baltimore, Md.: Johns Hopkins Univ. Press, 1992), 84–85.

78. William J. Simmons, *Men of Mark: Eminent, Progressive and Rising* (Cleveland, Ohio: Rewell and Co., 1887), 538–45; Hamilton, *Bright Side of Memphis,* 72–75; Willard B. Gatewood, *Aristocrats of Color: The Black Elite, 1880–1920* (Bloomington: Indiana Univ. Press, 1990), 21, 89.

79. *Memphis City Directory,* 1894, 5. See also Rauch, *Report on Medical Education, 1890,* 143; Rauch, *Medical Education, 1891,* 150.

80. Rauch, *Medical Education, 1891,* 151. On admission standards, see Ludmerer, *Learning to Heal,* 97.

81. Rauch, *Report on Medical Education, 1890,* 143; Rauch, *Medical Education, 1891,* 151; *Memphis City Directory,* 1893, 18.

82. Rauch, *Medical Education, 1891,* 151.

83. Bate, "*It's Been a Long Time,*" 110, lists several physicians who purportedly graduated from Hannibal. A closer look at the backgrounds of these physicians reveals that they graduated from other medical schools or that their medical alma maters cannot be confirmed through medical directories. Kenneth R. Manning of the Massachusetts Institute of Technology is compiling a database of African American physicians and kindly shared John J. Pullen's name with me in a personal communication, June 5, 1990.

84. Rauch, *Medical Education, 1891,* 151.

85. *American Medical Directory,* 1909, 40.

86. *Memphis City Directory,* 1896, 67, 210, 328, 724.

87. *Memphis City Directory,* 1893, 18; 1894, 5, and listings for Anderson, Chiles, Cottrell, Hall, Hickman, Jackson, Jeter, Morgan, and Settle; 1890, 121; 1893, 123.

88. *Medical and Surgical Observer* 1 (1893): 161.

89. *Transactions of the Medical Society of the State of Tennessee, Knoxville, 1900,* 23.

90. None of the available published annual reports of the state board, from 1890 through 1897, mention this action. Yet Hamer, *Centennial History of the Tennessee State Medical Association*, 107, states, without citation, that the board "on occasion . . . did refuse to recognize diplomas, for example, those from Hannibal Medical College in Memphis." The board may have taken that action later in the decade or in the next decade, when published reports are not available.

91. "Dr. Cottrell's Death," *The Christian Index* (Jackson, Tennessee), Nov. 18, 1899, 4.

92. Ibid.

93. *Memphis Commercial Appeal*, Oct. 28, 1899, 7; Nov. 5, 1899, 6.

94. "Charter of Incorporation for Chattanooga National Medical College," filed in Book J3, 118, Domestic Charters, Tennessee State Library and Archives, Nashville (hereafter cited as Charter of CNMC).

95. See *Polk's Medical Directory* and Chattanooga city directories for the 1890s and early twentieth century.

96. The manuscript United States Census for 1900 (Hamilton County, Tennessee, vol. 26, E.D. 67, sheet 17, line 84) reports Haigler's birthdate as July 1856. J. Bliss White, comp., *Biography and Achievements of the Colored Citizens of Chattanooga, 1904* (n.p.: n.p., 1904), 52, lists his birthdate as July 4, 1857.

97. White, *Biography and Achievements*, 52.

98. In 1886–87, Haigler studied medicine at the Northwestern Ohio Medical College (*Northwestern Ohio Medical College Catalogue*, 1887–88, 12 [list of matriculates for 1886–87], found in the National Library of Medicine, Bethesda, Md.). Northwestern Ohio Medical College did not list him as a student the following year, but a catalog from rival Toledo Medical College included his name, with the degree Ph.B. (bachelor of pharmacy) following it. His preceptor (all students at Toledo Medical College had a preceptor) that year was G. A. Collamore, an 1859 Harvard Medical College graduate practicing medicine in Chattanooga (*Toledo Medical College Catalogue*, 1888–89, 15, found in the National Library of Medicine, Bethesda, Md.; *Polk's Medical Directory*, 1890, 936). Haigler did not complete his medical studies at either Toledo school, however, but instead left Ohio in 1888 to enroll at two black medical schools for the 1888–89 term—Meharry Medical College in Nashville as a second-year student and the newly opened Louisville National Medical College in Kentucky as a senior (*Meharry Medical College Catalogue*, 1888–89, 6; *LNMC Catalogue*, 1889–90, 6).

99. White, *Biography and Achievements*, 53. See also *Polk's Medical Directory*, 1898, 1507; 1900, 1644; 1904, 1789; *Chattanooga City Directory*, 1899, 20, 304; 1902, 13, 323; 1903, 13.

100. White, *Biography and Achievements*, 53; Charter of CNMC.

101. White, *Biography and Achievements*, 50; Chattanooga city directories for 1890s and early 1900s.

102. Charter of CNMC.

103. White, *Biography and Achievements*, 53.

104. *Chattanooga City Directory*, 1902, 162, 323, 861–62; 1903, 176, 343, 950; 1904, 196, 368, 1003.

105. *Young and Co.'s Business Directory of the Principal Cities of Tennessee and Northern Alabama, for 1900* (Atlanta, Ga.: Young and Company, 1900), 29. Notes on this advertisement are found in the S. R. Bruesch Papers, University of Tennessee Health Sciences Library, Memphis.

106. *Polk's Medical Directory*, 1904, 832, 2125–26. Murdock also listed degrees from the University of Edinburgh in Scotland, the Kentucky School of Medicine in Louisville, the Michigan Medical College in Lansing, and the Michigan Homeopathic Medical College in Lansing.

107. *Polk's Medical Directory*, 1902, 165, states a faculty of eleven; 1904, 179, states a staff of nine for the 1902–3 term.

108. List of students copied by American Medical Association officials from "Announcement of the Chattanooga National Medical College, 7th Annual Session from September 2, 1904–April 27, 1905," in Medical Schools Alumni Files, vol. 44, Chattanooga National Medical College, AMA Archives, Chicago; Polk's and AMA medical directories, 1886–1912 (very few of the graduates of CNMC are listed in these directories, and those who are listed almost never identify CNMC as their medical alma maters); William L. Smith and Dan J. Smith, "The Extinct Black Medical Colleges of the United States: A History" (unpublished manuscript, Los Angeles, Calif., 1977), 22.

109. *Polk's Medical Directory*, 1904, 179.

110. "Biography of Isaac Henry Miller, By: Himself, Aug. 31, 1938," in WPA File, University of Louisville Health Sciences Library, Louisville, Ky. Miller claimed, in this autobiographical sketch, to have "spent two years at the Louisville National Medical College. One year interne Chattanooga National Medical College, Three years regular course, graduated in 1903." His name does not appear in any *LNMC Catalogues* nor in any medical directories through 1916.

111. Medical Schools Alumni Files, vol. 44, Chattanooga National Medical College, AMA Archives.

112. *Chattanooga City Directory*, 1906, 759; 1907, 821; 1905, 13; 1906, 12, 274; 1907, 13; *Polk's Medical Directory*, 1920, 1943; *American Medical Directory*, 1906, 1218; 1909, 1496; 1912, 1169; Arthur W. Hafner, Fred W. Hunter, and E. Michael Tarpey, eds., *Directory of Deceased American Physicians, 1804–1929* (Chicago: American Medical Association, 1993), 1:633.

113. *Memphis Tri-State Defender*, Jan. 1, 1955, 16; S. R. Bruesch, "Medical Education," in *The History of Medicine in Memphis*, ed. Marcus J. Stewart and William T. Black Jr. (Memphis, Tenn.: Memphis and Shelby County Medical Society, 1971), 325, states that UWT granted 216 M.D. degrees. The unidentified author of "Miles Vandahurst Lynk" in *Journal of the National Medical Association* 44 (1952): 475, claims 266 graduates, which probably includes law, pharmacy, nursing, and medicine.

114. Much of the information about Lynk's life comes from his autobiography, *Sixty Years of Medicine; or the Life and Times of Dr. Miles V. Lynk, An Autobiography* (Memphis, Tenn.: Twentieth Century Press, 1951). Lynk selects aspects of his life to include in this autobiography, focusing on certain achievements and omitting much detail between those high points.

115. *Meharry Medical College Catalogue*, 1888–89, 8.

116. Lynk, *Sixty Years*, 20–27.

117. Ibid., 27–28. Another Meharry graduate, John Edward Perry, had a very different response to this tactic in Columbia, Missouri, a few years later. See Perry's autobiography, *Forty Cords of Wood: Memoirs of a Medical Doctor* (Jefferson City, Mo.: Lincoln Univ. Press, 1947), 159–60, and Savitt, "Entering a White Profession," 521–22 (this article is reprinted in the current volume as chapter 19).

118. Lynk, *Sixty Years*, 28–29; *Jackson (Tennessee) City Directory*, 1891–92, 31, 36–37; M. V. Lynk, "The Afro-American Population of Jackson: Its Rise and Progress," *Jackson (Tennessee) Daily Sun*, Dec. 12, 1900.

119. *The Christian Index* (Jackson, Tenn.), Sept. 26, 1891.

120. Savitt, "'A Journal of Our Own,'" 58–59.

121. By 1900, Lynk had edited and published, through the Lynk Publishing House of Jackson, *The Afro-American School Speaker and Gems of Literature, For School Commencements, Literary Circles, Debating Clubs, and Rhetoricals Generally* (1896), a collection of black literature to acquaint African American schoolchildren with the greatest writings

of persons of color, and *The Black Troopers; Or, the Daring Heroism of the Negro Soldiers in the Spanish-American War* (1899), which sold more than fifteen thousand copies and gave readers a view of black accomplishments in the military. He had also edited and published several issues of an illustrated monthly journal for the general public called *Lynk's Magazine.* Lynk wrote of himself in the December 12, 1900, issue of the *Jackson Daily Sun,* "What Booker T. Washington is to industrial education, Dr. Lynk is to good, helpful race literature. . . . It is to his class of young colored men that his race must look for guidance and wholesome example." On his publications and reactions to them, see Lynk, *Sixty Years,* 6; Penelope L. Bullock, *The Afro-American Periodical Press, 1838–1909* (Baton Rouge: Louisiana State Univ. Press, 1981), 185–89; *Indianapolis Freeman,* Feb. 12, Nov. 5, and Dec. 10, 1898, and June 2, 1900; *Jackson Daily Sun,* Dec. 12, 1900; *Washington (D.C.) Colored American,* July 30, 1898.

122. Lakey, *CME Church;* Ralph G. Gay, "Christian Methodist Episcopal Church," in *Encyclopedia of World Methodism* (Nashville, Tenn.: United Methodist Publishing, 1974), 487–89; *Jackson Headlight,* Jan. 27, 1900.

123. Lynk, *Sixty Years,* 54–55.

124. Ibid., 55–59, quote on 54; Hamilton, *Bright Side of Memphis,* 71–72.

125. *University of West Tennessee Catalogue* (hereafter cited as *UWT Catalogue),* 1906–7, 5; 1909–10, 5, found in the National Library of Medicine, Bethesda, Md.

126. Lynk, *Sixty Years,* 64.

127. Ibid., 64–66; Hamilton, *Bright Side of Memphis,* 258.

128. Lynk, *Sixty Years,* 65; Deed, Ross Witherspoon & Wife To M.V. Lynk, Filed in Deed Book 60, 633, Aug. 13, 1901, Madison County, Tennessee, microfilm copy in Jackson/Madison County Library, Jackson, Tenn.

129. Lynk, *Sixty Years,* 65–66; *The Christian Index* (Jackson, Tenn.), Aug. 31, 1901.

130. Lynk, *Sixty Years,* 65.

131. Ibid., 66–67.

132. *Indianapolis Freeman,* Aug. 15, 1903; *UWT Catalogue,* 1906–7, frontispiece.

133. *Indianapolis Freeman,* Aug. 15, 1903. Before the start of the second year of classes, an additional story was added to the building. *The Christian Index* (Jackson, Tenn.), Sept. 13, 1902.

134. *Indianapolis Freeman,* Aug. 15, 1903; *Polk's Medical Directory;* local city directories; Meharry Medical College catalogs; Hamilton, *Bright Side of Memphis,* 258–59. A faculty picture with the caption "W. A. Cocolough, A.B., M.D." appears on the composite photo labeled "University of West Tennessee, Jackson, Tenn., 1901" in the Aug. 15, 1903, *Indianapolis Freeman* article. There is a discrepancy in dates here, as Cocolough did not receive his M.D. degree from Meharry until 1902.

135. *Polk's Medical Directory,* 1902, 165; 1904, 179.

136. *Polk's Medical Directory,* 1904, 179; *American Medical Directory,* 1906, 884.

137. *Polk's Medical Directory,* 1904, 179; *Indianapolis Freeman,* Aug. 15, 1903; *UWT Catalogue,* 1906–7, 8, 14.

138. *Indianapolis Freeman,* Aug. 15, 1903; *UWT Catalogue,* 1906–7, 8. On religious values of medical students at Leonard Medical School, see Savitt, "Training the 'Consecrated, Skillful, Christian Physician.'"

139. *UWT Catalogue,* 1906–7, 8–9.

140. *Indianapolis Freeman,* Aug. 15, 1903.

141. *UWT Catalogue,* 1906–7, 14–15. Lynk listed himself as a UWT law graduate, though his autobiography states that he graduated from the law school he established at Lane College, as described earlier.

142. *UWT Catalogue,* 1906–7, 5.

143. Madison County Deed Book 72, 97–99 (Jan. 23, 1907), 485–86 (June 29, 1907), 500–501 (July 10, 1907), microfilm copy in Jackson/Madison County Library, Jackson, Tenn.

144. *Memphis City Directory,* 1904, 87, 506; Lynk, *Sixty Years,* 70; *UWT Catalogue,* 1909–10, 7. Sanborn Fire Insurance Maps, Memphis, 1907, show the two vacant school buildings at the end of an unpaved street, South Phillips Place. Memphis city directories of the period contain full city maps with the streetcar lines marked.

145. *UWT Catalogue,* 1906–7, 5; Hamilton, *Bright Side of Memphis,* 257–58.

146. *UWT Catalogue,* 1906–7, 5; Hamilton, *Bright Side of Memphis,* 50–52, 47; *Polk's Medical Directory,* 1908, 2259 (advertisement). Hairston Hospital was located at 628 Orleans; Terrell-Patterson Infirmary at 159 Beale, then later at 698 Williams.

147. See lists of Memphis physicians in city and medical directories; biographical sketches and business cards of Memphis' African American physicians in Hamilton, *Bright Side of Memphis,* 26–54, 177–82. Of the forty physicians Hamilton listed, thirty-three were Meharry graduates, two from Knoxville Medical College (one of whom had attended Meharry for three years before transferring to Knoxville), one from Hannibal, three from the University of West Tennessee, and one from Howard.

148. Though catalogs and faculty lists are available for only a few of UWT's sixteen years in Memphis, Lynk's autobiography and the extant records indicate a trend toward using only African American faculty members. Lynk, *Sixty Years,* esp. 71–72; *UWT Catalogue,* 1906–7, 4; 1907–8, 1; 1909–10, 4.

149. *UWT Catalogue,* 1906–7, 3.

150. *American Medical Directory,* 1923, 33. The number of states not recognizing UWT's and other grade C medical schools was noted in each annual education issue of *JAMA.* See, for example, *JAMA* 79 (1922): 656. See also *Journal of the National Medical Association* 2 (1910): 306.

151. *UWT Catalogue,* 1906–7, 6–7; *Polk's Medical Directory,* 1908, 2259 (advertisement); *UWT Catalogue,* 1909–10, 7–9.

152. *UWT Catalogue,* 1906–7, 1909–10.

153. Flexner, *Medical Education in the United States,* 304–5.

154. *UWT Catalogue,* 1909–10, 9, 10.

155. Flexner, *Medical Education in the United States,* 305.

156. *UWT Catalogue,* 1909–10, 6; Flexner, *Medical Education in the United States,* 305, 309.

157. Savitt, "Abraham Flexner," 65–81 (this article is reprinted in the current volume as chapter 18).

158. Thomas Jesse Jones, *Negro Education: A Study of the Private and Higher Schools for Colored People in the United States,* U.S. Department of Interior, Bureau of Education, Bulletin no. 39, 1916 (Washington, D.C.: GPO, 1917), 2:565.

159. Ibid.

160. Oral history interview with Dr. George W. West, Aug. 4, 1976, tape at Fisk University Archives, Nashville, Tenn.

161. Oral history interview with Dr. George W. West, Aug. 4, 1976, tape at Fisk University Archives, Nashville, Tenn.

162. Lynk, *Sixty Years,* 67–68.

163. "A New Medical Practice Act for Tennessee," *Journal of the Tennessee State Medical Association* 7 (1914–15): 128–29; "Letters to the Editor," in ibid., 174–75, 210–14, 245–47, 331–32, 426; "The New Practice Act," in ibid., 8 (1915–16): 103–4.

164. *JAMA* 67 (1916): 606; 69 (1917): 551; 71 (1918): 551.

165. See, for example, *JAMA* 67 (1916): 590; 69 (1917): 561; *American Medical Directory,* 1923, 33.

166. *Memphis Tri-State Defender,* Jan. 1, 1955, 16; *Shaw University Catalogue,* 1914, 60–63.

167. *JAMA* 81 (1923): 551; Lynk, *Sixty Years.*

168. *Indianapolis Freeman,* Aug. 15, 1903; Hamilton, *Bright Side of Memphis,* 258; *Nashville Globe,* May 2, 1913, 1.

169. *Memphis Tri-State Defender,* Jan. 1, 1955, 16.

17. Money versus Mission at Knoxville College Medical Department, 1895–1900

This chapter was originally published as "Money versus Mission at an African-American Medical School: Knoxville College Medical Department, 1895–1900," *Bulletin of the History of Medicine* 75 (2001): 680–716.

I wish to thank the staff members of the History of Medicine Division at the National Library of Medicine in Bethesda for their collegiality and assistance on this project during the year I served there as Visiting Historical Scholar (1991–92). Thanks also go to Robert J. Booker of the James Beck Cultural Exchange Center Museum, Knoxville, Tennessee. Much of the information for this article came from the Knoxville College presidential letterbooks for 1895–97 and 1900–1902 (the presidential letterbook for 1897–1900 could not be located in the KC Archives or elsewhere). These letterbooks contain the president's monthly reports to Rev. J. W. Witherspoon, Corresponding Secretary of the Board of Control of the Board of Freedmen's Missions in Pittsburgh, Pa., and reveal some details about the inner workings of the medical college. Unfortunately, replies to these presidential letters have not survived, either at KC or at the Presbyterian Historical Society in Philadelphia. The manuscript materials that do remain help to fill out the otherwise sparse picture of the school's operations that is obtainable from official publications such as college catalogs and annual reports. Because much of the information that McCulloch and McGranahan present cannot be corroborated, the story of KCMD can be retold only through the eyes of these two admittedly biased participants in the events.

1. United Presbyterian Church of North America (hereafter UPCNA), *Minutes of the Thirty-Eighth General Assembly of the United Presbyterian Church of North America, Xenia, Ohio, May 27th to June 3d, 1896* 9, no. 1 (1896): appendix, 75.

2. Samuel Joseph Platt and Mary Louise Ogden, *Medical Men and Institutions of Knox County, Tennessee, 1789–1957* (Knoxville, Tenn.: Knoxville Academy of Medicine, 1969), 63–64, 277; Tennessee Medical College (hereafter TMC) catalogs, 1890–1900 (available at the National Library of Medicine, Bethesda, Md.).

3. Platt and Ogden, *Medical Men of Knox County,* 63–64; TMC catalogs, 1890–1900.

4. J. S. McCulloch to J. W. Witherspoon, May 1, 1895, in Knoxville College Presidential Letterbook Correspondence, 3:19–20, Knoxville College Archives, Knoxville, Tenn. (hereafter cited as KCC, followed by volume and page numbers).

5. McCulloch to Witherspoon, May 1, 1895, KCC, 3:20.

6. McCulloch to Witherspoon, May 1, 1895, KCC, 3:20.

7. McCulloch to Witherspoon, May 1, 1895, KCC, 3:20.

8. See, for example, Flexner, *Medical Education in the United States,* 307; *Polk's Medical Directory,* 1886, 399. On Hannibal Medical College, see Savitt, "Four African-American Proprietary Medical Colleges," 219–34 (this article is reprinted in the current volume as chapter 16).

9. Rothstein, *American Physicians,* 282–97.

10. McCulloch to Witherspoon, May 1, 1895, KCC, 3:20.

11. McCulloch to Witherspoon, May 1, 1895, KCC, 3:20.

12. McCulloch to Witherspoon, May 1, 1895, KCC, 3:20. The Industrial Building was a two-story structure with a large one-story rear extension that housed facilities for teaching agricultural and mechanical skills, including printing. *Catalogue and Announcement, Knoxville College, Knoxville, Tenn., 1897–98* (Knoxville: Press of Knoxville College, 1898), 7.

13. McCulloch to Witherspoon, May 1, 1895, KCC, 3:20.

14. McCulloch to Witherspoon, May 1, 1895, KCC, 3:21.

15. Du Bois, *Health and Physique of the Negro American,* 99.

16. McCulloch to Witherspoon, May 1, 1895, KCC, 3:21.

17. Hugh Alexander Kelsey, comp., *The United Presbyterian Directory: A Half-Century Survey, 1903–1958* (Pittsburgh, Pa.: Committee on Centennial Celebration and Pickwick Press, 1958), 215–16; Ralph W. McGranahan, "Early History of Knoxville College," in *Historical Sketch of the Freedmen's Missions of the United Presbyterian Church, 1862–1904* (Knoxville, Tenn.: Press of Knoxville College, 1904), 22–34; Cynthia G. Fleming, "Knoxville College: A History and Some Recollections of the First Fifty Years, 1875–1925," *East Tennessee Historical Society Publications,* nos. 58–59 (1986–87): 89–111; Cynthia G. Fleming, "A Survey of the Beginnings of Tennessee's Black Colleges and Universities, 1865–1920," *Tennessee Historical Quarterly* 39 (1980): 195–207; Robert J. Booker, *And There Was Light! The 120-Year History of Knoxville College, Knoxville, Tennessee, 1875–1995* (Virginia Beach, Va.: Donning, 1994), 10–45. On Knoxville's African American physicians, see Richard W. Hepler, "'The World Do Marvel': Health Care for Knoxville's Black Community, 1865–1940," *Journal of East Tennessee History* 63 (1991): 51–71.

18. Fleming, "Survey of the Beginnings," 205.

19. J. S. McCulloch, Annual Report, Apr. 24, 1897, KCC, 3:714–15.

20. Savitt, "Training the 'Consecrated, Skillful, Christian Physician,'" 250–76.

21. UPCNA, Board of Freedmen's Missions, Minutebook (hereafter cited as BFM, Minutebook), May 6, 1895, 2:11, Presbyterian Historical Society, Philadelphia, Pa.

22. BFM, Minutebook, May 6, 1895, 2:11.

23. McCulloch to Witherspoon, July 31, 1895, KCC, 3:113.

24. McCulloch to Witherspoon, June 26, 1895, KCC, 3:70; McCulloch to Witherspoon, July 31, 1895, KCC, 3:113–18.

25. Charles Clinton Yarborough, professor of chemistry, materia medica, and therapeutics, had recently (1893) graduated from and briefly taught medical chemistry, toxicology, and chemical hygiene at TMC. James M. Black had earned both his bachelor's and medical degrees from schools in Louisville, and had done additional medical studies in New York, before accepting the position of professor of principles and practice of surgery and clinical surgery at KCMD. Edwin L. Randall, KCMD secretary as well as professor of obstetrics and diseases of women and children, had graduated from Missouri Medical College in 1869 and moved to Knoxville about 1891. Hill, the dean, took on the professorship of clinical medicine. See McCulloch to Witherspoon, July 31, 1895, KCC, 3:113; Platt and Ogden, *Medical Men of Knox County,* passim; *Polk's Medical Directory,* 1896, 1393–94.

26. See catalogs and histories of these schools for faculty lists.

27. Joseph H. Cartwright, *The Triumph of Jim Crow: Tennessee Race Relations in the 1880s* (Knoxville: Univ. of Tennessee Press, 1976), 197–98.

28. McCulloch to Witherspoon, July 31, 1895, KCC, 3:113.

29. Meharry Medical College catalogs for 1892–93, 1893–94, and 1894–95; McCulloch to Witherspoon, July 31, 1895, KCC, 3:113.

30. McCulloch to Witherspoon, July 31, 1895, KCC, 3:113. The other African American physicians listed in Knoxville directories in 1895 were Alonzo A. Felding, trained in Ontario, Canada, and practicing in Knoxville since 1884; William L. Maples, an 1892 Howard University medical graduate who began seeing patients in Knoxville shortly

after graduation; and William Wallace Derrick, originally from Bell Factory, Alabama, who also arrived in Knoxville to practice medicine shortly after his graduation from Meharry Medical College in 1892. Derrick took courses at Knoxville College and received his A.B. in 1894. See *Knoxville City Directory,* 1895, 474–75; *Polk's Medical Directory,* 1896, 1393; Platt and Ogden, *Medical Men of Knox County,* 259, 260, 306. For more on Maples, see Lamb, *Howard University Medical Department,* 197. On Derrick, see *Polk's Medical Directory,* 1893, 1180; 1896, 1393; a newspaper clipping not otherwise identified, at James Beck Cultural Exchange Center Museum, Knoxville; and alumni lists printed in Knoxville College catalogs—e.g., 1900–1901, 47.

31. McCulloch to Witherspoon, July 31, 1895, KCC, 3: 13. Hill intended to fill a chair of medical jurisprudence with a lawyer (see ibid.).

32. Hill was able to replace James Black with Levi Jones Price, an 1877 graduate of the Hospital College of Medicine in Louisville, who had practiced medicine in Knoxville for several years: McCulloch to Witherspoon, Aug. 28, 1895, KCC, 3:140; Platt and Ogden, *Medical Men of Knox County,* 228, 325.

33. McCulloch to Witherspoon, Dec. 30, 1896, KCC, 3:617.

34. McCulloch to Witherspoon, Dec. 30, 1896, KCC, 3:617. See also an undated and unidentified newspaper article on Dr. Derrick in the Beck Cultural Exchange Center, Knoxville.

35. McCulloch to Witherspoon, Aug. 28, 1895, KCC, 3:140.

36. McCulloch to Witherspoon, July 31, 1895, KCC, 3:113.

37. *Knoxville College Catalogue,* 1896–97, 17.

38. McCulloch to Witherspoon, July 31, 1895, KCC, 3:113; *[Knoxville College] Aurora,* Oct. 1895; *Knoxville College Catalogue,* 1895–96, 37. Annual tuition and matriculation fees at other schools, as reported in their catalogs, were $29 at Louisville National Medical College, $30 at New Orleans University Medical Department, $30 at Meharry Medical College, and $65 at Leonard Medical School.

39. McCulloch to Witherspoon, Aug. 28, 1895, KCC, 3:140.

40. McCulloch to Witherspoon, May 1, 1895, KCC, 3:20.

41. *Knoxville College Catalogue,* 1896–97, 17. See also McCulloch to Witherspoon, Oct. 30, 1895, KCC, 3:196; McCulloch to Witherspoon, May 1, 1895, KCC, 3:20; and the Knoxville College Ledger Journal, Receipts/Disbursements 1890–1900, 138, Knoxville College Archives.

42. McCulloch to Witherspoon, Oct. 30, 1895, KCC, 3:196.

43. McCulloch to Witherspoon, Oct. 30, 1895, KCC, 3:196.

44. McCulloch to Witherspoon, Oct. 2, 1895, KCC, 3:166; Knoxville College Ledger Journal, Receipts/Disbursements 1890–1900, 138.

45. *[Knoxville College] Aurora,* Oct. 1895. It is possible that advertisements were published in regional and black newspapers, though no expense items to that effect appear in the college records.

46. McCulloch to Witherspoon, Oct. 30, 1895, KCC, 3:196.

47. McCulloch to [?], Nov. 1, 1895, KCC, 3:205.

48. McCulloch to Witherspoon, Nov. 26, 1895, KCC, 3:226. Tardy arrival for the start of classes was not an unusual occurrence in the unregulated atmosphere of late-nineteenth-century American medical education.

49. *Knoxville College Catalogue,* 1895–96, 40.

50. McCulloch to Witherspoon, Nov. 26, 1895, KCC, 3:227.

51. McCulloch to Witherspoon, Oct. 30, 1895, KCC, 3:196.

52. McCulloch to Dr. Robert M. C. Hill, Feb. 24, 1896, KCC, 3:[327?].

53. McCulloch to Witherspoon, Feb. 25, 1896, KCC, 3:330.

54. McCulloch to Hill, Feb. 24, 1896, KCC, 3:[327?].

55. McCulloch to Witherspoon, Feb. 25, 1896, KCC, 3:330.

56. McCulloch to Witherspoon, Apr. 2, 1896, KCC, 3:354.

57. See, e.g., McCulloch to Witherspoon, Dec. 2, 1896, KCC, 3:587.

58. McCulloch to Witherspoon, Oct. 30, 1895, KCC, 3:196.

59. McCulloch to Witherspoon, Feb. 25, 1896, KCC, 3:330.

60. McCulloch to Witherspoon, Apr. 2, 1896, KCC, 3:354.

61. UPCNA, *Minutes of Thirty-Eighth General Assembly,* appendix, 75.

62. McCulloch to Witherspoon, Jan. 1, 1896, KCC, 3:268.

63. McCulloch to Witherspoon, Feb. 25, 1896, KCC, 3:330.

64. McCulloch to Witherspoon, Apr. 29, 1896, KCC, 3:390.

65. McCulloch to Witherspoon, July 1, 1896, KCC, 3:445; McCulloch to Witherspoon, July 29, 1896, KCC, 3:470–71; *Polk's Medical Directory,* 1898, 1310; McCulloch to Witherspoon, Sept. 30, 1896, KCC, 3:532; McCulloch to Dear Brother [Witherspoon?], Oct. 30, 1896, KCC, 3:562; *Knoxville College Catalogue,* 1896–97; *[Knoxville College] Aurora,* June 1897; BFM, Minutebook, Nov. 3, 1896, 2:41.

66. McCulloch to Witherspoon, July 29, 1896, KCC, 3:471.

67. *[Knoxville College] Aurora,* Oct. 1896.

68. On the financial problems of medical students at Leonard Medical School, see Savitt, "Training the Consecrated Physician," 256–63.

69. McCulloch to Witherspoon, Sept. 10, 1896, KCC, 3:532.

70. McCulloch to Witherspoon, Dec. 2, 1896, KCC, 3:587.

71. McCulloch to Witherspoon, Oct. 28, 1896, KCC, 3:553.

72. But see, e.g., McCulloch to Witherspoon, Dec. 2, 1896, KCC, 3:587, for an instance of a missed lecture.

73. McCulloch to Witherspoon, Dec. 2, 1896, KCC, 3:587.

74. McCulloch to Witherspoon, Dec. 30, 1896, KCC, 3:617.

75. McCulloch to Witherspoon, Jan. 27, 1897, KCC, 3:644.

76. McCulloch to Witherspoon, Jan. 27, 1897, KCC, 3:644.

77. McCulloch to Witherspoon, Jan. 27, 1897, KCC, 3:644.

78. McCulloch to Witherspoon, Feb. 22, 1897, KCC, 3:664. No mention of this money appears in fiscal account books at the KC Archives or the Presbyterian Historical Society in Philadelphia.

79. McCulloch to Witherspoon, Apr. 29, 1897, KCC, 3:727.

80. McCulloch, Annual Report, Apr. 24, 1897, KCC, 3:714.

81. UPCNA, BFM, "Annual Report, 1897," in *Minutes of the General Assembly, 1897* 9, no. 2 (1897): appendix, 331.

82. See Hamer, *Centennial History of the Tennessee State Medical Association,* 90–103; minutes of the Medical Association of the State of Tennessee for the 1880s and 1890s, printed annually in the association's *Transactions* (esp. 1891, 231–36; 1900, 23–32; 1901, 18–20); T. J. Happel, "The Annual Report of the Secretary of the State Board of Medical Examiners of Tennessee," *Nashville Journal of Medicine and Surgery* 77 (1895): 264–75; T. J. Happel, "Seventh Annual Report of the Secretary and Treasurer of the State Board of Medical Examiners," *Nashville Journal of Medicine and Surgery* 81 (1897): 199–212; T. J. Happel, "A Sketch of Medical Legislation, and of the Work of the State Board of Medical Examiners of Tennessee," *State Board Health Bulletin* (1897): 165–75; T. J. Happel, "The Importance of Medical Organization in Securing and Enforcing Medical Laws," *JAMA* 42 (1904): 139–42.

83. McCulloch to Witherspoon, Sept. 29, 1897, KCC, 3:891; McCulloch to Witherspoon, Oct. 27, 1897, KCC, 3:910–11.

84. McCulloch to Witherspoon, Dec. 1, 1897, KCC, 3:937.

85. *Meharry Medical College Catalog,* 1900–1901, 29.

86. *Knoxville College Catalogue,* 1898–99, 31; 1899–1900, 37. Little information is available about events at the medical school during 1898, 1899, and the first few months of 1900, because the major source of information, the president's letterbook, cannot be located.

87. Kelsey, *United Presbyterian Directory,* 220.

88. R. W. McGranahan to Witherspoon, KCC, 5:37–38; "Two Doctors Graduated from Knoxville Colored College. First Commencement of Medical Department," *Knoxville Sentinel,* May 30, 1900.

89. McGranahan to Witherspoon, Sept. 24, 1900, KCC, 5:253–55, quotation on 253.

90. McGranahan to Witherspoon, Sept. 24, 1900, KCC, 5:253.

91. McGranahan to Witherspoon, Sept. 24, 1900, KCC, 5:253.

92. McGranahan to Witherspoon, Sept. 24, 1900, KCC, 5:253–55.

93. McGranahan to Witherspoon, Sept. 24, 1900, KCC, 5:255.

94. McGranahan to Witherspoon, Sept. 24, 1900, KCC, 5:260.

95. McGranahan to Witherspoon, Sept. 24, 1900, KCC, 5:260.

96. McGranahan to Witherspoon, Sept. 24, 1900, KCC, 5:254.

97. McGranahan to Witherspoon, Sept. 24, 1900, KCC, 5:254–55.

98. McGranahan to Witherspoon, Sept. 24, 1900, KCC, 5:254.

99. McGranahan to Witherspoon, Sept. 24, 1900, KCC, 5:256.

100. McGranahan to Witherspoon, Sept. 24, 1900, KCC, 5:256.

101. McGranahan to Witherspoon, Sept. 24, 1900, KCC, 5:256–57.

102. McGranahan to Witherspoon, Sept. 24, 1900, KCC, 5:257.

103. McGranahan to Witherspoon, Sept. 24, 1900, KCC, 5:257.

104. McGranahan to Witherspoon, Sept. 24, 1900, KCC, 5:257.

105. McGranahan to Witherspoon, Sept. 24, 1900, KCC, 5:257.

106. McGranahan to Witherspoon, Sept. 24, 1900, KCC, 5:257. Robert Green Ingersoll was a leading agnostic of the day.

107. McGranahan to Witherspoon, Sept. 24, 1900, KCC, 5:258.

108. McGranahan to Witherspoon, Sept. 24, 1900, KCC, 5:258.

109. McGranahan to Witherspoon, Sept. 24, 1900, KCC, 5:258.

110. McGranahan to Witherspoon, Sept. 24, 1900, KCC, 5:258.

111. According to the Knoxville College Financial Ledger, located in the KC Archives, the BFM made three donations of cash for medical equipment to the medical department: $50 on Apr. 14, 1899 (230), $25 on June 15, 1899 (239), and $50 on May 11, 1900 (274).

112. McGranahan to Witherspoon, Sept. 24, 1900, KCC, 5:259.

113. McGranahan to Witherspoon, Sept. 24, 1900, KCC, 5:259.

114. McGranahan to Witherspoon, Sept. 24, 1900, KCC, 5:259. After KCMD closed, the former faculty, according to McGranahan, published notices in the local Knoxville newspapers, accusing the KC administration of trying to impose its moral and religious values on both students and faculty. The president claimed that all he did was require medical students to attend chapel regularly and behave properly around the younger students. See McGranahan to Witherspoon, Oct. 31, 1900, KCC, 5:276–88.

115. McGranahan to Witherspoon, Sept. 24, 1900, KCC, 5:259.

116. McGranahan to Witherspoon, Sept. 24, 1900, KCC, 5:259.

117. BFM, Minutebook, Oct. 1, 1900, 2:122.

118. *Knoxville College Catalogue,* 1899–1900, 27.

119. *[Knoxville College] Aurora,* Oct. 15, 1900.

120. Ibid.

121. McGranahan to Witherspoon, Oct. 31, 1900, KCC, 5:277.

122. McGranahan to Witherspoon, Oct. 31, 1900, KCC, 5:277.

123. Because few published and no manuscript materials remain from Knoxville Medical College or its teachers or students, and because the school received scant public attention in contemporary local newspapers, not much information could be found about the school's history. What follows was gleaned from city and professional directories, contemporary local maps, American Medical Association (AMA) Council on Medical Education annual surveys, and a few other scattered sources.

124. McGranahan to Witherspoon, Sept. 24, 1900, KCC, 5:258.

125. McGranahan to Derrick, Nov. 21, 1900, KCC, 5:314.

126. *Polk's Medical Directory,* 1902, 2469.

127. *Knoxville City Directory,* 1901, 610, lists KMC at 1306 Clinton Road. The Knoxville Sanborn Insurance Maps for 1903 (a set may be found in the University of Tennessee Library, Special Collections Department) identify the exact building on Clinton Road near the intersection with Deaderick, but (ironically) mislabel it the "Medical Dept. of Knoxville College." For information on streetcar lines, see any city directory of the period—e.g., 1897, 9.

128. See Knoxville city directories for 1903 through 1910. The school's second address was 1320 Clinton Road, near the intersection with McGee Avenue. See also the Sanborn Insurance Maps of Knoxville for 1903.

129. American Medical Association Council on Medical Education, "Medical Schools of the United States," *JAMA* 49 (1907): 592–93; 53 (1909): 552–53; 55 (1910): 688–89.

130. American Medical Association Council on Medical Education, "Medical Schools of the United States," *JAMA* 51 (1908): 593.

131. See, for example, *Polk's Medical Directory,* 1900, 166; 1902, 2469; 1904, 179; *JAMA* 55 (1910): 684.

132. This and subsequent information about the instructional staff was gathered from published medical and city directories, unless otherwise noted.

133. McCulloch to Witherspoon, Dec. 30, 1896, KCC, 3:617.

134. A report from the KMC administration to the AMA, stamped "received July 27, 1907," names W. W. Derrick as dean. See *Medical Schools Alumni,* vol. 44, "Knoxville Medical College," in the AMA Archives, Chicago, Ill.

135. *Polk's Medical Directory,* 1902, 2469 (display advertisement for Knoxville Medical College). See also ibid., 1900, 166.

136. Known faculty members during the school's later years, in addition to Derrick, were two 1905 graduates of KMC, E. L. Watkins and Charles R. Wood; a 1907 graduate of Meharry, Ernest N. Ezidore; a 1905 graduate of Leonard Medical School, William H. Bryant; and Daniel W. Crawford, one of the small number who attended and graduated from (in 1901) Chattanooga National Medical College. See AMA, *American Medical Directory,* 1909, 1095, 1096; list of KMC alumni received at AMA, Chicago, on July 27, 1907, in *Medical Schools Alumni,* vol. 44, "Knoxville Medical College," in the AMA Archives, Chicago, Ill.; American Medical Association, Council on Medical Education, "Medical Schools of the United States," *JAMA* 55 (1910): 684; AMA, *American Medical Directory,* 1916, 1447; Platt and Ogden, *Medical Men of Knox County,* 365.

137. John F. Slater Fund, *Proceedings of the Trustees of the John F. Slater Fund for the Education of Freedmen* (New York: [The Fund], 1908), 73–74. Further information on Green may be found in Platt and Ogden, *Medical Men of Knox County,* 269; obituaries in unidentified newspaper clippings located at the Beck Cultural Exchange Center, Knoxville; Knoxville Sanborn Insurance Maps, 1903, in University of Tennessee Library, Special Collections Department; *Knoxville College Catalogue,* 1908–9, 26–27; Knoxville city directories for 1902–10; obituary notice in *Journal of the National Medical Association* 31 (1939): 225; Vanessa Northington Gamble, *Making a Place for Ourselves: The Black Hospital Movement, 1920–1945* (New York: Oxford Univ. Press, 1995).

138. H. F. Gamble, "Report of Committee on Medical Education and Negro Medical Schools," *Journal of the National Medical Association* 1 (1909): 257–58. See annual compilations of state licensing board results in *JAMA* for these years.

139. [News items], *Journal of the National Medical Association* 2 (1910): 28, 306.

140. Flexner, *Medical Education in the United States,* 303–4, quotation on 304.

141. Ibid., 304. See also Savitt, "Abraham Flexner and the Black Medical Schools," 65–81.

142. Gamble, "Report of Committee on Medical Education," 258.

18. Abraham Flexner and the Black Medical Schools

This chapter originally appeared as "Abraham Flexner and the Black Medical Schools," in *Beyond Flexner: Medical Education in the Twentieth Century,* ed. Barbara M. Barzansky and Norman Gevitz (Westport, Conn.: Greenwood Press, 1992), 65–81.

1. C. F. Meserve to W. Buttrick, May 25, 1907, General Education Board Papers, Box 103, Folder 929, Rockefeller Archive Center (hereafter cited as RAC), Sleepy Hollow, N.Y. (hereafter cited as GEB Papers).

2. For an example of the way these problems affected one black medical school, see Savitt, "Education of Black Physicians at Shaw University," 160–88.

3. See, for example, Hudson, "Abraham Flexner in Perspective," 545; Ludmerer, *Learning to Heal.* For a biography of Flexner, see Thomas Neville Bonner, *Iconoclast: Abraham Flexner and a Life in Learning* (Baltimore, Md.: Johns Hopkins Univ. Press, 2002).

4. *JAMA* 48 (1907): 1702.

5. *JAMA* 46 (1906): 1854–56; 47 (1906): 595.

6. *JAMA* 48 (1907): 1704–5.

7. See, for example, *JAMA* 47 (1906): 597–98; 48 (1907): 1702, 1706.

8. Catalogs of the various black medical schools give details of improvements each year, though, as Flexner, in *Medical Education in the United States,* stated in his report on Knoxville Medical College (304), the information was not always accurate. See also American Baptist Home Mission Society Trustees Minutes, May 6, 1904, in Minutebook, 1902–17, Shaw University Archives, Raleigh, N.C.

9. *JAMA* 48 (1907): 1603–4.

10. *JAMA* 48 (1907): 1702–3; 50 (1908): 1544.

11. *JAMA* 48 (1907): 1706.

12. See, for example, ibid. Ludmerer, *Learning to Heal,* 80–87, shows how many white schools of the time voluntarily made advances in their education program despite the cost. Black schools for the most part could not do this, though they did implement what reforms they felt feasible, as they did not have the financial strength to survive the several lean years until enrollments might grow again.

13. *JAMA* 48 (1907): 1702.

14. For more on LMS problems, see Savitt, "Education of Black Physicians at Shaw."

15. See faculty lists and other information in catalogs of these schools.

16. *JAMA* 48 (1907): 1702. For more on the history of African American proprietary medical schools, see Savitt, "Four African-American Proprietary Medical Colleges," 203–55.

17. *JAMA* 48 (1907): 1702; 63 (1914): 668.

18. C. F. Meserve to W. Buttrick, May 25, 1907, GEB Papers, Box 103, Folder 929.

19. No records of this school have been located. See Abrahams, *Extinct Medical Schools of Baltimore,* 324–25. Thanks to Ms. D. Wolverton, librarian at the Medical and Chirurgical Faculty of the State of Maryland, Baltimore, for her help in locating information on this school.

20. See catalogs of State University, LNMC, and correspondence and reports on State University in GEB Papers, Box 74, Folder 648. Information on Simmons College may be found in Williams, *Black Higher Education.*

21. On Chattanooga National Medical College, see Savitt, "Four African-American Proprietary Medical Colleges," 235–39.

22. Untitled Report, June 1, 1908, Abraham Flexner Papers, Box 21, "Professional Education—Misc.," Library of Congress, Washington, D.C (hereafter cited as Flexner Papers).

23. *JAMA* 50 (1908): 1543–46.

24. Flexner, *Medical Education in the United States.*

25. For an example of the manner in which a white medical journal ignored a black medical school, see issues of the *North Carolina Medical Journal* during the late nineteenth century. It mentions LMS only incidentally.

26. Flexner, *Medical Education in the United States,* 280.

27. Ibid., 305.

28. Ibid., 303–4.

29. Ibid., 280.

30. Ibid., 233.

31. Ibid., 304.

32. Ibid., 309.

33. Ibid., 303.

34. Ibid., 304.

35. Ibid., 280.

36. Ibid., 232.

37. Ibid., 305.

38. Ibid., 180–81.

39. Ibid., 180.

40. Ibid., 181.

41. *New Orleans University Catalogue,* 1911–12, 24.

42. *JAMA* 59 (1912): 639. See also Savitt, "Four African-American Proprietary Medical Schools," 218–19.

43. *Journal of the National Medical Association* 1 (1909): 257–58; 2 (1910): 23–29.

44. On the history of the school, see Savitt, "Four African-American Proprietary Medical Schools," 239–54; and Lynk, *Sixty Years.* Little more will be said about the University of West Tennessee in this chapter.

45. *JAMA* 59 (1912): 639.

46. W. P. Thirkield to H. S. Pritchett, Feb. 21, 1910, Flexner Papers. For more on Howard University's medical school during this period, see Epps, "Howard University Medical Department," 885–911.

47. [E. A. Balloch] to W. P. Thirkield, May 16, 1910, Carnegie Foundation for the Advancement of Teaching (CFAT)-Howard University Files, Carnegie Foundation Archives (hereafter cited as CFA), New York.

48. W. P. Thirkield to A. Carnegie, Oct. 31, 1910, Carnegie Corporation (hereafter cited as CC)-Howard University Files, CFA.

49. [A. Carnegie] to O. G. Villard, Dec. 9, 1910, CC-Howard University Files, CFA.

50. W. P. Thirkield to J. Bartram, May 9, 1911, CC-Howard University Files, CFA.

51. See letters in CC-Howard University Files, CFA, for 1911–20.

52. J. Bartram to H. S. Pritchett, May 10, 1911; Pritchett to G. W. Hubbard, May 11, 1911; Hubbard to Pritchett, Jan. 4, 1913, all in CC-Meharry Files, CFA.

53. A. Carnegie to H. S. Pritchett, Dec. 9, 1914, CC-Meharry Files, CFA.

54. See letters for this decade in both the CC and CFAT Files at CFA and the GEB Papers at RAC.

55. "Conditional Appropriation to Shaw University," Feb. 1, 1910, GEB Papers, Box 103, Folder 930.

56. Minutes of Council on Medical Education, June 21, 1914, 156, AMA Office of Medical Education, Chicago.

57. Ibid., Feb. 24, 1914, 109, 224.

58. See annual education issues of *JAMA* for this decade; for example, 63 (1914): 671; 65 (1915): 704; 67 (1916): 605; see also G. W. Hubbard to H. S. Pritchett, Jan. 29, 1915, CFAT-Meharry Files, CFA.

59. *JAMA* 65 (1915): 704.

60. See, for example, A. Flexner to E. A. Balloch, Oct. 6, 24, 1914, GEB Papers, Box 28, Folder 256; and E. C. Sage to W. C. McNeill, Feb. 8, 1915, GEB Papers, Box 28; Folder 257.

61. A. Flexner to H. S. Pritchett, Dec. 5, 1916; Pritchett to Flexner, Dec. 12, 1916; Flexner to Pritchett, Jan. 27, 1917; G. W. Hubbard to Flexner, Nov. 28, 1917; E. C. Sage to Hubbard, Dec. 10, 1917; Flexner to Pritchett, Dec. 9, 1918, all in GEB Papers, Box 133, Folder 1227.

62. A. Flexner to G. W. Hubbard, Dec. 16, 1914; Flexner to A. D. Bevan, Feb. 8, 1915, in GEB Papers, Box 133, Folder 1227. For a discussion of Flexner's position on "flexible standards" for black and Southern medical schools, see Daniel M. Fox, "Abraham Flexner's Unpublished Report: Foundations and Medical Education, 1909–1928," *Bulletin of the History of Medicine* 54 (1980): 488–89.

63. G. W. Hubbard to E. C. Sage, Nov. 20, 1917, GEB Papers, Box, 133, Folder 1227.

64. A copy of this appeal, "Crisis in Negro Medical Schools," dated Nov. 20, 1917, may be found in the Royster Family Papers, Folder "1915–1920," Southern Historical Collection, University of North Carolina at Chapel Hill. See also S. M. Newman to A. Flexner, Jan. 14, 1918, GEB Papers, Box 702, Folder 7220, and petition dated Dec. 30, 1917, enclosed with that letter.

65. N. P. Colwell to G. N. Brink, Feb. 23, 1918, GEB Papers, Box 702, Folder 7220.

66. N. P. Colwell to H. S. Pritchett, Mar. 12, 1918, CFAT-AMA Files, CFA; Colwell to E. C. Sage, Mar. 15, 1918, GEB Papers, Box 702, Folder 7220.

67. See enclosure with G. N. Brink to E. C. Sage, Mar. 11, 1918, GEB Papers, Box 702, Folder 7220.

68. H. S. Pritchett to N. P. Colwell, Apr. 3, 1918, CFAT-AMA Files, CFA.

69. A. McD. Moore to A. Flexner, May 22, 1918, GEB Papers, Box 702, Folder 7220. See also Palmetto Medical Association of South Carolina to E. C. Sage, Apr. 25, 1918, and W. T. B. Williams to W. Buttrick, May 13, 1918, in GEB Papers, Box 702, Folder 7220.

70. A. Flexner to H. D. Arnold, May 29, 1918; Flexner to N. P. Colwell, May 29, 1918; Colwell to Flexner, May 31, 1918, in GEB Papers, Box 702, Folder 7220.

71. A. Flexner to N. P. Colwell, May 29, 1918, GEB Papers Box 702, Folder 7220.

72. A. McD. Moore to G. N. Brink, Aug. 12, 1918, GEB Papers, Box 702, Folder 7220; "Memorandum Regarding Negro Medical Schools," Aug. 28, 1918, GEB Papers, Box 133, Folder 1228.

73. [H. S. Pritchett?] to Bishop Nicholson, Feb. 24, 1919, and W. Buttrick to Nicholson, Mar. 3, 1919, GEB Papers, Box 133, Folder 1228.

74. P. Bartsch to H. S. Pritchett, Apr. 11, 1919; Pritchett to Bartsch, Apr. 14, 1919, both in CFAT Files, CFA; A. Flexner to Pritchett, Apr. 27, 1921, Flexner Papers. See also Epps, "Howard Medical Department."

75. Hine, "Pursuit of Professional Equality," 173.

76. Raymond B. Fosdick, *Adventure in Giving: The Story of the General Education Board Established by John D. Rockefeller* (New York: Harper and Row, 1962), 177–85; Summerville, *Educating Black Doctors*, 60–105; Morais, *History of the Afro-American in Medicine*, 92–94.

77. A. Flexner to A. P. Stokes, "Memorandum on Medical Education," Feb. 17, 1920, in Anson Phelps Stokes Papers, addition, ser. 3, Box 76, Yale University Library.

78. Fosdick, *Adventure in Giving*, 174–77; Logan, *Howard University*, 256–57, 370–75; Morais, *History of the Negro in Medicine*, 90–92; Epps, "Howard Medical Department."

79. Helen E. Walker, *The Negro in the Medical Profession* (Charlottesville: Phelps-Stokes Fellowship Papers, University of Virginia, 1949), 24–29; Morais, *History of the Negro in Medicine*, 94.

19. Entering a "White" Profession, 1880–1920

This chapter originally appeared as "Entering a White Profession: Black Physicians in the New South, 1880–1920," *Bulletin of the History of Medicine* 61 (1987): 507–40.

The author gratefully acknowledges the helpful suggestions of Edward H. Beardsley of the University of South Carolina and of participants of several forums where he presented versions of this paper: the Johns Hopkins University Institute of the History of Medicine colloquium, Dec. 13, 1984; the annual meeting of the American Association for the History of Medicine, Rochester, N.Y., May 3, 1986; and the East Carolina University History Department seminar, Sept. 18, 1986. This publication was supported in part by a National Institutes of Health Grant (LM 03413) from the National Library of Medicine, 1980–82.

1. W. E. B. Du Bois, ed., *The College-Bred Negro: Report of a Social Study Made under the Direction of Atlanta University* (Atlanta, Ga.: Atlanta Univ. Press, 1900), 83.

2. *Medical World* 32 (1914): 65 (Charles Fremont Taylor was the editor).

3. On some black physicians' continued lack of concern for the health of African Americans in the early twentieth century, see Edward H. Beardsley, "Making Separate, Equal: Black Physicians and the Problems of Medical Segregation in the pre–World War II South," *Bulletin of the History of Medicine* 57 (1983): 382–96.

4. On the history of pre-1920 black medical schools, see chapter 11 of the current volume.

5. Examples of such complaints may be found in Gerald E. Markowitz and David Rosner, "Doctors in Crisis: Medical Education and Medical Reform during the Progressive Era, 1895–1915," in *Health Care in America: Essays in Social History*, ed. Susan Reverby and David Rosner (Philadelphia: Temple Univ. Press, 1979), 189–91.

6. *New Orleans University Department of Medicine and Surgery Catalogue*, 1895–96, 47. Similar pronouncements may be found in catalogs of the other black medical schools.

7. *African Expositor*, Apr. 1886, 3. This issue of Shaw University's newspaper may be found in the North Carolina Collection, Wilson Library, University of North Carolina, Chapel Hill.

8. *Howard University Journal*, 7 (Oct. 8, 1909): 2.

9. *The Workers* 2 (June–July 1906): 2. Issues of this college magazine are located at the Shaw University Archives, Raleigh, North Carolina.

10. W. R. Brown to Meserve, Apr. 26, 1897, Charles F. Meserve Letterbook 2, 287; P. H. Koon to Meserve, Mar. 12, 1898, Meserve Letterbook 3, 262, Shaw Archives. For other examples, see Meserve to A. D. Wimbs, Sept. 23, 1895, Meserve Letterbook 1, 704; C. G. Robinson to Meserve, Dec. 5, 1896, Letter File 1, Shaw Archives.

11. Meserve to W. B. [*sic*] Brown, Feb. 20, 1897, Meserve Letterbook 2, 70, Shaw Archives.

12. Booker T. Washington to Cornelius N. Dorsette, Feb. 28, 1883, in *The Booker T. Washington Papers*, ed. Louis R. Harlan and Raymond W. Smock (Urbana: Univ. of Illinois Press, 1972–1989), 2:219–20; Edward L. Wilkerson, *Struggling to Climb: A Biography* [of Frederick D. Sessoms, M.D.] (Cleveland, Ohio: n.p., 1958), 41.

13. See accounts of black medical school commencements in the *Christian Educator* 3 (1891–92): 363; 8 (1897): 85–88; 12 (1900–1901): 77–78; *The Workers* 2 (June–July 1906): 1–4; *Nashville (Tenn.) Daily American*, Feb. 23, 1883, 6; *New National Era* (Washington, D.C.), Mar. 9, 1871, 2; Mar. 7, 1872, 3.

14. T. J. Johnson, *From the Driftwood of Bayou Pierre* (Louisville, Ky.: Dunne, 1949), 28.

15. Perry, *Forty Cords of Wood*, 134. For more information on Dr. Perry, an important Kansas City physician, see Kaufman, Galishoff, and Savitt, *Dictionary of American Medical Biography*, 2:592.

16. On debts, see, for example, Caesar Bassette to Meserve, Sept. 1, 1905, Letter File 3; William A. Mapp to Meserve, Dec. 30, 1896, Letter File 1; Jeremiah M. Lloyd to Meserve, Nov. 23, 1896, Letter File 1; and John W. Jones to Meserve, Apr. 1, 1898, Meserve Letterbook 3, 402, all at Shaw Archives; Wilkerson, *Struggling to Climb*, 39; *Christian Educator* 1 (1889–90): 108. See also Savitt, "Training the 'Consecrated, Skillful, Christian Physician,'" 250–76.

17. See, for example, Meserve To Whom It May Concern, May 6, 1895, Meserve Letterbook 1, 485, Shaw Archives.

18. William E. Atkins to Meserve, Oct. 8, 1896, Letter File 1, Shaw Archives.

19. John H. G. Williams to Meserve, May 12, 1904, Letter File 2, Shaw Archives.

20. Wilkerson, *Struggling to Climb*, 39.

21. Perry, *Forty Cords of Wood*, 144–45.

22. William D. Johnson, *Biographical Sketches of Prominent Negro Men and Women of Kentucky* (Lexington, Ky.: n.p., 1897), 62.

23. Perry, *Forty Cords of Wood*, 145. The "orchard in Nashville" was Meharry Medical College, Perry's medical alma mater.

24. A. B. Caldwell, ed., *History of the American Negro and His Institutions* (Atlanta, Ga.: A. B. Caldwell, 1917–23); John A. Kenney, *The Negro in Medicine* (Tuskegee, Ala.: Tuskegee Institute Press, 1912); J. W. Gibson and W. H. Crogman, *Progress of a Race, or the Remarkable Advancement of the American Negro* (Naperville, Ill.: J. L. Nichols, 1912).

25. Mapp to Meserve, Dec. 30, 1896, Letter File 1, Shaw Archives.

26. Perry, *Forty Cords of Wood*, 144. See also John H. Tompkins to Meserve, Dec. 7, 1896, Letter File 1, Shaw Archives.

27. Tompkins to Meserve, Dec. 7, 1896, Letter File 1, Shaw Archives.

28. *Christian Educator* 1 (1889–90): 163.

29. Ibid.

30. See, for example, Luther T. Burbridge, "The Colored Man in Medicine," in *The Afro-American Encyclopedia; or The Thoughts, Doings, and Sayings of the Race*, comp. James T. Haley (Nashville, Tenn.: Haley and Florida, 1895), 72–73.

31. Thomas Jackson Woofter Jr., "The Negroes of Athens, Georgia," Phelps-Stokes Fellowship Studies, no. 1, *Bulletin of the University of Georgia* 14 (Dec. 1913): 40. Phelps-Stokes Fund fellowships, established in 1912, provided money for Southern white graduate students at major Southern universities to study race issues using social science methodology.

32. James W. Martin, "A Study of the Negro Physician with Particular Reference to Certain Tennessee Counties" (master's thesis, George Peabody College for Teachers [Nashville, Tennessee], 1921), 16. Thanks to James Summerville of Nashville for locating, obtaining, and sending me a copy of this thesis.

33. Unidentified article in the *Washington Post* reprinted in the *Journal of the National Medical Association* 2 (1910): 46–47.

34. Savitt, *Medicine and Slavery*, 171–80. Black self-care during enslavement is the subject of much of Fett, *Working Cures*.

35. Leonora Herron, "Conjuring and Conjure-Doctors," *Southern Workman* 24 (1895): 117–18; A. M. Bacon, "Conjuring and Conjure-Doctors," *Southern Workman* 24 (1895): 193–94; Wilbert C. Jordan, "Voodoo Medicine," in *Textbook of Black-Related Diseases*, ed.

Williams, 716–25. A comprehensive discussion and bibliography on the subject may be found in Gorn, "Black Magic," 295–326. See also Fett, *Working Cures*, 84–108.

36. J. A. Kumler, "Importance of Medical Schools for Colored People," *Christian Educator* 1 (1889–90): 22. See also F. Tipton, "The Negro Problem from a Medical Standpoint," *New York Medical Journal* 43 (1886): 571; Ambrose McCoy, "Voodooism in the South," *Louisville Medical News* 18 (1884): 380–81; Lawson A. Scruggs, "Medical Education as a Factor in the Elevation of the Colored Race," *African Expositor*, Apr. 1886, 3.

37. See references in note 35.

38. See, for example, I. A. Newby, *Black Carolinians: A History of Blacks in South Carolina from 1895 to 1968* (Columbia: Univ. of South Carolina Press, 1973), 115; Fett, *Working Cures*, 51–59.

39. George Campbell, *White and Black: The Outcome of a Visit to the United States* (London: Chatto and Windus, 1879), 339, quoted in George B. Tindall, *South Carolina Negroes, 1877–1900* (Columbia: Univ. of South Carolina Press, 1952), 147.

40. Perry, *Forty Cords of Wood*, 141.

41. Walter F. White, *The Fire in the Flint* (New York: Alfred A. Knopf, 1924), 48–49, 50.

42. Johnson, *From the Driftwood*, 30–31.

43. Meserve to Koon, May 8, 1897, Meserve Letterbook 2, 408, Shaw Archives.

44. *Medical World* 32 (1914): 65.

45. Ibid., 111–13, 147–49.

46. Edward T. Conner, M.D., to the Editor, *Medical World* 32 (1914): 148.

47. Perry, *Forty Cords of Wood*, 159–60.

48. Martin, "Study of the Negro Physician," 14–15.

49. Ibid., 59.

50. Carl R. Williams to the Editor, *Medical World* 32 (1914): 112.

51. Martin, "Study of the Negro Physician," 15.

52. White, *Fire in the Flint*, 56. The distinguished black physician Louis T. Wright wrote, in 1929, that *Fire in the Flint* "accurately depicted the life of the Negro doctor in the rural parts of the South." "The Negro Physician," *The Crisis* 36 (1929): 306.

53. Wilkerson, *Struggling to Climb*, 46–50.

54. White, *Fire in the Flint*, 57.

55. Burbridge, "Colored Man in Medicine," 72.

56. Beardsley, "Making Separate, Equal," 382–87. The daughter of an early-twentieth-century African American physician later recalled that her father, upon arriving in Bennettsville, South Carolina, in 1908, had to practice under the supervision of a white physician because the white doctors did not want him to have an independent practice. See Suzanne C. Linder, *Medicine in Marlboro County [S.C.], 1736 to 1980* (Baltimore, Md.: Gateway Press, 1980), 62, 186.

57. See source in note 23 and entries for black physicians in Kaufman, Galishoff, and Savitt, *Dictionary of American Medical Biography*. For descriptions of racial prejudice at postgraduate schools, see Perry, *Forty Cords of Wood*, 193–200; Martin, "Study of the Negro Physician," 32; Wright, "Negro Physician," 305; and Ward, *Black Physicians*, 82–92.

58. Perry, *Forty Cords of Wood*, 248.

59. Burbridge, "Colored Man in Medicine," 72.

60. Cobb, "Alexander Thomas Augusta," 327–29; Kaufman, Galishoff, and Savitt, *Dictionary of American Medical Biography*, 1:23.

61. W. Montague Cobb, *The First Negro Medical Society: A History of the Medico-Chirurgical Society of the District of Columbia, 1884–1939* (Washington, D.C.: Associated Publishers, 1939), 6–39; Morais, *History of the Negro in Medicine*, 52–58, 303; Herbert W. Nickens, "A Case of Professional Exclusion in 1870: The Formation of the First Black Medical Society," *Journal of the American Medical Association* 253 (1985): 2549–52.

62. *Medical Record* 21 (1882): 390.

63. Morais, *History of the Negro in Medicine*, 58, 133. See also Ward, *Black Physicians*, 191–212.

64. *Journal of the National Medical Association* 2 (1910): 323.

65. Ibid., 325.

66. Ibid., 324; W. E. B. Du Bois, *The Philadelphia Negro: A Social Study* (Philadelphia: Univ. of Pennsylvania, 1899), 117–18.

67. White, *Fire in the Flint*, 24, 25, 27.

68. Tompkins to Meserve, Dec. 7, 1896, Letter File 1, Shaw Archives.

69. Lilian Brandt, "The Negroes of St. Louis," *Publications of the American Statistical Association* 8 (1903): 234–35.

70. Burbridge, "Colored Man in Medicine," 71–72.

71. Du Bois, *College-Bred Negro*, 83.

72. Martin, "Study of the Negro Physician," 59.

73. Ibid., 42.

74. Ibid., 43.

75. Ibid., 60.

76. Some black physicians in the North encountered similar problems and acted in a similar manner. *Rochester (New York) Times-Union*, Feb. 12, 1980, 1B, article on Dr. Charles T. Lunsford.

77. White, *Fire in the Flint*, 63–64.

78. Ibid., 64–65.

79. Martin, "Study of the Negro Physician," 41–42.

80. Ibid. For an example from the North, see *Rochester (New York) Times-Union*, Feb. 12, 1980, 1B.

81. S. H. Wilson to Meserve, Apr. 14, 1904, Letter File 2, Shaw Archives.

82. Martin, "Study of the Negro Physician," 54, calculated the average black rural Tennessee physician's worth at about $7,700, compared with the average American black family's worth of about $500.

83. Williams to the Editor, *Medical World* 32 (1914): 112.

84. J. Edward Ashburn to Meserve, Oct. 8, 1896, Letter File 1, Shaw Archives.

85. Lloyd to Meserve, Nov. 23, 1896, Letter File 1, Shaw Archives. See also the *Indianapolis Freeman*, Dec. 24, 1910.

86. *Christian Educator* 1 (1889–90): 162.

87. Ibid., 163.

88. Ibid.

89. Ibid.

90. Ibid., 108.

91. "Slater Fund School Reports, 1903–04," in John F. Slater Fund, *Proceedings and Reports, 1904* (New York: John F. Slater Fund, 1904), 22.

92. Du Bois, *College-Bred Negro*, 83.

93. *Medical World* 32 (1914): 111–13, 148–49; *The Workers* 3 (Dec. 1906–Jan. 1907): 12; Harlan and Smock, *Booker T. Washington Papers*, 2:257; *Medical and Surgical Observer* 1 (Dec. 1892): 46.

94. Du Bois, *College-Bred Negro*, 83.

95. Benjamin F. Hutchins to Meserve, Apr. 26, 1904, Letter File 2, Shaw Archives.

96. J. Benton Dickson to Meserve, Oct. 2, 1896, Letter File 1, Shaw Archives.

97. *Christian Educator* 1 (1889–90): 108.

98. Ibid., 162–63; Du Bois, *College-Bred Negro*, 83; *The Workers* 1 (Jan. 1905): 15; 1 (Feb.–Apr. 1905): 5; 2 (Feb.–Mar. 1906): 23; 2 (Dec. 1905–Jan. 1906): 10; 3 (Dec. 1906–Jan.

1907): 11–12; *Augusta (Georgia) Chronicle*, Sept. 30, 1919, front page of "Colored Section." See also references in note 23 herein.

99. Dr. Robert F. Boyd in *Christian Educator* 1 (1889–90): 163.

100. See, for example, Perry, *Forty Cords of Wood*, 159–60; Tompkins to Meserve, Dec. 7, 1896, Letter File 1, Shaw Archives.

101. See city and medical directories of the period, and John M. Matthews, "Studies in Race Relations in Georgia, 1880–1935" (Ph.D. diss., Duke University, 1970), 270.

102. James Summerville, "Formation of a Black Medical Profession in Tennessee, 1880–1920," *Journal of the Tennessee Medical Association* 10 (1983): 646; *Indianapolis Freeman*, May 13, 1911, 4.

103. Williams to Meserve, May 12, 1904, Letter File 2, Shaw Archives.

104. Perry, *Forty Cords of Wood*, 280–81.

105. Martin, "Study of the Negro Physician," 60.

106. Ibid., 31; Perry, *Forty Cords of Wood*, 276, 279ff. See also Gamble, *Making a Place for Ourselves*, 3–34.

107. Robert E. Perdue, *The Negro in Savannah, 1865–1900* (New York: Exposition Press, 1973), 126–28; Sara W. Brown, "Colored Women Physicians," *Southern Workman* 52 (1923): 582–83.

108. *Columbia (S.C.) Palmetto Leader*, Nov. 23, 1935.

109. Report of W. T. B. Williams on Hospital and Training School for Nurses, Nov. 28, 1905, 6–7, 11, in General Education Board Papers, Box 200, Folder 1899, RAC. The Waring Historical Library, Medical University of South Carolina, Charleston, also has a file of materials on the school. See also Todd L. Savitt, "Walking the Color Line: Alonzo McClennan, *The Hospital Herald*, and Segregated Medicine in Turn-of-the-Twentieth-Century Charleston, South Carolina," *South Carolina Historical Magazine* 104 (2003): 228–57.

110. S. P. Wadsworth, "The Burruss Sanitariam [*sic*]," *Voice of the Negro* 3 (1906): 339. See also *Augusta (Georgia) Chronicle*, Nov. 3, 1907.

111. Wadsworth, "Burruss Sanitariam," 339.

112. Martin, "Study of the Negro Physician," 31.

113. Ibid.

114. Robert C. Burt Papers, Fisk University, Nashville, Tennessee (hereafter Burt Papers).

115. John W. Lawlah, "George Cleveland Hall, 1864–1930, Profile," *Journal of the National Medical Association* 46 (1954): 207–10; Daniel Hale Williams to Booker T. Washington, Sept. 7, 1898, in Booker T. Washington Papers, Library of Congress, Washington, D.C.; Martin, "Study of the Negro Physician," 31–32.

116. Annual editions of Monroe N. Work, ed., *The Negro Year Book* (Tuskegee, Ala.: Negro Year Book Publishing, 1912–52).

117. See, for example, Martin, "Study of the Negro Physician," 32; Certificates of postgraduate education, in Burt Papers; Wadsworth, "Burruss Sanitariam," 341.

118. Morais, *History of the Negro in Medicine*, 68; W. Montague Cobb, "The Black American in Medicine," *Journal of the National Medical Association*, suppl., 73 (Dec. 1981): 1225–26. For more on the founding of the National Medical Association, see W. Michael Byrd and Linda A. Clayton, *An American Health Dilemma*, vol. 1, *A Medical History of African-Americans and the Problem of Race, Beginnings to 1900* (New York: Routledge, 2000), 401–2.

119. See list in each issue of Monroe Work's *Negro Year Book*; see also Summerville, "Formation of a Black Medical Profession in Tennessee," 646; Morais, *History of the Negro in Medicine*, 67; Cobb, "Black American in Medicine," 1225; Ward, *Black Physicians*, 191–213.

120. *Jackson (Miss.) Daily Clarion-Ledger*, Apr. 27, 1905, 8. (Thanks to Mr. Thomas N.

Boschert of Duncan, Mississippi, for this reference.) See also Summerville, "Formation of a Black Medical Profession in Tennessee," 644–46.

121. Lynk, *Sixty Years*; Morais, *History of the Negro in Medicine*, 64.

122. *Medical and Surgical Observer* 1 (July 1893): back cover.

123. Monroe A. Majors to the Editor, Nov. 29, 1892, *Medical and Surgical Observer* 1 (Dec. 1892): 47.

124. *Journal of the National Medical Association* 44 (1952): 475–76; Kaufman, Galishoff, and Savitt, *Dictionary of American Medical Biography*, 1:466; Morais, *History of the Negro in Medicine*, 64–65, 67. For a history of the *Medical and Surgical Observer*, see Savitt, "Journal of Our Own," 52–59, 115–22.

125. Cobb, "Black American in Medicine," 1230–32, 1235–36. For a history of the *Hospital Herald*, see Savitt, "Walking the Color Line."

126. *Journal of the National Medical Association* 12 (1920): 32–33.

127. See Beardsley, "Making Separate, Equal."

20. "A Journal of Our Own"

This chapter originally appeared as "'A Journal of Our Own': The *Medical and Surgical Observer* at the Beginnings of an African-American Medical Profession in Late Nineteenth-Century America," *Journal of the National Medical Association* 88 (1996): 52–59, 115–22.

1. "List of Serials Received at the Library of the Surgeon General's Office," located in the History of Medicine Division, National Library of Medicine, Bethesda, Md., manuscript folder 149:566.

2. "Our Golden Anniversary Volume," *Journal of the National Medical Association* 50 (1958): 55; Bullock, *Afro-American Periodical Press*, 185–89, 253–54.

3. On the establishment of medical schools for African Americans in the late nineteenth and early twentieth centuries, see chapter 11 of the current volume.

4. Savitt, "Entering a White Profession," 507–40.

5. On the Reconstruction era, see C. Vann Woodward, *Origins of the New South, 1877–1913* (Baton Rouge: Louisiana State Univ. Press, 1951), and Ayers, *Promise of the New South.* On the history of late-nineteenth-century medical education, see Ludmerer, *Learning to Heal.* On white responses to the entry of African Americans into the medical profession, see Beardsley, *History of Neglect;* Morais, *The History of the Negro in Medicine;* Savitt, "Entering a White Profession"; Ward, *Black Physicians.*

6. Morais, *History of the Negro in Medicine,* 52–58, 133, 303; Savitt, "Entering a White Profession"; Cobb, *First Negro Medical Society;* Nickens, "Case of Professional Exclusion," 1549–52; *Medical Record* 21 (1882): 390; Summerville, "Formation of a Black Medical Profession," 644–46; Ward, *Black Physicians.*

7. Lynk's *Sixty Years of Medicine* is not a complete biography. Lynk is selective in the aspects of his life he discusses in the book, focusing on certain achievements and omitting much detail between those high points. Unfortunately, his papers are not extant, and there are few other sources of information about his life.

8. *Meharry Medical College Catalogue,* 1888–89, 8.

9. Lynk, *Sixty Years,* 20–27; *Meharry Medical College Catalogue,* 1890–91, 5.

10. United States, Department of the Interior, Census Office, *Report on Population of the United States at the Eleventh Census: 1890,* vol. 1, pt. 1 (Washington, D.C.: GPO, 1895), 384, 481.

11. Lakey, *CME Church;* Gay, "Christian Methodist Episcopal Church," 487–89.

12. Lynk, *Sixty Years,* 27.

13. Ibid., 27–29.
14. Lynk, "Afro-American Population of Jackson."
15. Bullock, *Afro-American Periodical Press,* 185–89, 253–54; Lynk, *Sixty Years;* Lynk, "Afro-American Population of Jackson"; *Indianapolis Freeman,* Feb. 12, Nov. 5, and Dec. 10, 1898, and June 2, 1900.
16. *Medical and Surgical Observer* [hereafter *MSO*] 1 (Jan. 1893): 55.
17. Advertisement in the *MSO* 1 (Dec. 1892).
18. *MSO* 1 (Dec. 1892): 15.
19. Ibid., 17.
20. "To Contributors and Correspondents," *MSO* 1 (Dec. 1892): 14.
21. *MSO* 1 (Mar. 1893): 103.
22. *MSO* 1 (June 1893): 148–49.
23. J. T. Walton, "The Importance of Physical Examination in the Disorders of the Pelvic Viscera, in Females, with Special Observations as to the Influence of Local Disturbing Factors, in the Associated Conditions of Dysmenorahoea [*sic*], Mennorrhagia [*sic*], and Mettorrhagia [*sic*]," *MSO* 1 (Apr. 1893): 107–12.
24. C. Royal Alexander, "Treatment of Summer Complaint," *MSO* 1 (June 1893): 131–33.
25. H. H. Hall, "Prevention of Some Diseases from a Practical Hygienic Standpoint," *MSO* 1 (June 1893): 133–40.
26. S. C. Snelson, "Practical Hints in the Practice of Medicine," *MSO* 1 (Feb. 1893): 65–68.
27. *MSO* 1 (Dec. 1892): 15–16.
28. *MSO* 1 (Dec. 1893): 214.
29. *MSO* 1 (Feb. 1893): 84.
30. *MSO* 1 (Dec. 1893): 214.
31. Ibid., 213–14.
32. *MSO* 1 (Feb. 1893): 81.
33. Ibid.
34. *MSO* 1 (July 1893): 158.
35. *MSO* 1 (Sept. 1893): 180.
36. *MSO* 1 (May 1893): 127.
37. *MSO* 1 (Sept. 1893): 180.
38. *MSO* 1 (Dec. 1893): 214.
39. *MSO* 1 (Jan. 1893): 49, 53–54.
40. *MSO* 1 (Feb. 1893): 84; 1 (Mar. 1893): 104.
41. *MSO* 1 (Mar. 1893): 104–5.
42. *MSO* 1 (Dec. 1892): 17.
43. *MSO* 1 (Jan. 1893): 48. It was not the same Dr. Snead. William Joseph Sneed, cofounder of Meharry Medical College, died in Asheville, N.C., on Mar. 17, 1907. See Summerville, *Educating Black Doctors,* 19, 225n31.
44. *MSO* 1 (Feb. 1893): 85–86; 2 (Jan. 1894): 13.
45. *MSO* 1 (Dec. 1893): 214.
46. *MSO* 1 (Jan. 1893): 50.
47. *MSO* 1 (July 1893): 161.
48. *MSO* 1 (Dec. 1892): 16; 1 (May 1893): 128; 1 (July 1893): 157. For more on Hannibal Medical College and Louisville National Medical College, see Savitt, "Four African-American Proprietary Medical Colleges," 203–55.
49. *MSO* 1 (Mar. 1893): 104; Joseph A. Chatman, *The Lone Star State Medical, Dental, and Pharmaceutical [Association] History* (Lubbock, [Tex.?]: n.p., 1959).

50. *MSO* 1 (Dec. 1892): 17; 1 (Mar. 1893): 99–100; 1 (June 1893): 149.

51. "The Colored Medical Association, of Arkansas," *MSO* 1 (Sept. 1893): 180.

52. "Salutory [*sic*]," *MSO* 1 (Dec. 1892): 14.

53. Cobb, *First Negro Medical Society;* Nickens, "Case of Professional Exclusion."

54. *MSO* 1 (Dec. 1892): 17.

55. Lynk, *Sixty Years,* 45.

56. Ibid., 45–52; *MSO* 1 (Dec. 1892): 17; Francis L. Broderick and August Meier, eds., *Negro Protest Thought in the Twentieth Century* (Indianapolis, Ind.: Bobbs-Merrill, 1965), 4–8; Byrd and Clayton, *An American Health Dilemma,* vol. 1, *Medical History of African-Americans,* 401–2.

57. L. L. Burwell, "Consumption among the Colored Race," *MSO* 1 (Aug. 1893): 167–69.

58. John S. Haller, "The Physician versus the Negro: Medical and Anthropological Concepts of Race in the Late Nineteenth Century," *Bulletin of the History of Medicine* 44 (1970): 154–67; Haller, "Race, Mortality, and Life Insurance: Negro Vital Statistics in the Late Nineteenth Century," *Journal of the History of Medicine and Allied Sciences* 25 (1970): 247–61; Savitt, *Medicine and Slavery.*

59. *MSO* 1 (Mar. 1893): 104–5.

60. Furman J. Shadd, "Sarcoma," *MSO* 1 (Feb. 1893): 57–64.

61. Photograph, "Enormous Sarcoma of Buttock," in *An American Text-book of Surgery, for Practitioners and Students,* ed. William W. Keen and J. William White (Philadelphia: W. B. Saunders, 1892).

62. Shadd, "Sarcoma," 61.

63. Ibid.

64. Ibid.

65. S. C. Snelson, "Surgery in General," *MSO* 1 (Aug. 1893): 163–67.

66. Ibid., 164.

67. *MSO* 1 (June 1893): 146.

68. *MSO* 1 (May 1893): 127.

69. S. C. Snelson [to Lynk], *MSO* 1 (Jan. 1893): 46.

70. M. W. Alston [to Lynk], *MSO* 1 (Jan. 1893): 47.

71. J. H. Wilkins [to Lynk], *MSO* 1 (Jan. 1893): 48.

72. D. E. Caldwell [to Lynk], *MSO* 1 (Sept. 1893): 177.

73. Monroe A. Majors [to Lynk], *MSO* 1 (Jan. 1893): 47.

74. L. L. Burwell [to Lynk], *MSO* 1 (July 1893): 159.

75. *MSO* 1 (Dec. 1892): 15.

76. *JAMA* 20 (1893): 49.

77. *MSO* 1 (Dec. 1892): 16.

78. Ibid., 17, 15.

79. "Our Splendid Success," *MSO* 1 (July 1893): 158.

80. *MSO* 1 (Jan. 1893): 54–55.

81. *MSO* 1 (June 1893): 144.

82. *MSO* 1 (July 1893): 158–59.

83. Ibid., 160.

84. Ibid.

85. *MSO* 1 (Aug. 1893): 169.

86. Ibid., 171.

87. *MSO* 1 (Dec. 1893).

88. *MSO* 1 (Mar. 1893): 103.

89. *MSO* 1 (May 1893): 127.
90. Ibid., 127–28.
91. "List of Serials," 149:566.
92. Lynk, *Sixty Years*, 40.
93. Ibid., 40–41.
94. For more information on the *Hospital Herald*, see Savitt, "Walking the Color Line," 228–57.

21. Walking the Color Line

This chapter originally appeared as "Walking the Color Line: Alonzo McClennan, *The Hospital Herald*, and Segregated Medicine in Turn-of-the-Twentieth-Century Charleston, South Carolina," *The South Carolina Historical Magazine* 104 (2003): 228–57.

The author wishes to thank Jane Brown, curator of the Waring Historical Library, Medical University of South Carolina, Charleston, and Dr. Thomas L. Johnson at the South Caroliniana Library, University of South Carolina, Columbia, for their help in locating materials relating to the *Hospital Herald*. He also wishes to thank the Wildacres Residency Program at Wildacres Retreat, Little Switzerland, North Carolina, for allowing him a week's peaceful and productive residence in their "Scholar's Cabin."

1. *The Hospital Herald* [hereafter cited as *HH*] 1, no. 5 (Apr. 1899): 6, and 1, no. 9 (Aug. 1899): 3–7. See also, *HH* 2, no. 2 (Feb. 1900): 4; Newby, *Black Carolinians*, 61–62; Tindall, *South Carolina Negroes*, 255–56.
2. Savitt, "Journal of Our Own," 52–60, 115–22.
3. Savitt, "Journal of Our Own"; Savitt, "Entering a White Profession," 507–40; Ward, *Black Physicians;* Cobb, *First Negro Medical Society;* Nickens, "Case of Professional Exclusion," 1549–52; Summerville, "Formation of a Black Medical Profession," 644–46; Beardsley, "Making Separate, Equal," 382–96; Beardsley, *History of Neglect;* Gamble, *Making a Place for Ourselves;* Hine, *Black Women in White.* On the histories of various African American medical schools, see references in chapter 11 of the current volume.
4. Census figures for 1890 and 1900. Alabama in 1890 had one black physician for every 24,232 black citizens; South Carolina had one for every 22,964. See also Savitt, "Entering a White Profession," 511.
5. Meserve to P. H. Koon, May 8, 1897, Meserve Letterbook 2, 408, Shaw Archives, Shaw University, Raleigh, NC.
6. The Charleston *Sunday News*, Apr. 25, 1897, 9. This article by McClennan recounts his early education and describes in detail the problems he faced as a black naval cadet in Annapolis. Also on McClennan's life, see Edward Beardsley, "McClennan, Alonzo Clifton," in *American National Biography*, ed. John A. Garrity and Mark C. Carnes (New York: Oxford Univ. Press, 1999), 14:871–73; Willard B. Gatewood Jr., "Alonzo Clifton McClennan: Black Midshipman from South Carolina, 1873–1874," *South Carolina Historical Magazine* 89 (1988): 24–39; Robert J. Macbeth, "Dr. A. C. McClennan," *HH* 1, no. 1 (Dec. 1898): 5–6.
7. Lamb, *Howard University Medical Department*, 194.
8. Gatewood, "McClennan," 25–26; Beardsley, "McClennan," 872; Gatewood, *Aristocrats of Color*, 81.
9. On the history of the South Carolina Medical Association and the county medical societies, see Joseph Ioor Waring, *A Brief History of the South Carolina Medical Association, To Which Are Added Short Historical Sketches of Various Medical Institutions of South Carolina* (Columbia: South Carolina Medical Association, 1948).

10. On the importance of medical societies and black physicians' exclusion from them, see Savitt, "Entering a White Profession," 524–25, and Ward, *Black Physicians*, 191–212.

11. Suggested name change was mentioned in *HH* 2, no. 3 (Mar. 1900): 5. Though an informal report of the association's annual meeting published in *HH* 2, no. 4 (May 1900): 3–4, did not mention a formal vote on the matter, the masthead on page 3 of that same issue carried the new name.

12. *MSO* 1 (Mar. 1893): 104; Chatman, *Lone Star State Medical, Dental, and Pharmaceutical [Association] History.*

13. *MSO* 1 (Dec. 1892): 17; 1 (Mar. 1893): 99–100; 1 (June 1893): 149.

14. *MSO* 1 (Sept. 1893): 180.

15. *MSO* 1 (Dec. 1892): 17.

16. Johnson constructed a series of survey questions published in the *MSO* for a paper he was scheduled to present at the May 1893 North Carolina Medical Association meeting in Raleigh titled "The Professional Relation between Physicians of the Opposing Races in the South." The program for the N.C. Medical Association on which his name and paper are listed is published in *MSO* 1 (Mar. 1893): 100. Neither the results of his survey nor the completed paper itself are extant, but the questions he asked black physicians to answer were published in *MSO* 1 (Mar. 1893): 104–5, and reproduced in Savitt, "Journal of Our Own," 115–16.

17. McClennan and two other South Carolina physicians—W. D. Crum of Charleston and C. L. Walton of Columbia—attended and presented papers at that same 1893 N.C. Medical Association meeting in Raleigh where Johnson presented the results of his survey and where a proposal to establish an interstate association of black physicians from Virginia, North Carolina, and South Carolina was discussed. *MSO* 1 (Mar. 1893): 100. Early records of the Palmetto Medical Association are not extant. See Barbara A. Woods and Tracy D. Tisdale-Clawson, *A Golden Century of Black Medicine: An Historical Overview of the Palmetto Medical, Dental and Pharmaceutical Association, 1896–1996* (N.P.: n.p., 1996). I am indebted to Professor Barbara A. Woods of South Carolina State University in Orangeburg for providing me with a copy of this publication.

18. On the early history of African American nurses and nurse-training schools, see Hine, *Black Women in White.* On race, nursing, and nursing care in Charleston during this time period, see Karen Buhler-Wilkerson, *No Place Like Home: A History of Nursing and Home Care in the United States* (Baltimore, Md.: Johns Hopkins Univ. Press, 2001), 69–82. The Charleston school's predecessors included programs at Spelman College (Atlanta, 1886), Provident Hospital (Chicago, 1891), Dixie Hospital (Hampton, Va., 1891), Tuskegee Institute (Tuskegee, Ala., 1892), Freedmen's Hospital (Washington, D.C., 1894), Lincoln School for Nurses (New York, N.Y., 1896), St. Agnes Hospital (Raleigh, N.C., 1896), and the Phillis Wheatley Sanitarium (New Orleans, 1896).

19. "Editorial," *HH* 2, no. 2 (Feb. 1900): 3.

20. The physician faculty included McClennan, Dr. Lucy Hughes Brown, Dr. John M. Thompson, Dr. Thomas D. Rankin, and Dr. T. N. Roberts (white). Robert J. Macbeth, an African American dentist, also taught. See "An Interesting Experiment," *Charleston News and Courier*, Jan. 16, 1897, 8.

21. "Editorial," *HH* 2, no. 2 (Feb. 1900): 3.

22. "An Interesting Experiment," *Charleston News and Courier*, Jan. 16, 1897, 8.

23. "A Credit to the Race," *Charleston Sunday News*, June 20, 1902, 3; L. C. Downing, "Early Negro Hospitals, with Special Reference to Nurse's Training Schools," *Journal of the National Medical Association* 33, no. 1 (Jan. 1941): 15; Hine, *Black Women in White*, 15.

24. *HH* 1, no. 7 (June 1899): 7; *Charleston, S.C. City Directory for 1900* (Charleston: Lucas and Richardson, 1900), 45, 46.

25. "Editorial," *HH* 2, no. 2 (Feb. 1900): 3–4.

26. Ibid.; "A Credit to the Race," *Charleston Sunday News,* June 20, 1902, 3.

27. "In the Colored Hospital," *Charleston News and Courier,* Nov. 5, 1897, 8.

28. A full run of the *Hospital Herald* may be found at the Waring Historical Library, Medical University of South Carolina, Charleston, and at the South Caroliniana Library, University of South Carolina, Columbia.

29. *HH* 1 (Dec. 1898): [1–2].

30. Ibid., [1].

31. Ibid., [2]. In practice, the promised sketches appeared sporadically, not monthly.

32. For example, one reader wrote to the president of the Hospital Association, "I received a copy of the *Hospital Herald* and was much interested in the work of your Association. I inclose [*sic*] you a check to your order for $10.00, to be devoted to such part of the work as you may deem be fit." *HH* 1, no. 9 (Aug. 1899): 8.

33. *HH* 1, no. 9 (Aug. 1899): 10.

34. *HH* 1, no. 4 (Mar. 1899): [9]. The March 1899 list declared, in part, "$15.00 will support a free bed for one month. $200.00 will complete water supply in building including sanitary water closets, hot water, etc. $250.00 will furnish the equipments needed for the operating room. $300.00 will pay the salary of our Head Nurse for one year. $1,500 will pay the yearly running expenses of the hospital. $3,000 will pay the remaining indebtedness on the Hospital building."

35. *HH* 1, no. 11 (Oct. 1899): 5–6, 12.

36. *HH* 2, no. 3 (Mar. 1900): 3–5.

37. *HH* 1, no. 8 (July 1899): 15; 1, no. 9 (Aug. 1899): 7.

38. *HH* 1, no. 12 (Nov. 1899): 3.

39. For example: "Messrs. J. A. Bell and L. J. Hollings, contractors, have done work at the hospital only making a charge for material. Thanks." *HH* 1, no. 2 (Jan. 1899): 4. "Mrs. Gordon, 16 Water Street, has very kindly donated bedding. Thanks." *HH* 1, no. 2 (Jan. 1899): 4. "Mrs. C. L. Riley . . . sent down six cash subscribers [to the *Hospital Herald*] from Lincolnville. Mrs. Riley is a thorough race woman and takes advantage of every opportunity to do something for the Hospital." *HH* 1, no. 4 (Mar. 1899): [8]. "Mr. James Wheeler makes us indebted to him again for the hat rack in the hospital. He has few, if any, equals as an upholsterer and wood worker." *HH* 1, no. 9 (Aug. 1899): 8. "The newspapers received in exchange for the *Herald* will serve to make a reading room for the girls [student nurses] at the Hospital." *HH* 1, no. 2 (Jan. 1899): 4.

40. *HH* 1, no. 9 (Aug. 1899): 7–8.

41. Ibid., 8, 12; *HH* 2, no. 2 (Feb. 1900): 12; *HH* 1, no. 10 (Sept. 1899): 7.

42. *HH* 1, no. 12 (Nov. 1899): 5. In this same article, he wrote of another white board member: "Hon. George I. Cunningham does not forget to give a substantial donation whenever we have our fairs. . . . We regret very much that he forbids us to make known the amount that he usually contributes, as it would probably influence others equally as able to give to our hospital."

43. *HH* 1, no. 12 (Nov. 1899): 6.

44. *HH* 1, no. 9 (Aug. 1899): 11–12. See also "Nurse Training in Charleston," *Southern Workman* 28 (June 1899): 224.

45. *HH* 1, no. 3 (Feb. 1899): 8.

46. *HH* 2, no. 2 (Feb. 1900): 11. Other examples include, "Miss Whaley, through the kindness of Dr. [Lane] Mullally [a white physician in Charleston], has gone to North Carolina with one of his patients." *HH* 2, no. 2 (Feb. 1900): 11. "[Student] Nurse Droze was highly complimented and was given five dollars [to keep for herself?] where she recently nursed in the family of Mrs. Jervey, Tradd Street." *HH* 2, no. 2 (Feb. 1900): 11. "Five

[student] nurses are at the Catholic Infirmary every night doing faithful work. The sisters are kind to them and give them valuable points of information." *HH* 1, no. 1 (Dec. 1898): 2–3. "Miss Daniel, one of our senior nurses, was sent to Darlington last week to nurse a case of pneumonia." *HH* 1, no. 6 (May 1899): 11.

47. *HH* 1, no. 6 (May 1899): 11; 1, no. 8 (July 1899): 13.

48. *HH* 2, no. 4 (May 1900): 5.

49. *HH* 1, no. 9 (Aug. 1899): 11.

50. For example: "A patient was sent into the hospital through Mrs. Heins, the trained nurse. Thanks." *HH* 1, no. 2 (Jan. 1899): 4. "Dr. R[obert] J. Macbeth and friends had Mr. Gilbert Johnson, who was sick at the Old Folks' Home, removed to the hospital." *HH* 1, no. 4 (Mar. 1899): [8]. "Dr. [C. Wainwright] Birnie [an African American physician] brought with him a patient from Sumter. This makes the third case Dr. Birnie has sent since he has located in Sumter. Thanks." *HH* 2, no. 4 (May 1900): 4. "Dr. R. S. Cathcart, one of our young white physicians, has a surgical case in the hospital." *HH* 1, no. 11 (Oct. 1899): 6. "Dr. R. J. Kirk, [a white] surgeon to the Atlantic Coast Line R.R., visited our hospital recently, and was so much impressed with what he saw, and also our facilities and equipments for caring for the sick, that he has made arrangements to send all his railroad cases to our hospital. Dr. Kirk has had several of our nurses in cases of his at Mt. Pleasant and Sullivan's Island, and speaks in the highest terms of their faithful service." *HH* 2, no. 2 (Feb. 1900): 12. "Dr. Kirk, as promised, brought in a case of accident on the A[tlantic] C[oast] L[ine] Railroad. Dr. Kirk promises to do all he can for our work." *HH* 2, no. 4 (May 1900): 5. "Mr. Potter, Superintendent of Vesta Cotton Mills, sent us a man who had his hand injured and required surgical attention. Thanks." *HH* 2, no. 4 (May 1900): 4.

51. *HH* 1, no. 12 (Nov. 1899): 6–7; 2, no. 1 (Jan. 1900): 11; 1, no. 2 (Jan. 1899): 5.

52. *HH* 2, no. 4 (May 1900): 5.

53. See, for example, *HH* 1, no. 2(Jan. 1899): 5; 1, no. 4(Mar. 1899): 7. The list of visitors to the hospital published occasionally in the journal also included Northerners whom Hospital Association members presumably were cultivating for donations. See, for example, lists in *HH* 1, no. 3 (Feb. 1899): 8; 1, no. 6 (May 1899): 11–12.

54. *HH* 1, no. 8 (July 1899): 4–5.

55. *HH* 1, no. 10 (Sept. 1899): 7.

56. *HH* 2, no. 2 (Feb. 1900): 4–6.

57. *HH* 1, no. 1 (Dec. 28, 1898): 4–5.

58. *HH* 1, no. 5 (Apr. 1899): 5–6.

59. *HH* 1, no. 6 (May 1899): 3–6.

60. *HH* 2, no. 1 (Jan. 1900): 6–7.

61. *HH* 2, no. 2 (Feb. 1900): 7. National statistics for that period show that the failure rate on state licensing exams was significantly higher for graduates of African American medical schools than for graduates of predominantly white medical schools. See Savitt, "Education of Black Physicians at Shaw University," 181–83.

62. *HH* 1, no. 8 (July 1899): 15.

63. *HH* 1, no. 9 (Aug. 1899): 7. On conditions for African Americans at the asylum, see Peter McCandless, *Moonlight, Magnolias, and Madness: Insanity in South Carolina from the Colonial Period to the Progressive Era* (Chapel Hill: Univ. of North Carolina Press, 1996): 259–61, 283–87.

64. *HH* 1, no. 7 (June 1899): 5.

65. *HH* 1, no. 3 (Feb. 1899): 3–4 (editorial), 9 (news item).

66. Newby, *Black Carolinians*, 47; Walter Edgar, *South Carolina: A History* (Columbia: Univ. of South Carolina Press, 1998), 448.

67. *HH* 1, no. 3 (Feb. 1899): 5–6.

68. Ibid., 4.

69. *HH* 1, no. 11 (Oct. 1899): 13.

70. *HH* 2, no. 2 (Feb. 1900): 13.

71. See, for example, *HH* 1, no. 1 (Dec. 1898): 2, 3; 1, no. 2 (Jan. 1899): [4]; 1, no. 3 (Feb. 1899): 10; 1, no. 4 (Mar. 1899): 8; 1, no. 6 (May 1899): 11.

72. *HH* 1, no. 8 (July 1899): 12.

73. Ibid., 7–8 (Scruggs's article), 14 (McClennan's editorial endorsement). For more on Scruggs and Pickford, see Murray, "Scruggs, Lawson Andrew," 307–8.

74. *HH* 2, no. 1 (Jan. 1900): 9–10 (Scruggs's letter), 5 (McClennan's editorial endorsement).

75. *HH* 1, no. 4 (Mar. 1899): 7.

76. *HH* 1, no. 12 (Nov. 1899): 4.

77. *HH* 1, no. 9 (Aug. 1899): 14–16.

78. *HH* 2, no. 1 (Jan. 1900): 10.

Index

Abbreviations

AMA = American Medical Association
CF = Carnegie Foundation
CME = Council on Medical Education
GEB = General Education Board
HH = *Hospital Herald*
HUMD = Howard University Medical Department
KCMD = Knoxville College Medical Department
KMC = Knoxville Medical College
LMS = Leonard Medical School
LNMC = Louisville National Medical College
LUMD = Lincoln University Medical Department
MSO = *Medical and Surgical Observer*
SUMD = Straight University Medical Department

www.ingramcontent.com/pod-product-compliance
Lightning Source LLC
LaVergne TN
LVHW090258210926
848480LV00001B/58